Surgery of the Cervical Spine

Surgery of the Cervical Spine

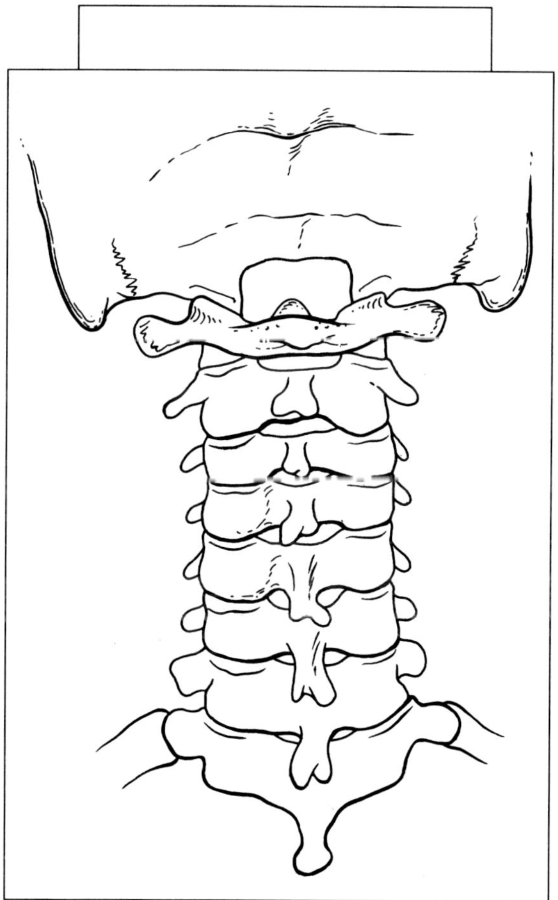

Edited by

Howard S An
MD
Associate Professor of Orthopaedic Surgery
Director of Reconstructive Spine Surgery
Department of Orthopaedic Surgery
The Medical College of Wisconsin
Milwaukee, Wisconsin 53226
United States of America

J Michael Simpson
MD
Clinical Assistant Professor
Department of Orthopaedic Surgery
The Medical College of Virginia
Director of Spine Surgery
Tuckahoe Orthopaedic Associates Ltd
Glen Allen, Virginia 23060
United States of America

with illustrations by
Carole Hilmer and Anita Hylton

Williams & Wilkins
BALTIMORE • PHILADELPHIA • HONG KONG
LONDON • MUNICH • SYDNEY • TOKYO
A WAVERLY COMPANY

MARTIN DUNITZ

Distributed by Williams & Wilkins, 428 East Preston Street, Baltimore, Maryland 21202, USA, in North America (United States and Canada)

First published in the United Kingdom in 1994 by Martin Dunitz Ltd, The Livery House, 7–9 Pratt Street, London NW1 0AE

Library of Congress Cataloging in Publication Data
An, Howard S.
Surgery of the cervical spine/Howard S. An, J. Michael Simpson: with illustrations by Carole Hilmer and Anita Hylton.
p. cm.
Includes bibliographical references and index.
ISBN 0–683–00128–0
1. Cervical vertebrae—Surgery. 2. Cervical vertebrae—Diseases. 3. Cervical vertebrae—Wounds and injuries. I. Simpson, J. Michael. II. Title.
[DNLM: 1. Cervical Vertebrae—physiopathology. 2. Cervical vertebrae—surgery. 3. Spinal Diseases—physiology. WE725 A531s 1994]
RD533.A5 1994
617.3'75—dc20
DNLM/DLC 93–47689
for Library of Congress CIP

Composition by Scribe Design, Gillingham, Kent, UK
Origination by Imago Publishing Ltd
Printed and bound in Singapore by
Toppan Printing Company (S) Pte Ltd

Contents

List of contributors

Howard S An MD
Associate Professor
Director of Reconstructive Spine Surgery
Department of Orthopaedic Surgery
The Medical College of Wisconsin
Milwaukee
Wisconsin 53226
United States of America

Thomas G Andreshak MD
Spine Fellow
Department of Orthopaedic Surgery
The Medical College of Wisconsin
Milwaukee
Wisconsin 53226
United States of America

Brian E Black MD
Assistant Professor
Department of Orthopaedic Surgery
Section of Pediatric Orthopaedics
The Medical College of Wisconsin
Milwaukee
Wisconsin 53226
United States of America

Scott D Boden MD
Assistant Professor of Orthopaedic Surgery
Emory University School of Medicine
Emory Clinic Spine Center
Decatur
Georgia 30033
United States of America

Henry H Bohlman MD
Professor and Vice-Chairman
of Orthopaedic Surgery
Case Western Reserve University of Medicine
Chief of Reconstructive and Traumatic Spine Surgery
Center and Spinal Cord Injury Service
Department of Veteran Affairs Medical Center
Cleveland
Ohio 44106
United States of America

Guillermo F Carrera MD
Professor and Chief of Diagnostic Radiology
Department of Radiology
The Medical College of Wisconsin
Milwaukee
Wisconsin 53226
United States of America

John B Catalano MD
Resident
Department of Orthopaedic Surgery
Thomas Jefferson University
Philadelphia
Pennsylvania 19107
United States of America

Jerome M Cotler MD
Professor and Vice Chairman
Department of Orthopaedic Surgery
Thomas Jefferson University
Philadelphia
Pennsylvania 19107
United States of America

Jeffrey Fischgrund MD
Spine Fellow
Department of Orthopaedic Surgery
William Beaumont Hospital
Royal Oak
Michigan 48073
United States of America

Steven R Garfin MD
Professor of Surgery
Division of Orthopaedics and Rehabilitation
University of California
San Diego Medical Center
San Diego
California 92103
United States of America

Steven Gnatz MD
Assistant Professor and Vice Chairman
Department of Physical Medicine and Rehabilitation
University of Missouri
Columbia
Missouri 65203
United States of America

Daniel A Green MD
Assistant Professor of Surgery
Division of Orthopaedics and Rehabilitation
University of California
San Diego Medical Center
San Diego
California 92103
United States of America

John G Heller MD
Assistant Professor
Department of Orthopaedic Surgery
Emory University
Atlanta
Georgia 30322
United States of America

Harry N Herkowitz MD
Chairman
Department of Orthopaedic Surgery
William Beaumont Hospital
Royal Oak
Michigan 48073
United States of America

Martin H Krag MD
Department of Orthopaedics and Rehabilitation
College of Medicine
University of Vermont
Burlington
Vermont 05405
United States of America

Peter D Pizzutillo MD
Professor
Chief of Pediatric Orthopaedics
Department of Orthopaedic Surgery
Thomas Jefferson University
Philadelphia
Pennsylvania 19107
United States of America

Thomas Reinsel MD
Spine Fellow
Department of Orthopaedics and Rehabilitation
College of Medicine
University of Vermont
Burlington
Vermont 05405
United States of America

Steven J Rizzolo MD
Department of Orthopaedic Surgery
Thomas Jefferson University
Philadelphia
Pennsylvania 19107
United States of America

Christopher P Silveri MD
Orthopaedic Resident
Long Island Jewish Hospital
Long Island
New York
New York
United States of America

Frederick A Simeone MD
Professor of Neurosurgery
The University of Pennsylvania School of Medicine
Director
Elliot Neurological Center
Pennsylvania Hospital
Philadelphia
Pennsylvania 19107
United States of America

J Michael Simpson MD
Clinical Assistant Professor
Department of Orthopaedic Surgery
The Medical College of Virginia
Director of Spine Surgery
Tuckahoe Orthopaedic Associates Ltd
Glen Allen
Virginia 23060
United States of America

Douglas Sutton MD
Orthopaedic Resident
Department of orthopaedic Surgery
Thomas Jefferson University
Philadelphia
Pennsylvania 19107
United States of America

Alexander R Vaccaro MD
Assistant Professor
Department of Orthopaedic Surgery
Thomas Jefferson University
Philadelphia
Pennsylvania 19107
United States of America

William R White MD
Assistant Professor
Clinical Professor of Neurosurgery
Department of Neurosurgery
Medical College of Virginia
Richmond
Virginia
United States of America

Thomas A Zdeblick MD
Assistant Professor
Division of Orthopaedic Surgery
University of Wisconsin Medical Center
Madison
Wisconsin 53226
United States of America

Forewords

To carry out any operation on the cervical spine, the surgeons involved have to be familiar with normal and abnormal anatomy. This textbook concentrates on illustrating those anatomical variations, so we can care for our patients more appropriately.

Dr An's initial chapter starting out with the anatomy of the cervical spine is an exhaustive review of the various bony, muscular, ligamentous, and neuro structures. The drawings are represented in such a fashion that we can remember all these structural variations. With this knowledge one can then concentrate on the best surgical approaches to correct the various pathological processes without significant disruption of the normal anatomical structures. This initial chapter is followed by the biomechanics of the normal cervical spine. By understanding both function and form, one can fully appreciate the seven neck bones and their attaching structures before considering operative care for diseases.

In patients with spinal disorders, the clinical evaluation is the next most important step. Every patient needs radiological evaluation and our techniques now have sophisticated x-rays, computerized tomographies, and magnetic resonating images. There is no longer any exploratory surgery of the cervical spine; we know exactly what's wrong and what has to be fixed when we plan an operation.

Not every patient has to be treated surgically, and these individuals need to be identified. Once one decides on surgical treatment, picking the operation is where the art of medicine still applies. We have to appreciate the congenital anomalies that may occur normally and how that may influence the pathology. One has to be fully cognizant of the capabilities and limitations of either an anterior, posterior, and even the rare lateral approaches.

Traumatic injuries provide us with a different spectrum of diseases. The huge experience from Thomas Jefferson Hospital of these injured patients is fully documented in this book. Certainly, rapid alignment and restoration of the normal anatomy is the first goal. At the same time, we have to keep the neuro structures free and uncompressed. The skeletally immature spine has to be treated differently, and the information to do so has been provided.

Tumors of the bone and nervous system can alter neck and spinal cord function. An untreated tumor will continue to grow. If at all possible, the lesion needs to be removed. Spinal stability, as well as a freed nervous system, is a goal of each of these therapies. Chapters 14 and 15 are devoted to this.

Infection involving the cervical spine is still a challenge. While they are not common, they can be devastating. Rapid drainage and correction of any instability can now be achieved. Fortunately, we have antibiotics to control infection and promote healing.

Rheumatoid arthritis has always provided us with quite a challenge. Long experience of Dr Boden and Dr Bohlman, with respect for the space required for a functioning nervous system, has been clearly outlined for atlas-axis disease as well as subaxial disease. The former presents with unique neurologic problems, while the latter fits more into the standard spondylitic myelopathy cases.

Ankylosing spondylitis and other diseases will lead to excessive cervical kyphosis. This has to be treated in certain patients, and the techniques are outlined.

Finally, with any treatment, certain equipment of a specific nature is required in select cases. The last two chapters of the book deal with the instrumentation needed in some of these cases. At the same time, the complications of cervical spine surgery are also addressed. The importance of carrying out the right amount of surgery, not too much or too little, cannot be over stressed.

This textbook will give the reader who is honestly interested in problems of the cervical spine a better perspective on how to handle individual cases. Obviously no one cookbook can advise a single formula where we just simply add the ingredients and put our patient on the proper assembly line. Only by understanding all of the aspects of normal anatomy and of pathophysiology can one treat in a rational fashion. The drawings provided in this textbook should aid those surgeons responsible for cases of the cervical spine disease.

Thomas B Ducker, MD
Clincal Professor, Neurosurgery
University of Maryland,
Associate Professor of Neurosurgery
Johns Hopkins University School of Medicine
Baltimore, Maryland 21205
United States of America

The management of disorders of the cervical spine, whether caused by disease, trauma, or congenital malformation, has changed dramatically over the last two decades. In fact, it was just 20 years ago in 1973 that some 18 orthopaedists and neurosurgeons met in New York at the invitation of J William Fielding to discuss clinical problems related to the cervical spine. These founding members of the Cervical Spine Research Society felt that the group would remain small and there would not be more than 25 or 30 people in the country interested in an annual meeting to discuss such an isolated clinical area as the cervical spine. The annual meetings have provided a forum for learning the intricacies of the anatomy, biomechanics, physiology and the clinical nuances of the neurologic and orthopaedic complexities of this unique area. The Cervical Spine Research Society now lists some 165 members, including orthopaedic surgeons, neurologic surgeons, radiologists, anatomists, biomedical engineers and rehabilitation specialists. A wealth of knowledge has evolved from the formal presentations as well as the informal discussions during the meetings. Entire issues of the journal Spine have been devoted to the cervical spine. Monographs, symposiums, texts, concentrating on various aspects of cervical spine surgery, have appeared.

The editors have compiled in one text authors who represent the current state of management of cervical spine disorders. This all–encompassing text explains the basic aspects of anatomy, biomechanics, and surgical approaches as well as the more controversial areas of types of surgical management from a broad range of clinicians. This text will provide an invaluable basis of knowledge for those of us who are called to evaluate and treat patients with cervical spine disorders. It will also be an excellent reference book for students, residents, and fellows learning about the special concerns of cervical spine surgery.

E Shannon Stauffer, MD
Professor and Chairman
Division of Orthopaedics and Rehabilitation
Southern Illinois University School of Medicine
Springfield, Illinois 62794
United States of America

Preface

As knowledge of the cervical spine, pathophysiology, and biomechanics evolve, our approach to treatment changes accordingly. In this text on surgery of the cervical spine, an updated review of cervical anatomy, pathophysiology, biomechanics, radiologic techniques, and clinical evaluation is provided. Ensuing chapters address specific disorders and their treatment, both non–surgical and surgical. However, the emphasis of this text, and thus its primary purpose and interest, is on specific surgical techniques of the cervical spine. We are thankful to contributing authors who have shared their expertise in these various areas, and thus broadened the scope and value of the text itself.

There currently exist a wide range of acceptable philosophies concerning the treatment of cervical spine disorders. The rampage of technology, availability of multiple instrumentation forms, and complexities of the individual case, coupled with these existing philosophical differences, render no text complete or dogmatic. The main stream of this text, however, reflects the editors' training at the Rothman Institute at Thomas Jefferson University Hospital under the tutelage of Drs Jerome M Cotler, Frederick A Simeone, and Richard A Balderston. We are grateful to these physicians for their dedication, stimulation, wisdom, and guidance in pursuit of excellence in the field of cervical spine surgery.

While we have strived to provide the details of the variously described operative procedures, the surgeon must remember that no perfectly performed procedure fares well under improper circumstances. Attention to detail, preoperative evaluation, and application of the principles set forth in this text, followed by proper, attentive operative execution, render surgery of the cervical spine successful and rewarding.

Howard S An, MD
J Michael Simpson, MD

1 Anatomy of the cervical spine

Howard S. An

The success of cervical spine surgery depends on careful patient selection, performance of an appropriate operative procedure, and precise surgical technique. Correct approach and meticulous exposure are essential in performing surgery with minimal complications. Thorough knowledge of normal cervical spine anatomy is imperative to an understanding of pathologic anatomy and completion of excellent surgical exposures. In this chapter, the basic anatomy of the cervical spine will be presented. The anatomy of the osseous structures, joints, intervertebral disc, ligaments, muscles, neurovascular structures, and related soft tissue structures will be described.

OSSEOUS STRUCTURES AND ARTICULATIONS OF THE CERVICAL SPINE

The cervical spine consists of the first seven vertebrae in the spinal column (Fig. 1.1); the bony anatomy of the atlas and axis is unique (Fig. 1.2). The atlas has no centrum, but is simply a ring-like structure in which the thick anterior arch blends into the two bulky lateral masses. The truncated balls of the occipital condyles articulate with the concave superior aspects of the atlas lateral masses (Fig. 1.3).[7] The occipital condyles project downward and laterally, whereas the kidney-shaped superior facets of the atlas face upward and inward to support the occiput (Figs 1.3 and 1.4).[10] This atlanto-occipital articulation is supported by the anterior and posterior occipital membranes, which are a continuation of the anterior longitudinal ligament and ligamentum flavum, respectively (Fig. 1.5).

The atlanto-occipital articulation mostly allows flexion, extension, and some lateral bending motions. To allow for rotatory motion at the atlantoaxial articulation, the inferior facets of the atlas are flatter and more circular than the superior facets, and face downward and laterally to articulate with the axis (Fig. 1.6).[16] The anterior tubercle of the anterior arch serves as an attachment for the longus coli muscle, whereas the posterior tubercle of the atlas serves as the bony attachment site for the rectus minor muscle and suboccipital membrane. The atlas has large transverse processes, where the superior and inferior oblique muscles attach. The transverse foramen is located within the transverse process, through which the vertebral artery passes before coursing posteriorly along the lateral masses. On the posterior aspect of the anterior arch of the atlas there are prominent tubercles for attachment of the strong transverse ligament, which confines the odontoid process of the axis to the anterior third of the atlantal ring although allowing free rotation about the atlantoaxial joint. Developmentally, the posterior neural arch fuses at 3 years, and the anterior neural arch at 7 years.

In the axis, the odontoid process projects upward anteriorly, articulating with the posterior aspect of the anterior arch of the atlas as a synovial joint. The transverse ligament, which spans the arch of the atlas, holds the odontoid process against the anterior arch of the atlas (Fig. 1.7). This transverse ligament is the principal stabilizing structure for atlantoaxial articulation. The transverse ligament has superior and inferior extensions, which form the cruciform ligament of the atlas. Secondary stabilizers of this articulation include the thick alar ligaments, which arise from the sides of dens to the condyles of the occipital bone, and the apical ligament, which arises from the apex of the dens to the foramen magnum as a remnant of the notochord.[18] The tectorial membrane is a continuation of the posterior longitudinal ligament (Fig. 1.7). Posteriorly, the axis has the large lamina and bifid spinous process, which serve as attachments for the rectus major and inferior oblique muscles. The zone between the lamina and the lateral mass of the axis is indistinct. The pedicle of the axis is large and projects medially and superiorly in a posteroanterior direction. Developmentally, the synchondrosis between the dens and the body of the axis, as well as the neurocentral

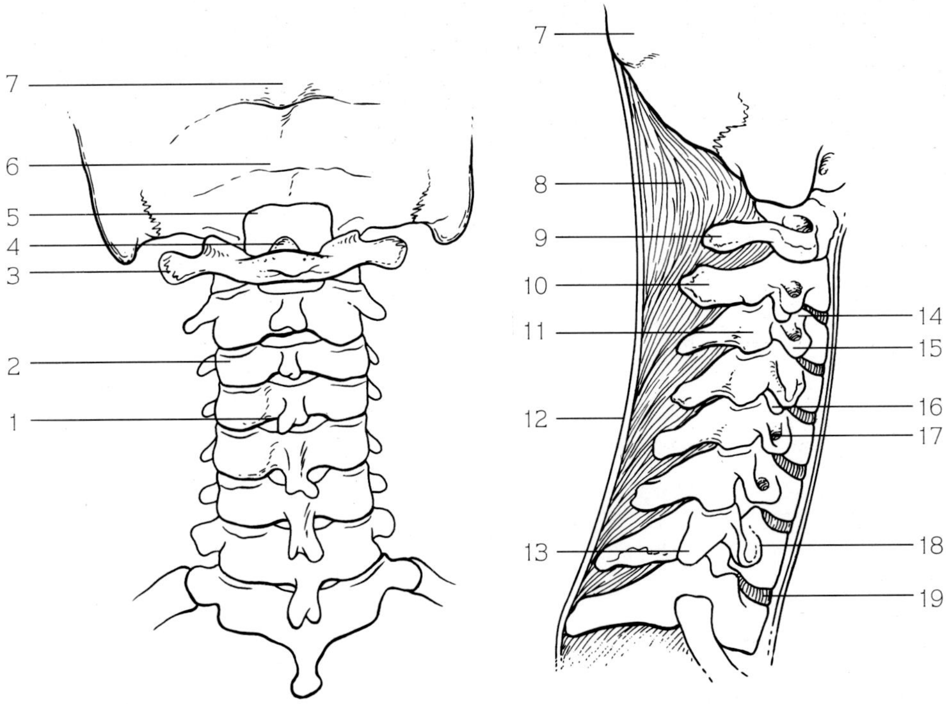

Figure 1.1
Posterior and lateral views of the occiput and cervical spine showing the basic bony anatomy

1 Spinous process
2 Lateral articular process or lateral mass
3 Transverse process of C1
4 Odontoid process of C2
5 Foramen magnum
6 Inferior nuchal line
7 Inion
8 Ligamentum nuchae
9 Posterior arch of C1
10 Spinous process of C2
11 Lateral mass
12 Supraspinous ligament
13 Lateral articular process
14 Uncinate process
15 Anterior tubercle of transverse process
16 Neural foramen
17 Transverse foramen
18 Carotid tubercle
19 Intervertebral disc

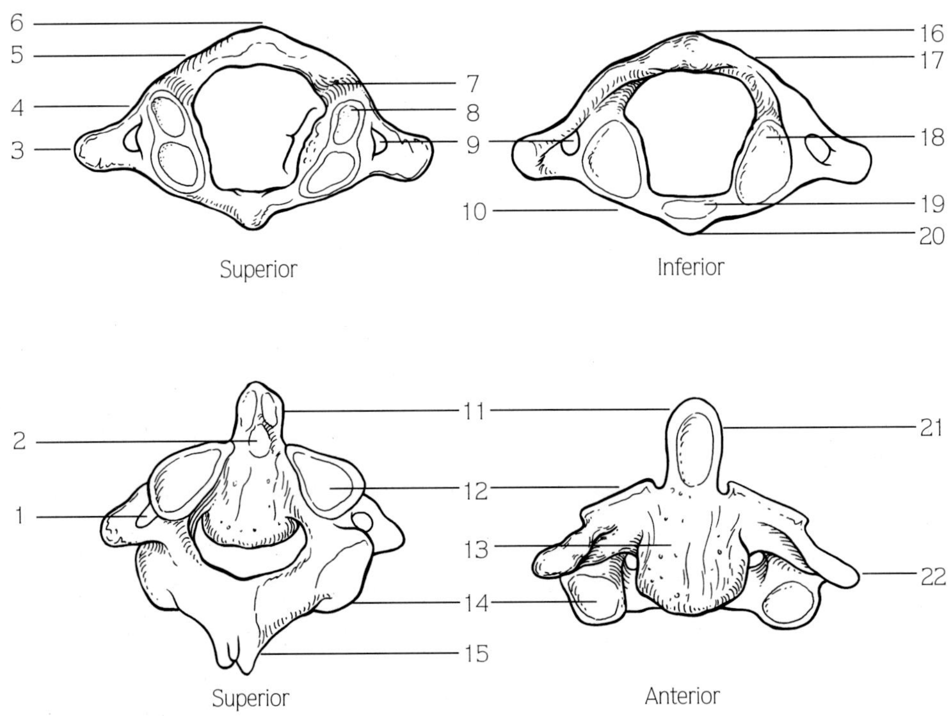

1 Transverse foramen
2 Posterior articular facet
3 Transverse process
4 Lateral mass
5 Posterior arch
6 Posterior tubercle
7 Groove for vertebral artery
8 Superior articular facet
9 Transverse foramen
10 Anterior arch
11 Dens (odontoid process)
12 Superior articular facet
13 Body
14 Inferior articular facet
15 Spinous process
16 Posterior tubercle
17 Posterior arch
18 Inferior articular process
19 Fovia dentis
20 Anterior tubercle
21 Anterior articular facet
22 Transverse process

Figure 1.2
The bony anatomy of the atlas and axis. The atlas is a ring-like structure, in which the thick anterior arch blends into the lateral masses. The atlas has large transverse processes through which the vertebral artery passes. The axis has a distinct large spinous process and the odontoid process that articulates with the anterior arch of the atlas

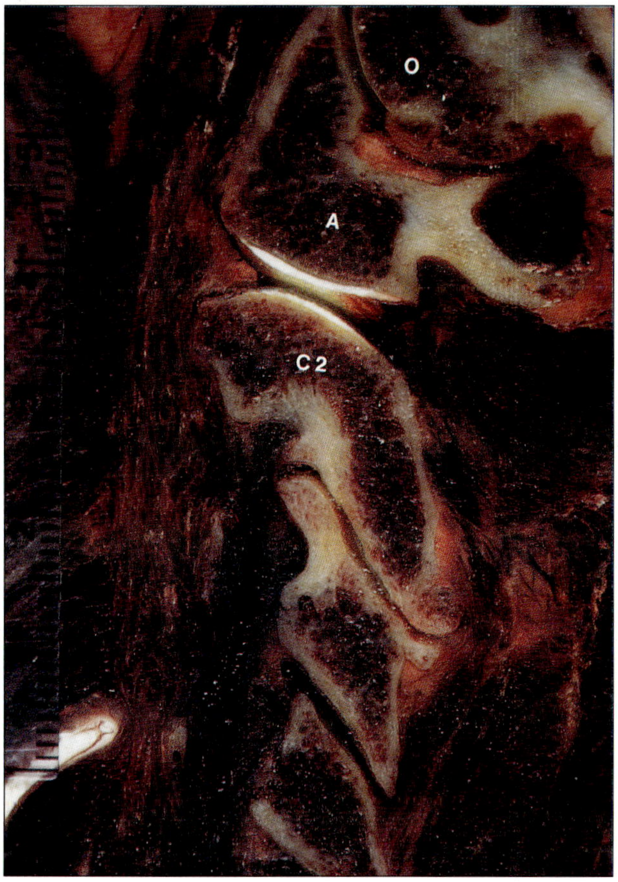

Figure 1.3
A freezing microtome section of the occiput–C4 region in a parasagittal plane, showing the occipital condyles articulating with the concave superior aspects of the lateral masses. The superior facet of the atlas faces upward anteriorly and posterior to support the occipital condyle. The inferior facets of the atlas are flatter and more circular than the superior facets to articulate with the axis below. Occipital condyle (O), atlas (A), axis (C2)

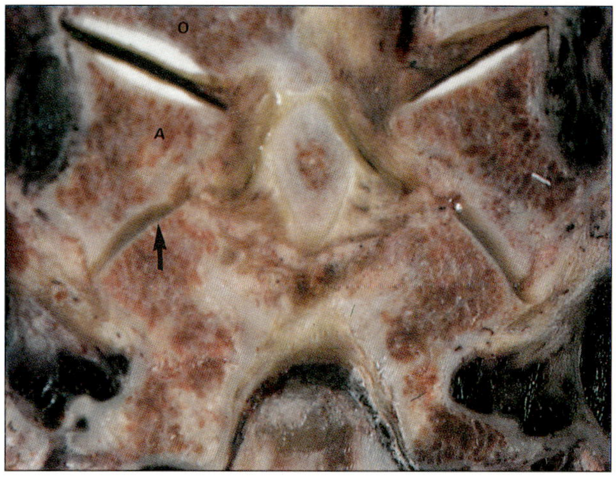

Figure 1.4
A freezing microtome section of the occiput–C2 region in a coronal plane, showing the occipital condyles project upward laterally whereas the superior facet of the atlas faces upward laterally to support the occiput. The articulation between C1 and C2 is flatter to allow rotation. Occipital condyle (O), lateral mass of the atlas (A), and C1–C2 articulation (arrows)

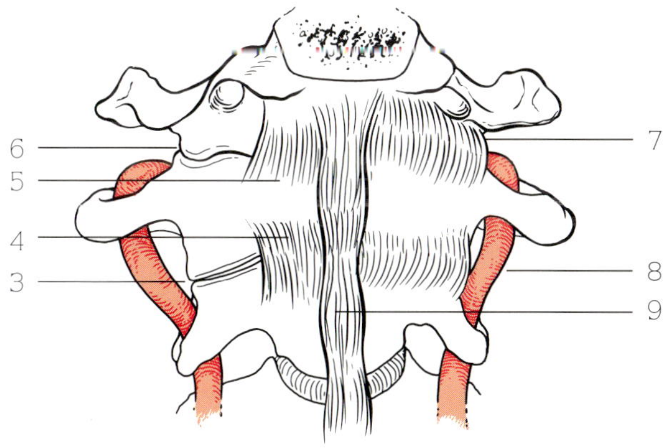

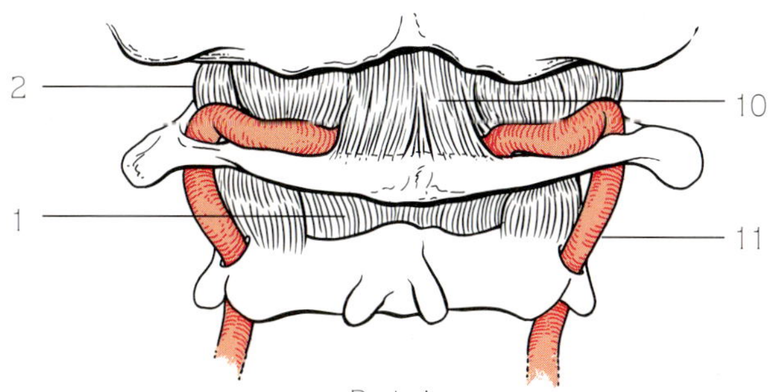

Figure 1.5
Anterior and posterior views of the occiput–C2 articulation, showing the atlanto-occipital articulation supported by anterior and posterior occipital membranes, which are continuations of anterior longitudinal ligament and ligamentum flavum, respectively

1 Ligamentum flavum
2 Atlanto-occipital joint capsule
3 Atlantoaxial articulation
4 Atlantoaxial membrane
5 Anterior atlanto-occipital membrane
6 Atlanto-occipital articulation
7 Atlanto-occipital joint capsule
8 Vertebral a.
9 Anterior longitudinal ligament
10 Posterior atlanto-occipital membrane
11 Vertebral a.

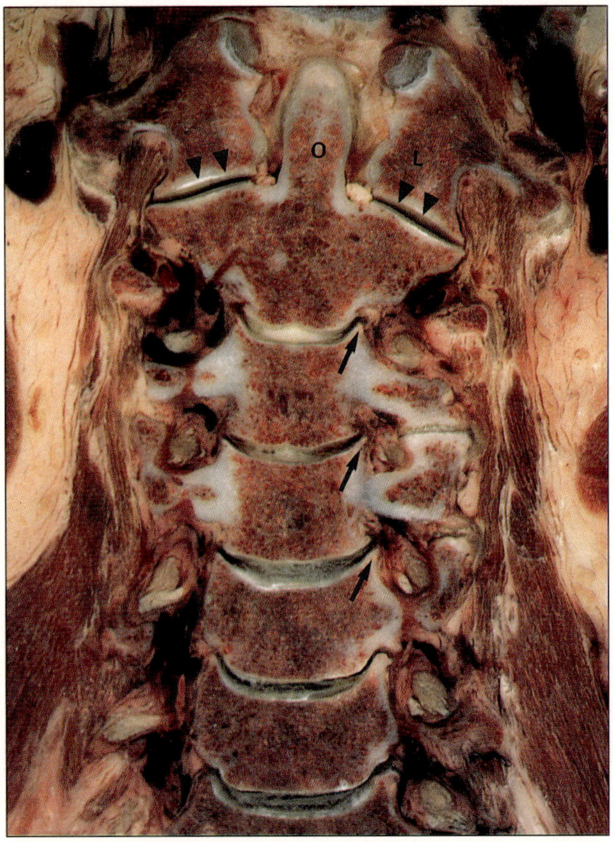

Figure 1.6
A freezing microtome section of the occiput–C7 region in a coronal plane, showing the inferior facets of the atlas that are flatter and facing downward laterally to articulate with the axis (arrow heads). Lateral projections of the uncinate processes of the lower cervical spine are well appreciated. Odontoid (O), lateral mass of C1 (L), uncinate process (arrows)

Figure 1.7 (below)
Diagrams of ligamentous anatomy of the upper cervical region. The odontoid process projects upward anteriorly, articulating with the posterior aspect of the anterior arch of the atlas as a synovial joint. The transverse ligament which spans across the arch of the atlas holds the odontoid process against the anterior arch of atlas. The transverse ligament has superior and inferior extensions, which form the cruciate ligament of the atlas. Secondary stabilizers of this articulation are alar ligament, which arises from the sides of dens to the condyles of the occipital bone and the apical ligament, which arises from the apex of the dens to the foramen magnum as a remnant of the notocord. The tectoral membrane is a continuation from the posterior longitudinal ligament

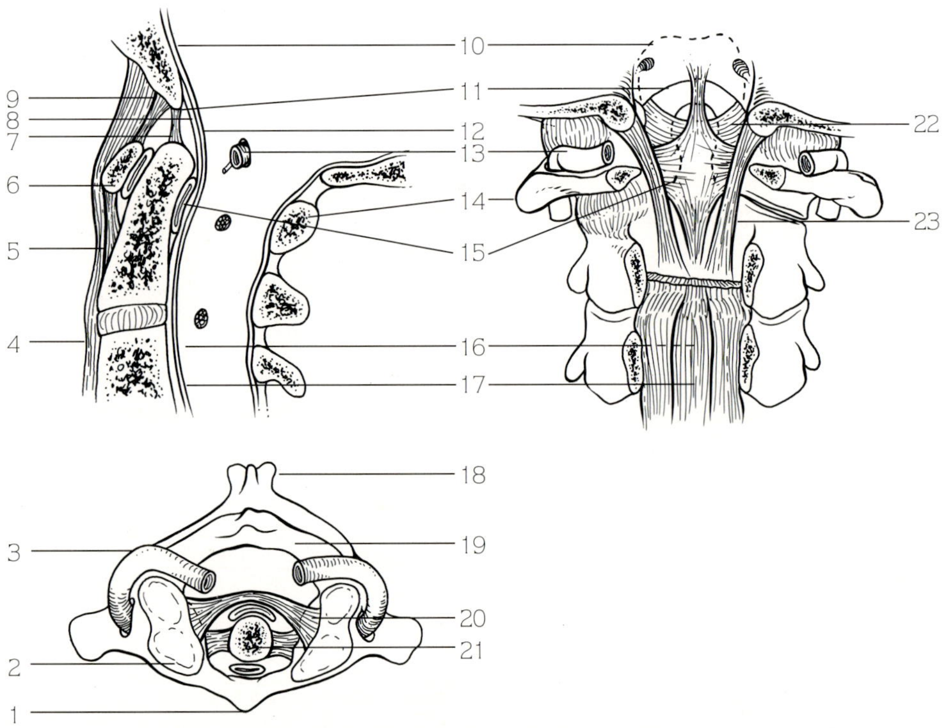

1 Anterior tubercle
2 Superior articular facet
3 Vertebral a.
4 Anterior longitudinal ligament
5 Anterior atlas–axis membrane
6 Anterior arch of atlas
7 Apical ligament
8 Vertical cruciform ligament
9 Anterior atlas–occipital membrane
10 Attachment of tectorial membrane
11 Anterior edge of foramen magnum
12 Tectorial membrane
13 Vertebral a.
14 Atlas
15 Transverse ligament
16 Origin of tectorial membrane
17 Posterior longitudinal ligament
18 Spinous process (axis)
19 Atlas
20 Transverse ligament
21 Dens (odontoid process)
22 Alar ligament
23 Deep tectorial membrane

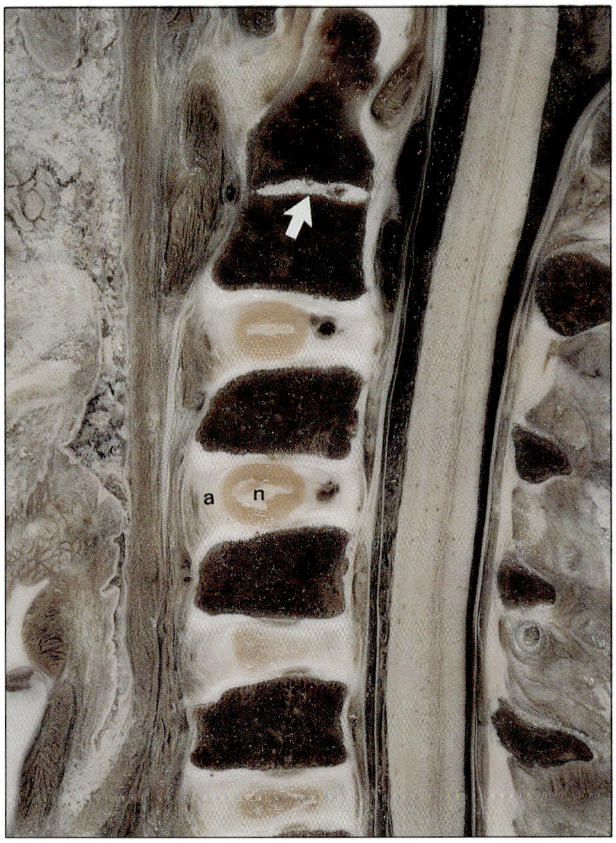

Figure 1.8
A midsagittal freezing microtome section of an immature cervical spine, showing the synchondrosis (arrow) between the odontoid process and the body. The margin between the nucleus pulposus (n) and annulus fibrosis (a) of the intervertebral disc is distinct

cleft between the body and the arch, fuse at 3–6 years, and the dens begins to fuse to the ossific nucleus of the C2 vertebral body at the age of 4 years (Fig. 1.8). These developmental lines should not be confused on radiographs with fractures in the skeletally immature patient.

The atlantoaxial articulation provides about 50% of rotatory motion of the cervical spine. The spinal canal at the upper cervical spine is more capacious than the lower cervical spine with saggital diameters averaging about 23 mm at C1 and 20 mm at C2 (Fig. 1.9). When approaching the posterior aspect of the atlas and axis surgically, the surgeon must avoid injuries to the associated neurovascular structures, such as the vertebral artery, spinal ganglion of C2, and the spinal cord (Fig. 1.10).

The bony anatomy of the lower cervical spine from C3 to C6 is similar, with slight dimensional increases on proceeding in a cranial-to-caudal direction. C7 is unique because it represents the transitional vertebra of the cervicothoracic region (Fig. 1.11). Posteriorly, the spinous processes are bifid structures from C3 to C6, and project posteriorly and inferiorly. The C7 spinous process is large and not bifid, and is often called the vertebra prominens. The junction between the spinous process and lamina is distinct from C3 to C6, but not well defined at the C7 level. This junction is anatomically important during spinous process wiring because, when the wire penetrates anterior to the spinolaminar line,

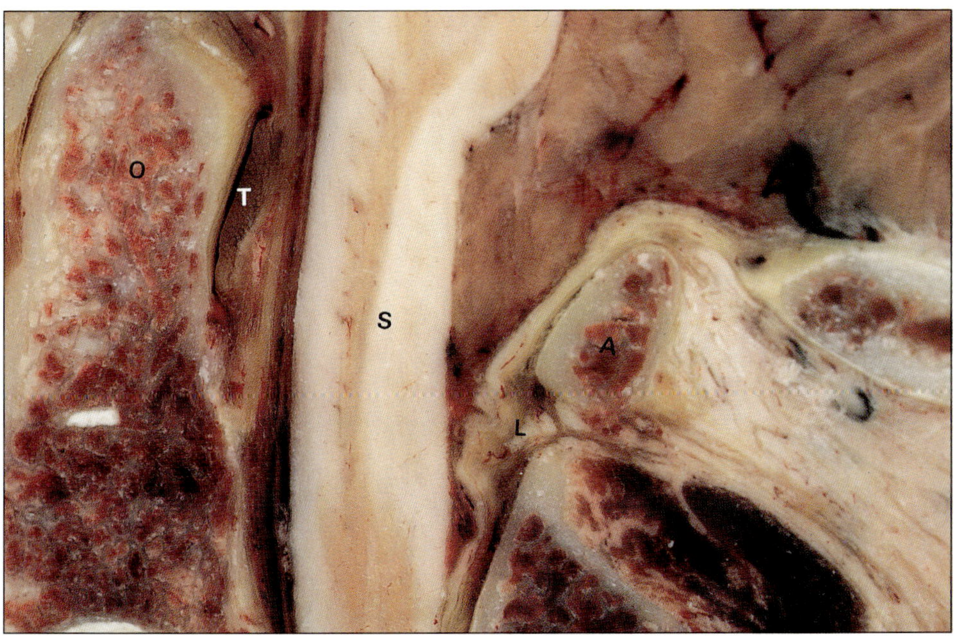

Figure 1.9
A midsagittal freezing microtome section of the upper cervical spine, showing a capacious spinal canal. Odontoid process (O), posterior ring of the atlas (A), ligamentum flavum (L), transverse ligament (T), and spinal cord (S)

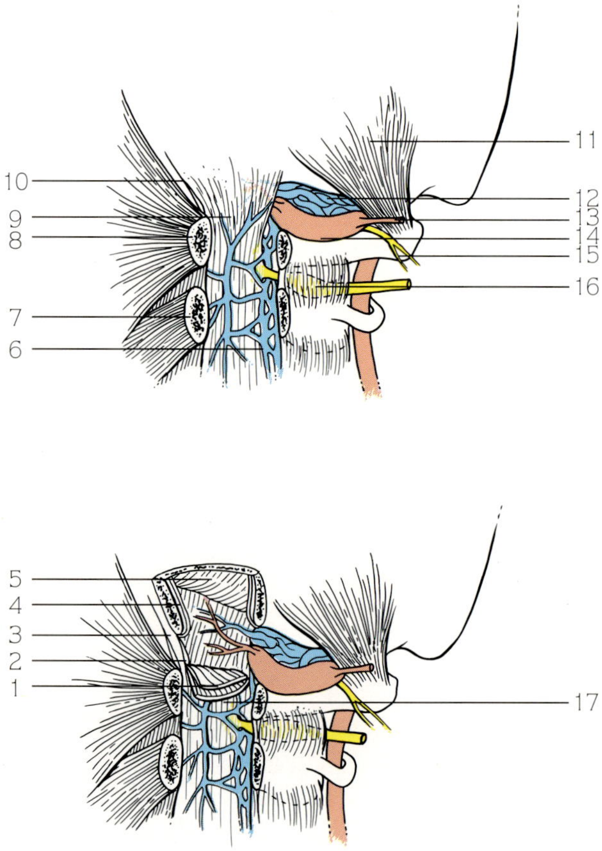

Figure 1.10
Neurovascular anatomy of posterior upper cervical spinal region. The vertebral artery, spinal ganglion of C2, and the spinal cord are in close proximity to the osseous structures

1 Line of incision between spinal dura mater and cranial dura mater
2 Spinal dura mater (cut edge)
3 Cut edge of spinal dura mater
4 Cranial dura mater (cut edge)
5 Arachnoid over cerebellum
6 Anteroinferior vertebral venous plexus
7 Axis
8 Atlas
9 Spinal dura mater
10 Posterior atlanto-occipital membrane (removed on right)
11 Oblique capitis superior m.
12 Suboccipital venous plexus
13 Muscular branch of vertebral a.
14 Right vertebral a.
15 Suboccipital a.
16 Spinal ganglion C2
17 Line of incision of reflected spinal dura mater along occipital bone

Table 1.1 Interfacet or inter-screw-hole distances from C3 to T1 from 22 cadaveric specimens

	Interfacet of inter-screw-hole distances (mm) for						
	C3–C4	*C4–C5*	*C5–C6*	*C6–C7*	*C6–C7p**	*C7–T1p*	*C7p–T1p*
Average	12.8	13.1	13.1	13.5	8.9	10.7	15.3
Median	13	13	13	13	9	11	15
Range	10–16	9–16	10–16	10–16	7–12	7–14	13–18
Standard deviation	1.7	1.9	1.7	1.9	1.3	1.9	2.0

*p designates pedicle.

it may impinge on the spinal cord. The lamina blends into the lateral mass, which is the bone between the superior and inferior articular processes. The articular processes themselves oppose each other to form the facet joint. The normal cervical facet joint has articular cartilage and menisci surrounded by a capsular ligament and lined by a synovial membrane (Fig. 1.11). Most adult cervical facet joints undergo changes with aging which consist of a thin layer of cartilage and irregularly thickened subarticular cortical bone.[12] Yu et al[23] reported four distinct types of menisci in the cervical facet joints (Fig. 1.12). The joint capsules are richly innervated by proprioceptive and pain receptors which may be important in the pathogenesis of neck pain.

When viewing the facet joint posteriorly, the facet joint line is horizontal and slightly circular inferiorly. The interfacet distances are relatively constant at different levels, but individual variations exist from 9 mm to 16 mm with an average of 13 mm (Table 1.1).[1] For this reason, most lateral

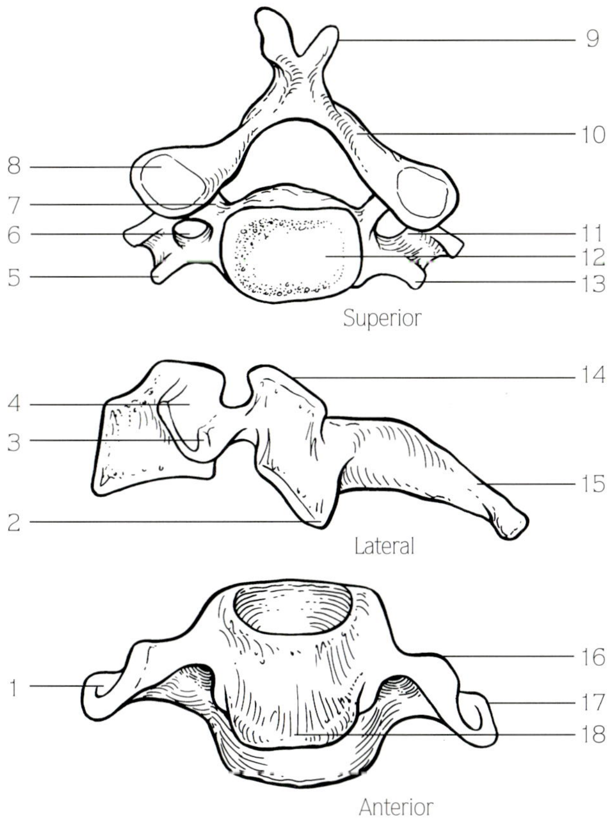

Figure 1.11
Superior, lateral, and anterior views of a middle cervical vertebra

1 Sulcus for nerve
2 Inferior articular process
3 Posterior tubercle
4 Sulcus for spinal n.
5 Anterior tubercle
6 Transverse foramen
7 Pedicle
8 Superior articular process
9 Spinus process
10 Lamina
11 Sulcus for spinal n.
12 Body
13 Costal process
14 Sup. articular process
15 Spinous process
16 Anterior tubercle
17 Posterior tubercle
18 Body

Figure 1.12 (below)
(a) Diagram of the four types of menisci. Type 1 is a structure of dense connective tissue that covers 50% or more of a joint surface. Type 2 in the sagittal section has a triangular cross-section and covers less than half of the joint surface. Type 3 has no meniscus-like tissue in the joint. Type 4 has an irregular mass of collagen, fat, and cartilage within the joints. (From Yu S, Sether L, Haughton VM: Facet joint menisci of the cervical spine: correlative MR imaging and cryomicrotomy study. *Radiology* 1987; 164: 79–82.) (b) A freezing microtome section of the facet joint and type 4 meniscus (arrow). Nerve root (N)

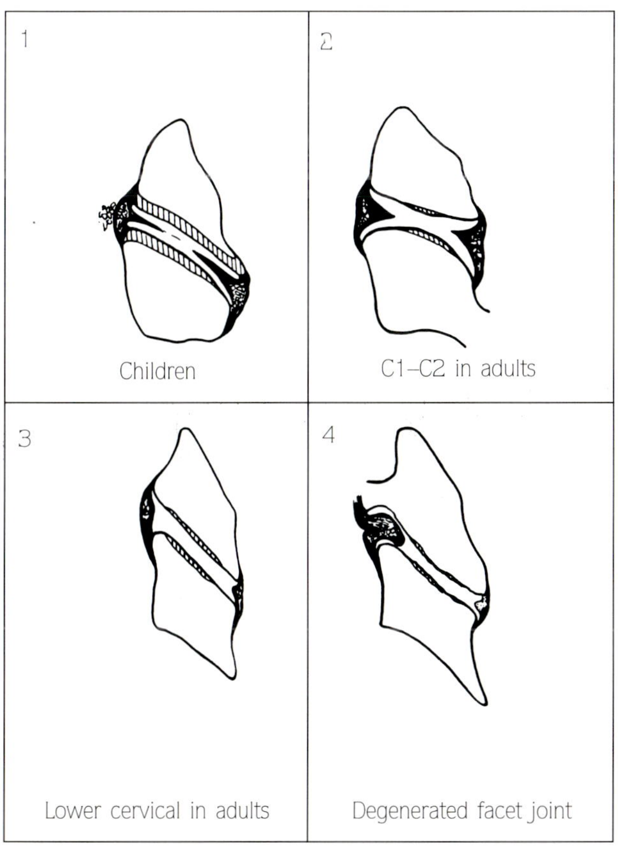

a

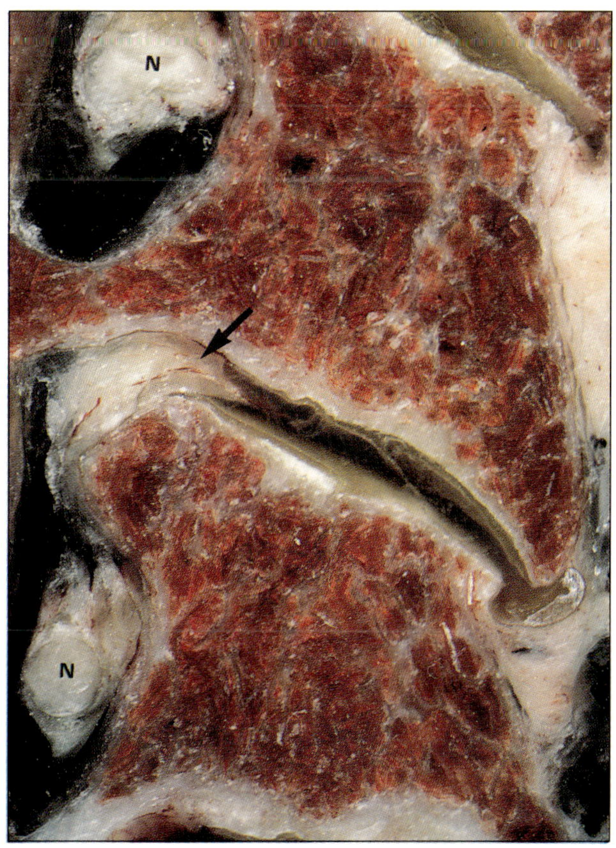

b

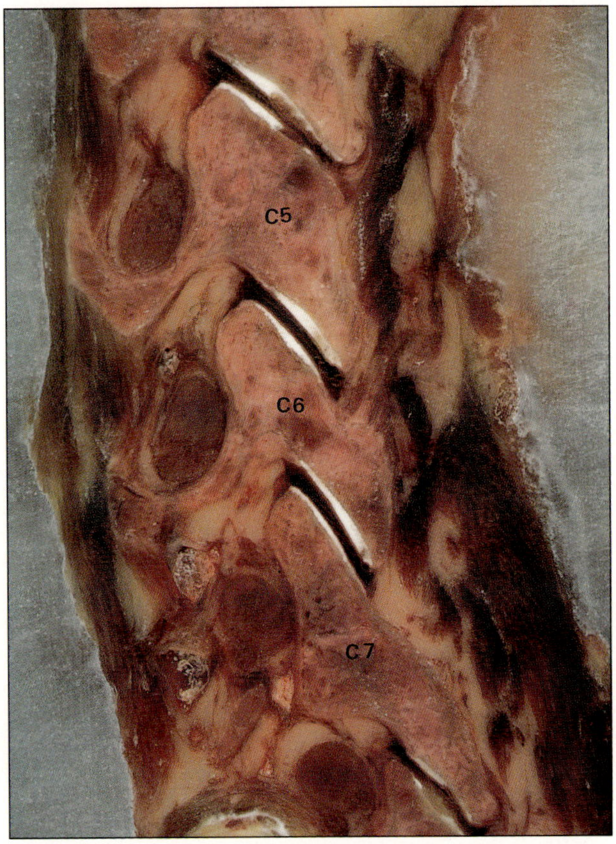

Figure 1.13
A parasagittal freezing microtome section of the facet joint showing an angle about 45° cephalad from the transverse plane in the middle cervical region and a greater angle in the lower cervical region. The lateral mass of C7 is more elongated from superior to inferior and thinner from anterior to posterior

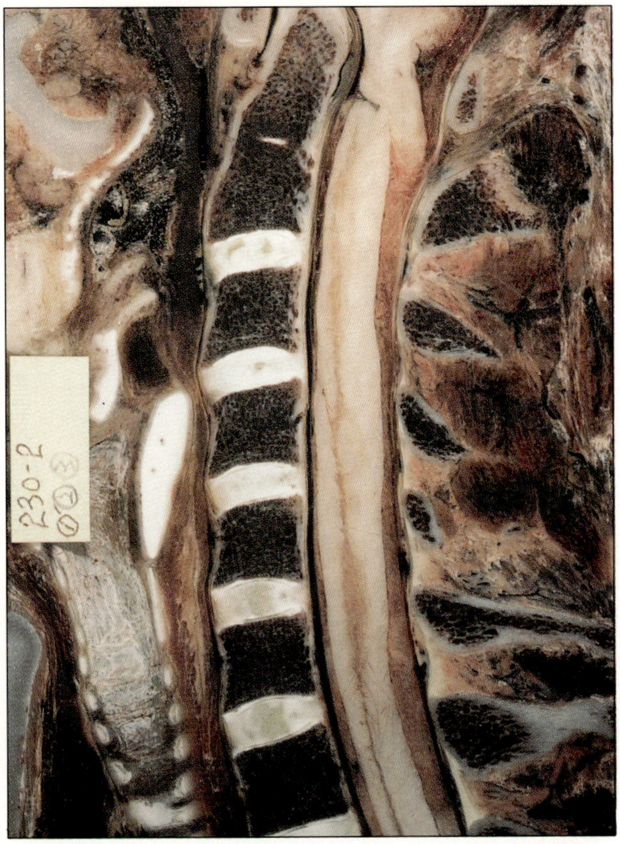

Figure 1.14
A midsagittal freezing microtome section, showing the vertebral body, intervertebral disc, spinal canal, and posterior elements. The superior surface of the body is slightly convex or straight with the corresponding concave inferior surface of the upper vertebral body

mass plate-screw systems are designed to have screw hole distances of 13 mm. Important anatomic landmarks for posterior plate-screw instrumentation include the facet joint lines, medial and lateral margins of the lateral mass, and joint inclination. Medially, from C3 to C6, there is a definite junction between the lamina and lateral mass. The lateral edge of the lateral mass forms a ridge down to the transverse process. The facet joint itself is typically angled 45° cephalad from the transverse plane (Fig. 1.13). The lateral mass of C7 is more elongated in a superoinferior and thinner in an anteroposterior direction (Fig. 1.13).

Anterolaterally, a typical cervical vertebra consists of a body, transverse processes, and pedicles. The body is relatively small and oval in shape with the medial–lateral diameter more than the anteroposterior diameter. In the coronal plane, the superior surface of the vertebral body is concave, and the inferior surface of the body is correspondingly convex (see Fig. 1.6). However, in the saggital plane, the superior surface of the body is slightly convex or straight with the corresponding concave inferior surface of the upper vertebral body (Fig. 1.14), the anteroinferior edge of the vertebral body is lipped inferiorly, and the lateral surfaces of the superior vertebral body project upward, conforming to small grooves in the inferolateral borders of the cephalad vertebra, forming the unconvertebral joints or joints of Luschka (see Fig. 1.6).

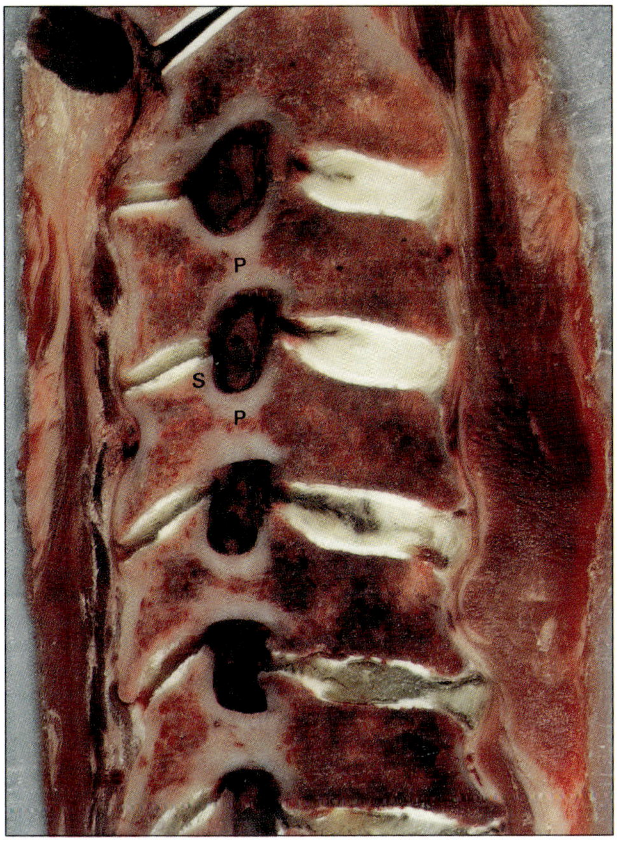

Figure 1.15
A 45° oblique freezing microtome showing the intervertebral foramina that are bounded anteriorly by the vertebral bodies and intervertebral discs, posteriorly by the facets and superior articular process (S), cephalad and caudad by the pedicles (P)

The width and depth of the vertebral surfaces average 17 mm and 15 mm respectively, from C2 to C6, and increase to about 20 mm and 17 mm respectively, at C7.[15] Vertebral heights on the posterior wall in the midsaggital plane range from 11 mm to 13 mm. The anterior tubercle of the transverse process projects laterally from the cephalad aspect of the vertebral body. This joins the posterior tubercle of the transverse process (see Fig. 1.11). The anterior tubercle is a costal element and is most prominent at C6; it is also known as the carotid tubercle, which is commonly used as a palpable surgical landmark. Between the posterior and anterior tubercles lies the groove or costotransverse lamella, which projects inferiorly for passage of the spinal nerve. The vertebral artery and venous system pass through the transverse foramen, which is located medial to the tubercles of the transverse process and lateral to the vertebral body. The transverse processes increase significantly in size at C6 and C7, with the pedicles projecting posterolaterally from the vertebral body at a 30–45° angle, and joining the lamina to form the vertebral arch (see Fig. 1.11).

The spinal canal or vertebral foramen is triangular in shape with rounded angles. The lateral width of the canal is significantly greater than the anteroposterior depth at all levels. Normal sagittal diameters of the cervical spine are 17–18 mm at C3 through C6, and 15 mm at C7.[15] The cross-sectional area of the spinal canal is largest at C2 and smallest at C7, with the height of the pedicle about 7 mm, and the width 5–6 mm with a slight increase from C3 to C7.[15] As mentioned earlier, the C2 pedicle is larger, with a height of 10 mm and width of 8 mm. From C3 to C7, angulation of the pedicles varies from 8° below to 11° above the transverse plane. The pedicle angle in the sagittal plane decreases from 45 to 30° for C3 down to C7. The intervertebral foramina are bounded anteriorly by the vertebral bodies and intervertebral discs, posteriorly by the facets, and cephalad and caudad by the pedicles (Fig. 1.15). The cervical foramina measure 9–12 mm in height and 4–6 mm in width for passage of the spinal nerves.[4,5] The cervical foramina are aligned in a 45° oblique direction in the sagittal plane. Oblique radiographs and oblique magnetic resonance images (Fig. 1.16) are helpful in assessing the bony dimensions and/or soft tissue contents of the intervertebral foramen. During anterior exposures of the vertebral body and intervertebral discs, dissection carried too far laterally on the inferior half of the vertebral body and unconvertebral joints endangers the vertebral artery and spinal nerve around the intervertebral foramen.

The cervicothoracic junction is a transition region with C7 having similar anatomic characteristics to T1 and T2. The dimensions of the vertebral body, and transverse and spinous processes, are larger at C6 and C7, whereas the dimensions of the spinal canal decrease at C6 and C7, representing a distinct transition to the thoracic region. The articulating facet joint between C7 and T1 resembles the thoracic facet joint. The lateral mass of C7 is quite thin when compared to the mid-cervical spine. Morphologic characteristics of C7, T1, and T2 pedicles have been obtained with respect to diameter, depth, and angulation (Table 1.2).[1] Inner diameters of the pedicles at C7, T1, and T2, in a medial–lateral plane, average 5.2, 6.3, and 5.5 mm, respectively. From a posteroanterior direction, the pedicles were found to angulate medially 34, 30, and 26° at C7, T1, and T2, respectively. These morphologic characteristics should be borne in mind when performing transpedicular procedures in the cervicothoracic region.

Table 1.2 Morphological characteristics of C7, T1, and T2 pedicles in their diameters, depths, and medial angulation

		*Pedicle measurements (mm)**					
		Diameter$_O$	*Diameter$_I$*	*Diameter$_{S/I}$*	*Depth$_P$*	*Depth$_B$*	*Angulation$_M$*
C7	Average	5.2	6.9	6.4	9.1	33	34
	Median	5	7	7	9	33	35
	Range	4–6	6–8	5–8	7–12	29–37	27–40
	s.d.	0.6	0.8	1.0	1.5	2.3	4.3
T1	Average	6.3	8.5	8.8	9.9	34.3	31.8
	Median	6	9	9	10	35	30
	Range	5–9	7–12	8–10	7–15	28–39	27–37
	s.d.	1.4	1.6	0.6	2.2	3.6	3.6
T2	Average	5.5	7.5	10.7	10.4	38.2	26.5
	Median	5	7	11	10	37	25
	Range	5–7	6–9	9–12	7–14	33–45	20–35
	s.d.	0.7	0.9	1.0	2.4	4.2	4.4

*Diameter$_O$ = medial–lateral outer diameter; Diameter$_I$ = medial–lateral inner diameter; Diameter$_{S/I}$ = superoinferior outer diameter; Depth$_P$ = pedicle depth; Depth$_B$ = body depth; Angulation$_M$ = medial pedicle angulation.
s.d. = standard deviation.

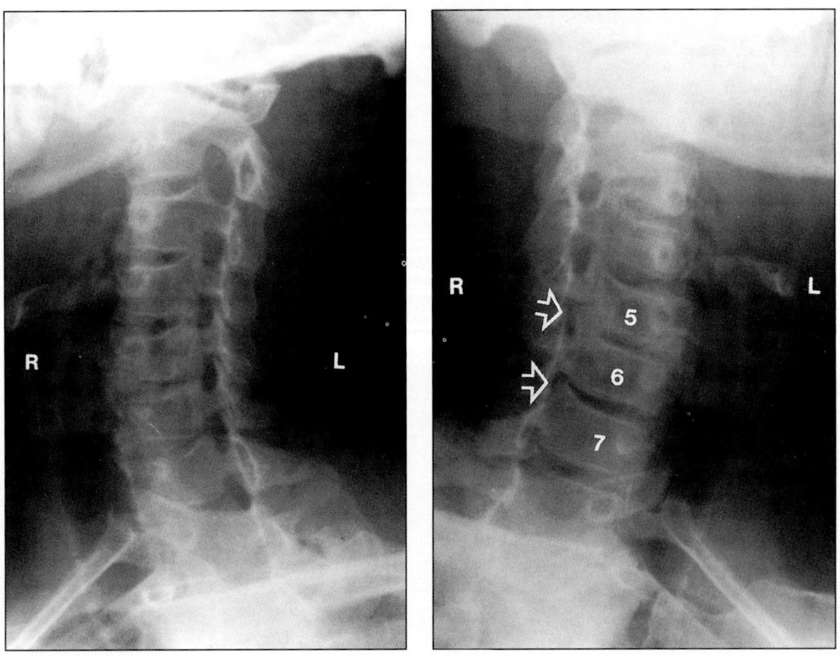

a b

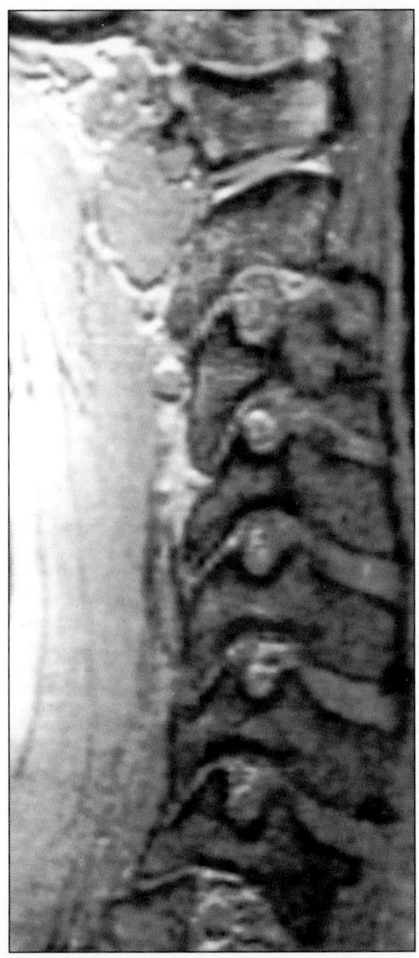

c

Figure 1.16
Oblique radiographs showing left cervical foramina (a), and right cervical foramina (b) that align in a 45° oblique direction in the sagittal plane. (c) Oblique MRI. Right C5–C6 and C6–C7 foramina narrowed (arrows) (b)

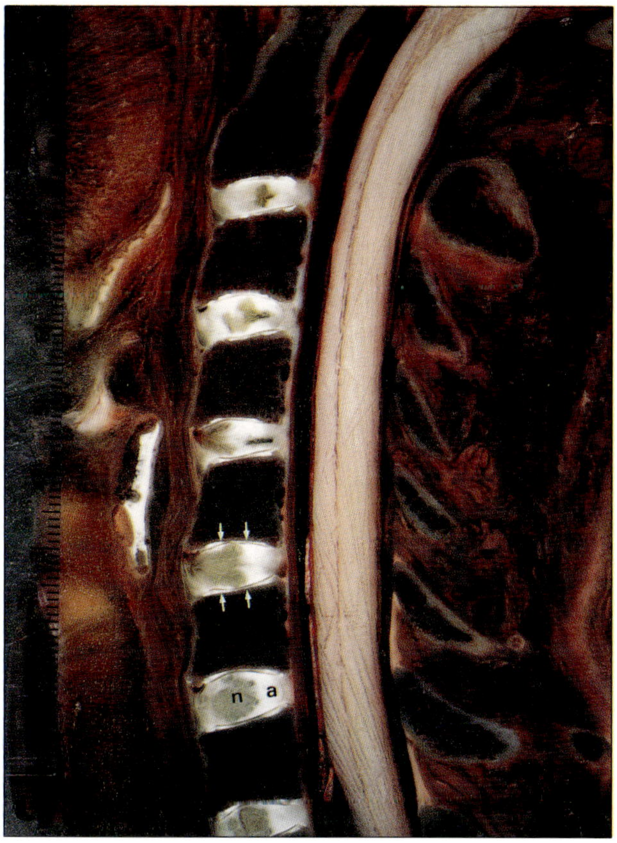

Figure 1.17
A midsagittal freezing microtome of cervical spine showing the intervertebral disc consisting of the nucleus pulposus (n) at the interior of the disc, the outer annulus fibrosis (a), and the cartilaginous end-plates (arrows) adjacent to the vertebral surfaces

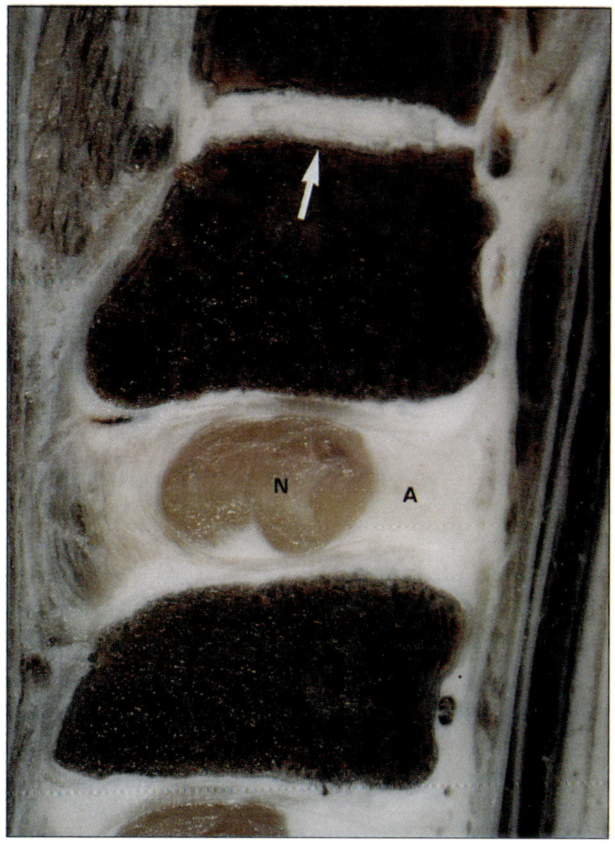

Figure 1.18
A midsagittal freezing microtome of an infant cervical spine with a clear border between the annulus fibrosis (A) and annulus (N). The synchondrosis (arrow) between the odontoid process and the body is demonstrated at C2

INTERVERTEBRAL DISC AND LIGAMENTS

Intervertebral discs are present between vertebrae except at the atlantoaxial level. Each intervertebral disc is essentially an avascular structure which consists of an inner nucleus pulposus, an outer annulus fibrosis, and the cartilaginous end-plates adjacent to the vertebral surfaces (Fig. 1.17). The nucleus pulposus is derived from the primitive notochord and functions as a shock absorber, whereas the annulus fibrosis aids the stability of the motion segment together with the ligamentous structures and posterior articulations. The nucleus pulposus is clearly bordered by the annulus fibrosis in infancy, but the margin between the nucleus pulposus and annulus fibrosis becomes less distinct in the adult (Fig. 1.18).[2] After 50 years of age, the nucleus pulposus is difficult to distinguish from the annulus fibrosis, as the nucleus pulposus becomes a fibrocartilaginous mass similar to the inner zone of the annulus fibrosis.

The annulus has an outer collagenous layer, in which the fibers are arranged in concentric oblique layers of lamellae, with the fibers of each lamella running perpendicular to the fibers of the adjacent lamella. The collagen fibers in the posterior portion of the disc run in a more vertical than an oblique direction, which could account for the relative frequency of radial tears seen clinically in the annulus fibrosis. From birth to adolescence, the cervical disc increases in height from 7.6 to 17.8 mm (0.3 to 0.7 inches).[22] The vertebral bodies grow in height more than the discs. At birth, one-third of the length of the spine comes from the intervertebral discs, whereas after the age of 7 years, the

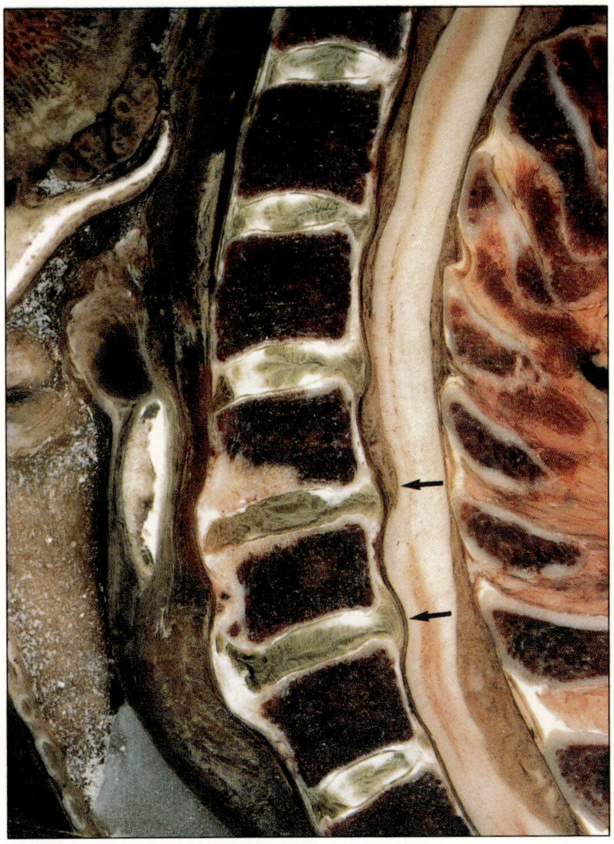

Figure 1.19
A midsagittal freezing microtome of a degenerative cervical spine showing degeneration of the annulus fibrosis and herniation of nucleus pulposus at C5–C6 and C6–C7 levels with spinal cord impingement (arrows)

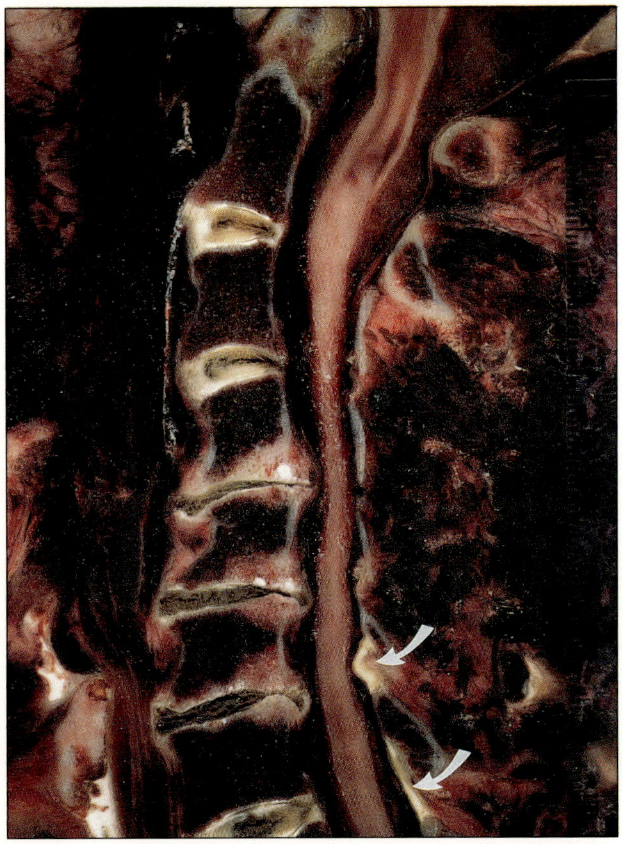

Figure 1.20
A midsagittal freezing microtome of a severe cervical spondylotic spine showing narrowing of the disc spaces and spinal canal narrowing at C4–C5, C5–C6, and C6–C7 levels. Ligamentum flavum (arrow) buckling is shown as well

discs account for only one-fifth of the total spinal length. The discs are shaped to conform to the surface of the vertebral bodies, so the superior surface of the disc is concave, and the inferior surface of the disc is correspondingly convex in the coronal plane (see Fig. 1.6). The discs are also slightly thicker anteriorly than posteriorly, which contributes to the lordotic posture of the cervical spine (Fig. 1.17). The cervical intervertebral discs allow some translation in the sagittal plane, but lateral movement is resisted by the uncinate processes. The uncinate process, which is located in the posterolateral aspect of the disc, may help prevent disc herniation in this area.

Degeneration of the annulus fibrosis in the cervical spine is similar to the lumbar region, in which concentric, transverse, and radial tears of the annulus occur over time. Radial tears in the posterior aspect of the disc are thought to be more clinically significant as they may allow for herniation of the nucleus pulposus (Figs 1.19 and 1.20).[21] The annulus fibrosis is firmly attached to the adjacent vertebral end-plates. The cartilaginous end-plate represents a layer of hyaline cartilage resting on the subchondral bone of the vertebral body, and serves as a barrier to distribute stress over the nucleus pulposus and adjacent vertebral bodies. This cartilage is a growth plate and is responsible for endochondral ossification during growth. The cartilaginous end-plates also allow for the insertion of the inner fibers of the annulus fibrosis and diffusion of nutrients from the subchondral bone to the disc.

The outermost fibers of the annulus fibrosis are contiguous with the anterior and posterior longitudinal ligaments. The anterior longitudinal ligament is a strong band that attaches from the skull as the anterior atlanto-occipital

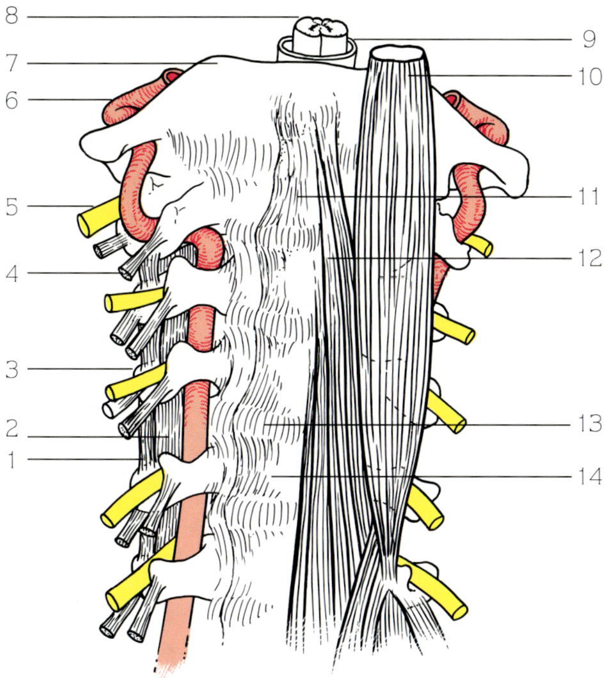

Figure 1.21
Anterior aspect of the cervical spine showing the anterior longitudinal ligament and longus colli muscle. The anterior longitudinal ligament is a strong band that attaches from the skull and continues caudally over the entire length of the spine down to the sacrum. The anterior longitudinal ligament is thinner and more closely attached at the intervertebral disc margins than at the concave anterior vertebral surfaces. Also shown are the spinal nerves and the vertebral artery on the lateral aspect of the cervical spine

1 Intertransversus ligament
2 Posterior inter-transversus m.
3 Posterior tubercle
4 Anterior scalenus m.
5 Spinal n.
6 Vertebral a.
7 Atlas
8 Spinal cord
9 Dura mater
10 Longus capitus m.
11 Anterior longitudinal ligament
12 Longus colli m.
13 Intervertebral disc
14 Vertebral body

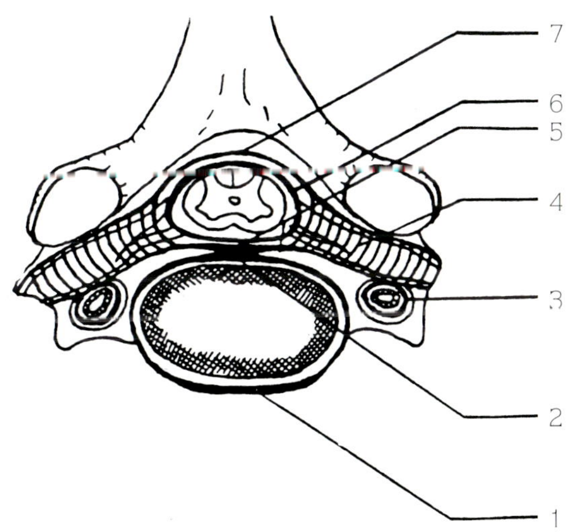

Figure 1.22
Diagram of layers of the posterior longitudinal ligament. The posterior longitudinal ligament is double-layered, and the deep layer sends fibers to the annulus fibrosis and continues laterally to the intervertebral foramina. The anterior longitudinal ligament extends laterally to merge with the deep layer of the posterior longitudinal ligament in the region of the intervertebral foramina. The superficial or more dorsal layer of the posterior longitudinal ligament is adjacent to the dura mater and continues as a connective tissue membrane which envelops the dura mater, nerve roots and the vertebral artery. (From Hayashi K, Yabuki T, Kurokawa T, Seki H, Hogaki M, Minoura S: The anterior and the posterior longitudinal ligaments of the lower cervical spine. *J Anat* 1977; 124: 633–6

1 Anterior long. ligament
2 Deep layer of the post. long. ligament
3 Epiarterial sheath
4 Epiradicural sheath
5 Superficial layer of the post. long. ligament
6 Dura mater
7 Epidural membrane

membrane, and continues caudally over the entire length of the spine down to the sacrum. The anterior longitudinal ligament is thinner and more closely attached at the intervertebral disc margins than to the concave anterior vertebral body surfaces (Fig. 1.21). The posterior longitudinal ligament is wider in the upper cervical spine than in the lower cervical spine, and wider over the intervertebral discs than over the vertebral bodies.[16] According to Hayashi et al[14] the posterior longitudinal ligament is double-layered, with the deep layer sending fibers into the annulus fibrosis and continuing laterally to the region of the intervertebral foramina (Fig. 1.22). The anterior longitudinal ligament also sweeps around and envelops the lateral aspect of the vertebral bodies under the longus colli muscle. This lateral extension of the anterior longitudinal ligament is continuous with the deep layer of the posterior longitudinal ligament in the

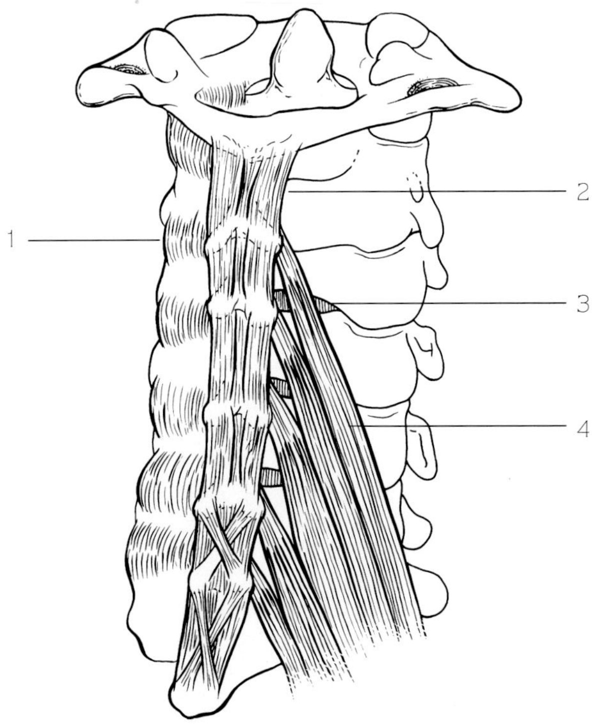

Figure 1.23
Posterior aspect of the cervical spine showing the interspinous ligament, articular capsule, and the ligamentum flavum

1 Articular capsule
2 Interspinous m.
3 Ligamentum flavum
4 Semispinalis cervicis m.

region of the intervertebral foramina.[14] The superficial or more dorsal layer of the posterior longitudinal ligament is adjacent to the dura mater and continues as a connective tissue membrane which envelops the dura mater, nerve roots, and vertebral artery, suggesting that this membrane may serve as a protective barrier.

The ligamentum flavum of the cervical spine attaches to the anterior surface of the lamina above, and to the superior margin of the lamina below (see Fig. 1.19). The ligamentum flavum extends laterally to the articular processes and contributes to the boundary of the intervertebral foramen. The ligamentum flavum primarily consists of elastic fibers, although this elasticity diminishes with age. Thickening and anterior buckling of the ligamentum flavum may contribute to symptoms of spinal cord compression. In the midline, there is a gap in the ligamentum flavum which allows for the exit of veins. The interspinous ligament of the cervical spine is thin and less well developed than in the lumbar region. The interspinous ligaments attach in an oblique orientation from the posterosuperior aspect to the anteroinferior aspect of the spinous process below (Fig. 1.23). The supraspinous ligament of the thoracolumbar spine extends into the cervical region as the ligamentum nuchae, which spans from the external occipital protuberance to the seventh cervical vertebra. There is no separate supraspinous ligament in the cervical region.[18] The ligamentum nuchae is a fibroelastic septum for the attachment of adjacent muscles.

MUSCLES AND FASCIA

The posterior muscles of the neck are divided into superficial, intermediate, and deep groups. The most superficial muscle is the trapezius, which originates from the external occipital protuberance and the medial nuchal line of C7 to T12 spinous processes and inserts onto the spine of the scapula, acromion, and the lateral aspect of the clavicle. The trapezius is innervated by the eleventh cranial nerve and functions to extend the head.

The intermediate muscles beneath the trapezius muscle include the splenius capitis and splenius cervicis, which originate from the spinous processes of the lower cervical and upper thoracic spine, and insert on the transverse processes of the upper cervical spine and the mastoid process (Fig. 1.24).

In the deep layer, the erector spinae muscles from the thoracolumbar spine continue into the cervical region and include iliocostalis laterally, longissimus cervicis and longissimus capitis centrally, and spinalis cervicis, semispinalis capitis, and semispinalis cervicis medially (Figs 1.25 and 1.26). Beneath the semispinalis muscles lie the multifidus from C4 to C7 and rotatores muscles, which cross only one segment of the spine and extend from the transverse process to the spinous process. In the upper cervical spine, suboccipital muscles attach from the occiput to the second vertebra. Rectus capitis posterior major originates from the C2 spinous process, and inserts on the inferior nuchal line of the occiput. Rectus capitis posterior minor originates from the posterior tubercle of the atlas, and inserts on the occiput (Fig. 1.26). Obliquus capitis inferior originates from the C2 spinous process and inserts on the transverse process of the atlas, whereas the obliquus capitis superior originates from the transverse process of the atlas and inserts on the occiput between the superior and inferior nuchal lines. Most posterior muscles are involved in producing extension of the neck and head, whereas some produce rotation and lateral flexion (Table 1.3).[16] The posterior deep muscles are innervated by the posterior primary rami and blood supply is via the deep cervical vessels (Fig. 1.27).

Table 1.3 The muscles that are involved in extension, flexion, and rotation and lateral bending

Extension	
	Splenius capitis
	Splenius cervicis
	Semispinalis capitis
	Semispinalis cervicis
	Longissimus capitis
	Longissimus cervicis
	Trapezius
	Interspinalis
	Rectus capitis posterior major
	Rectus capitis posterior minor
	Obliquus capitis superior
	Sternocleidomastoid (posterior fibers)
Flexion	
	Sternocleidomastoid (anterior fibers)
	Longus colli
	Longus capitis
	Rectus capitis anterior
Rotation and lateral bending	
	Sternocleidomastoid
	Scalene group
	Splenius capitis
	Splenius cervicis
	Longissimus capitis
	Levator scapulae
	Longus colli
	Iliocostalis cervicis
	Multifidi
	Intertransversarii
	Obliquus capitis inferior
	Obliquus capitis superior
	Rectus capitis lateralis

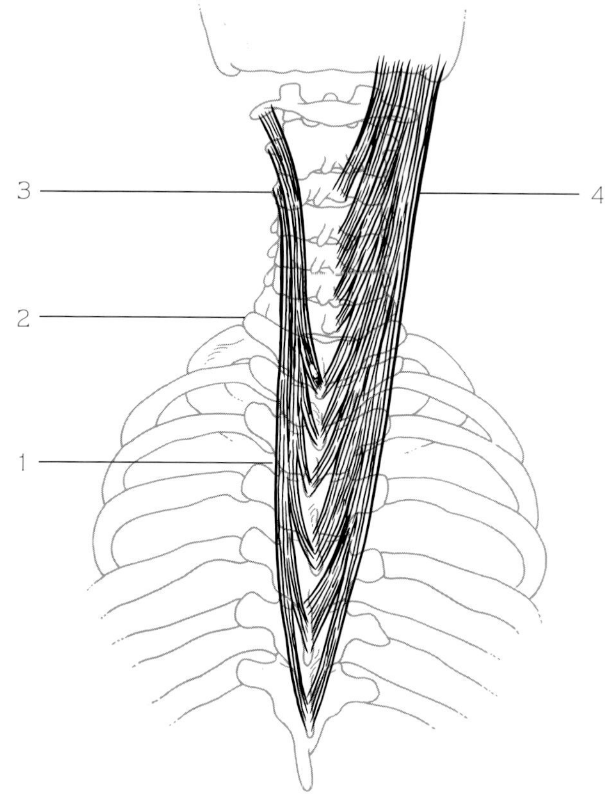

Figure1.24
The superficial layer of muscle consisting of splenius capitis and splenius cervicis, which originate from the spinous processes of the lower cervical and upper thoracic spines and insert on the transverse processes of the upper cervical spine and the mastoid process

1 Splenius cervicis m.
2 T1
3 Posterior C3 tubercle
4 Splenius capitis m.

The anterolateral muscles of the neck include the platysma, sternocleidomastoid, hyoid muscles, strap muscles of the larynx, scalenes, longus colli, and longus capitis (Fig. 1.28). The platysma is a thin muscle just beneath the subcutaneous tissues, and spans the deltoid to the upper pectoral fascia, crosses over the clavicle, and passes obliquely upward and medially to insert on to the mandible, muscles of the lip, and skin of the lower part of the face. The platysma functions to depress the lower jaw and lip, and both tenses and ridges the skin of the anterior neck. The sternocleidomastoid originates from the sternum and the medial clavicle and attaches to the mastoid process and the lateral half of the superior nuchal line of the occipital bone. The sternocleidomastoid is innervated by both the second cervical nerve and spinal accessory nerve, and functions to draw the head toward the ipsilateral shoulder while rotating it so that the chin points cranially and toward the opposite side. When contracting synchronously, the sternocleidomastoids can either flex the head or raise the thorax, with the head held in a fixed position.

Muscles that attach to the hyoid bone include the digastric, stylohyoid, mylohyoid, geniohyoid, and omohyoid muscles. The strap muscles of the larynx include the sternohyoid and sternothyroid muscles. These muscles do

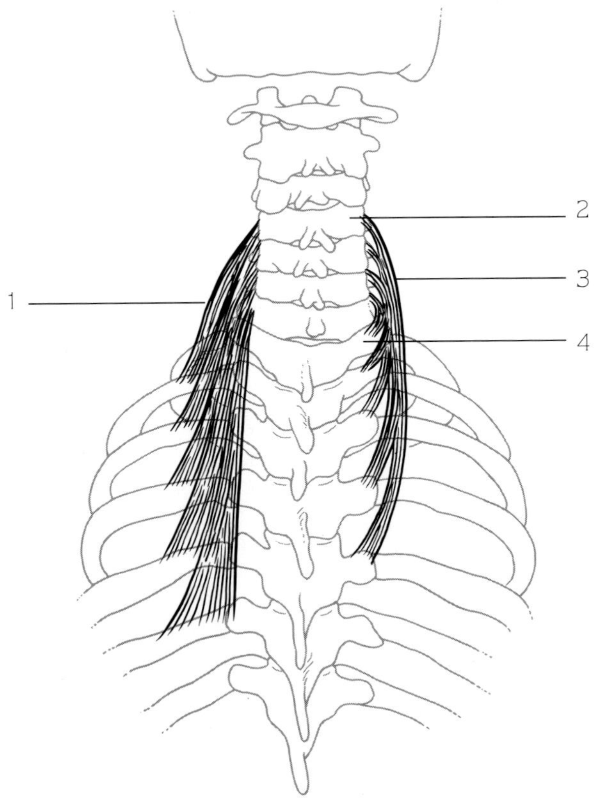

Figure 1.25
The deep layer of the cervicothoracic region showing the iliocostalis and longissimus cervicis laterally

1 Iliocostalis cervicis m.
2 C4
3 Longissimus cervicis m.
4 T1

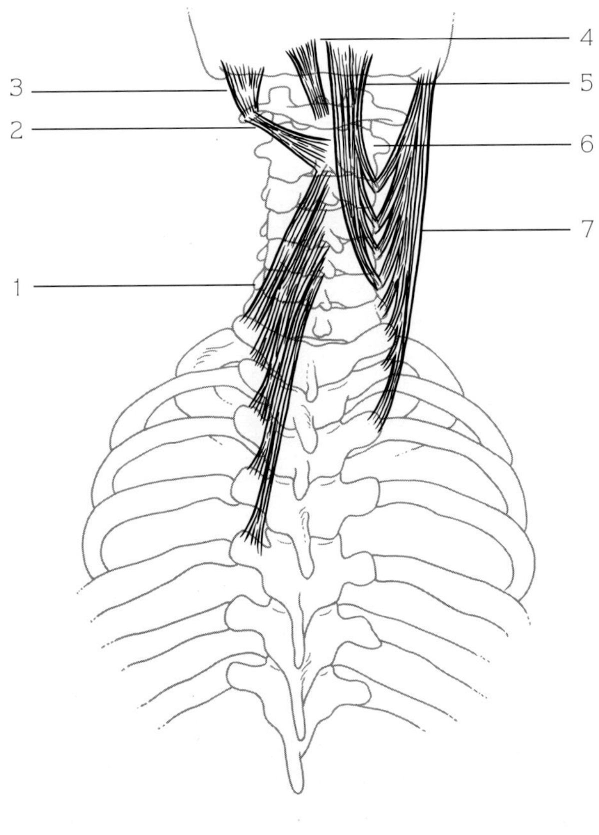

Figure 1.26
The deeper layer of muscles consisting of longissimus capitis laterally, and semispinalis capitis, and semispinalis cervicis medially. Suboccipital muscles attach at the occiput to second vertebrae. Rectus capitis posterior major originates from the C2 spinous process and inserts to the inferior nuchal line of the occiput (not shown), and rectus capitis posterior minor originates from the posterior tubercle of the atlas and inserts to the occiput, obliquus capitis inferior originates from the C2 spinous process and inserts on the transverse process of atlas, and obliquus capitis superior originates from the transverse process of the atlas and inserts on the occiput between the superior and inferior lines

1 Semispinalis cervicis m.
2 Oblique capitis inferior m.
3 Oblique capitis superior m.
4 Rectus capitis posterior minor m.
5 Semispinalis capitis m.
6 C2
7 Longissimus capitis m.

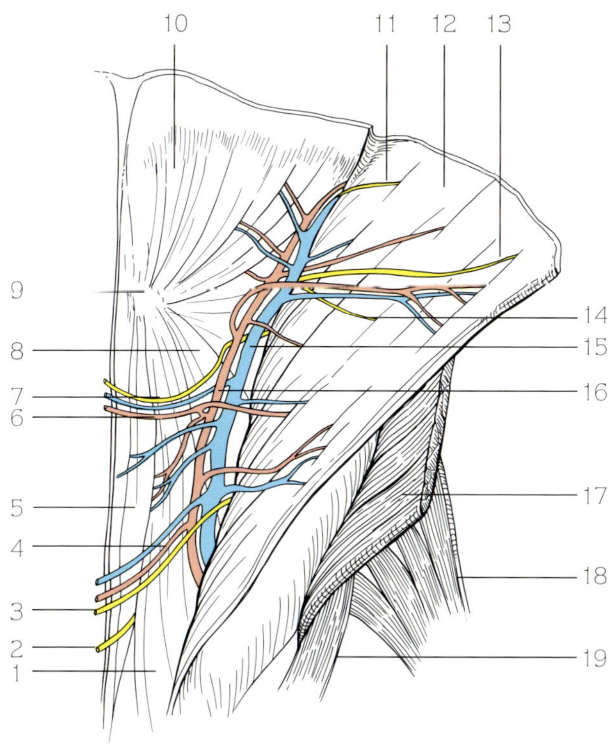

a

Figure 1.27

(a) Blood supply and innervation of the posterior deep muscles showing the deep cervical artery and branches and the posterior primary rami. (b) Suboccipital muscles are innervated by the suboccipital nerve (posterior primary ramus of C1) and blood supply is by muscular branch of the vertebral artery and branches from the deep cervical artery

1 Semispinalis cervicis m.
2 Medial branch ot posterior primary ramus of C5
3 Medial branch of posterior primary ramus of C4
4 Cutaneous branches of deep cervical a.
5 Spinalis cervicis m.
6 Cutaneous branches of deep cervical a.
7 Medial branch of posterior primary ramus of C3 (third occipital n.)
8 Multifidus m.
9 Spinous process of axis
10 Rectus capitis posterior major m.
11 Muscular branch of posterior primary ramus of C1
12 Semispinalis capitis m.
13 Greater occipital n.
14 Muscular branch of posterior primary ramus of C2
15 Deep cervical v.
16 Deep cervical a.
17 Longissimus cervicis and capitis mm.
18 Levator scapulae m.
19 Iliocostalis cervicis m.

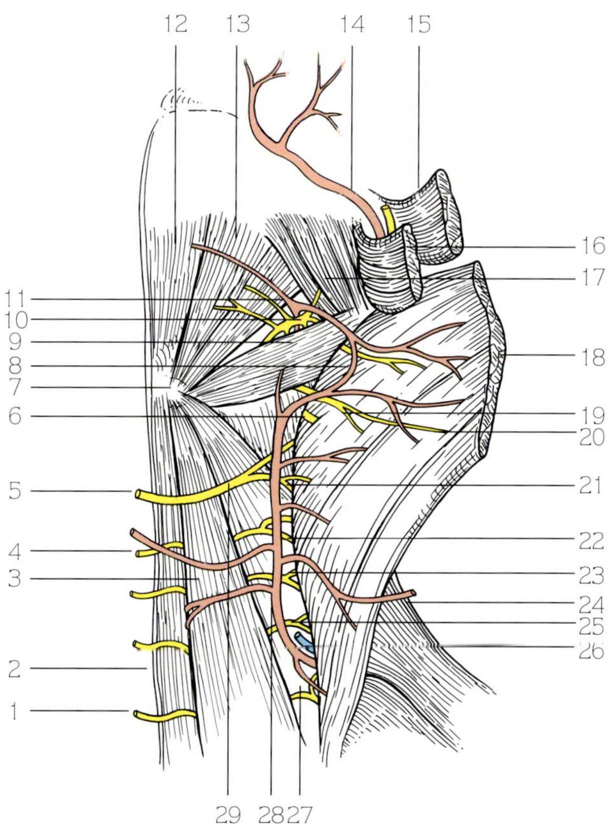

b

1 Medial cutaneous branch of posterior primary ramus of C8
2 Spinalis cervicis m.
3 Semispinalis cervicis m.
4 Medial cutaneous branch of posterior primary ramus of C5
5 Third occipital n. (medial cutaneous branch of posterior primary ramus of C3 and C4)
6 Posterior primary ramus of C3
7 Spinous process of axis
8 Anastomotic branch of deep cervical a.
9 Oblique capitis inferior m.
10 Suboccipital n. (posterior primary ramus C1)
11 Muscular branch of vertebral a.
12 Rectus capitis posterior minor m.
13 Rectus capitis posterior major m.
14 Occipital a.
15 Splenus capitis m.
16 Longissimus capitis m.
17 Oblique capitis superior m.
18 Semispinalis capitis m.
19 Muscular branch of posterior primary ramus of C2
20 Greater occipital n. (medial cutaneous branch of posterior primary ramus of C2)
21 Posterior primary ramus of C4
22 Deep primary ramus of C5
23 Posterior primary ramus of C6
24 Levator scapulae m.
25 Posterior primary ramus of C7
26 Deep cervical vein
27 Multifidus
28 Deep cervical a.
29 Cutaneous branch of deep cervical a.

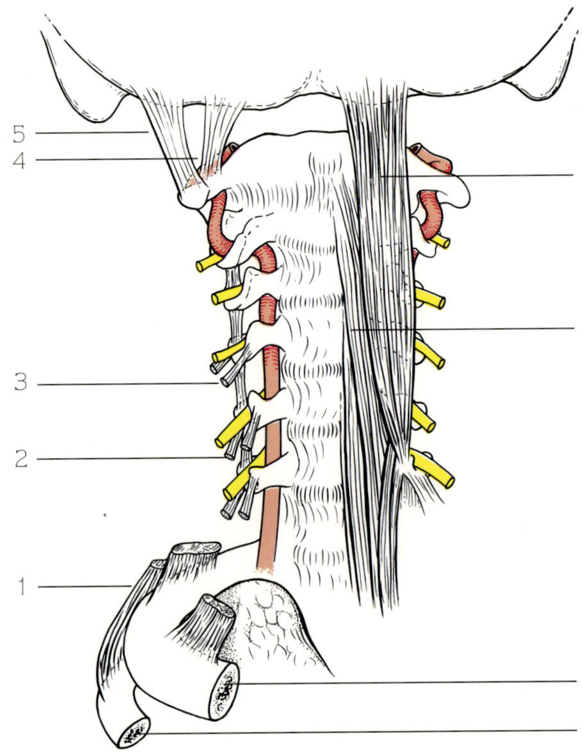

Figure 1.28
Longus colli and muscle attachments on the anterior aspect of the cervical spine. The longus colli spans from C1 to T3 and extends laterally to attach to the anterior tubercles of the transverse processes of C3, C4, C5, and C6. The longus capitis originates from the anterior tubercles of the transverse processes of C3, C4, C5, and C6, and attaches on the inferior surface of the basilar part of the occipital bone. Underneath the longus capitis the rectus capitis anterior spans from the lateral mass of the atlas to the base of the occipital bone, and the rectus capitis lateralis spans laterally from the transverse process of the atlas to the inferior surface of the jugular process of the occipital bone. The scalenus anterior originates from the anterior tubercles of the transverse processes of C3 to C6 and inserts on the first rib, and the scalenus medius originates from the posterior tubercles of the transverse processes of C2 to C7 and inserts on the first rib

1 Posterior scalenus m.
2 Middle scalenus m.
3 Ant. scalenus m.
4 Rectus capitis anterior m.
5 Rectus capitis lateral m.
6 Longus capitus m.
7 Longus colli m.
8 First rib
9 Second rib

not control motion of the cervical spine, but are important in controlling movement of the hyoid and larynx, and are important surgical landmarks during an anterior approach to the cervical spine.

The longus colli and longus capitis muscles are the prevertebral muscles of the neck (Fig. 1.28). The longus colli spans C1 to T3 and extends laterally to attach to the anterior tubercles of the transverse processes of C3, C4, C5 and C6. The longus capitis originates on the anterior tubercles of the transverse processes of C3, C4, C5, and C6 and attaches to the inferior surface of the basilar part of the occipital bone. Beneath the longus capitis muscle, the rectus capitis anterior muscle is found to span the lateral mass of the atlas to the base of the occipital bone, whereas the rectus capitis lateralis extends laterally from the transverse process of the atlas to the inferior surface of the jugular process of the occipital bone. The scalenus anterior originates from the anterior tubercles of the transverse processes of C3–C6 and inserts on the first rib. The scalenus medius originates from the posterior tubercles of the transverse processes of C2–C7 and inserts on the first rib. A vascular impingement of the subclavian artery may occur as it runs between scalenus anterior and scalenus medius as seen in the thoracic outlet syndrome. The scalenus posterior originates from the posterior tubercles of the transverse processes of C4–C6 and inserts on the second rib.

The anterolateral neck muscles and their relationships to the vital structures of this region are also described anatomically as forming various triangles (Fig. 1.29a). The posterior triangle of the neck is formed by the sternocleidomastoid, clavicle, and trapezius muscles. The posterior triangle is divided by the omohyoid muscle into the supraclavicular and the occipital triangles.[16] The anterior triangle is bounded by the midline of the neck anteriorly, the lower border of the mandible superiorly, and the sternocleidomastoid posteriorly. The anterior triangle can be subdivided into the submental, muscular, digastric, and carotid triangles. These triangles serve as important landmarks during anterior approaches to the cervical spine.

The fascial layers of the anterior neck invest the muscles and viscera of this region to form separate compartments, and generally facilitate surgical exposure (Fig. 1.29b). The superficial fascia contains the subcutaneous fat and areolar tissue, the platysma muscle, external jugular vein, and the cutaneous sensory nerves. The structures deep to the superficial fascia are compartmentalized by the deep fascia including the outer investing layer of deep fascia, middle cervical fascia, and the prevertebral fascia. The outer layer of the deep fascia extends from the trapezius muscle over

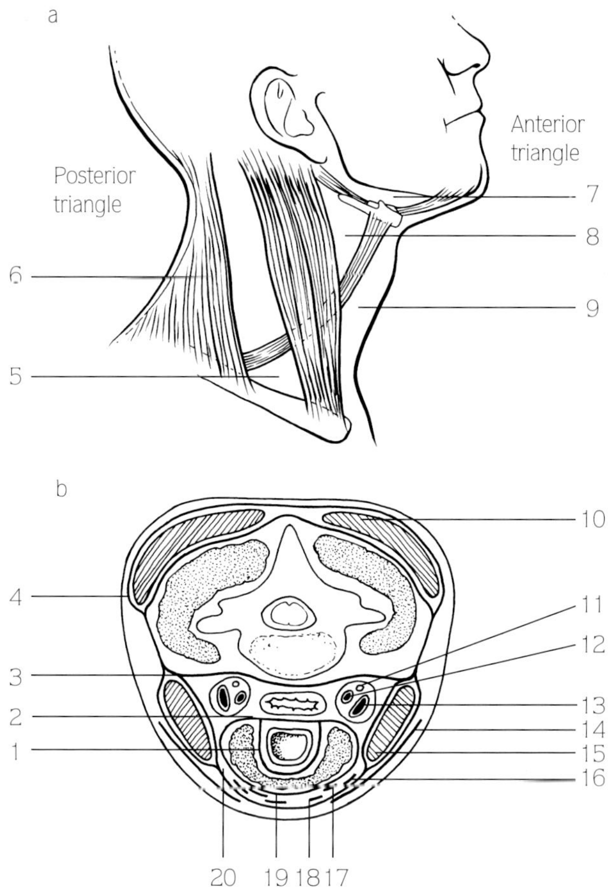

Figure 1.29
(a) Triangles of the neck bordered by muscles. The posterior triangle is formed by the sternocleidomastoid, clavicle, and the trapezius muscles, and the omohyoid muscle divides it into the supraclavicular and the occipital triangles. The anterior triangle is bounded by the midline of the neck anteriorly, the lower border of the mandible superiorly, and the sternocleidomastoid posteriorly. The anterior triangle is subdivided by the submental triangle, the muscular triangle, the digastric triangle, and the carotid triangle. (b) The fascia of the anterior part of the neck invest the muscles and viscera in separate compartments. The superficial fascia contains fat and areolar tissue including the platysma muscle, external jugular vein, and the cutaneous sensory nerves. The structures deep to the superficial fascia are compartmentalized by the deep fascia including the outer investing layer of deep fascia, middle cervical fascia (pre-tracheal fascia), and the prevertebral fascia. The outer layer of the deep fascia extends from the trapezius muscle over the posterior triangle and splits to enclose the sternocleidomastoid muscle. The middle layers of the deep cervical fascia enclose the strap muscles and omohyoid and extend as far laterally as the scapula. The deeper middle layer is the visceral fascia that surrounds the thyroid gland, larynx, trachea, pharynx, and esophagus. The carotid sheath encloses the carotid artery, internal jugular vein, and vagus nerve. The deepest layer of the deep fascia is the prevertebral fascia, which covers the scalenus muscles, longus colli muscles, and the anterior longitudinal ligament

1 Pre-tracheal lamina
2 Prevertebral (middle)
3 Prevertebral (deep)
4 Superficial (investing)
5 Supraclavicular
6 Occipital triangle
7 Digastric triangle
8 Carotid triangle
9 Muscular triangle
10 Trapezius
11 Vagus n.
12 Common carotid a.
13 Jugular v.
14 Platysma m.
15 Sternocleidomastoid m.
16 Omohyoid m.
17 Sternothyroid m.
18 Sternohyoid m.
19 Pre-thyroid lamina
20 Posterior thyroid space

the posterior triangle, and then splits to enclose the sternocleidomastoid muscle. The middle layer of the deep cervical fascia encloses the strap muscles and omohyoid, and extends as far laterally as the scapula. A deeper portion of middle layer is the visceral fascia, which surrounds the thyroid gland, larynx, trachea, pharynx, and esophagus. The alar fascia spreads behind the esophagus and surrounds the carotid sheath structures laterally. The carotid sheath encloses the carotid artery, internal jugular vein, and vagus nerve. The deepest layer of the deep fascia is the prevertebral fascia, which covers the scalenus muscles, longus colli muscles, and the anterior longitudinal ligament.

NEUROVASCULAR STRUCTURES

Neurovascular structures of the cervical spine include the spinal cord, nerve roots, carotid artery, vertebral artery, laryngeal nerves, sympathetic chain, veins, and vessels to the spinal cord. The cervical cord emerges from the foramen magnum as a continuation of the medulla. The cervical cord enlarges from C3 and becomes maximal at C6 with a circumference of 38 mm.[16] This enlargement results from the increased nerve supply to the upper limbs. The spinal cord includes the outer white matter and the inner gray matter, which can be distinguished by magnetic

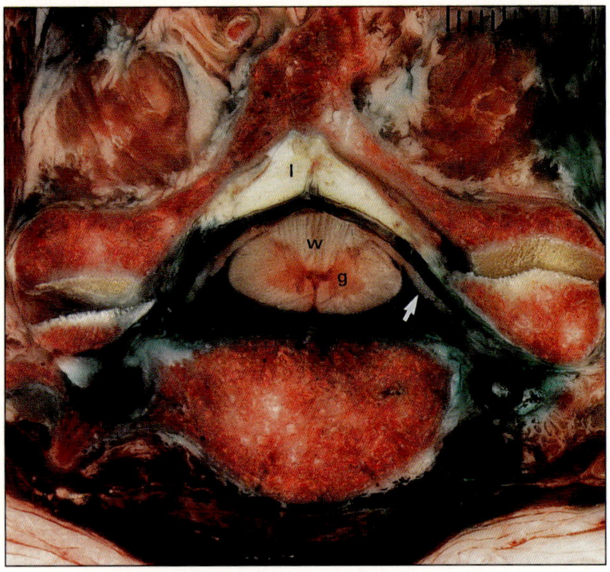

Figure 1.30
An axial freezing microtome section of the cervical spine showing the white (w) and gray matter (g) of the spinal cord, dorsal root (arrow), and ligamentum flavum (l)

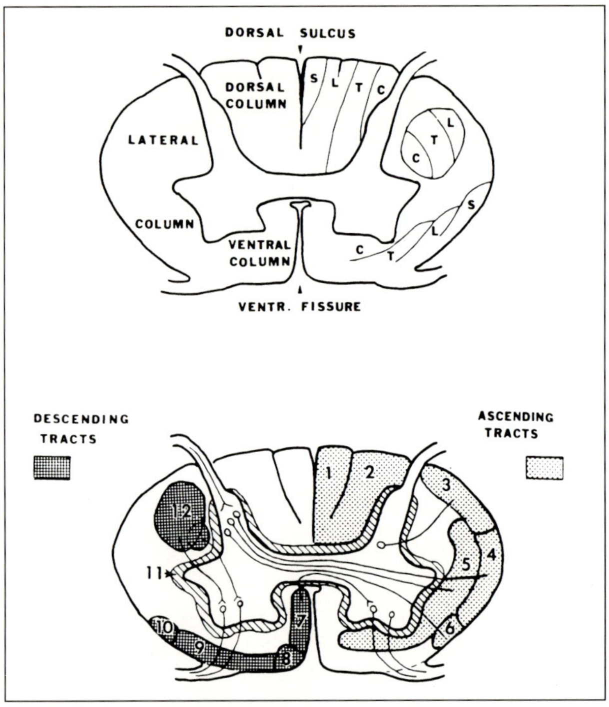

Figure 1.31
Cross-sectional anatomy of the spinal cord at C5 level with columns and tracts of the white matter. Top: columns or funiculi are shown on the left, and segmental arrangement of ascending and descending longitudinal tracts on the right: sacral (S), lumbar (L), thoracic (T), and cervical (C). Bottom: tracts of the spinal cord at C5 level with the ascending tracts on the right and descending tracts on the left: (1) fasciculus gracilis, (2) fasciculus cuneatus, (3) dorsal spinocerebellar tract, (4) ventral spinocerebellar tract, (5) lateral spinothalamic tract, (6) spino-olivary tract, (7) anterior corticospinal tract, (8) tectospinal tract, (9) vestibulospinal tract, (10) olivospinal tract, (11) intersegmental or propriospinal tract, and (12) lateral corticospinal tract. (From Parke WW, Sherk HH: Normal Adult Anatomy. In *Cervical Spine*, 2nd ed., eds, Sherk HH et al., Philadephia: JB Lippincott, 1989: 22.)

resonance imaging (Fig. 1.30).[6] The white matter of the spinal cord contains nerve fibers and glia, and is divided into three columns: posterior, lateral, and anterior. The posterior column includes the fasciculus cuneatus laterally and fasciculus gracilis medially, mediating proprioceptive, vibratory, and tactile sensations (Fig. 1.31). The lateral column contains the descending motor lateral corticospinal and lateral spinothalamic fasciculi, and the anterior funiculus contains the ascending anterior spinothalamic tract and other descending tracts. The lateral spinothalamic tracts cross through the ventral commissure to the contralateral side of the cord, conveying pain and temperature sensations. The anterior spinothalamic tract conveys crude touch sensation.

The gray matter of the spinal cord contains cell bodies of efferent and internuncial neurons. The somatosensory

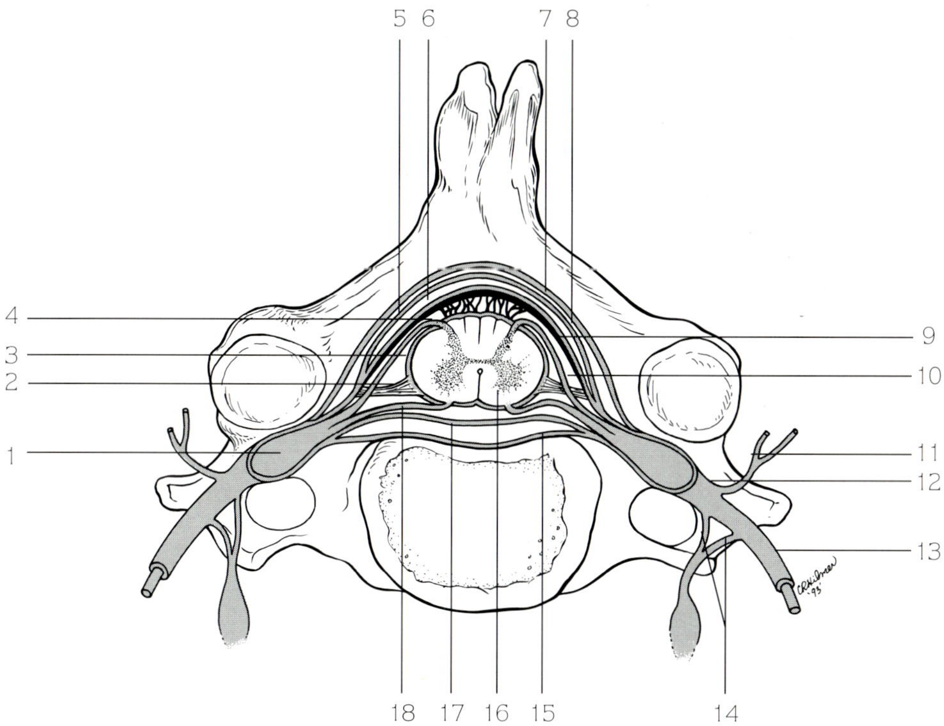

1 Spinal ganglion
2 Dentate ligament
3 Pia mater
4 Dorsal root of spinal n.
5 Dura mater
6 Subdural space
7 Periosteum
8 Epidural space
9 Arachnoid membrane
10 Subarachnoid space
11 Dorsal ramus
12 Spinal n.
13 Ventral ramus of spinal n.
14 Ramus communicans
15 Periosteum
16 Medulla spinalis
17 Dura mater
18 Ventral root of spinal n.

Figurc 1.32
Cross-sectional diagram of the cervical spine showing the spinal cord, nerve root, dorsal root ganglion, and spinal nerve. The spinal cord is covered by the pia mater and suspended in the cerebrospinal fluid contained by the arachnoid membrane. The dentate ligament secures the spinal cord within the spinal canal

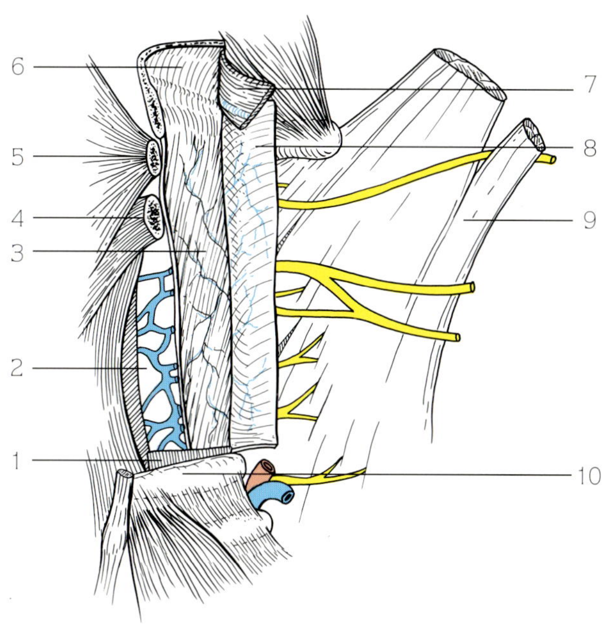

Figure 1.33
The dura mater is the outer covering of the spinal cord, which is continuous at the foramen magnum with the inner layer of the cranial dura. The arachnoid membrane is underneath the dura mater and contains the cerebrospinal fluid

1 Ligamentum flavum
2 Posteroinferior vertebral venous plexus
3 Arachnoid
4 Axis
5 Atlas
6 Cerebellum
7 Dura mater of brain
8 Spinal dura mater
9 Semispinalis capitis m.
10 Vertebral arch C7

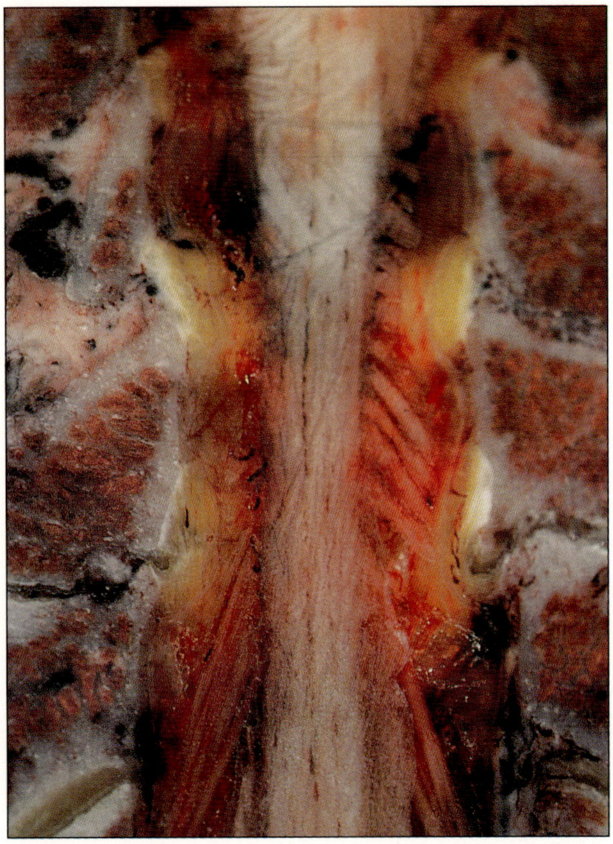

Figure 1.34
A coronal freezing microtome section showing the dorsal sensory rootlets entering the cord through the lateral longitudinal sulcus

neurons are located in the posterior horn, and the somatomotor neurons are found in the anterior horn of the gray matter. The visceral center of the gray matter is found in the intermediolateral horn. In the center of the spinal cord is the central ependymal canal for the passage of cerebrospinal fluid.

The spinal cord is covered by the pia mater, which is the outer lining of the cord, and the transparent arachnoid membrane which contains the cerebrospinal fluid (Fig. 1.32). The dura mater is the outer covering of the spinal cord, which is continuous at the foramen magnum with the inner layer of the cranial dura (Fig. 1.33). The cervical cord is anchored to the dura by the dentate ligaments which project laterally from the lateral side of the cord to the arachnoid and dura, at points midway between exiting spinal nerves. By suspending the spinal cord in the cerebrospinal fluid, the dentate ligaments cushion and protect the cord while minimizing movement of the cord during range of motion (Fig. 1.32). The epidural space contains fat, the internal vertebral venous plexus, and loose connective tissue. This venous plexus may be involved in the spreading of infection or neoplasm. There is a potential space between the dura and arachnoid; the subarachnoid space exists between the arachnoid and pia and contains the cerebrospinal fluid, spinal blood vessels, and nerve rootlets from the spinal cord.

The dorsal sensory rootlets enter the cord through the lateral longitudinal sulcus, whereas the ventral motor rootlets exit the cord through the ventral lateral sulcus (Fig. 1.32). The six or eight rootlets at each level leave the spinal cord laterally to lie in the lateral subarachnoid space bathed in the cerebrospinal fluid (Fig. 1.34). The rootlets join to form the dorsal and ventral roots respectively, which together enter a narrow sleeve of arachnoid and pass through the dura to become a nerve root at each level. The cervical nerve roots forming from the ventral and dorsal nerve rootlet complex then extend anterolaterally at a 45° angle to the coronal plane and inferiorly at 10° to the axial plane. The nerve roots enter the intervertebral foramina by passing directly in a lateral direction from the spinal canal adjacent to the corresponding disc and over the top of the corresponding pedicle (Fig. 1.35). The anterior root lies anteroinferiorly adjacent to the uncovertebral joint, whereas the posterior root approximates the superior articular process (Fig. 1.36). The nerve root is positioned at the tip of the superior articular process in the medial aspect of the neural foramen, and then courses more inferiorly to position itself over the pedicle in the lateral aspect of the neural foramen (Figs 1.37 and 1.38).[8] Each cervical spinal nerve root exits over the pedicle bearing the same number, except for the C8 cervical nerve, which lies between the C7 and T1 pedicles (Fig. 1.39).

The roots occupy about one-third of the foraminal space in the normal spine, although this increases in the degenerative spine. Normally, the roots are located in the inferior half of the neural foramen, but when the neck is extended, the nerve roots tend to occupy the more cranial portion of the foramina, whereas the volume of the foramen itself is diminished.[18] The upper half of the neural foramen contains fat and small veins,[11] the whole neural foramen being approximately 9–12 mm in height, 4–6 mm in width, and 4–6 mm in length.[5] It is bounded superiorly and inferiorly by pedicles, anteriorly by the uncinate process, the posterolateral aspect of the intervertebral disc, and the inferior portion of the vertebral body above the disc level, and posteriorly by the facet joint and superior articular process of vertebral body below (Fig. 1.40 and see Fig. 1.16). The nerve root becomes enlarged in the distal aspect of the intervertebral foramen, and the dorsal root ganglion is located just distal to it.[17] The dorsal root ganglion is located between the vertebral artery and a small concavity in the superior articular process (Fig. 1.40). The anterior and

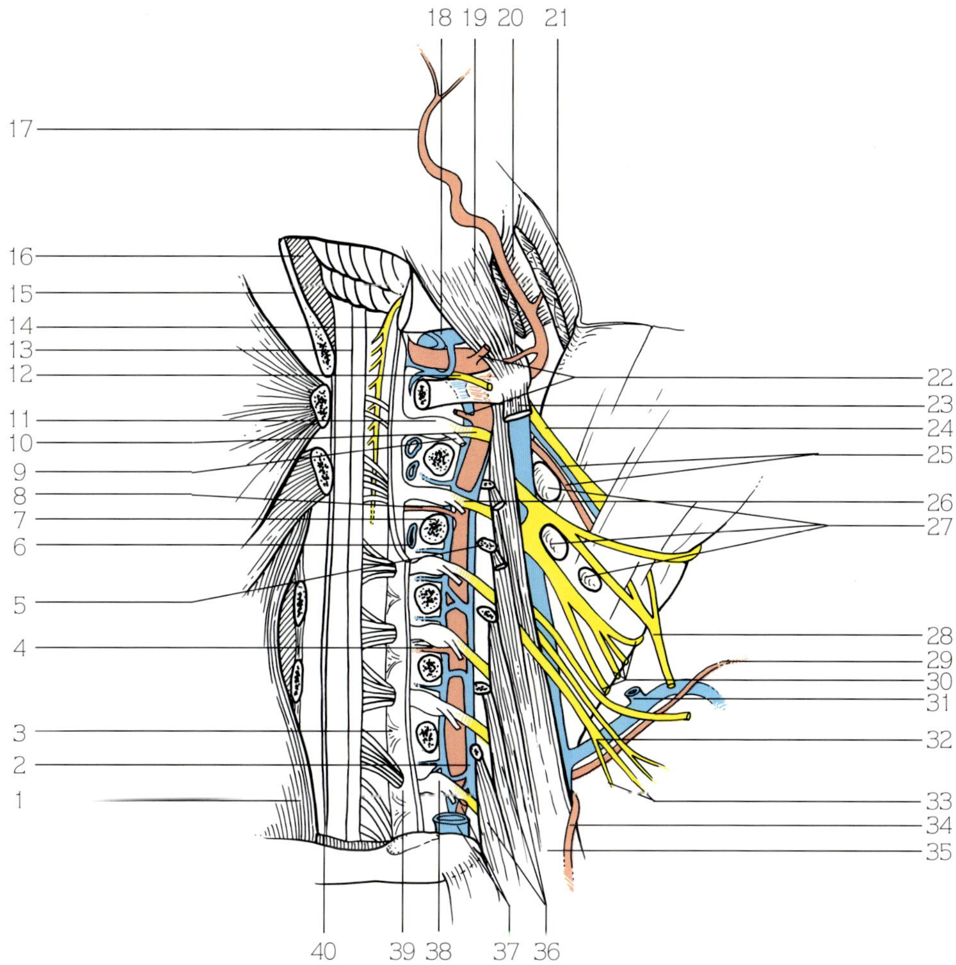

Figure 1.35
Spinal cord and neural structures of the cervical spine showing six or eight rootlets at each level leaving the spinal cord. The rootlets join to form the dorsal and ventral root, which together enter a narrow sleeve of arachnoid and pass through the dura to become a nerve root at each level. The cervical nerve roots that form from the ventral and dorsal nerve rootlet extend anterolaterally at a 45° angle to the coronal plane and inferiorly at about 10° to the axial plane. The nerve roots enter the intervertebral foramina by passing directly laterally from the spinal canal adjacent to the corresponding disc and over the top of the corresponding pedicle

1 Left erector spinae m.
2 Vertebral v.
3 Ligamentum denticulatum
4 Spinal branch of vertebral a.
5 Transverse process C3
6 Vertebral venous plexus
7 Pedicle, vertebral arch C3
8 Spinal branch vertebral a.
9 Posterior primary ramus, C2
10 Anterior primary ramus, C2
11 Spinal gang, C2
12 Suboccipital n.
13 Lateral intermediate sulcus
14 Spinal roots of accessory n.
15 Occipital bone
16 Cerebellomedullary cisterna
17 Occipital a.
18 Vertebral v.
19 Oblique cupitis superior m.
20 Longissimus capitis m.
21 Splenius capitis m.
22 Muscular branches of vertebral a.
23 Levator scapulae m. (first digitation)
24 Accessory n.
25 Sternocleidomastoid a. and v.
26 Anterior primary ramus C3
27 Deep cervical lymph nodes
28 Accessory n.
29 Superior cervical a.
30 Cutaneous branches of cervical plexus
31 External jugular v.
32 Dorsal scapulae n.
33 Branches to trapezius
34 Transverse cervical a. (deep branch)
35 Scalenus medius m.
36 Scalenus posterior m.
37 Deep cervical a. v.
38 Spinal ganglion C7
39 Spinal dura mater
40 Lig. flavum

posterior roots join to form the spinal nerve just distal to the ganglion and outside the intervertebral foramen.

The spinal nerve divides into dorsal primary rami and ventral primary rami branches (see Fig. 1.32). The gray rami from the sympathetic cervical ganglion join the ventral primary rami. There are interconnections between gray rami, the perivascular plexus around the vertebral artery, and the sympathetic trunk, all of which give contributions to the ventral nerve plexus to innervate the anterior longitudinal ligament, outer annulus fibrosis, and the anterior vertebral body (Fig. 1.41).[3,13] The dorsal nerve plexus receives contributions from the sinovertebral nerves. The sinovertebral nerve originate from the gray rami and perivascular plexus of the vertebral artery. The dorsal nerve

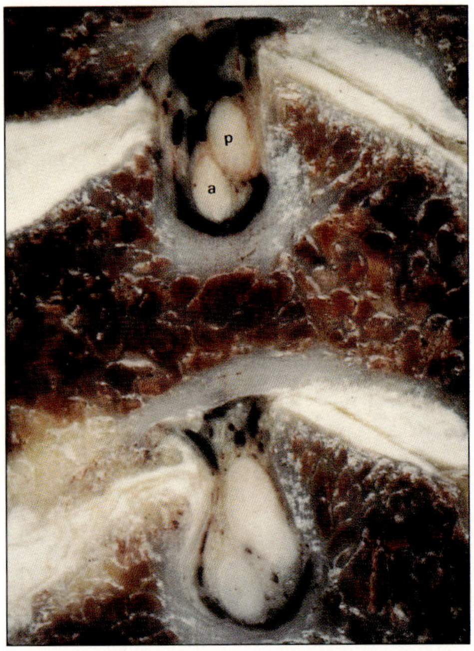

Figure 1.36
A 45° oblique freezing microtome showing the intervertebral foramen and the nerve root. The anterior root (a) lies anteroinferiorly, adjacent to the uncovertebral joint, and the posterior root (p) is close to the superior articular process

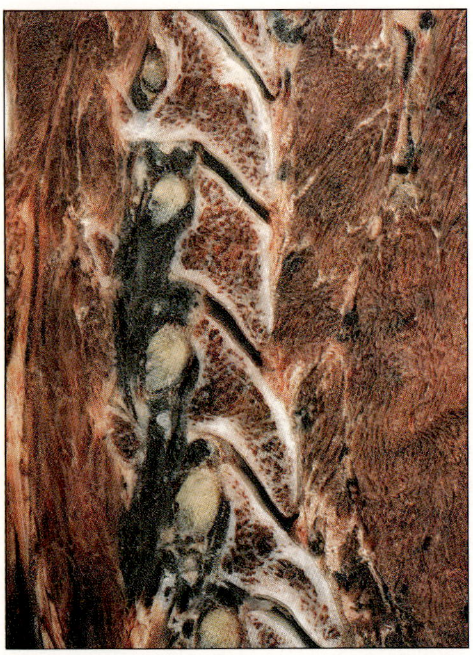

Figure 1.37
A parasagittal freezing microtome showing the nerve root positioned just anterior to the tip of the superior articular process in the medial aspect of the neural foramen

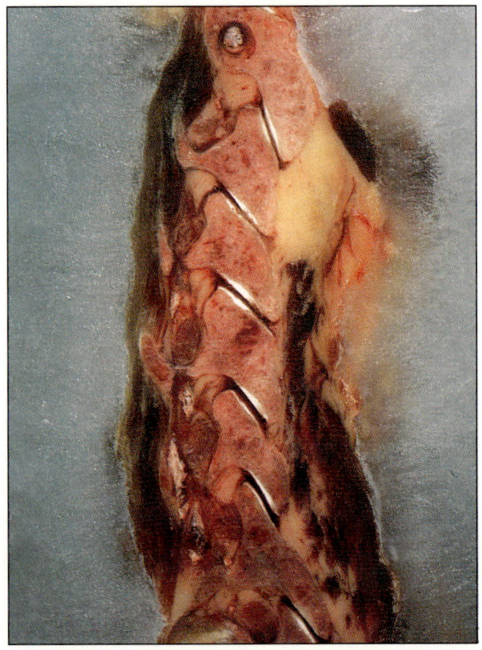

Figure 1.38
A parasagittal freezing microtome showing the nerve root courses more inferiorly to position over the pedicle in the lateral aspect of the neural foramen

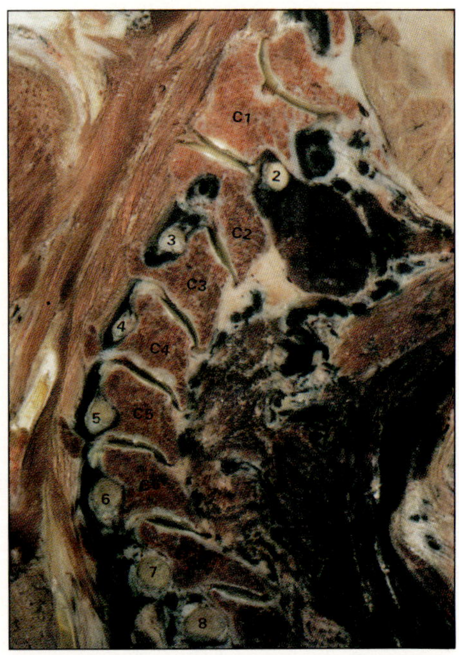

Figure 1.39
A parasagittal freezing microtome section of the cervical spine showing the nerve root from C2 to C8. The cervical nerve exits over the pedicle that bears the same number, except C8 cervical nerve lies between the C7 and T1 vertebrae

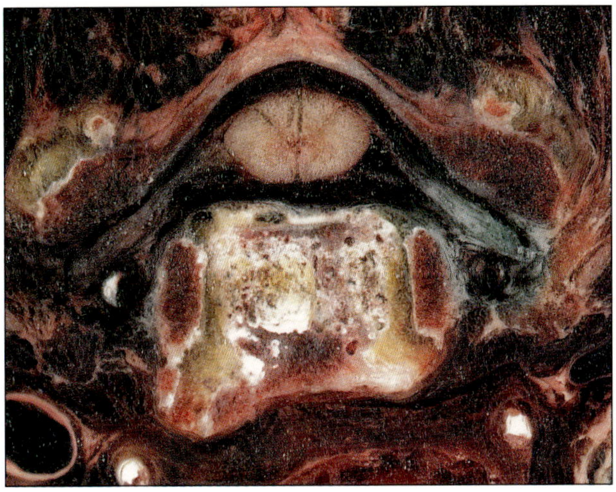

Figure 1.40
An axial freezing microtome section showing the spinal cord and nerve root exiting in the neural foramen that is bound anteriorly by the uncinate process, the posterolateral aspect of the intervertebral disc, and inferior portion of the vertebral body above the disc level, and posteriorly by the facet joint and superior articular process of the vertebral body below

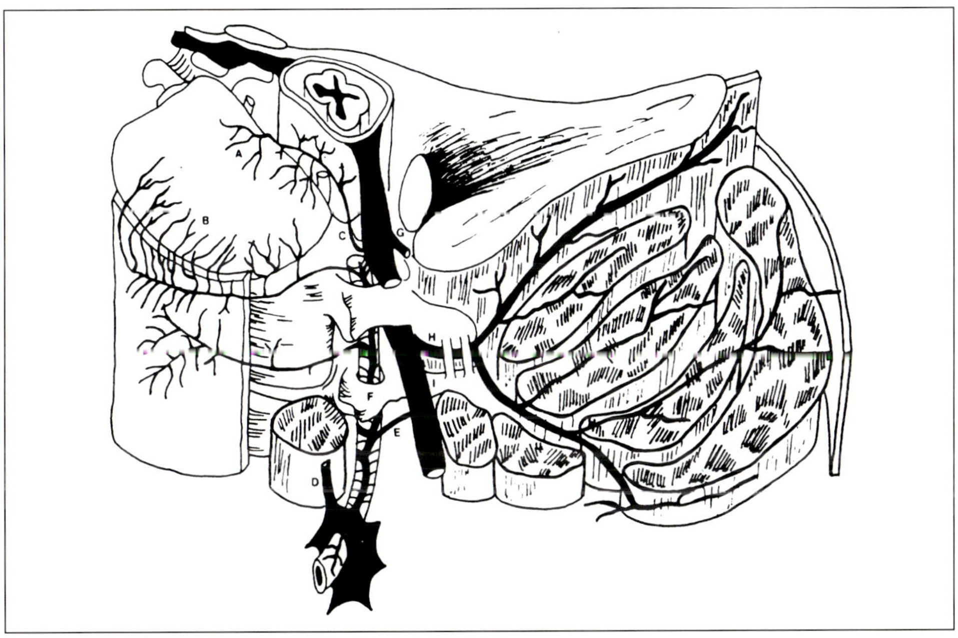

Figure 1.41
Innervation of the cervical spine: (a) dorsal nerve plexus, (b) ventral nerve plexus, (c) sinovertebral nerve, (d) sympathetic trunk, (e) gray ramus communicantes, (f) vertebral perivascular plexus, (g) dorsal root ganglion, (h) dorsal ramus, and (i) ventral ramus. (From Young PA, Young PH: Surgical anatomy of the cervical spine surrounding structures. In *Microsurgery of the Cervical Spine*, Young PH, ed., New York: Raven Press, 1991: 33.)

plexus innervates the posterior longitudinal ligament, whereas the sinovertebral nerves supply branches to the posterior part of the annulus and the ventral portion of the dura. The sinovertebral nerves also innervate two or more discs or motion segments.

The first cervical nerve or suboccipital nerve exits from the vertebral canal above the posterior arch of the atlas and posteromedial to the lateral mass, lying between the vertebral artery and the posterior arch (Fig. 1.42). The posterior primary ramus of the first cervical nerve enters the suboccipital triangle and sends motor fibers to the deep muscles (Fig. 1.43). The anterior primary ramus of the first cervical nerve forms a loop with the second anterior primary ramus, and sends fibers to the hypoglossal nerve.

The cervical plexus receives fibers from the anterior primary rami of C1 through C4. The cervical plexus is located opposite C1 through C3, ventral and lateral to the levator scapulae and middle scalene muscles. The cervical plexus has distributions to the skin and muscles, including rectus capitis anterior and lateralis, longus capitis and cervicis, levator scapulae, and middle scalene. The cervical

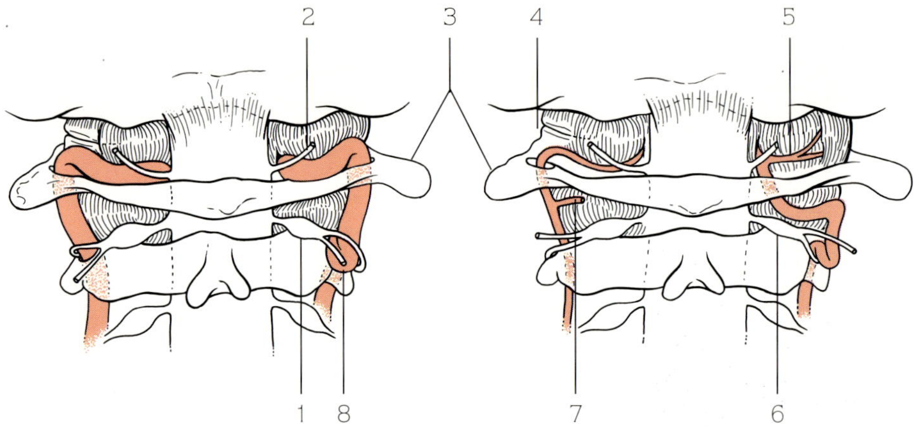

1 Spinal ganglion C2
2 Suboccipital n.
3 Transverse process of atlas
4 Bony ridge on superior articular process of atlas
5 Muscular branch right vertebral a.
6 Spinal ganglion
7 Muscular branch left vertebral a.
8 Right vertebral a. with loop formation

Figure 1.42
Posterior aspect of the upper cervical spine showing the suboccipital nerve (C1) and spinal nerve of C2 and the normal position of the left vertebral artery. Anomalies of the vertebral artery at C1–C2 are shown for the right vertebral artery. The first cervical nerve or suboccipital nerve exits the vertebral canal above the posterior arch of the atlas and posteromedial to the lateral mass and lies between the vertebral artery and the posterior arch. The second cervical nerve lies on the lamina of the axis posterior to the lateral mass. (Modified from Rickenbacher J, Landolt AM, Theiler K: *Applied Anatomy of the Back*, Berlin: Springer Verlag, 1982.)

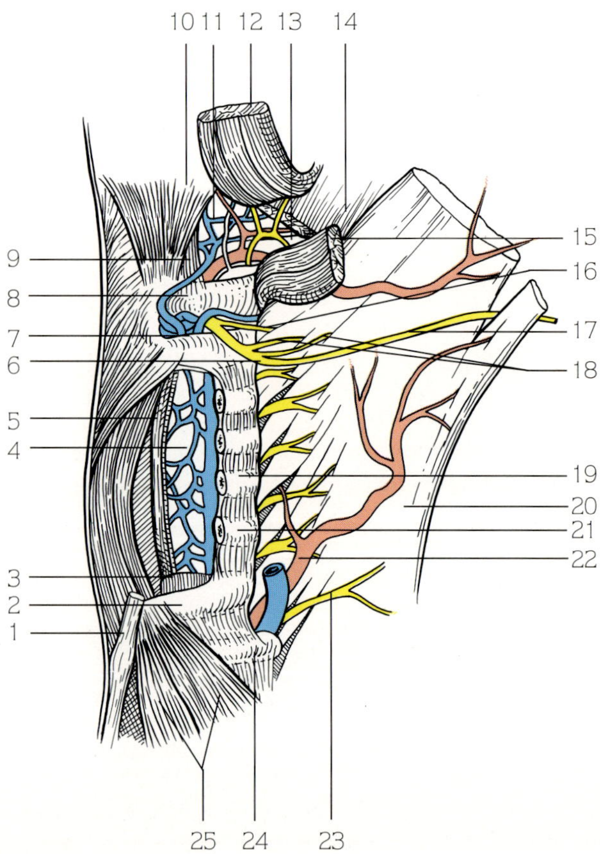

Figure 1.43
The suboccipital nerve enters the suboccipital triangle and sends motor fibers to the deep muscles. Posterior primary rami of cervical nerves innervate the posterior musculature. The deep cervical artery and venous plexus in the epidural space are also depicted

1 Supraspinus ligament
2 Vertebral arch C7
3 Ligamentum flavum
4 Posterior internal vertebral venous plexus
5 Ligament of spinal dura mater
6 Posterior primary ramus of spinal n. C2
7 Axis
8 Atlas
9 Posterior atlanto-occipital membrane
10 Rectus capitis posterior minor m.
11 Suboccipital venous plexus
12 Rectus capitis posterior major m.
13 Suboccipital n.
14 Oblique capitis superior m.
15 Oblique capitis inferior m.
16 Anterior primary ramus of spinal n. C2
17 Greater occipital n.
18 Posterior muscular branches of C2
19 C5
20 Semispinalis capitis m.
21 C6
22 Deep cervical a.
23 Anterior primary ramus of spinal n. C8
24 Transverse process of T1
25 Transverso-spinalis m.

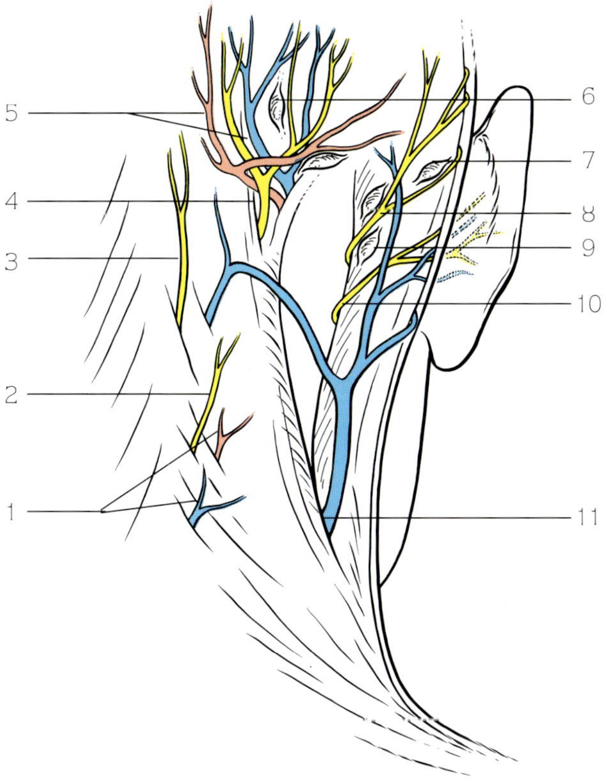

Figure 1.44

Superficial nerves of the posterior neck. The second cervical nerve or the greater occipital nerve pierces the trapezius about 2 cm below the external occipital protuberance and 2–4 cm from the midline. Cutaneous branches of the posterior primary rami of C2–C5 are consistently present in the skin of nuchal region, and the largest cutaneous nerve in this region is the greater occipital nerve. The lesser occipital nerve is a branch of the anterior cervical plexus and runs upwards and lateral to the greater occipital nerve. The posterior primary ramus of C3 or third occipital nerve pierces the trapezius more inferiorly and about 1 cm medial from the midline

1 Cutaneous branches of superior cervical a. and v.
2 Medial branch of posterior primary ramus of C5
3 Medial branch of post. primary ramus of C3 and C4 (third occipital nerve)
4 Greater occipital n.
5 Occipital a. and v.
6 Occipital lymph nodes
7 Retroauricular lymph node
8 Lesser occipital n.
9 Superficial cervical lymph node
10 Great auricular n.
11 External jugular v.

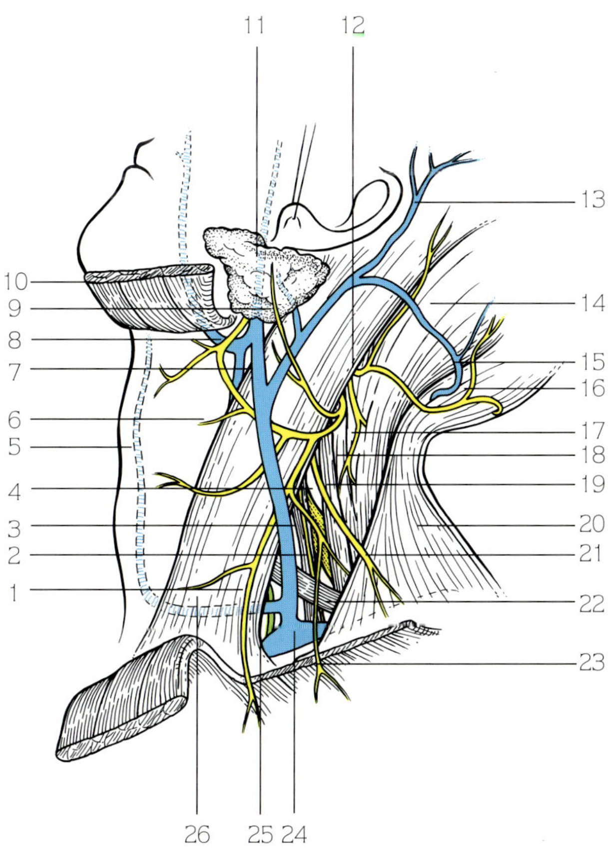

Figure 1.45

The lateral aspect of the neck showing the superficial nerves. The external jugular vein and branches are also depicted

1 Med. supraclavicular n.
2 Phrenic n.
3 Ant. scalenus m.
4 Mid. scalenus m.
5 Ant. jugular v.
6 Trans. cervical n.
7 Ext. jugular v.
8 Cervical br. facial n.
9 Greater auricular n.
10 Platysma m.
11 Retromandibular n.
12 Lesser occipital n.
13 Post. auricular v.
14 Splenius capitus m.
15 Gr. occipital v.
16 Gr. occipital n.
17 Accessory n.
18 Levator scapulae n.
19 Post. scalenus m.
20 Trapezius m.
21 Lat. suprascapulae n.
22 Post. belly omohyoid m.
23 Intermediate supraclavicular n.
24 Subclavian v.
25 Thoracic duct
26 Sternocleidomastoid m.

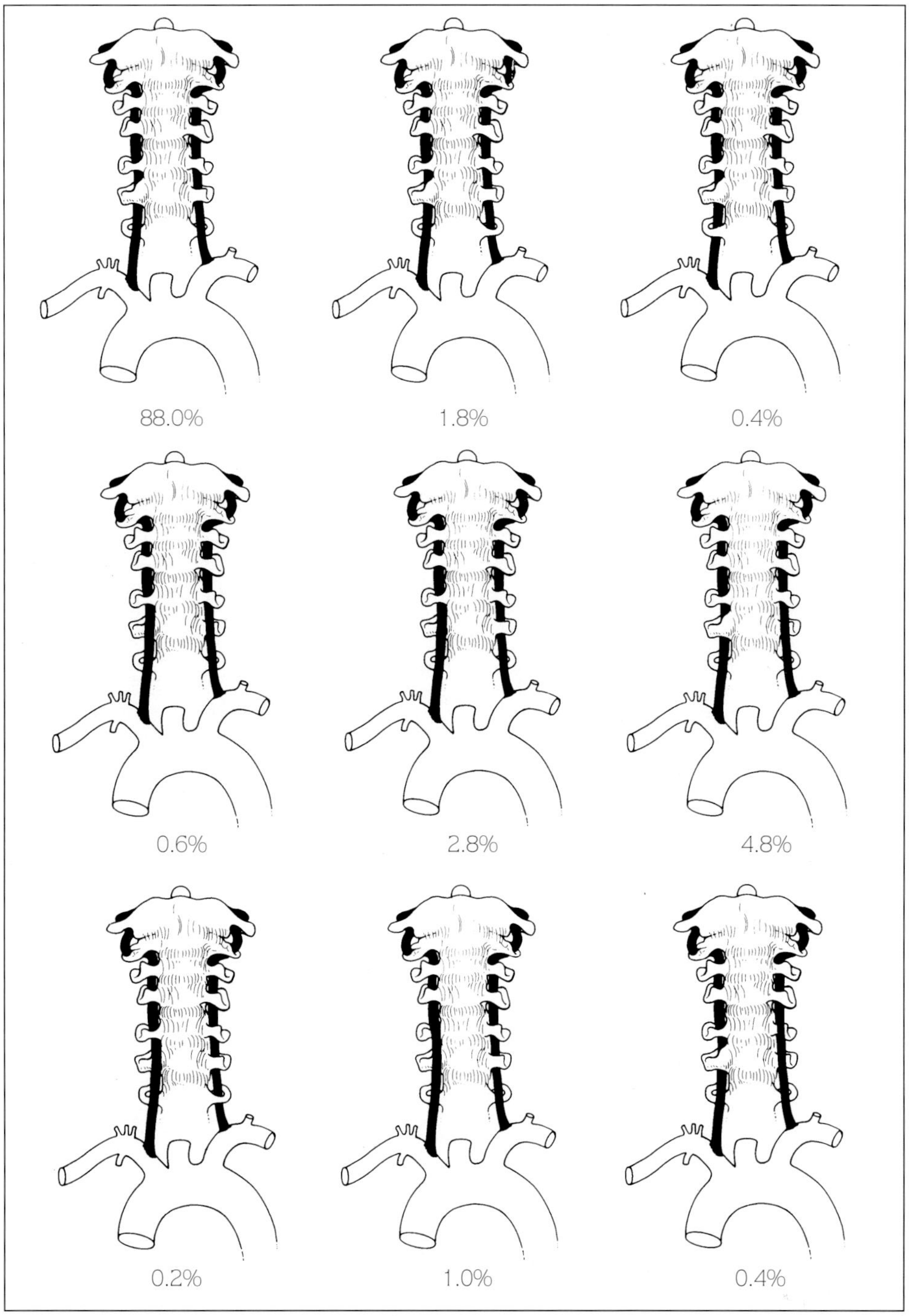

Figure 1.46
Variations of the course of the vertebral artery. (Modified from Rickenbacher J, Landolt AM, Theiler K: *Applied Anatomy of the Back*, Berlin: Springer Verlag, 1982.)

plexus forms loops and branches to supply the sternocleidomastoid and trapezius muscles, and has communications with the hypoglossal nerve from C1 and C2; then it leaves this trunk as the descending branch and unites with the descending cervical nerve (C2 and C3) to form the ansa cervicalis.

The posterior primary ramus of the second cervical nerve lies on the lamina of the axis posterior to the lateral mass. The greater occipital nerve is a branch of the C2 posterior primary ramus, and pierces the trapezius about 2 cm below the external occipital protuberance and 2–4 cm from the midline (Fig. 1.43). This is the largest cutaneous nerve of the cervical region. Cutaneous branches of the posterior primary rami of C2–C5 are consistently present in the skin of the nuchal region. The lesser occipital nerve is a branch of the anterior cervical plexus, and runs upwards and lateral to the greater occipital (Fig. 1.44). The posterior primary ramus of C3, or the

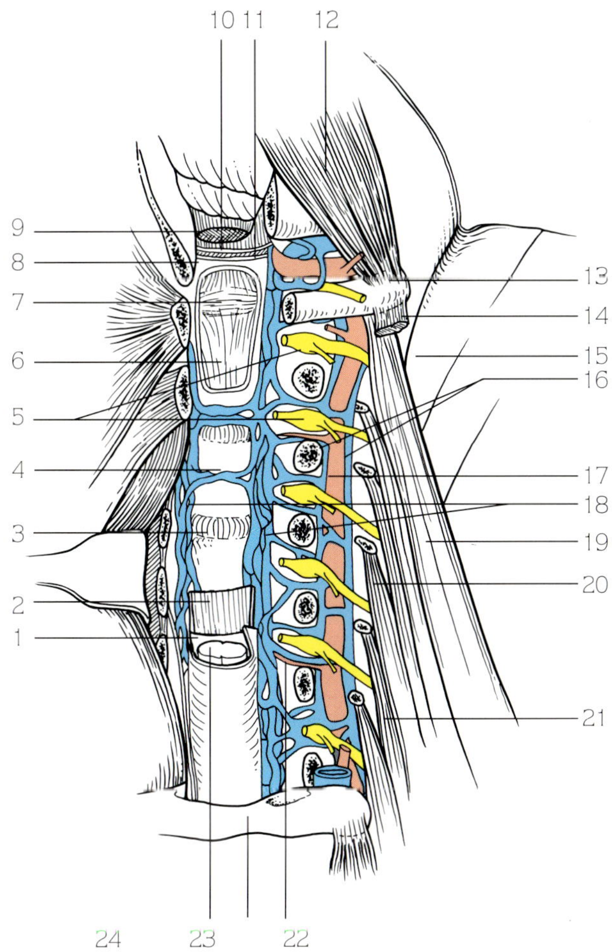

Figure 1.47
The vertebral artery and extensive venous network around the vertebral foramen and spinal canal

1 Spinal dura mater
2 Posterior longitudinal ligament
3 Intervertebral disc C3 and C4
4 Basivertebral v.
5 Spinal ganglia
6 Longitudinal fibers of cruciform ligament of atlas
7 Transverse ligament of atlas
8 Tectorial membrane
9 Medulla
10 Cranial dura mater
11 Posterior longitudinal ligament
12 Oblique capitis m.
13 Transverse process of atlas
14 Levator scapulae m.
15 Semispinalis capitis m.
16 Vertebral v.
17 Vertebral a.
18 Anteroinferior vertebral venous plexus
19 Scalenus medius m.
20 Anterior cervical intertransverse m.
21 Scalenus posterior m.
22 Spinal branch
23 Spinal cord
24 Vertebral arch T1

third occipital nerve, pierces the trapezius more inferiorly and about 1 cm medial from the midline (Fig. 1.44). The posterior primary rami of cervical nerves send motor fibers to the deep muscles and sensory fibers to the skin, but the first cervical nerve has no cutaneous branches. The anterior primary rami of C1–C4 form the cervical plexus, and of C5–T1 form the brachial plexus. Laterally, the musculature and skin are innervated by branches of the cervical plexus such as the accessory nerve, the greater auricular nerve, transcervical nerve, supraclavicular nerves, and lesser occipital nerve (Fig. 1.45).

BLOOD SUPPLY TO THE CERVICAL SPINAL CORD

The major blood supply of the cervical cord and the cervical spine is the vertebral artery, which originates from the subclavian arteries and enters the transverse foramen at C6 in most cases. Variations in the course of the vertebral artery have been reported (Fig. 1.46).[19] The vertebral artery courses cephalad within the transverse foramen of each vertebra and winds around the lateral mass and posterior arch of the atlas, and then passes through the posterior atlanto-occipital membrane into the foramen magnum (Fig. 1.47). The vertebral arteries join together to form the basilar artery beyond the foramen magnum (Fig. 1.48). In the foramen magnum region, the vertebral arteries give branches anteriorly that join together to form the single anterior spinal artery. The posteroinferior cerebellar arteries send branches on the posterolateral aspect of the spinal cord called posterior spinal arteries. These are paired and give rise to plexiform channels which are arranged transversely on the dorsum of the spinal cord. The anterior and posterior spinal arteries are the major blood supplies of the spinal cord (Fig. 1.49).[9] The anterior spinal artery supplies most of the spinal cord except for the posterior columns.

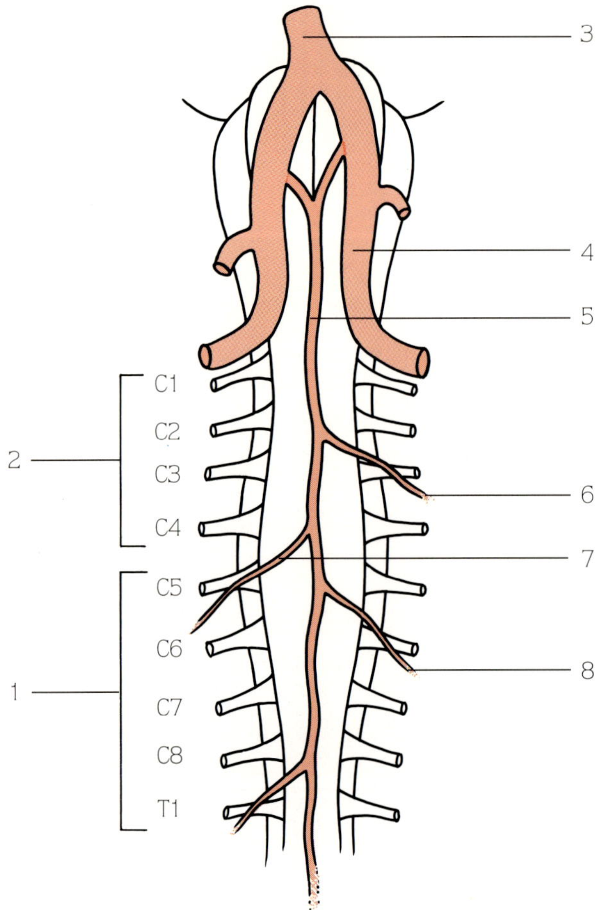

Figure 1.48
The vertebral arteries join together to form the basilar artery beyond the foramen magnum. In the foramen magnum region, the vertebral arteries give branches anteriorly that join together to form the single anterior spinal artery

1 Cervico-thoracic
2 Cervico-intracranial
3 Basilar a.
4 Vertebral a.
5 Anterior spinal a.
6 Second most frequent level of major cervical medullary artery
7 Third most frequent level of major cervical medullary a.
8 Most frequent level of major cervical medullary a.

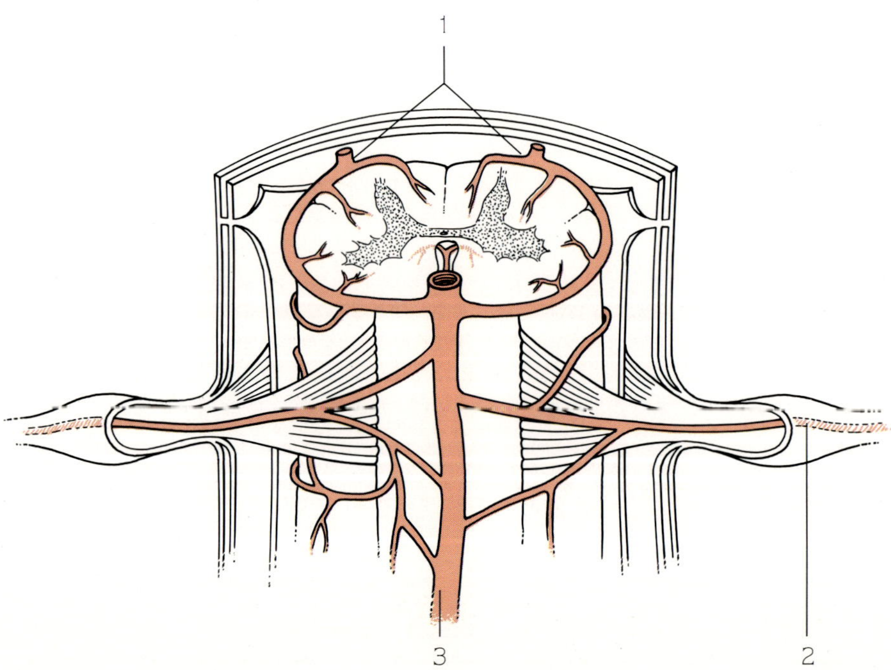

Figure 1.49
The anterior spinal artery and posterior paired spinal arteries supply blood to the spinal cord. A segmental artery may also contribute to the vascularity of the spinal cord as a medullary feeding artery

1 Posterior spinal aa.
2 Segmental a.
3 Anterior spinal a.

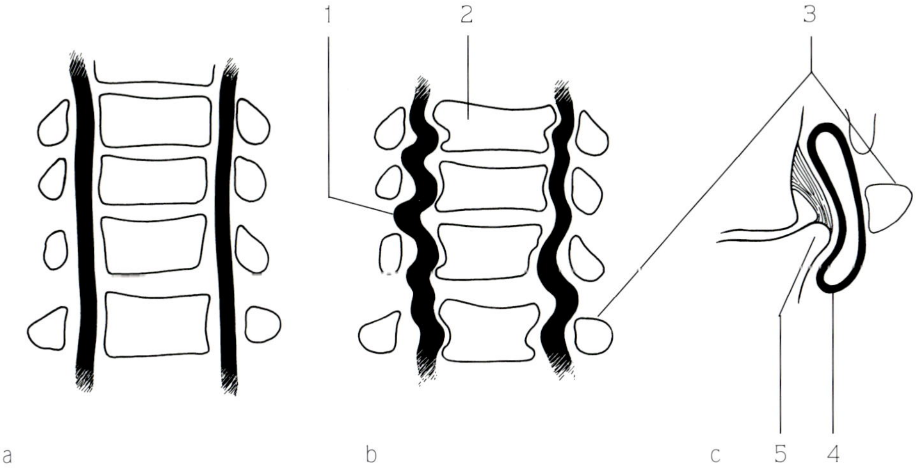

Figure 1.50
(a) Normal vertebral artery; (b) the vertebral artery may form loops due to disc collapses in cervical spondylosis; (c) the vertebral artery may be impinged by an osteophyte anteriorly. (Modified from Rickenbacher J, Landolt AM, Theiler K: *Applied Anatomy of the Back*. Berlin: Springer Verlag, 1982)

1 Loop formation
2 Bone erosion
3 Transverse process
4 Vertebral a.
5 Uncinate process

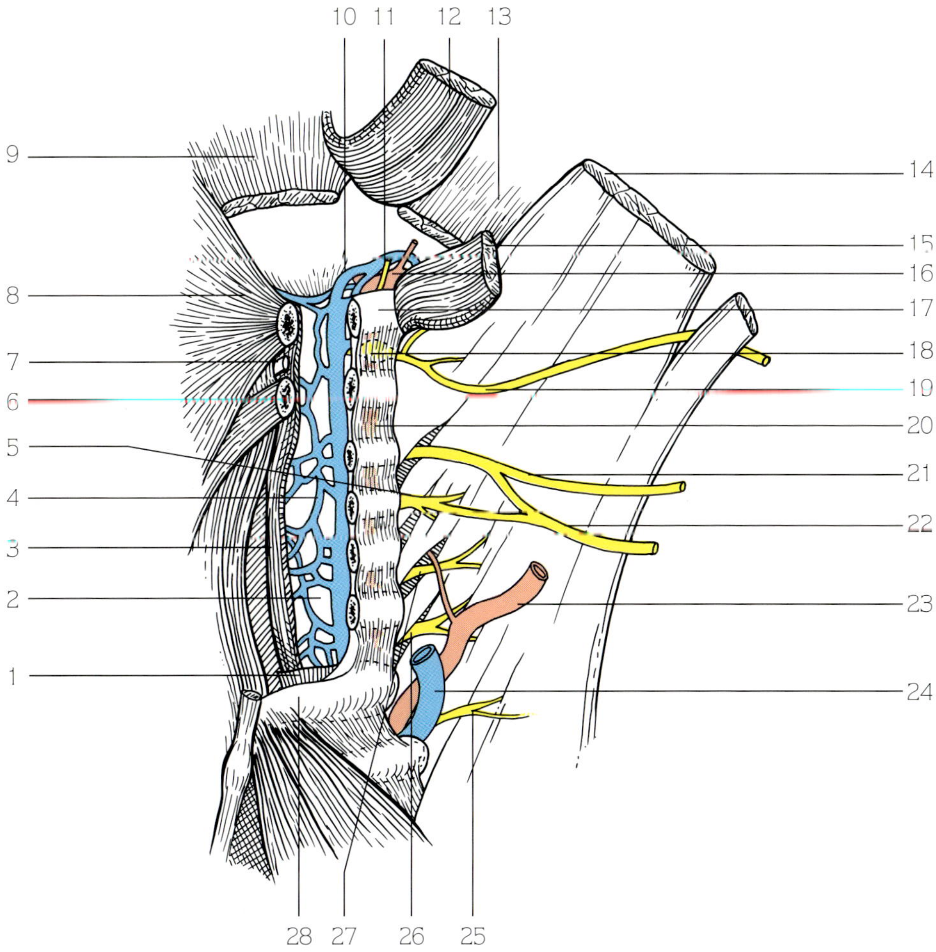

Figure 1.51
Posterior aspect of the cervical spine showing the epidural valveless venous network that connects with suboccipital venous plexus, the anterior basivertebral venous plexus, and veins in the foramen. Posterior primary rami of the cervical nerves are also shown innervating the posterior musculature

1 Ligamentum flavum
2 Spinal dura mater
3 Cranial ligament of dura mater
4 Posterior int. vertebral venous plexus
5 Posterior primary ramus C5
6 Axis
7 Anastomotic branch of posterior external vertebral venous plexus
8 Ligamentum nuchae
9 Rectus capitis posterior minor m.
10 Suboccipital venous plexus
11 Suboccipital n.
12 Rectus capitis posterior major m.
13 Obliquus capitis superior m.
14 Semispinalis m.
15 Obliquus capitis inferior m.
16 Vertebral a.
17 Posterior arch of atlas
18 Spinal ganglion C2
19 Greater occipital n.
20 Vertebral a.
21 Third occipital n.
22 Medial cutaneous branch posterior primary ramus, C3 and C4
23 Deep cervical a.
24 Deep cervical v.
25 Posterior primary ramus C8
26 Posterior primary ramus C7
27 Posterior primary ramus C6
28 Arch of C7

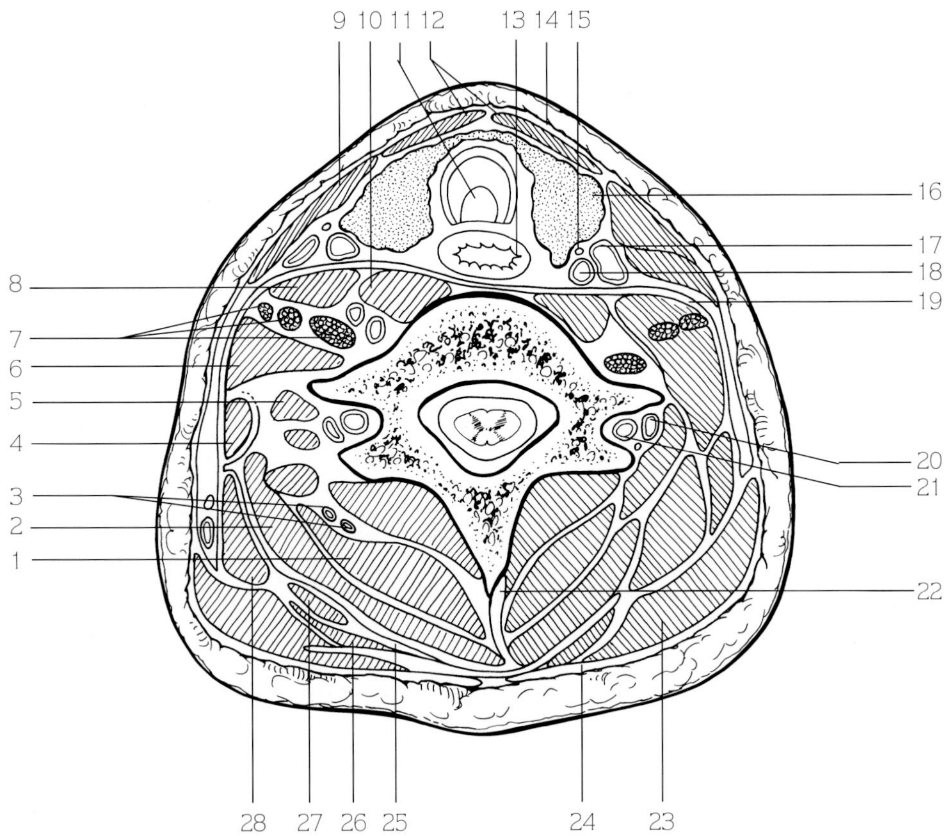

1 Transversospinal m.
2 Splenius m.
3 Deep cervical a. and v.
4 Scalenus posterior m.
5 Cervical inter-transverse mm.
6 Scalenus medius m.
7 Brachial plexus
8 Scalenus anterior m.
9 Sternocleidomastoid m.
10 Longus colli m.
11 Trachea
12 Infrahyoid m.
13 Esophagus
14 Superficial layer of cervical fascia
15 Vagus nerve
16 Thyroid
17 Internal jugular v.
18 Common carotid a.
19 Prevertebral layer of cervical fascia
20 Vertebral v.
21 Vertebral a.
22 Ligamentum nuchae
23 Trapezius m.
24 Fascia of trapezius m.
25 Nuchal fascia
26 Rhomboid m.
27 Serratus postero-superior m.
28 Levator scapulae m.

Figure 1.52
Cross-sectional view of the middle cervical spine showing the musculature and associated vital structures

The spinal cord also receives blood supply from radicular arteries or medullary feeders from the vertebral arteries and ascending cervical arteries.[9] The segmental arteries, which are branches of the vertebral artery present at each level of the spine, supply the vertebrae and surrounding tissues, but only a few segmental vessels give rise to radicular arteries or medullary feeders to the spinal cord. These vessels have a variable distribution, but medullary feeders are more commonly present at C6 and C3 from the left and C5 and T1 from the right (Fig. 1.48).[16] The vertebral artery may be compromised in severe cervical spondylosis patients, in which an osteophyte impinges on the artery (Fig. 1.50).[19] Additionally, complications of vertebral artery laceration during the anterior cervical surgical approach have been reported. The surgeon should remember that the vertebral artery is located lateral to the uncinate process and in line with the middle one-third of the vertebral body just anterior to the nerve root (see Fig. 1.39).

Venous blood returns from the cord through three veins posteriorly and three veins anteriorly (Fig. 1.51). The venous system within the spinal canal consists of valveless sinuses in the epidural space. The venous plexus is most apparent anteriorly just medial to the pedicles over the midportion of the vertebral bodies, and anastomoses with the veins from the opposite side as well as with the basivertebral sinus. The basivertebral sinus is located in the space between the posterior longitudinal ligament and the posterior aspect of the vertebral body.

RELATED STRUCTURES

Anterior surgical approaches of the cervical spine involve dissections of related vital structures around the neck (Fig. 1.52). Anatomic knowledge of these structures is obviously

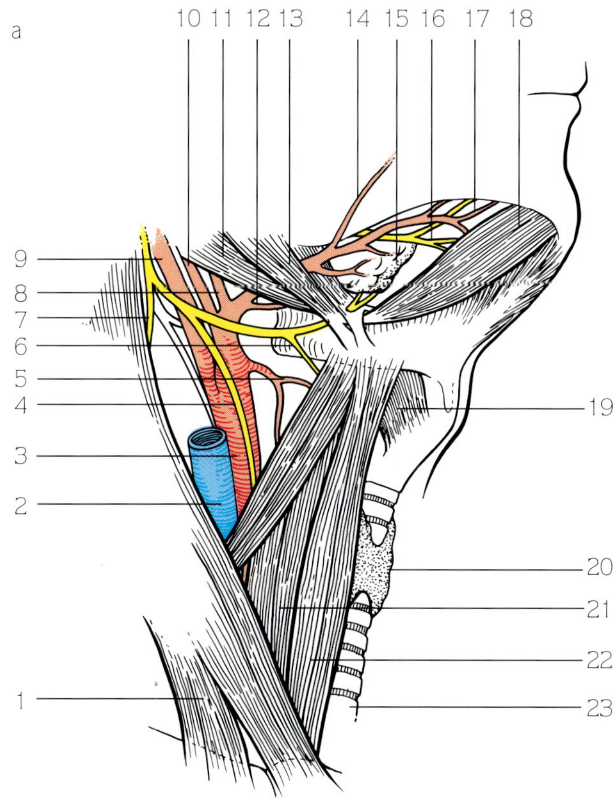

Figure 1.53

(a) Related structures during anteromedial exposures of the cervical spine. The carotid sheath contains the common carotid artery, the internal jugular vein, and the vagus nerve. It is adherent to the thyroid sheath and the fascia under the sternocleidomastoid. The ansa cervicalis is on the surface of the carotid sheath and the cervical sympathetic trunk is in the dorsomedial aspect of the sheath. The superior laryngeal nerve and the hypoglossal nerve (not shown) and the laryngeal artery are frequently encountered during the upper cervical exposure. (b) Related structures during anterolateral exposures of the cervical spine. Great auricular nerve and spinal accessory nerve may be encountered posterior to the sternocleidomastoid muscle

1 Sternocleidomastoid m.
2 Internal jugular v.
3 Common carotid a.
4 Superior root ansa cervicalis
5 Laryngeal a.
6 Superior laryngeal n.
7 Accessory n.
8 External carotid a.
9 Internal carotid a.
10 Occipital a.
11 Digastric m.
12 Lingual a.
13 Stylohyoid m.
14 Facial a.
15 Submandibular gland
16 Mylohyoid n.
17 Submental a.
18 Digastric m.
19 Thyrohyoid m.
20 Thyroid
21 Sternothyroid m.
22 Sternohyoid m.
23 Trachea

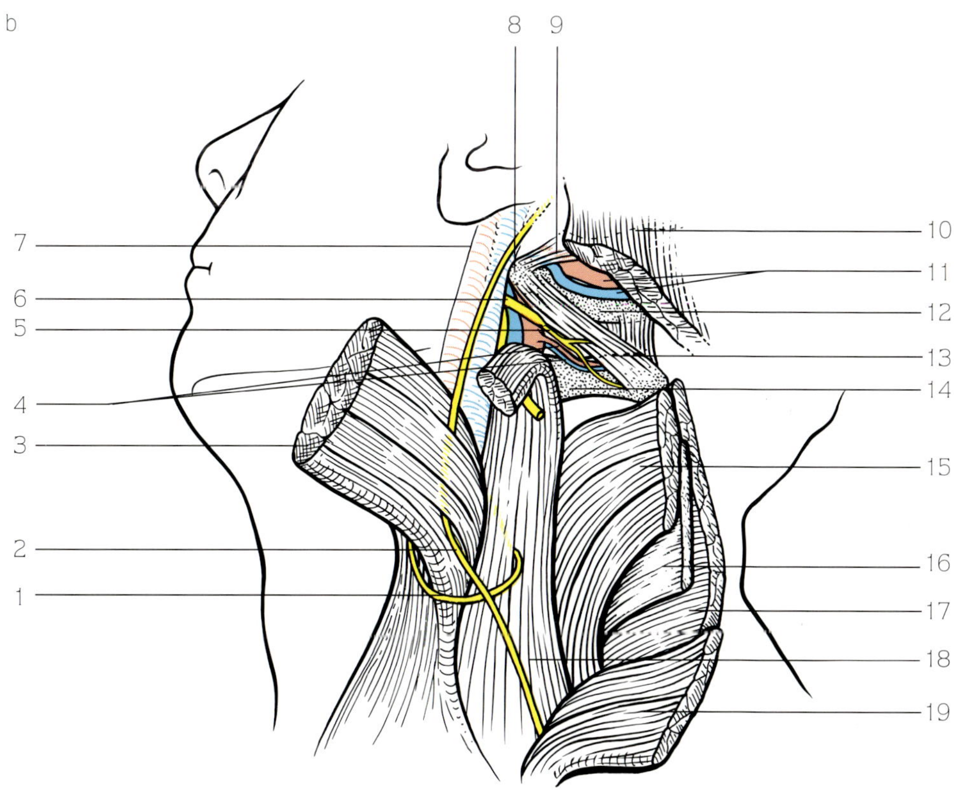

1 Great auricular n.
2 Spinal accessory n.
3 Sternocleidomastoid m.
4 Muscular branches of vertebral a. and v.
5 Posterior primary ramus of C2
6 Anterior primary ramus of C2
7 Carotid sheath
8 Transverse process of atlas
9 Oblique capitis superior m.
10 Sternocleidomastoid m.
11 Vertebral a. and v.
12 Posterior arch of atlas
13 Oblique capitis inferior m.
14 Lamina of arch of axis
15 Semispinalis capitis m.
16 Nuchal fascia
17 Splenus capitis m.
18 Levator scapulae m.
19 Longissimus capitis m.

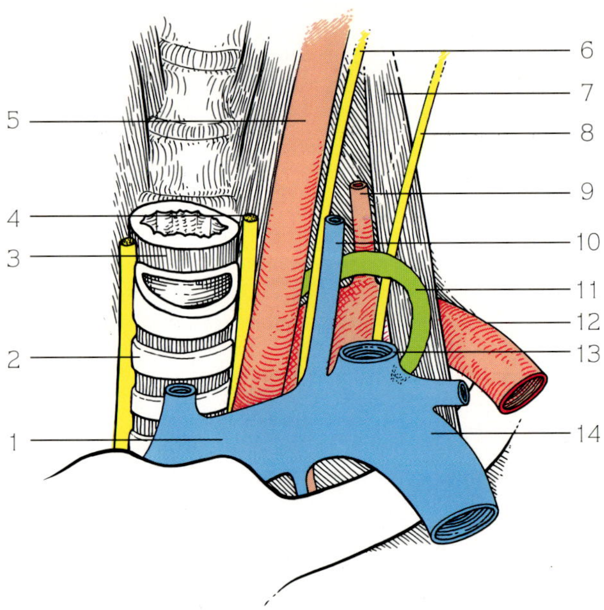

Figure 1.54
Structures on the left cervicothoracic junction. The thoracic duct lies behind the left common carotid artery, internal jugular vein, and the vagus nerve, and terminates at the junction of the left internal jugular and subclavian veins. The thoracic duct lies ventral to the subclavian artery, vertebral artery, thyrocervical trunk and the prevertebral fascia, which separates the duct from the phrenic nerve and anterior scalene muscle. The phrenic nerve on the ventral surface of the anterior scalene muscle

1 Brachiocephalic v.
2 Trachea
3 Esophagus
4 Recurrent laryngeal n.
5 Common carotid a.
6 Vagus n.
7 Anterior scalene m.
8 Phrenic n.
9 Vertebral a.
10 Vertebral v.
11 Thoracic duct
12 Subclavian a.
13 Internal jugular v.
14 Subclavian v.

important in preventing injury during exposure. The carotid sheath is an investment of the internal and common carotid arteries, the internal jugular vein, and the vagus nerve (Fig. 1.53). It is adherent to the thyroid sheath and the fascia under the sternocleidomastoid. Proximally, it is attached to the bone around the jugular foramen and carotid canal, and distally it continues into the thorax. The ansa cervicalis is on the surface of the carotid sheath and the cervical sympathetic trunk in the dorsomedial aspect. The carotid artery can be palpated and retracted, but should not be entered during anterior exposure of the cervical spine. During the left side approach to the lower cervical spine, the thoracic duct may be encountered. The thoracic duct lies behind the left common carotid artery, internal jugular vein, and the vagus nerve, and terminates at the junction of the left internal jugular and subclavian veins (Fig. 1.54). The thoracic duct lies ventral to the subclavian artery, vertebral artery, thyrocervical trunk, and the prevertebral fascia. The prevertebral fascia separates the duct from the phrenic nerve and anterior scalene muscle.

The phrenic nerve lies on the ventral surface of the anterior scalene muscle, and is crossed by the inferior belly of the omohyoid muscle, transverse cervical and suprascapular arteries, and then passes between the subclavian artery and vein to reach the thorax (Fig. 1.55). The phrenic nerve originates from C4 but receives fibers from C3 and C5.

The spinal accessory nerve emerges under the posterior aspect of the sternocleidomastoid muscle between the lesser and greater auricular nerves. The spinal accessory nerve and the cervical plexus innervate the sternocleidomastoid and trapezius muscles. Both the spinal accessory nerve and the phrenic nerve are at risk of injury during anterolateral approach to the cervical spine.

The larynx is an important structure for respiration and vocalization. The cricothyroid muscle is innervated by the external laryngeal branch of the superior laryngeal nerve of the vagus nerve, and the other intrinsic muscles of the larynx are innervated by the recurrent laryngeal nerve. For surgical landmarks, the anterior thyroid cartilage is located at C4–C5, and the cricoid cartilaginous ring is located at C6 (Fig. 1.56).

The superior laryngeal nerve is a branch of the inferior ganglion of the vagus nerve, and travels along with the superior thyroid artery to innervate the cricothyroid muscle. Damage to this nerve may result in hoarseness, but often produces only minor symptoms such as easy fatiguing of the voice.[6] The inferior laryngeal nerve is a recurrent branch of the vagus nerve which innervates all laryngeal muscles except the cricothyroid. On the left side, the recurrent laryngeal nerve loops under the arch of the aorta and is protected in the left tracheoesophageal groove (Fig. 1.57). On the right side, the recurrent laryngeal nerve travels around the subclavian artery, passing dorsomedial to the side of the trachea and esophagus. It is vulnerable

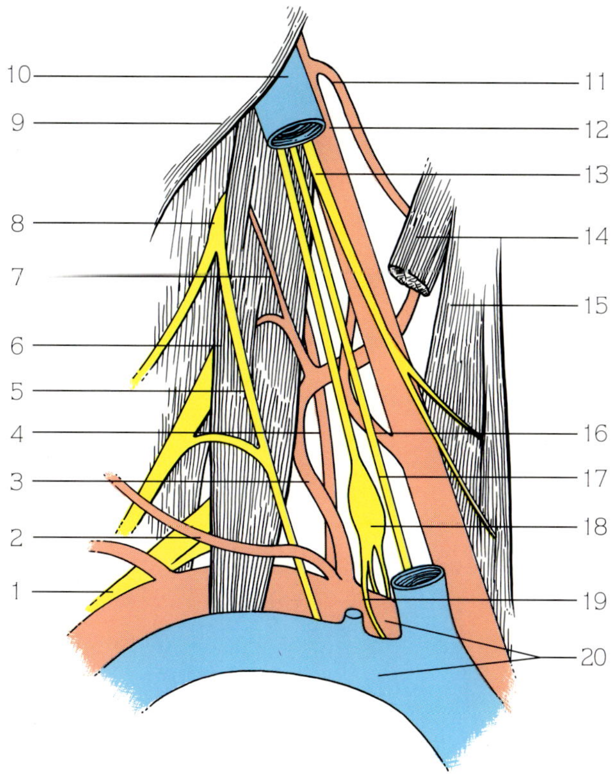

Figure 1.55

The phrenic nerve and arterial system of the anterior neck. The phrenic nerve is on the ventral surface of the anterior scalene muscle and is crossed by the inferior belly of the omohyoid muscle, transverse cervical and suprascapular arteries, and passes between the subclavian artery and vein to reach the thorax

1 Bracheal plexus
2 Suprascapular artery
3 Thyrocervical trunk
4 Vertebral a.
5 Phrenic n.
6 Anterior scalene m.
7 Ascending cervical a.
8 C4
9 Sternocleidomastoid m.
10 Internal jugular v.
11 Superior thyroid a.
12 Common carotid a.
13 Superior root ansa cervicalis
14 Omohyoid m.
15 Sternothyroid m.
16 Inferior thyroid a.
17 Vagus n.
18 Middle cervical ganglion
19 Ansa subclavian
20 Subclavian a. and v.

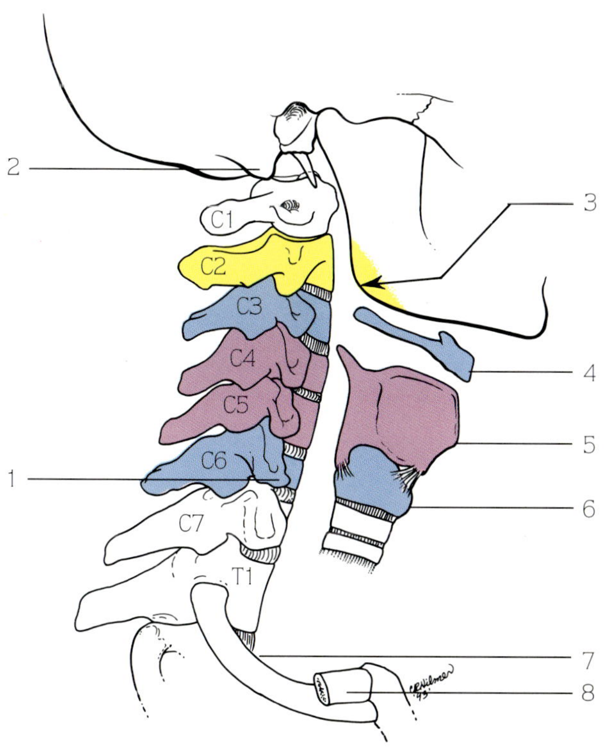

Figure 1.56

The larynx in relation to the cervical spine. The anterior thyroid cartilage is located at C4–C5, and the cricoid cartilaginous ring and the carotid tubercle is located at C6. The angle of the mandible is at C2, and anterior hyoid bone is at C3.

1 Carotid tubercle C6
2 Mastoid process
3 Angle of mandible (C2)
4 Anterior hyoid (C3)
5 Anterior thyroid cartilage (C4–C5)
6 Anterior cricoid cartilage ring (C6)
7 First rib
8 Clavicle

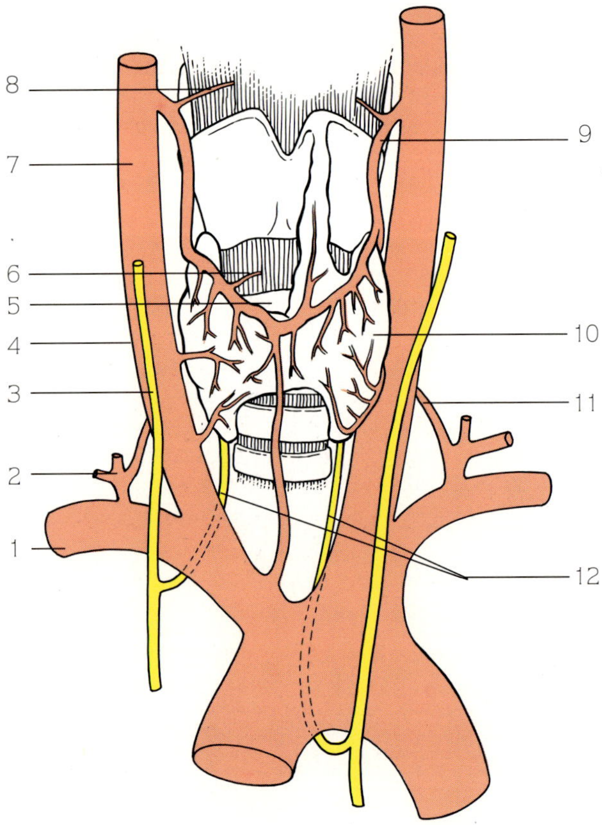

Figure 1.57
Anatomy of recurrent laryngeal nerve. On the left side, the recurrent laryngeal nerve loops under the arch of the aorta and is protected in the left tracheoesophageal groove. On the right side, the recurrent nerve travels around the subclavian artery, passing dorsomedial to the side of the trachea and esophagus

1 Subclavian a.
2 Thyrocervical trunk
3 Vagus n.
4 Common carotid a.
5 Cricoid cartilage
6 Cricothyroid a.
7 External carotid a.
8 Superior laryngeal a.
9 Superior thyroid a.
10 Thyroid
11 Inferior thyroid a.
12 Recurrent laryngeal n.

Figure 1.58 (see opposite)
The cervical sympathetic system consists of three ganglia with intervening cords, and variations exist. The sympathetic trunk is located ventral to the transverse processes and embedded in dorsal aspect of the carotid sheath. (Modified from Richenbacher J, Landolt AM, Theiler K: *Applied Anatomy of the Back*, Berlin: Springer Verlag, 1982.)

1 Cardiac branches of thoracic ganglion
2 Second thoracic gang.
3 Internal thoracic a.
4 Superior internal a.
5 T1
6 Thyrocervical trunk
7 Rami communicantes
8 Middle cervical ganglion
9 Vertebral a.
10 Common carotid a.
11 Carotid tubercle
12 C6
13 Carotid n.
14 Middle cervical ganglion and cardiac branch
15 Inferior cervical ganglion
16 First thoracic ganglion
17 Ansa subclavia
18 Cardiac br. of inf. cervical ganglion
19 Cardiac branch of inferior cervical ganglion
20 Cervical plexus
21 Vertebral a.
22 Inferior cervical ganglion
23 Thyrocervical trunk
24 First thoracic ganglion
25 Superior intercostal a.
26 Second thoracic ganglion
27 Cardiac branches of thoracic ganglion
28 Cardiac branches of inferior cervical ganglion
29 Third thoracic ganglion
30 Second thoracic ganglion
31 C8
32 C7
33 C6
34 C5
35 C4
36 Internal carotid n.
37 Superior cervical ganglion
38 Pharyngeal plexus
39 C3
40 Superior thyroid plexus
41 Superior cervical ganglion
42 C4
43 Esophageal branches
44 Inferior thyroid plexus
45 Middle cervical gang.
46 Inferior cervical ganglion } Crevico-thoracic (stellate) ganglion
47 Ansa subclavia }
48 First thoracic ganglion }
49 Cardiac branch of superior cervical ganglion
50 Cardiac branch of middle cervical ganglion
51 Internal carotid n.
52 External carotid ganglion
53 Cardiac branches of superior cervical ganglion
54 Middle cervical ganglion
55 Cardiac branch of middle cervical ganglion
56 Inferior cervical ganglion } Cervico-thoracic (stellate) ganglion
57 First thoracic ganglion }
58 Cardiac branch of inferior cervical ganglion
59 Second thoracic ganglion

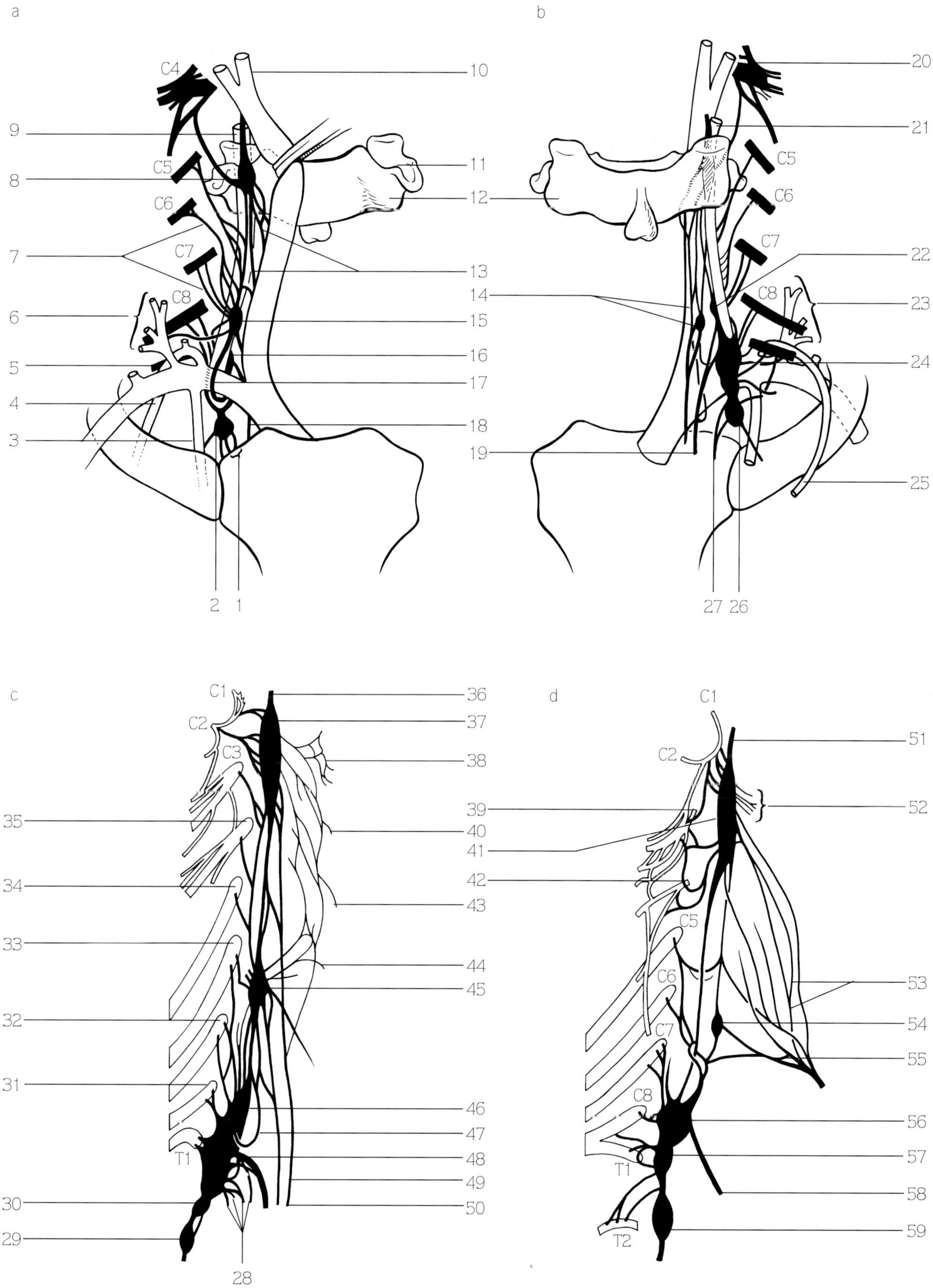
a
b
C4
C5
C6
C7
C8
1
2
3
4
5
6
7
8
9
10
11
12
13
14
15
16
17
18
19
20
21
22
23
24
25
26
27
c
d
C1
C2
C3
T1
T2
28
29
30
31
32
33
34
35
36
37
38
39
40
41
42
43
44
45
46
47
48
49
50
51
52
53
54
55
56
57
58
59

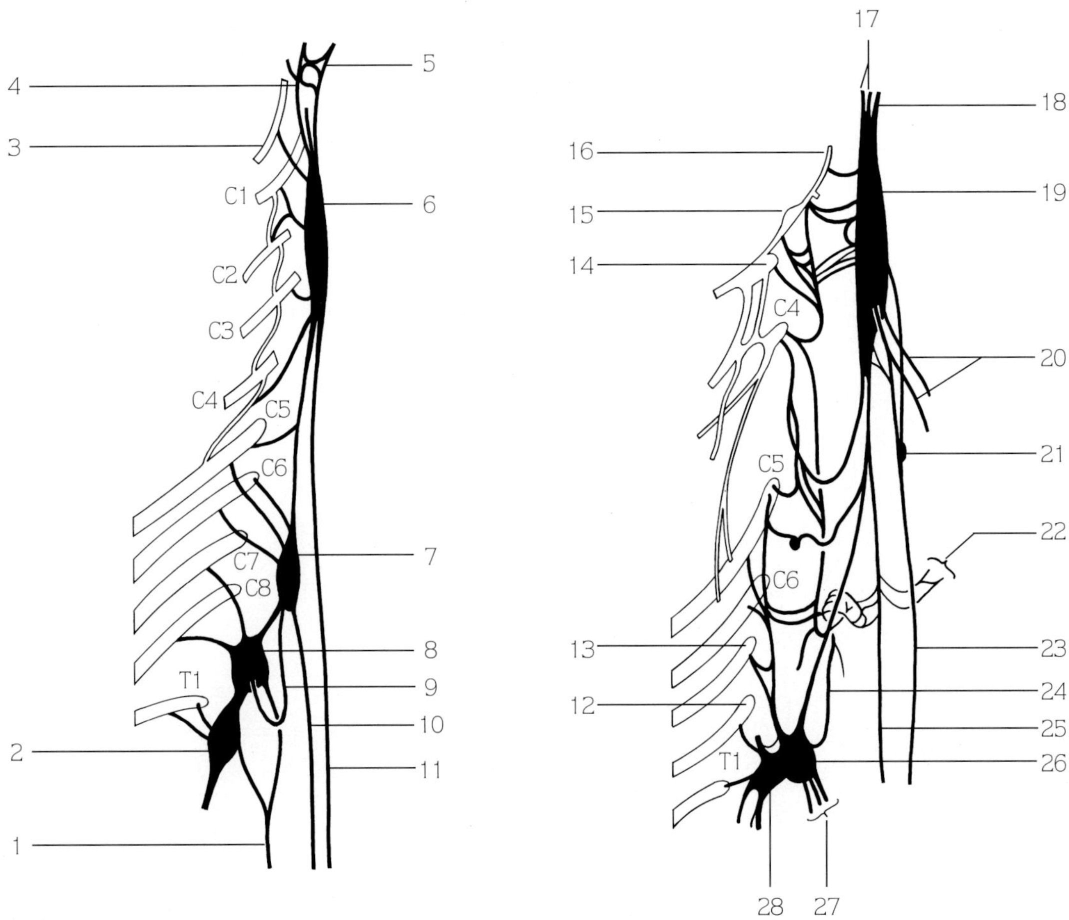

Figure 1.59
Stellate ganglion: when the inferior cervical and the first thoracic ganglia are fused, this mass is referred to as the cervicothoracic or stellate ganglion. (Modified from Rickenbacher J, Landolt AM, Theiler K: *Applied Anatomy of the Back*, Berlin: Springer Verlag, 1982.)

1 Cardiac branch of inferior cervical ganglion
2 Thoracic ganglion
3 Vagus n.
4 Jugular n.
5 Internal carotid n.
6 Superior cervical ganglion
7 Middle cervical ganglion
8 Inferior cervical ganglion
9 Ansa subclavia
10 Cardiac branch of middle cervical ganglion
11 Cardiac branch of superior cervical ganglion
12 C8
13 C7
14 C3
15 C2
16 C1
17 Jugular n.
18 Internal carotid n.
19 Superior cervical ganglion
20 Superior thyroid plexus
21 Accessory ganglion on cardiac branch of superior cervical ganglion
22 Inferior thyroid plexus
23 Cardiac branch of superior cervical ganglion
24 Ansa subclavia
25 Cardiac branch of mid-cervical ganglion
26 Inferior cervical ganglion
27 Cardiac branches of inferior cervical ganglion
28 First thoracic ganglion

as it passes from the subclavian artery to the right tracheoesophageal groove. The recurrent laryngeal nerve should be located when working at C6 or below. The best guideline to its location is the inferior thyroid artery. The nerve usually enters the tracheoesophageal groove where the inferior thyroid artery enters the lower pole of the thyroid. It is also more common for the right inferior laryngeal nerve to be non-recurrent where it travels directly from the vagus nerve and carotid sheath to the larynx. The incidence of non-recurrent inferior laryngeal nerve on the right side is reported as 1%.[20]

The cervical sympathetic system consists of three ganglia with intervening cords, and is highly variable anatomically (Fig. 1.58).[19] The sympathetic trunk is located ventral to the transverse processs, and embedded in the dorsal aspect of the carotid sheath. The cervical sympathetic system consists of pre- and post-ganglionic autonomic fibers. The origin of preganglionic fibers is from the intermediolateral gray column of the T1–T5 spinal cord segments. White rami communicantes leave the ventral roots of corresponding thoracic nerves and ascend into the trunk. The largest ganglion is the superior ganglion, which is located on the transverse processes of C2–C3. The middle ganglion is smallest at C6 and C7, and the inferior ganglion lies between the transverse process of C7 and the neck of the first rib. When the inferior cervical and the first thoracic ganglia are fused, this mass is referred to as the cervicothoracic or stellate ganglion (Fig. 1.59). Injury to the sympathetic system may result in a Horner's syndrome, which consists of ptosis, meiosis, and anhidrosis. Subperiosteal dissection is important to prevent damage to these nerves. The esophagus courses anterior to the cervical vertebrae and longus colli muscles, and posterior to the trachea. The recurrent laryngeal nerve ascends in the groove between the trachea and the esophagus. Vigorous retraction during surgery should be avoided to avoid injury to these structures.

REFERENCES

1 An HS, Gordin R, Renner K. Anatomic considerations for plate-screw fixation of the cervical spine. *Spine* **16**(suppl): S548–S551, 1991.

2 Bland JH, Boushey DR. Anatomy and physiology of the cervical spine. *Semin Arthrit Rheumat* **20**: 1–20, 1990.

3 Bogduk N. The clinical anatomy of the cervical dorsal rami. *Spine* **7**: 319 320, 1982.

4 Czervionke LF, Daniels DL. Cervical spine anatomy and pathologic processes. Applications of new MR imaging techniques. *Radiol Clin North Am* **26**: 921–947, 1988.

5 Czervionke LF, Daniels DL, Ho PSP, Yu S, et al. Cervical neural foramina: correlative anatomic and MR imaging study. *Neuroradiology* **169**: 753–759, 1988.

6 Czervionke LF, Daniels DL, Ho PSP, et al. MR appearance of gray and white matter in the cervical spinal cord. *Am J Neuroradiol* **9**: 557–562, 1988.

7 Daniels DL, Williams AL, Haughton VM. Computed tomography of the articulations and ligaments at the occipito-atlantoaxial region. *Radiology* **146**: 709–716, 1983.

8 Daniels DL, Hyde JS, Kneeland JB, et al. The cervical nerves and foramina: Local-coil MR imaging. *Am J Neuroradiol* **7**: 129–133, 1986.

9 Dommisse GF. The blood supply of the spinal cord. *J Bone Joint Surg Br* **56**: 225, 1974.

10 Ellis JH, Martell W, Lillie JH, Aisen AM. Magnetic resonance imaging of the normal craniovertebral junction. *Spine* **16**: 105–111, 1991.

11 Flannigan BD, Lufkin RB, McGlade C, et al. MR imaging of the cervical spine: Neurovascular anatomy. *Am J Radiol* **148**: 785–790, 1987.

12 Fletcher G, Haughton VM, Ho KC, Yu S. Age related changes in the cervical facet joints: Studies with cryomicrotomy, MR, and CT. *Am J Neuroradiol* **11**: 27–30, 1990.

13 Gerbrand JG, Baljet B, Drukker J. Nerves and nerve plexuses of the human vertebral column. *Am J Anat* **188**: 282–296, 1990.

14 Hayashi K, Yabuki T, Kurokawa T, Seki H, Hogaki M, Minoura S. The anterior and the posterior longitudinal ligaments of the lower cervical spine. *J Anat* **124**: 633–636, 1977.

15 Panjabi MM, Duranceau J, Goel V, Oxland T, Takata K. Cervical human vertebrae. Quantitative three-dimensional anatomy of the middle and lower regions. *Spine* **16**: 861–874, 1993.

16 Parke WW, Sherk HH. Normal adult anatomy. In Sherk HH, Dunn EJ, Eismont FJ, et al. (eds) *The Cervical Spine*, 2nd ed. (Cervical Spine Research Society), 11–32. Philadelphia: JB Lippincott 1988.

17 Pech P, Daniels DL, Williams AL, Haughton VM. The cervical neural foramina: correlation of microtomy and CT anatomy. *Radiology* **155**: 143–146, 1985.

18 Rauschning W. Anatomy and Pathology of the Cervical Spine. In Frymoyer JW (ed.), *The Adult Spine*. New York: Raven Press, 907–929, 1991.

19 Rickenbacher J, Landolt AM, Theiler K. *Applied Anatomy of the Back*. Berlin: Springer Verlag 1982.

20 Sanders G, Uyeda RY, Karlan MS. Nonrecurrent inferior laryngeal nerves and their association with a recurrent branch. *Am J Surg* **146**: 501–503, 1983.

21 Sether LA, Yu S, Haughton VM, Wagner M. Ruptures of the annulus fibrosus of cervical intervertebral discs studied by cryomicrotomy and magnetic resonance. *Clin Anat* **2**: 1–8, 1989.

22 Yeager VL, Cooper MH. Surgical anatomy of the cervical spine surrounding structures. In Young PH (ed.) *Microsurgery of the Cervical Spine*, 1–17. New York: Raven Press 1991.

23 Yu S, Sether L, Haughton VM. Facet joint menisci of the cervical spine: Correlative MR imaging and cryomicrotomy study. *Radiology* **164**: 79–82, 1987.

2 Surgical approaches to the cervical spine

Howard S. An

Surgical approaches to the cervical spine are well described in the literature. The anteromedial approach, first described by Smith–Robinson, and the posterior approach are commonly used and familiar to most spinal surgeons. However, less commonly used exposures, such as anterior approaches to the upper cervical and cervicothoracic regions, often require a review of pertinent anatomic structures by the surgeon. Preoperative cadaveric dissection is advised for more difficult exposures by the inexperienced surgeon. In this chapter, anterior and posterior operative approaches from the occiput to the cervicothoracic junction will be described in detail. Additionally, application of the halo vest and other external orthotic devices will be reviewed at its conclusion.

POSTERIOR APPROACHES TO THE CERVICAL SPINE

Lower Cervical Spine (C3–C7)

Any surgical approach to the cervical spine requires complete and thorough preoperative planning which includes both anesthetic and positioning considerations. Careful positioning of the patient will minimize the potential for iatrogenic injury and facilitate the proper surgical procedure.

Endotracheal intubation of the patient can be completed by one of several methods. The neurologic status of the patient and the potential for neurological injury with positioning of the head are of the greatest concern. In cases of radiculopathy secondary to degenerative disc disease, the patient is not at undue risk for injury, so special intubation techniques are not necessary. However, for patients with myelopathy, acute spinal cord injury, or cervical instability, conscious fiberoptic intubation is required to prevent excessive movement of the head, and to minimize potential for neurologic injury. Somatosensory evoked potentials should be used for any patient with intraspinal lesions, myelopathy, or significant neurologic deficits. We often position leads on the patient before the intubation process, and monitor the labile patient throughout the intubation and positioning process.

Once intubated, the patient must be carefully turned into the prone position. For degenerative conditions requiring foraminotomy or laminectomy, it is preferable to secure the patient's head with a Mayfield pin-holder headrest (Fig. 2.1). The headrest is first secured to the patient's head with the patient supine. The Mayfield pin-holder can then be used by the surgeon to control the head during the turning process. Once the patient is prone, the device is attached to the operative table, rigidly securing the head and neck (Fig. 2.2). A few surgeons prefer simply to rest the patient's face on a padded horseshoe-shaped headrest; however, excessive pressure may develop on the eyes or facial structures with imperfect positioning or prolonged operative time. The pin-holder headrest avoids all such pressure points.

For cases of cervical instability secondary to fracture, ligamentous disruption, or tumor, use of a Stryker bed may facilitate turning of the patient from the supine to the prone position. The Stryker frame is particularly useful in cases requiring combined anterior and posterior surgical approaches. For many of these cases, it is, in addition, preferable to have the patient immobilized and secured with a halo vest. The patient's head may be stabilized through the use of a C-shaped halo ring while permitting surgical access. Alternatively, cranial tongs can be applied, and traction used to maintain stability and correct deformity (Fig. 2.3).

Whatever technique is used to stabilize and position the patient's head for a posterior surgical approach, extremes of neck flexion or extension should be avoided. For degenerative conditions requiring laminectomy or foraminotomy, many surgeons prefer the sitting position to minimize epidural venous bleeding and improve exposure. This position, however, does increase the risk of air embolism. The author's group prefer a reverse Trendelenburg position with the patient's head elevated at 30–45° above

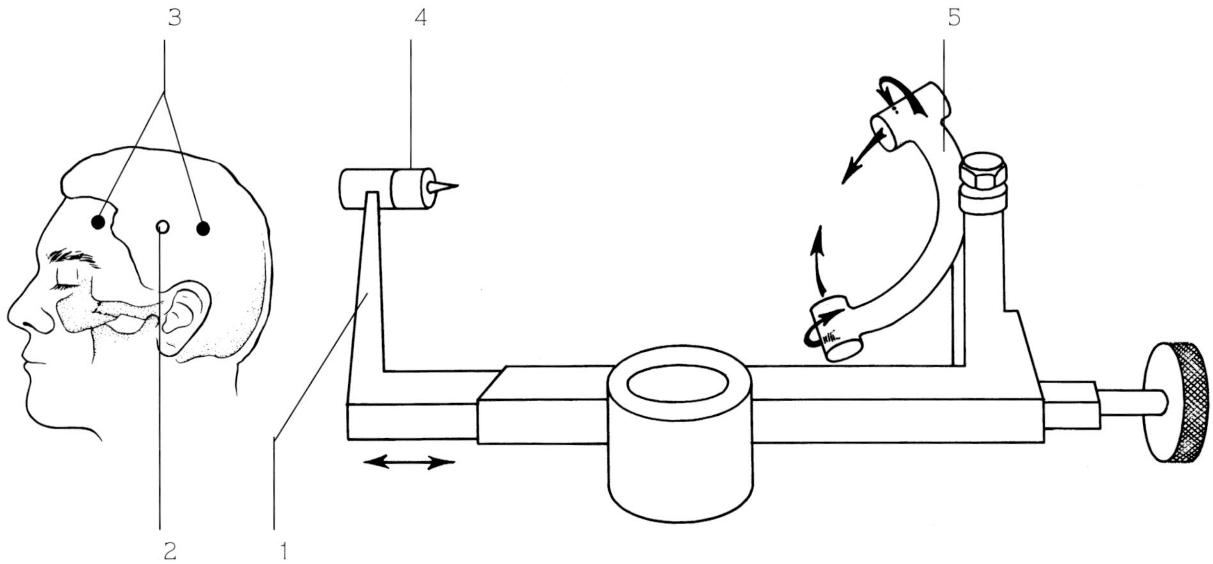

Figure 2.1
A diagram of a Mayfield pin-holder headrest with pin hole sites on the head

1 Side arm
2 Site for 'single' pin
3 Sites for 'double' pins
4 Pin
5 Movable yoke

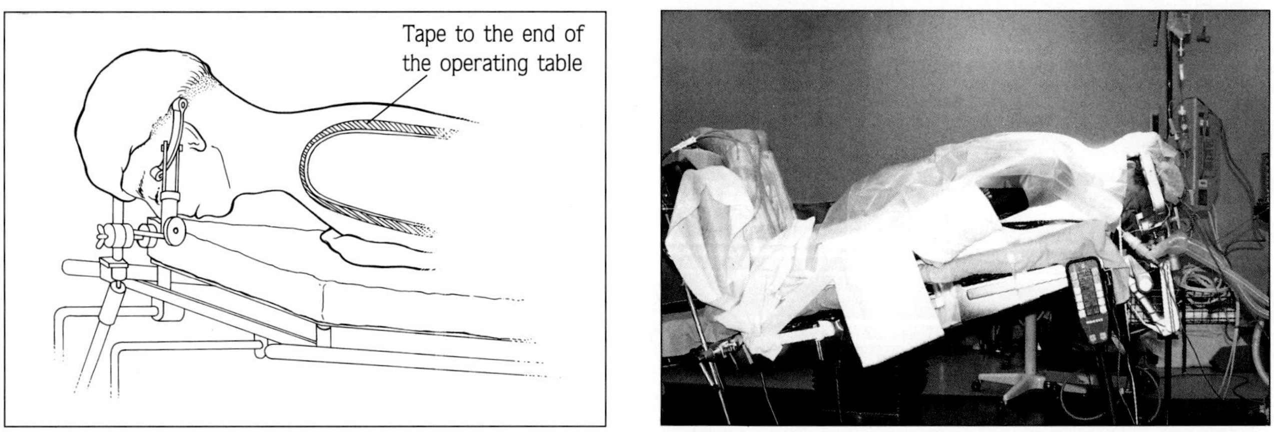

a b

Figure 2.2
(a) A diagram of prone positioning with the Mayfield pin holder. (b) Intraoperative photograph of the prone position for posterior cervical approaches

the parallel. If the table is positioned in this manner, the posterior aspect of the neck parallels the floor, and venous congestion and cerebrospinal fluid pressure are reduced (see Fig. 2.2). The elbows are well padded to prevent pressure on the ulnar nerve, and chest rolls used to avert pressure on the brachial plexus. In the lower extremities, the knees must also be protected from excessive pressure points.

The posterior approach uses a longitudinal midline incision, which extends above and below the vertebral

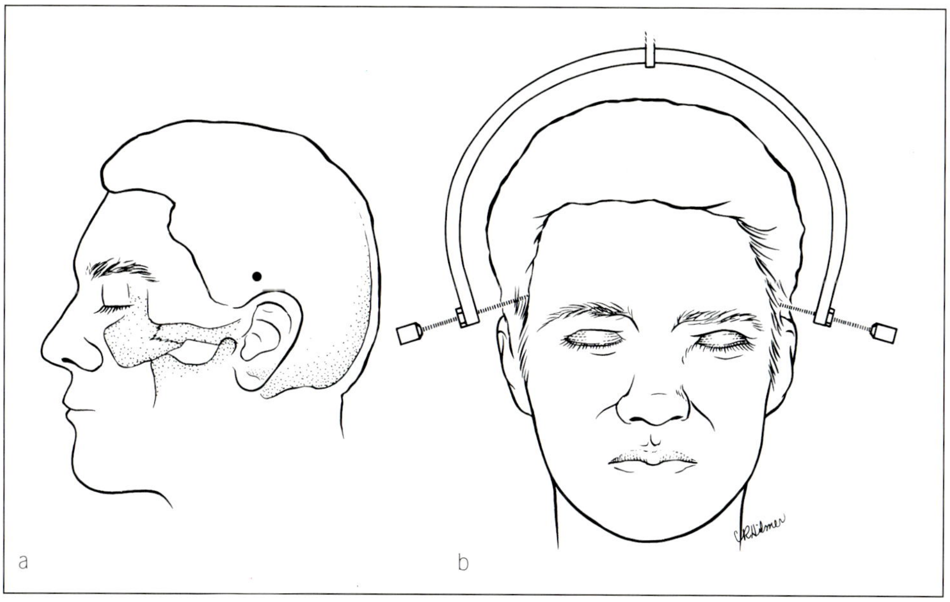

Figure 2.3
(a) Mayfield tong pin site which is just above the ear. (b) Mayfield tongs should be applied above the ears but below the equator of the head

segments required for the procedure. This extension of the skin incision and subcutaneous tissues is necessary for retraction, because the skin of the posterior neck is thicker and less mobile. The skin and subcutaneous tissues are incised sharply. Cutaneous nerves are usually well protected if dissection does not deviate from the midline (Fig. 2.4). Electrocautery is used to obtain meticulous hemostasis. The ligamentum nuchae is incised in the midline with electrocautery, and dissection continued subperiosteally along the spinous processes. Care should be taken to stay in the subperiosteal plane, because the bifid nature of the spinous processes may result in a bulbous expanse and force dissection to err into the paraspinal musculature. A superficial plexus of veins may be encountered and should be cauterized as needed (Fig. 2.4). A wide flat periosteal elevator, such as a Cobb, should be used to dissect the paraspinal muscles carefully off the spinous processes. Electrocautery is used as the knife for severing these muscular attachments from the spinous process and interspinous ligaments. The surgeon should examine preoperative radiographs for any evidence of spina bifida or other bony defect to avoid inadvertent entry of an instrument into the spinal canal. In the cervical spine, the laminae do not override each other as much as in the thoracic spine; the interlaminar space can, therefore, be inadvertently penetrated if care is not taken during exposure of the laminae. When approaching the junction of the lamina to the lateral mass, care is taken not to disrupt the facet capsule, except in fusion cases. The capsule is a stabilizing structure, and can easily be damaged during dissection.

In addition, care should be taken when dissecting to the lateral edge of the joint, because the nerve root and vertebral artery lie anterior to the spinolamellar membrane of the adjoining transverse processes. Vigorous decortication or stripping may damage the thin bone, and subsequently result in injury to the nerve root or vertebral artery. The segmental artery at the lateral edge of the facet joints may be cauterized as it exits between the transverse processes. Various commercially available, self-retaining retractors may be used to facilitate exposure. For fusion cases, only the levels to be fused should be exposed because creeping fusion extension is common. Various wiring and fusion techniques are discussed in Chapter 19.

For degenerative disease requiring foraminotomy or laminectomy, loupe magnification of × 3.5 and headlamp illumination are recommended. Alternatively, the operating microscope can be used, and is especially useful in foraminotomy cases and intradural procedures. Somatosensory evoked potentials are monitored routinely in myelopathic and intradural procedures. As mentioned earlier, however, the author prefers the prone position with the table placed in a 45° reverse Trendelenburg position. The head is positioned in slight flexion unless the patient has cervical spondylotic myelopathy, in which case the head is placed in the neutral position. This prevents further cord compression from spondylotic bars.

Unilateral foraminotomy is completed by exposing the lamina and facet joint to the lateral edge of the articular masses (Fig. 2.5). A Taylor retractor is then placed lateral to the lateral mass without placing it too deeply, thereby safeguarding the nerve root. A small Kerrison rongeur is

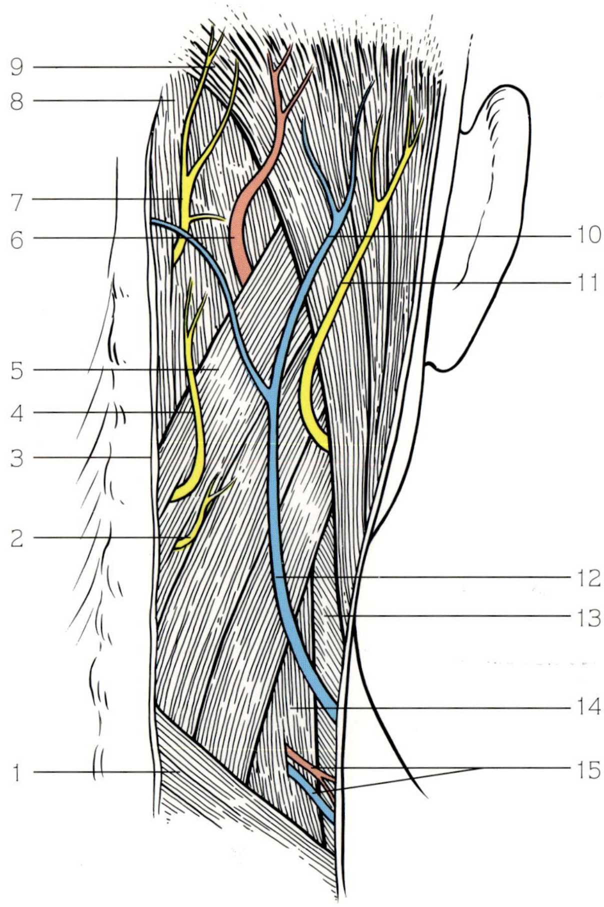

Figure 2.4
Anatomy of cutaneous nerves and superficial vessels in the posterior neck

1 Rhomboid
2 Medial branch of posterior primary ramus of C5
3 Cut edge of trapezius
4 Third occipital n.
5 Splenius capitis m.
6 Occipital a.
7 Greater occipital n.
8 Semispinalis capitis m.
9 Sternocleidomastoid m.
10 Retroauricular v.
11 Lesser occipital n.
12 External jugular v.
13 Levator scapulae m.
14 Splenius cervicis m.
15 Deep branch of cervical a. and v.

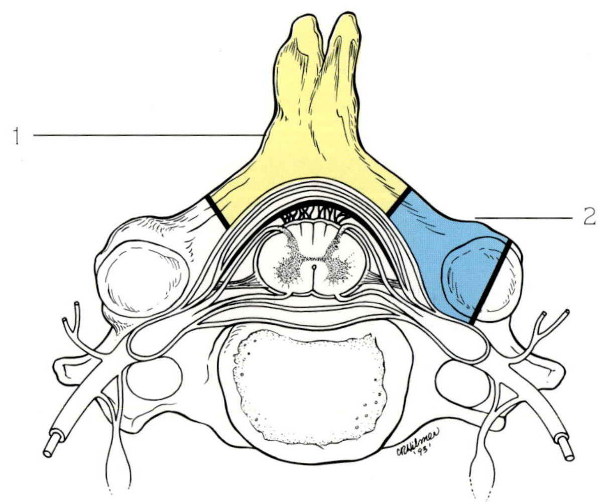

Figure 2.5
Laminectomy involves removal of the spinous process and lamina, and foraminotomy requires about 50% resection of the facet joint

1 Laminectomy
2 Foraminotomy

used to remove a portion of the inferior and superior laminae directly over the affected nerve root. Partial facetectomy or foraminotomy is performed by thinning the facets with a power burr. The author's preferred method is to use an air-powered, high-speed burr to thin the cortex over the foramen, and then complete the thinning with a diamond-tip burr (Fig. 2.6). The surgeon should hold the instrument with both hands, carefully resting the wrists and forearms on the patient, providing proprioceptive feedback to the surgeon and averting unexpected deviation of the instrument. The thinned bone is then gently lifted off the nerve root with small angled curettes.

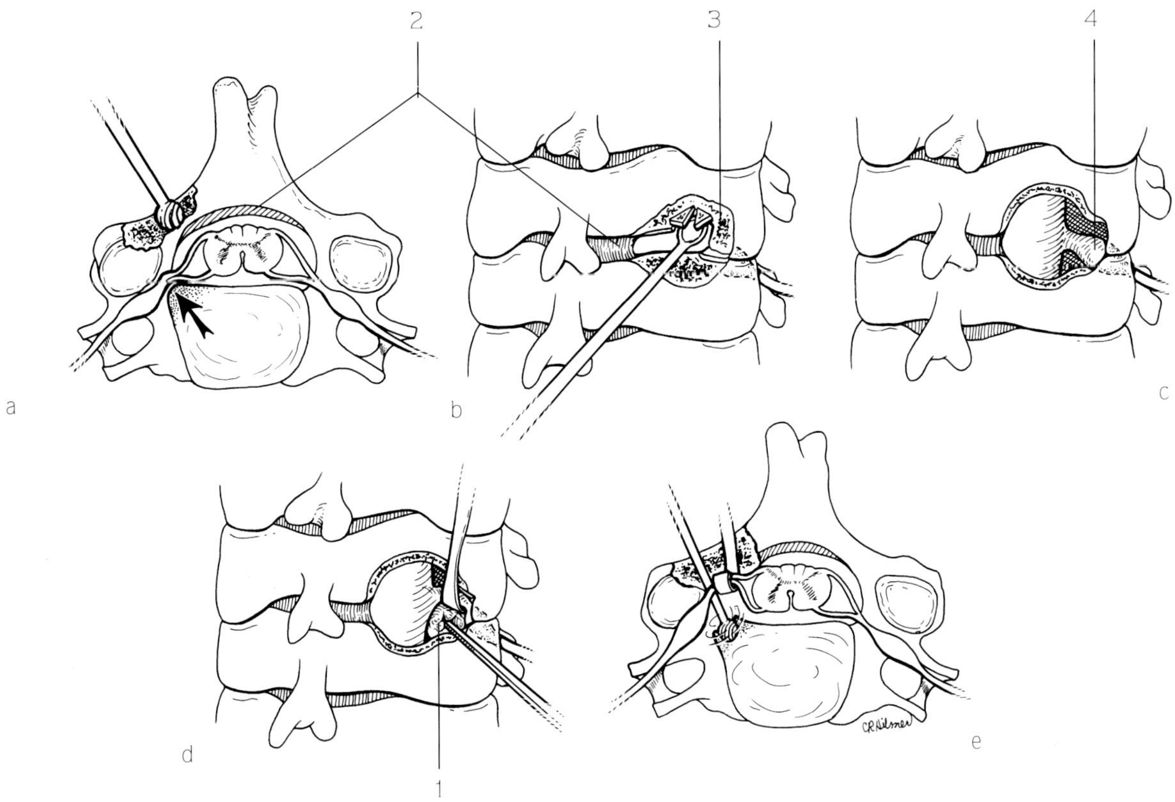

Figure 2.6

Unilateral foraminotomy steps: (a) after exposure of the lamina and facet joint, a Taylor retractor is placed lateral to the lateral mass. A small Kerrison rongeur is used to remove a portion of the inferior and superior laminae directly over the affected nerve root. Partial facetectomy or foraminotomy is performed by thinning the facets with a power burr. (b) An air-powered, high-speed burr is used to thin the cortex of the foramen, and then the thinned bone is gently lifted off the nerve root with small angled curettes. (c) Once the bone is removed, the dura and nerve root are exposed. (d) If the underlying disc or osteophyte is to be removed, the venous plexus overlying the nerve root may need to be cauterized with the bipolar cautery to control bleeding. (e) The nerve root may be gently retracted for removal of the disc or osteophyte

1 Disc fragment
2 Ligamentum flavum
3 Facet
4 Nerve root

Placement of a Kerrison rongeur under the lamina or the foramen may result in injury to the neural elements. Once the bone is removed, the dura and nerve root are exposed. The venous plexus overlying the nerve root may need to be cauterized with bipolar cautery to control bleeding. The nerve root can be gently retracted if necessary, but manipulation of the spinal cord is prohibited. The nerve root is usually well decompressed by removal of the lamina and 50% of the facet joint. Attempted retraction of the nerve root for removal of an underlying osteophyte or disc material is not routinely done, unless the nerve root is felt to be 'tight' after completion of the foraminotomy.

Laminectomy is performed by thinning of the cortices at the lateral margins of the lamina with a power burr (Fig. 2.7). A small Kerrison rongeur may be used to finish the cut, but it is safer to use a small angled curette to finish the cut and lift the lamina away from the spinal cord. In order to prevent laminectomy-associated instability, several authors reported laminoplasties as alternatives to laminectomy of the cervical spine (Fig. 2.8). The 'keyhole' foraminotomy, laminectomy, and laminoplasty techniques are more thoroughly reviewed in Chapter 10.[26,42]

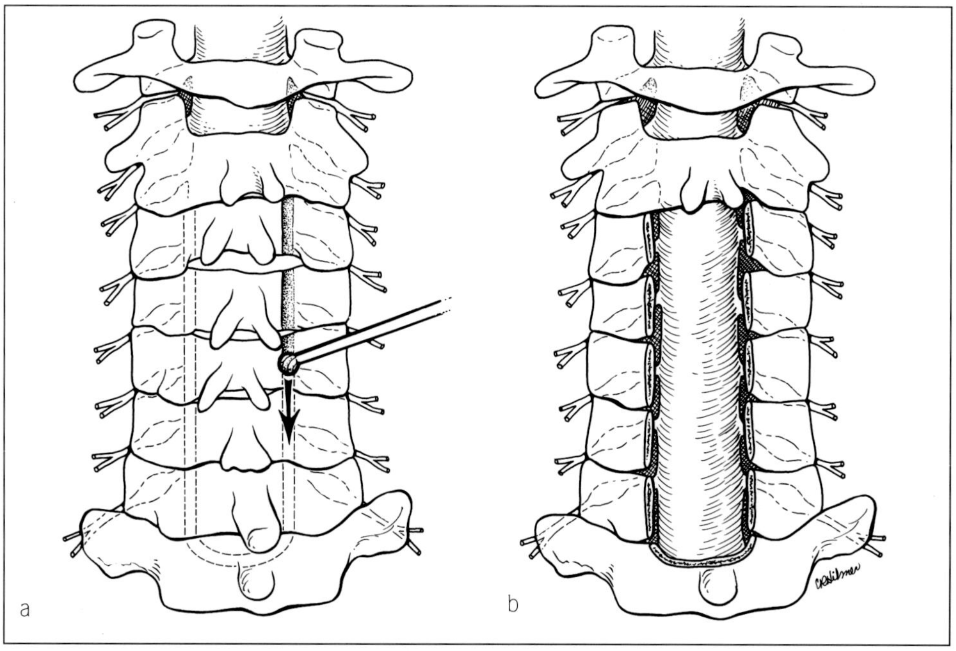

Figure 2.7
(a) Laminectomy is performed by thinning of the cortices at the lateral margins of the lamina with a power burr. A small Kerrison rongeur may be used to finish the cut, but it is safer to use a small angled curette to finish the cut and lift the lamina away from the spinal cord. (b) Laminectomy exposes the underlying spinal cord

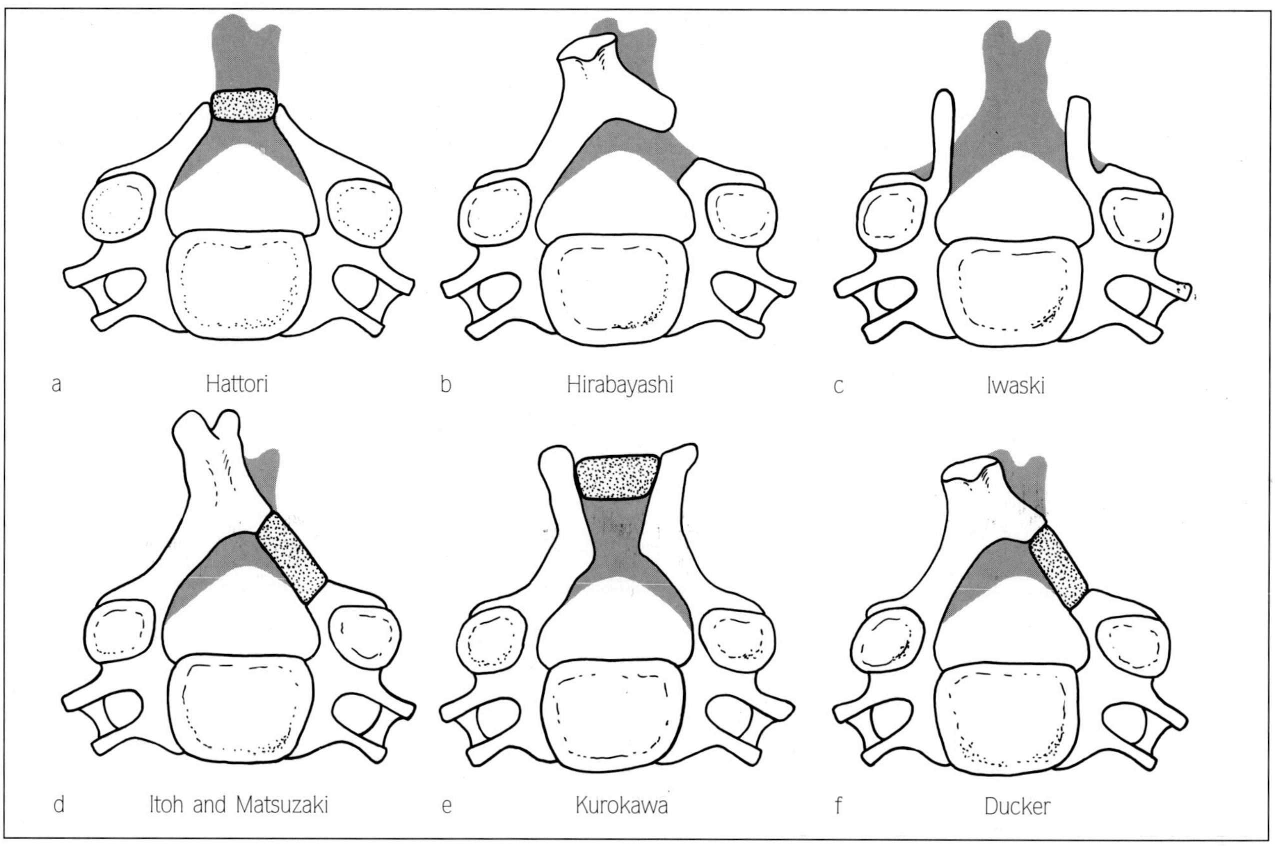

Figure 2.8
Different techniques of laminoplasty

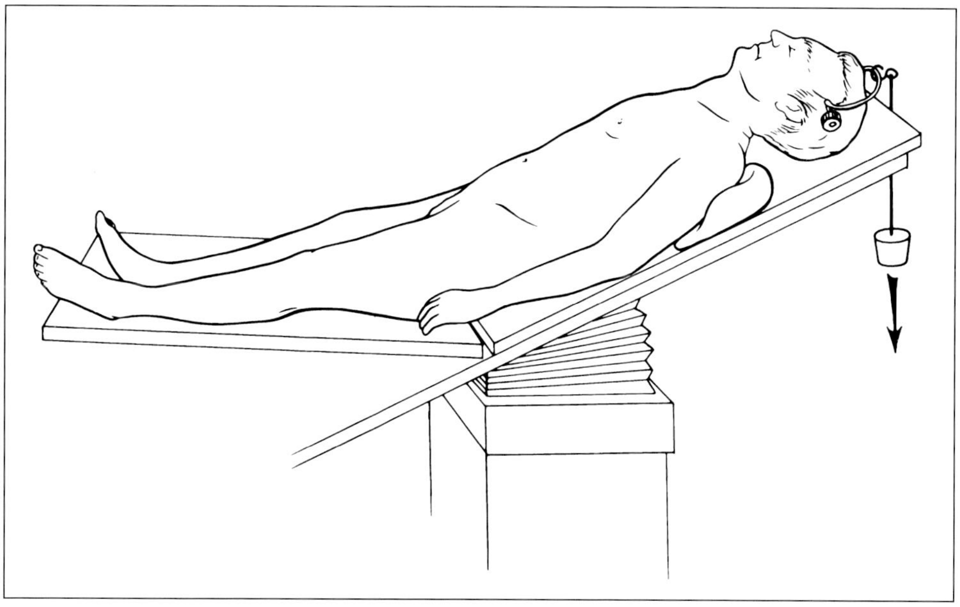

Figure 2.9
The patient is placed in a supine and reverse Trendelenburg positions with Gardner–Wells traction applied to the head

Upper Cervical Spine (C1–C2)

Posterior approaches to the upper cervical spine are commonly performed for occipitocervical and atlantoaxial arthrodeses, spinal cord decompression, and tumors. Intubation and patient positioning considerations are identical to those of the lower cervical spine. For cases of cervical instability, it is preferable to immobilize the patient before the operation with a halo vest. A halo ring with a posterior opening (C ring) allows surgical access. Alternatively, cranial tongs may be used, permitting application of traction forces during the operative procedure. A Stryker frame is often used to facilitate turning of the patient as well as maintaining traction during the procedure.

Once the patient is turned into the prone position, the head is usually positioned in slight flexion to open the space between the ring of C1 and the occiput. The external occipital protuberance and the spinous process of C2 can be palpated, and the incision made from the inion caudally for a distance of approximately 8 cm. The dissection is continued through the ligamentum nuchae, and the paraspinal muscles then stripped from C3 to the occiput. Palpation of the large C2 spinous process and the posterior C1 ring confirms the correct level. A large broad elevator and electrocautery are used to aid dissection of the posterior paracervical muscles from the arches of C1 and C2. Care should be taken to avoid inadvertent plunging of instruments into the spinal canal. A small curette can be helpful to remove the muscular attachments on the bifid spinous process of C2, while stabilizing the arch of C2. However, muscular insertions on the spinous process of C2 should be preserved as much as possible to prevent instability at C2–C3. Lateral dissection on the posterior arch of C1 should not exceed 1.5 cm in the adult and 1 cm in the child to avoid injury to the vertebral artery. Dissection must remain subperiosteal in this region to prevent injury. The vertebral artery courses over the arch of the atlas and pierces the lateral angle of the posterior atlanto-occipital membrane.

The removal of the atlantoaxial ligament or atlanto-occipital membrane is not required, except in cases of laminectomy. Careful separation of the membrane or ligament from the bone is all that is usually required to pass sublaminar wires; this can be performed with a small angled curette or a small periosteal elevator. It is necessary to be cautious when dissecting at the inferior edge of the foramen magnum, because uncontrollable bleeding may be encountered.

The spinal cord should never be retracted at this level, because death from respiratory paralysis can result. The greater occipital nerve (C2) and the third occipital nerve cross the field and course laterally in the paracervical muscles. Subperiosteal dissection and avoidance of excessively vigorous lateral dissection should prevent injury to these nerves.

The spinal canal at C1–C2 is capacious, and allows extensive motion. Passage of sublaminar wires at the C1–C2 level is common and relatively safe when done correctly. Passage at lower cervical levels is associated with increased risk of neurologic injury caused by the narrow canal. The Brooks-type C1–C2 arthrodesis, which involves sublaminar wiring of both C1 and C2, is preferred in extension injuries, whereas the Gallie-type fusion is adequate for flexion instabilities, and avoids passage of sublaminar wires at C2 by using the spinous process.[6,17,20] The key to fusion success is thorough decortication of the bone surfaces and application of sufficient autogenous bone grafts. Various wiring and internal fixation techniques are discussed in Chapter 19.

The approach to the occipitocervical junction is used for stabilization of basilar impression, tumor, or fractures of the odontoid with a concurrent fracture of C1. A posteriorly opening halo is usually used before the operation to stabilize the head. A midline incision is made from the inion to the spinous process of C2. Capsular ligaments of the facets should be preserved to maintain stability. Sharp subperiosteal dissection of the external occipital protuberance and lamina is performed, and care taken to protect the vertebral arteries at the lateral border of the atlas. The external occipital protuberance is thick, and allows adequate purchase with unicortical passage of wires, without the inherent difficulties and risks of wire passage through both tables. The exposed bone must be cleaned of all soft tissues, and a power burr can be used to decorticate the surfaces to be fused. For the purpose of fusion, autogenous iliac crest bone graft material is preferable, but allograft material can be supplemented if the pelvic bone is insufficient or osteoporotic. Fusion is usually extended from the occiput to C2, but, in some cases, may require extension to C3 or C4. There are various techniques of occipitocervical fusion which will be described fully in Chapter 19.[19,22,33,51]

Cervicothoracic Junction

Lesions of the cervicothoracic junction are generally anterior, and require extensive anterior approaches for decompression with or without some form of posterior fixation. Those lesions that may require posterior stabilization include tumors, trauma, postlaminectomy instability, or infection. If the posterior elements are intact, the simple and safe triple-wiring technique, used commonly in the lower cervical spine, can be completed for short segment fusions. More commonly, however, longer fusions with hook–rod constructs are required. Pedicle screw fixation is an alternative technique which is used when the posterior elements are deficient. The transpedicular technique at the cervicothoracic junction is an exacting procedure with very little margin for error.

As a result of cadaveric studies, the pedicle landmarks and anatomic characteristics of the cervicothoracic region have been described. A standard posterior approach is used with the dissection extending laterally to expose the lateral mass and the tips of the transverse processes of the upper thoracic vertebrae. The facet joint to be fused is cleaned of its capsule, and the articular margins identified. The entry point of the pedicle lies at the intersection of a horizontal line at the midportion of the transverse processes and a vertical line at the lamina–transverse process junction. This pedicle entrance point is 1 mm inferior to the facet joint and the middle point from the medial to the lateral margins of the facet joint. The outer cortex is decorticated at this point with a small burr, and a small Penfield elevator or straight curette is used to probe and enter the pedicle in a blunt fashion. Once the pedicle is identified a 2.5 mm drill may be used for this entry. Medial angulation is required for entry of the pedicle into the vertebral body, and averages 34° at C7, 31.8° at T1, and 26.5° at T2.[1] When compared to the pedicles of the lumbar spine, the superoinferior diameter of the thoracic pedicle is relatively greater than its mediolateral diameter. This leaves little margin for error in the mediolateral plane.

Associated Complications

Complications associated with posterior approaches to the upper and lower cervical spine may be catastrophic. Care is required during passage of wires or insertion of screws to prevent injury to the brain or spinal cord. Dissection on the ring of the atlas must be done in a gentle manner, because direct pressure may result in fracture or slippage of an instrument. The arch of the atlas should be dissected laterally to only about 1.5 cm, because the vertebral artery is at risk. Dissection of the foramen magnum from the inferior edge of the foramen should be avoided to prevent uncontrollable venous bleeding. The author's group recommend halo vest immobilization after surgery for most upper cervical spine cases to prevent construct failure, and to lessen the likelihood of pseudoarthrosis. The exposures of the lower cervical spine and the cervicothoracic junctions are less risky, but spinal cord injury, nerve root injury, cerebrospinal fluid leakage, vertebral artery injury, and fusion failures can on the whole be prevented with careful and meticulous surgical technique. Laminoplasty or concomitant fusion may prevent laminectomy-associated instability of the cervical spine.[25,26,58] Complications of cervical spine surgery are reviewed in detail in Chapter 20.

ANTERIOR APPROACHES TO THE CERVICAL SPINE

Anterior approaches often use horizontal incisions with dissection anterior to the sternocleidomastoid and carotid

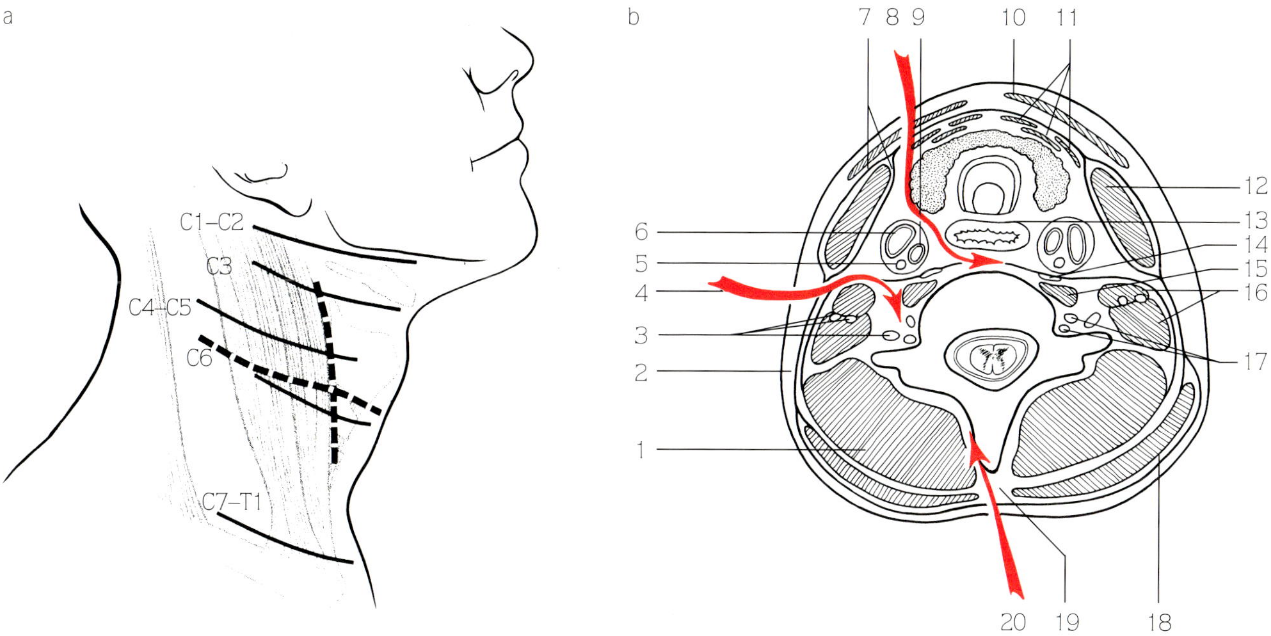

Figure 2.10
(a) The hyoid bone overlies C3, the thyroid cartilage overlies C5, the cricoid ring at C6, and supraclavicular level for C7–T1 region. (b) Anteromedial approaches involve dissection anterior to the carotid sheath between the sternocleidomastoid and viscera, whereas anterolateral approaches involve dissection posterior to the sternocleidomastoid and carotid sheath

1 Erector spinae and transversospinalis mm.
2 Prevertebral layer of cervical fascia
3 Brachial plexus
4 Anterolateral approach
5 Vagus n.
6 Internal jugular v.
7 Superficial layer of cervical fascia
8 Anteromedial approach
9 Common carotid a.
10 Platysma m.
11 Infrahyoid mm.
12 Sternocleidomastoid m.
13 Esophagus
14 Sympathetic trunk
15 Prevertebral mm.
16 Paravertebral mm.
17 Vertebral vessels
18 Trapezius
19 Ligamentum nuchae
20 Posterior approach

sheath. Surgical landmarks are the submandibular area for C1–C2, the hyoid bone for C3, the thyroid cartilage for C4–C5, the cricoid ring for C6, and the supraclavicular area for C7–T1 (Fig. 2.10a). The most commonly used anterior approach to the cervical spine is the Smith–Robinson approach for exposure of the middle and lower cervical spine. Anterior exposure of the upper cervical spine and the cervicothoracic junction is only occasionally required. Additionally, anterolateral approaches with dissection posterior to the sternocleidomastoid and carotid sheath are rarely encountered but are described and reviewed in detail in this chapter (Fig. 2.10b).

Upper Cervical Spine

Anterior approaches to the upper part of the cervical spine include the commonly described anterior retropharyngeal approaches[12,35,57] and transoral approaches,[10,11,14] but may, in rare circumstances, require extension to include dislocation of the temporomandibular joint[39] or osteotomy of the mandible.[21] Each procedure has inherent advantages and disadvantages. The surgeon should be thoroughly familiar with the anatomy and potential for complications associated with the particular procedure before undertaking this formidable task.

DeAndrade and MacNab[12] described an anteromedial retropharyngeal approach to the upper cervical spine, which is, in essence, an extension of the Smith–Robinson approach to the lower cervical spine. The patient is positioned supine with Gardner–Wells traction applied to the head (see Fig. 2.9). The reverse Trendelenburg position allows for venous drainage and, hence, less bleeding during surgery. The neck is hyperextended, and the chin turned to the opposite side. The degree of neck hyperextension should be assessed before the operation because too much can produce myelopathic or radicular signs and

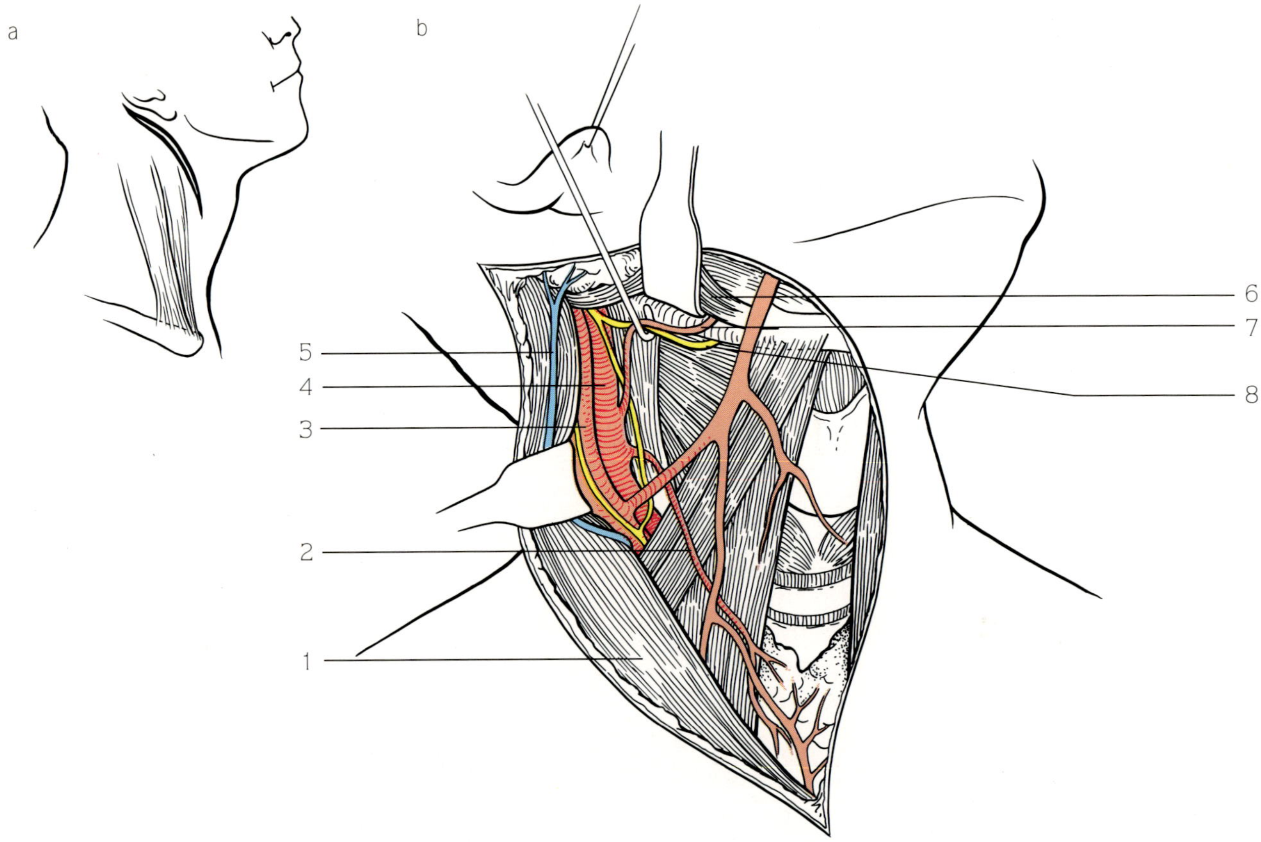

Figure 2.11

(a) A skin incision is made along the anterior aspect of the sternocleidomastoid muscle, and curved toward the mastoid process. (b) The platysma and the superficial layer of the deep cervical fascia are divided in line with the incision to expose the anterior border of the sternocleidomastoid. The sternocleidomastoid muscle is retracted anteriorly, and the carotid artery laterally. The superior thyroid artery and lingual vessels may require ligation, but this should not be done until the hypoglossal nerve is identified. The facial artery is identified at the upper portion of the incision, which is adjacent to the hypoglossal nerve along with the digastric muscle. The prevertebral fascia is bluntly dissected and the longus colli muscles are elevated and a Cloward retractor inserted under the muscle

1 Sternocleidomastoid m.
2 Superior thyroid a.
3 Internal carotid a.
4 External carotid a.
5 Superficial temporal v.
6 Digastric m.
7 Hypoglossal m.
8 Facial a.

symptoms. A skin incision is made along the anterior aspect of the sternocleidomastoid muscle, and curved toward the mastoid process (Fig. 2.11). The platysma and the superficial layer of the deep cervical fascia are divided in line with the incision to expose the anterior border of the sternocleidomastoid.

The greater auricular nerve and anterior cervical nerve are branches of the ansa cervicalis which course from the posterior edge of the sternocleidomastoid, crossing over for distribution to the auricular and mandibular skin. It is important that these nerves should be preserved whenever possible. The sternocleidomastoid muscle is retracted anteriorly, and the palpable carotid artery laterally. The superior thyroid artery and lingual vessels may require ligation, but this should be left until the hypoglossal nerve is identified. The superior thyroid artery branches from the external carotid artery at the level of the hyoid bone, and then crosses the carotid triangle deep to the strap muscles, entering the superolateral aspect of the thyroid gland. The facial artery is identified at the upper portion of the incision, which is adjacent to the hypoglossal nerve, along with the digastric muscle.

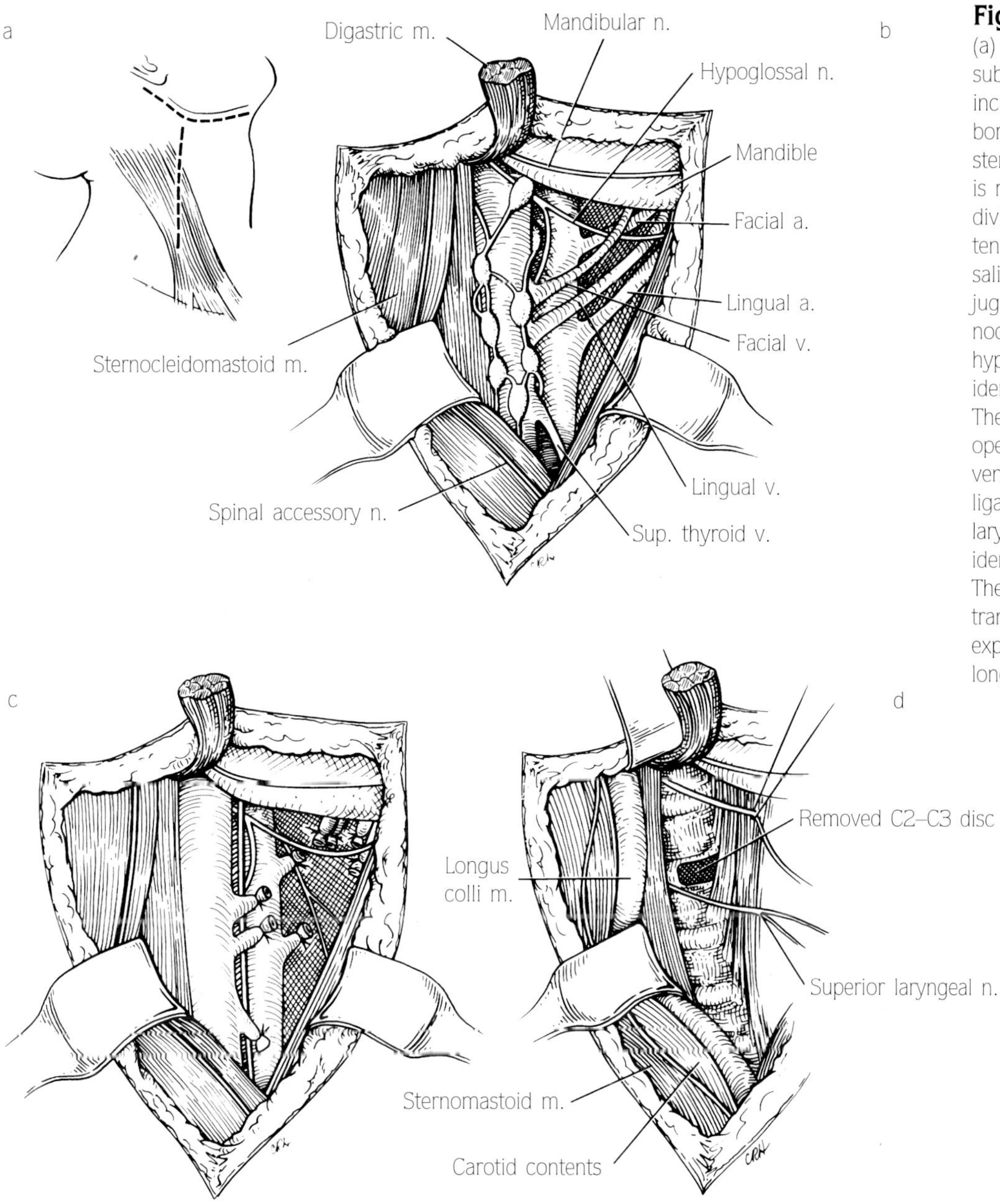

Figure 2.12
(a) A right-sided submandibular transverse incision. (b) The anterior border of the sternocleidomastoid muscle is mobilized, followed by division of the digastric tendon. The submandibular salivary gland and the jugular digastric lymph nodes are resected. The hypoglossal nerve is identified and mobilized. (c) The carotid sheath is opened and arterial and venous branches are ligated. (d) The superior laryngeal nerve is also identified and protected. The prevertebral fascia are transected longitudinally to expose and dissect the longus colli muscles

The hypoglossal nerve is found passing lateral to medial and superficial to the external carotid, lingual, and facial arteries. It is a superficial structure, coursing in a vertical fashion parallel to the carotid sheath; it then passes horizontally and medially over the carotid artery and its branches. It is best retracted in a cephalad direction to prevent traction injury. The superior laryngeal nerve is in close proximity to the superior thyroid artery. Excessive retraction of this nerve may cause hoarseness or inability to sing high notes.

Once these neurovascular structures are identified and retracted or ligated appropriately, the prevertebral fascia is bluntly dissected with a Kitner dissector. Radiographic confirmation of the operative level is completed. The longus colli muscles are elevated and a Cloward retractor inserted beneath them.

Another anterior retropharyngeal exposure of the upper cervical spine has been described by McAfee and associates (Fig. 2.12).[35] A right-sided submandibular transverse incision and division of the platysma lead to the

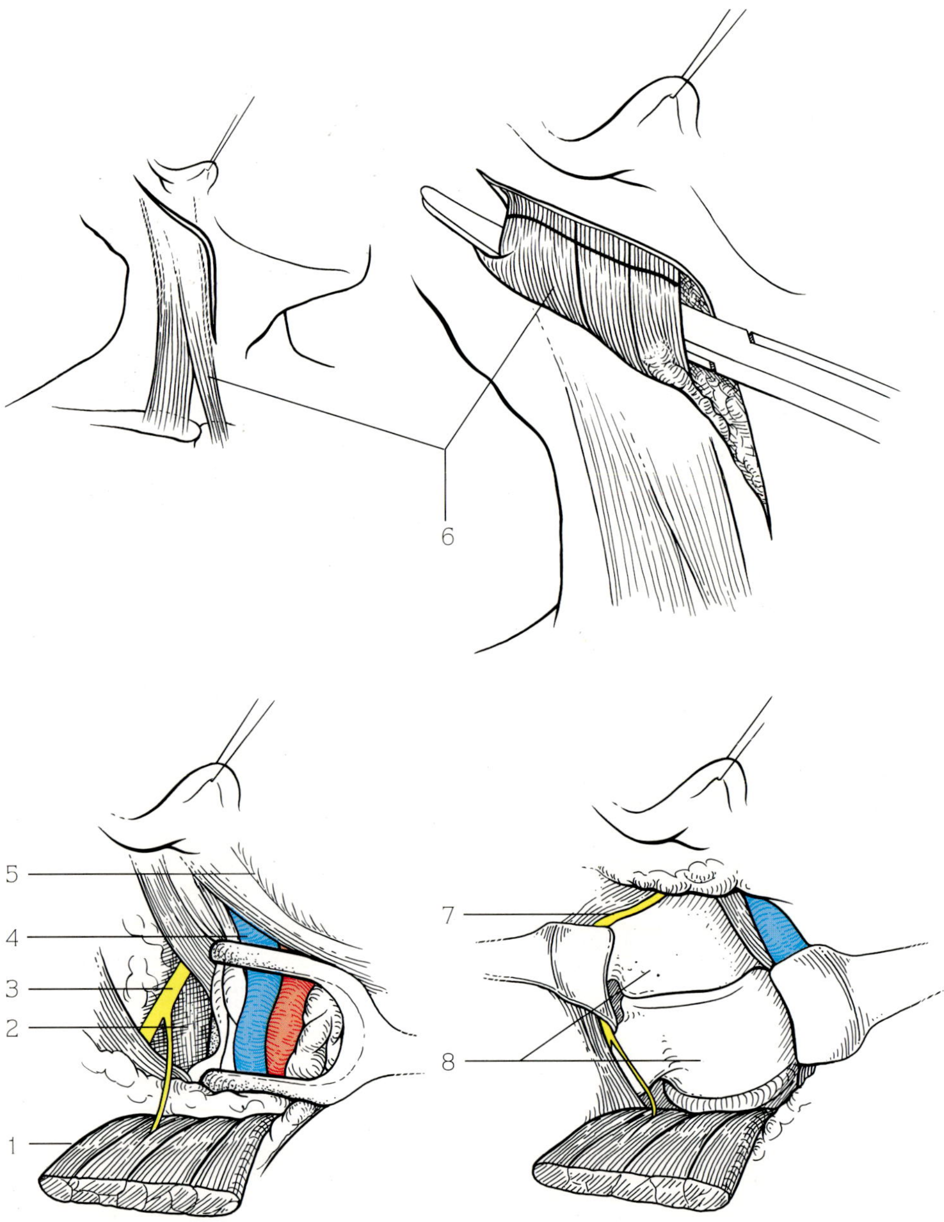

Figure 2.13
The anterolateral retropharyngeal approach described by Whitesides and Kelley. (a) The skin incision is made from the mastoid along the anterior aspect of the sternocleidomastoid. (b) The sternocleidomastoid and splenius capitus muscles are detached from the mastoid. (c) Dissection is posterior to the carotid contents leading to the transverse processes and anterior aspect of C1–C3. (d) Prevertebral fascia is divided and the anterior C1–C2 exposed

1 Sternocleidomastoid m.
2 Retrovisceral space
3 Spinal accessory n.
4 Internal jugular v.
5 Mandible
6 Sternocleidomastoid m.
7 Spinal accessory n.
8 Vertebral body

sternocleidomastoid muscle and its deep cervical fascia. The mandibular branch of the facial nerve should be identified with the aid of a nerve stimulator, and initially the retromandibular vein is ligated. The anterior border of the sternocleidomastoid muscle is then mobilized, and the submandibular salivary gland and jugular digastric lymph nodes resected. Care should be taken to suture the salivary gland's duct to prevent a salivary fistula. The digastric tendon is divided and tagged for later repair. Then the hypoglossal nerve is identified and mobilized. For lateral mobilization of the carotid contents, the carotid sheath is opened and the arterial and venous branches ligated, including the superior thyroid artery and vein, lingual artery and vein, ascending pharyngeal artery and vein, and facial artery and vein. The superior laryngeal nerve is also identified with the aid of a nerve stimulator and mobilized. The prevertebral fasciae are transected longitudinally to expose and dissect the longus colli muscles.

The anterolateral retropharyngeal approach described by Whitesides and Kelley[57] also provides exposure of the upper cervical spine but not the basiocciput (Fig. 2.13). This approach involves dissection anterior to the sternocleidomastoid, but posterior to the carotid sheath, with the skin incision being made from the mastoid along the anterior

a

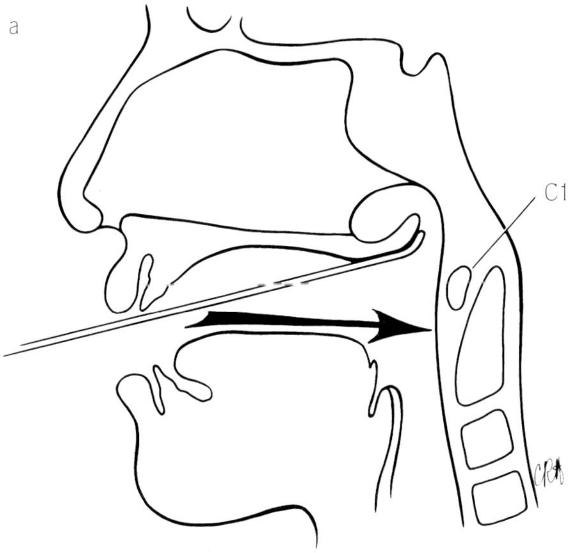

b

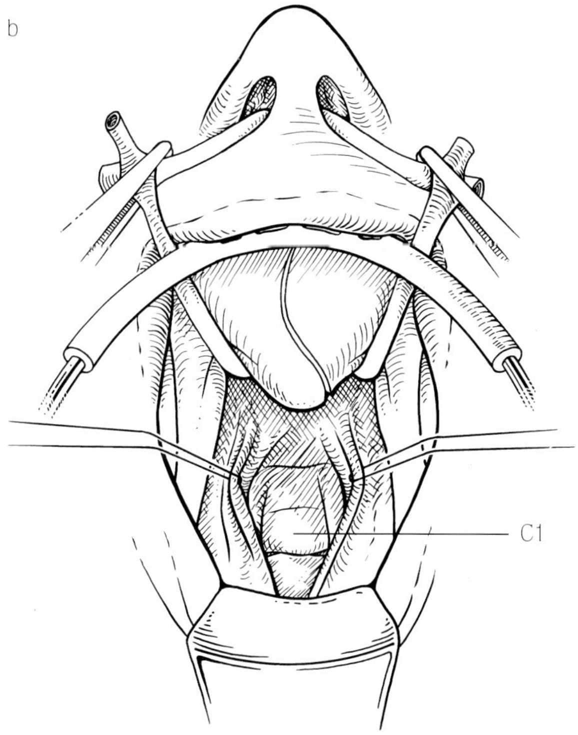

Figure 2.14
The transoral approach: (a) a diagram showing a direct approach to the anterior C1–C2; (b) a special ENT retractor is placed, and the pharynx is divided in the midline

aspect of the sternocleidomastoid. The external jugular vein is ligated, and the greater auricular nerve spared if possible. The sternocleidomastoid and splenius capitis muscles are detached from the mastoid, leaving a fascial edge for later repair. The spinal accessory nerve should be identified and protected: it enters the sternocleidomastoid muscles 3–4 cm below the tip of the mastoid. The internal jugular vein lies just medial to the nerve, and must also be avoided. The nerve should be dissected proximally to allow retraction of the sternocleidomastoid, and the carotid contents are retracted along with the hypoglossal nerve medially and anteriorly, whereas the sternocleidomastoid is retracted posteriorly. Blunt dissection leads to the transverse processes and allows development of the retropharyngeal space anterior to the spine and posterior to the visceral fascia. The prevertebral fascia and anterior longitudinal ligament are identified in the midline. Potential complications of this approach include injuries to the spinal accessory nerve, sympathetic ganglion, and vertebral artery.

Limited anterior exposure from the occiput to C2 may be achieved by the transoral technique of Fang and Ong (Fig. 2.14).[14] This involves splitting the soft palate and posterior pharyngeal wall, but carries a high risk of infection. Fang and Ong[14] reported on six patients who underwent an anterior transoral approach to the upper cervical spine. Four patients developed infections of the pharyngeal wall, including one patient who died of meningitis.

Fortunately, other series have not reported such high rates of complications. Crockard and colleagues[10,11] reported on 68 rheumatoid arthritis patients undergoing one-stage transoral decompression and posterior fixation. Four patients died after the operation, but no major wound complications were noted; cerebrospinal fluid leaks were seen in six patients, including two non-fatal cases of meningitis. After completion of intubation a tracheotomy is carried out, and the patient positioned supine with the head held in a slightly flexed position. Control of the head with the Mayfield pin-holder headrest is advised. A McIver ENT self-retaining retractor is used to depress the tongue and retract the walls of the oral cavity. The soft palate is retracted by placing small, soft, rubber tubes through the nasal cavity and out via the oral cavity; these are tied over sufficient padding. The oropharynx is prepped with povidone-iodine (Betadine) solution. A vertical incision is made from 1 cm cephalad to the tip of the odontoid to 2 cm distal to the anterior tubercle of C1. Radiographic confirmation of the operative level is required. The soft tissues anterior to the bone structures are incised sharply right to the bone, and include the posterior pharyngeal mucosa, the superior constrictor muscle of the pharynx,

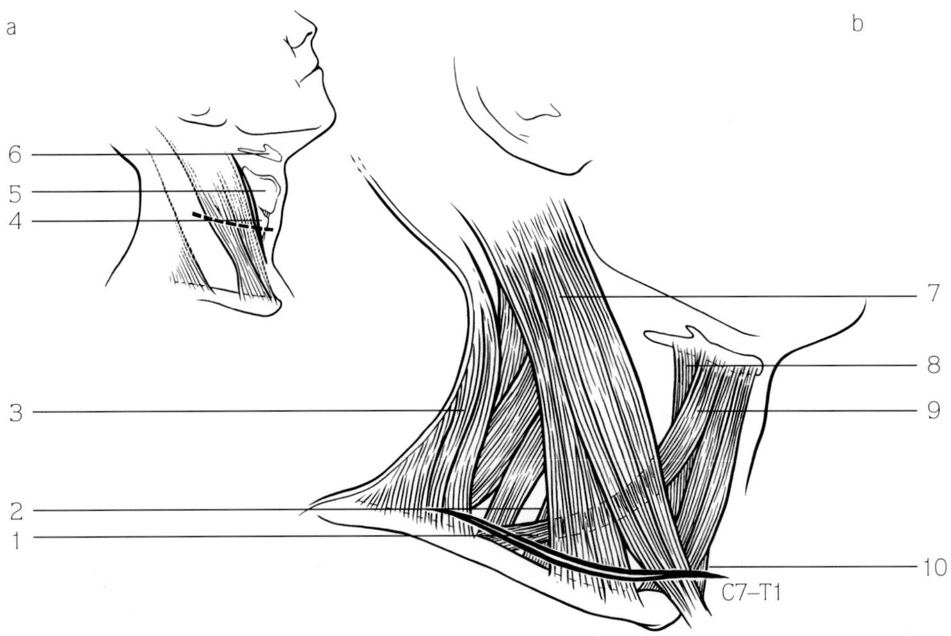

Figure 2.15
Smith-Robinson anteromedial approach to the middle and lower cervical spine. (a) The cricoid ring corresponds to the C6 level, the thyroid cartilage for C4–C5, the hyoid bone for C3. (b) Supraclavicular incision is for the C7–T1 region

1 Omohyoid m. inferior belly
2 Anterior scalene
3 Trapezius
4 Cricoid ring
5 Thyroid cartilage
6 Hyoid bone
7 Sternocleidomastoid m.
8 Sternothyroid m.
9 Omohyoid m. superior belly
10 Sternohyoid m.

the prevertebral fascia, and the anterior longitudinal ligament. Blunt dissection with an elevator is used to complete exposure of the odontoid and anterior tubercle of C1. Dissection may be carried laterally to expose the lateral masses of C1–C2 when required. After completion of the procedure, closure is completed as a single layer with absorbable suture.

Lower Cervical Spine

Anterior approaches to the lower cervical spine have been well described in the literature.[39,40] Meticulous and careful surgical technique is again paramount in the prevention of complications associated with surgical exposure. The patient is placed in a supine and slightly reversed Trendelenburg position to minimize venous pooling in the surgical area. Traction is applied to the head using Gardner–Wells tongs or a halter device, and caudal traction to the shoulders is applied using adhesive tape. In order to minimize injury to the recurrent laryngeal nerve, the cervical spine is often approached from the left, particularly at the C6–T1 region. Although right-handed surgeons prefer the right-sided approach, the recurrent laryngeal nerve is at greater risk of injury because it may leave the carotid sheath at a higher level on the right side.

Several palpable anterior structures in the midline of the neck help identify the vertebral level in the neck. It should be remembered that the hyoid bone overlies the third vertebra, the thyroid cartilage the C4–C5 intervertebral disc space, and the cricoid ring the C6 vertebra (Fig. 2.15). An alternative method that may be of use involves measuring the distance from the clavicle to the appropriate level on a routine preoperative anteroposterior chest radiograph.

The anteromedial Smith-Robinson approach to the midcervical spine is started with a horizontal incision in most cases, but a vertical incision anterior to the sternocleidomastoid may be necessary in cases where multiple levels are exposed (Fig. 2.16). A transverse incision in line with the skin crease is made from the midline beyond the anterior aspect of the sternocleidomastoid muscle. The skin and subcutaneous tissue are undermined slightly, and division of the platysma muscle is completed, division being either horizontal or vertical. Retraction of the divided muscle exposes the sternocleidomastoid muscle laterally and the strap muscles medially. The deep cervical fascia is divided between the sternocleidomastoid muscle and strap muscles, and blunt finger dissection is completed through the pre-tracheal fascia during lateral palpation and retraction of the carotid sheath (Fig. 2.17). Hand-held Cloward retractors are used to expose the prevertebral fascia and longus colli muscles (Fig. 2.18). Care must be taken not to enter the carotid sheath laterally to avoid injury to the carotid artery, internal jugular vein, or vagus nerve. Great

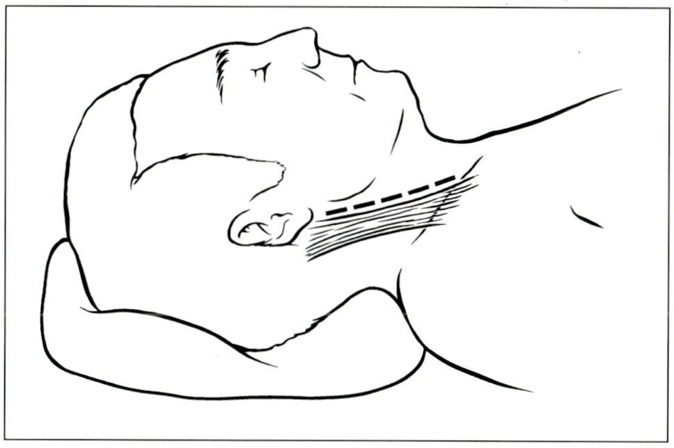

Figure 2.16
A vertical incision just anterior to the sternocleidomastoid is occasionally used for multi-level exposure

Figure 2.17 (below)
Dissection is along the anterior aspect of the sternocleidomastoid muscle. The deep cervical fascia is divided between the sternocleidomastoid muscle and strap muscles, and blunt dissection is done through the pre-tracheal fascia while retracting the carotid contents laterally

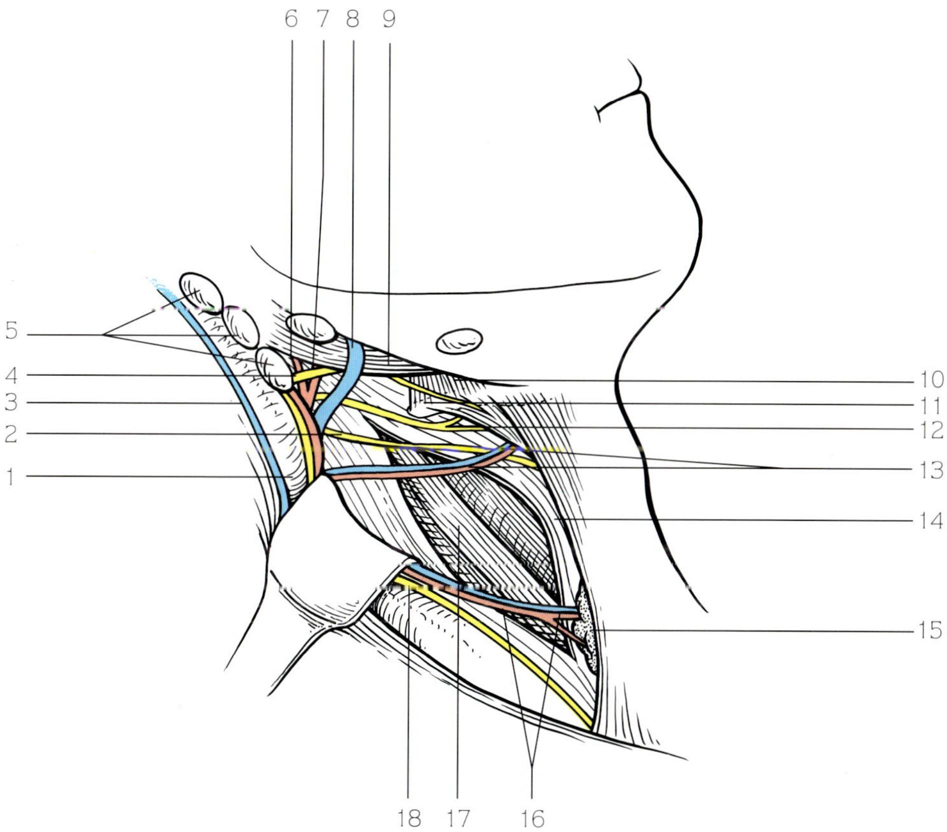

1 Carotid sheath
2 External branch of superior laryngeal
3 External jugular v.
4 Hypoglossal n.
5 Medial deep cervical lymph nodes
6 Facial a.
7 Lingual a.
8 Linguofacial v.
9 Digastric m. posterior belly
10 Thyrohyoid branch
11 Right greater cornu of hyoid bone
12 Inferior branch of superior laryngeal n.
13 Superior laryngeal a. and v.
14 Prevertebral layer of cervical fascia
15 Thyroid
16 Superior thyroid a. and v.
17 Right longus colli m.
18 Cervical root of ansa cervicalis

care should also be taken medially, because the strap muscles surround the thyroid gland, trachea, and esophagus. In addition, surgical dissection should not enter the plane between the trachea and esophagus, because the recurrent laryngeal nerve is at risk.

The superior thyroid artery may be encountered above C4, and the inferior thyroid artery below C6, and they should be identified and ligated as necessary. There should also be awareness of the thoracic duct below C7 during the left-sided approach. Further dissection is performed by palpating the prominent disc margins ('hills') and concave anterior vertebral bodies ('valleys'). A bent, 18-gauge needle is placed in the disc space, and a lateral radiograph taken to confirm the correct level (Fig. 2.19). Use of a bent needle prevents inadvertent penetration to the spinal cord. Once the appropriate level is identified, the longus colli

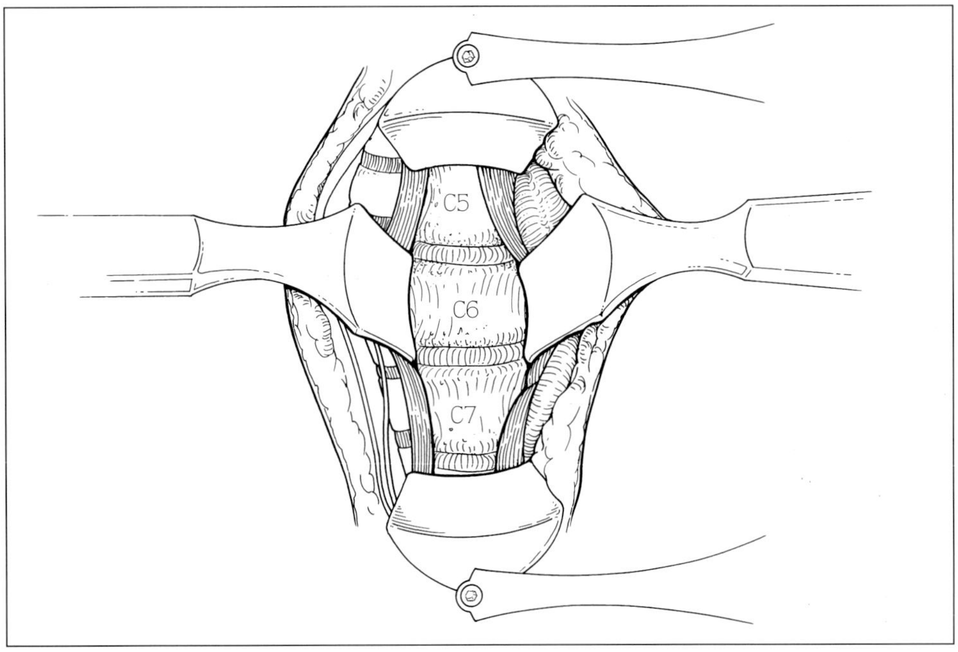

Figure 2.18
Division of the prevertebral fascia and dissection of longus colli lead to the vertebral bodies and the intervertebral discs

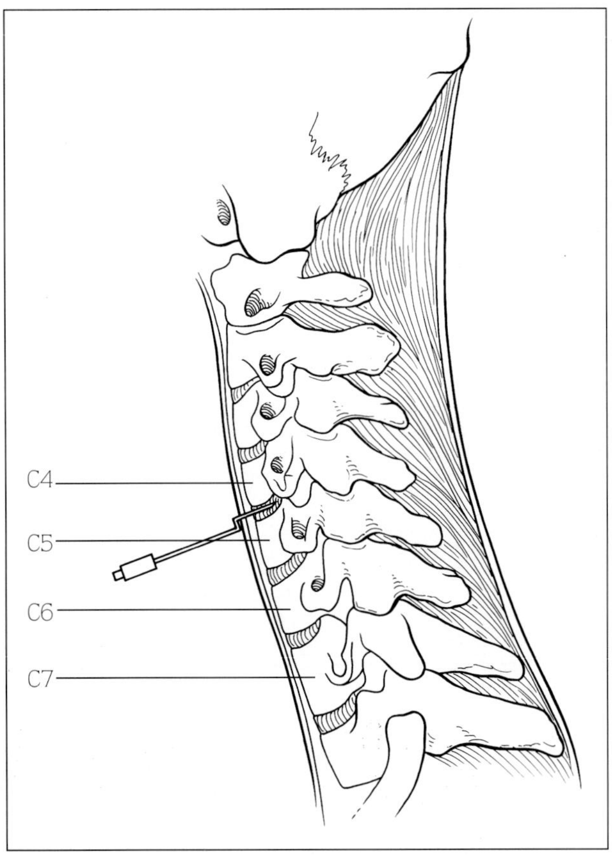

Figure 2.19
A bent needle is placed into the intervertebral disc for radiographic confirmation of the level. This prevents inadvertent penetration of the needle into the spinal canal

muscles are elevated, and the Cloward self-retaining retractor placed. The sharp Cloward blades should be avoided to prevent medial perforation of the esophagus. It is also important to check the temporal artery pulse once the retractor is spread, because prolonged occlusion of the carotid artery may cause brain ischemia and stroke. To minimize bleeding and prevent injury to the sympathetic chain, the pre-tracheal fascia and the anterior longitudinal ligament must be divided in the midline and subperiosteal mobilization of the longus colli muscles completed. Excessively vigorous lateral dissection may damage the vertebral artery or nerve roots.

This anteromedial approach to the cervical spine is used in most cervical cases. In special circumstances, however, lateral approaches may be used as described by Henry, Hogson, and Verbiest.[24,27,48]

Hogson[27] described an approach to the lower cervical spine in which dissection is carried posterior to the carotid sheath, exposing the anterior and lateral aspect of the cervical spine (Fig. 2.20). This approach avoids the thyroid vessels, vagus nerve, and superior laryngeal nerve, and to carry it out, a transverse or oblique skin incision is made from the right side. The subcutaneous tissue and the platysma muscle are divided, and branches of the external jugular vein ligated. The cutaneous nerves should be spared if possible (Fig. 2.21). The posterior border of the sternocleidomastoid muscle is identified, and blunt finger dissection carried through the fat pad of the posterior triangle of the cervical spine. The dissection should stay anterior to the anterior scalene muscle and anterior tubercle of the transverse process to avoid injuries to the vertebral artery or nerve root. If retraction of the sternocleidomastoid

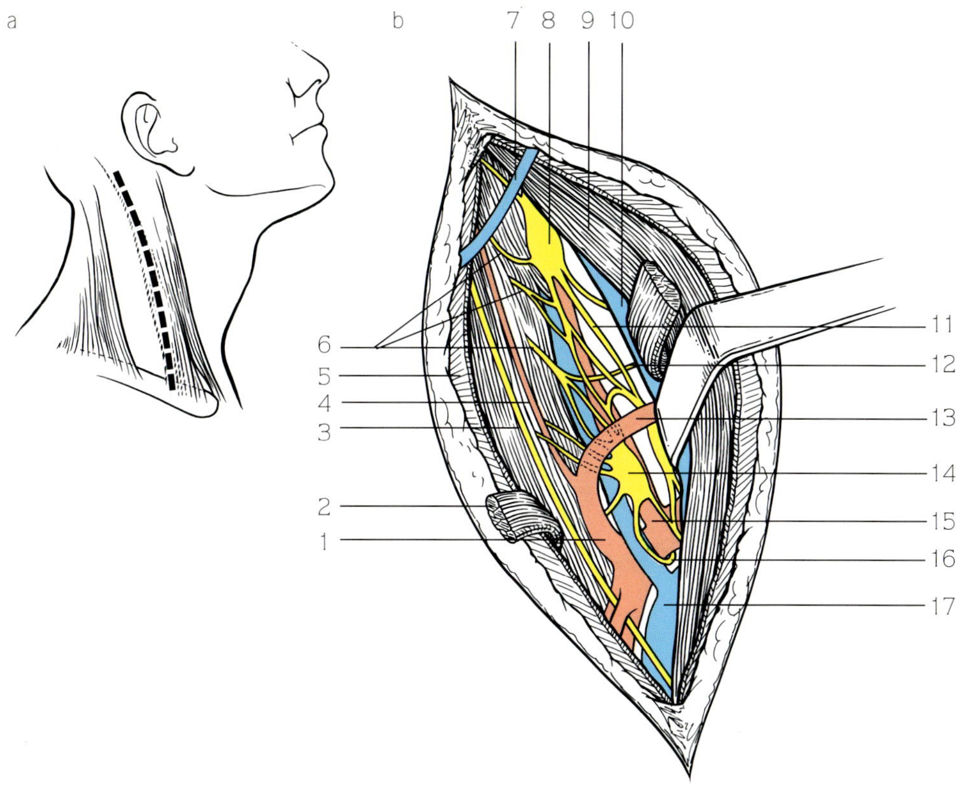

1 Thyrocervical trunk
2 Omohyoid m.
3 Phrenic n.
4 Ascending cervical a.
5 Platysma
6 Gray rami communicantes C4–C6
7 External jugular v.
8 Middle cervical gang.
9 Sternocleidomastoid m.
10 Internal jugular v.
11 Cervical br. of middle cervical gang.
12 Inferior thyroid n.
13 Inferior thyroid a.
14 Inferior cervical ganglion
15 Subclavian a.
16 Ansa subclavia
17 Subclavian v.

Figure 2.20
Hogson's lateral approach: a transverse or oblique skin incision is made from the right side. The subcutaneous tissue and platysma muscle are divided, and branches of the external jugular vein ligated. The posterior border of the sternocleidomastoid muscle is identified, and blunt finger dissection carried through the fat pad of the posterior triangle of the cervical spine. The dissection should stay anterior to the anterior scalene muscle and the anterior tubercle of the transverse process to avoid injuries to the vertebral artery or nerve root. The prevertebral fascia is incised in the midline, and subperiosteal dissection completed for exposure of the cervical spine

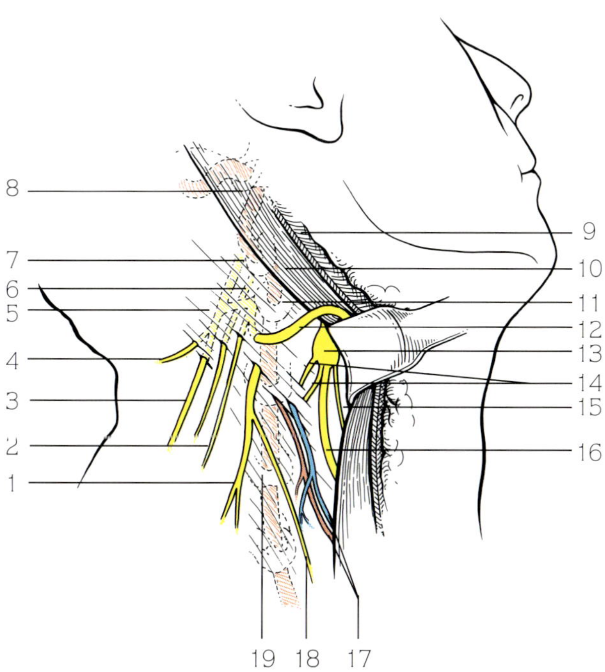

Figure 2.21
Potential structures of injury during Hogson's lateral approach include cutaneous nerves posterior to sternocleidomastoid muscle including the greater auricular nerve, supraclavicular nerves, spinal accessory nerve, and lesser occipital nerve. Deep to the sternocleidomastoid muscle, phrenic nerve and sympathetic trunk may be encountered

1 Medial and intermediate supraclavicular nn.
2 Lateral supraclavicular n.
3 Branch to trapezius
4 Lesser occipital n.
5 Prevertebral layer of cervical fascia
6 Spinal accessory n.
7 C2
8 Transverse process of C1
9 Plastysma m.
10 Sternocleidomastoid m.
11 C3
12 Great auricular n.
13 Superior cervical gang.
14 Rami communicantes
15 Cardiac branch of superior cervical gang.
16 Sympathetic trunk
17 Ascending cervical a. and v.
18 Phrenic n.
19 C6

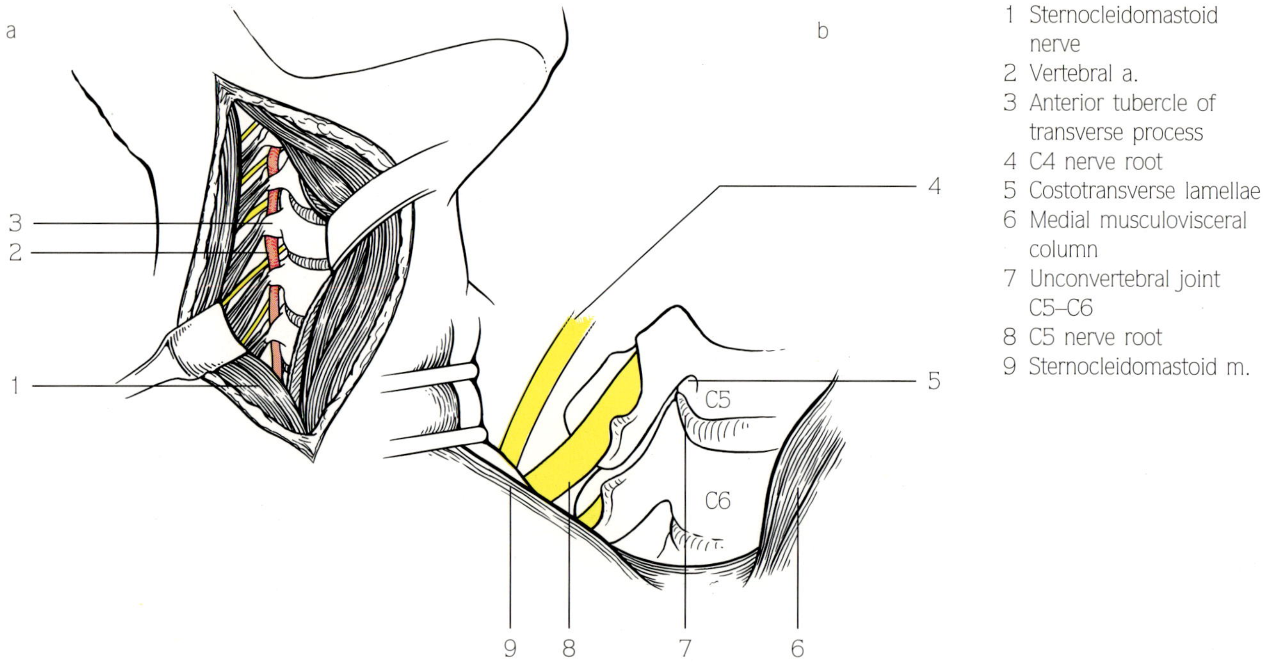

Figure 2.22
Verbiest's lateral approach: sternocleidomastoid muscle is identified and retracted laterally. The carotid sheath is identified by finger palpation, and the middle cervical fascia dissected bluntly between the sternocleidomastoid and carotid sheath laterally and the visceral structures medially. A hand-held Cloward retractor is used to retract the medial structures. The anterior tubercle of the transverse process, which is the key to this dissection, is then identified by palpation. The muscular insertions onto the anterior tubercle, including longus colli, longus capitis, and anterior scalene, are dissected sharply to the bone. Once the anterior tubercle is cleared of soft tissues, it is removed with a narrow-tipped rongeur, exposing the vertebral artery. The costotransverse lamellae are resected as well. The spinal nerve lies posterior to the vertebral artery

muscle is difficult, the posterior third of this muscle can be divided to enhance exposure. The cervical sympathetic plexus on the lateral aspect of the prevertebral musculature should be identified and protected. The prevertebral fascia is incised in the midline, and subperiosteal dissection completed for exposure of the cervical spine.

Verbiest's[48] lateral approach to the cervical spine is a direct approach to the spinal nerve and vertebral artery in the intervertebral foramen (Fig. 2.22). The skin incision and platysma dissection are carried out in an identical fashion to the Smith-Robinson technique: the sternocleidomastoid muscle is identified and retracted laterally; the carotid sheath is identified by finger palpation; and the middle cervical fascia dissected bluntly between the sternocleidomastoid and carotid sheath laterally and the musculovisceral structures medially. A hand-held Cloward retractor is used to retract the medial structures. The anterior tubercle of the transverse process, which is the key to this dissection, is then identified by palpation. The muscular insertions on to the anterior tubercle, including the longus colli, longus capitis, and anterior scalene, are dissected sharply to the bone. Care must be taken to avoid the nerve root laterally and the vertebral artery medially. Venous hemostasis should be controlled with bipolar electrocautery. Once the anterior tubercle is cleared of soft tissues, it is removed with a narrow-tipped rongeur, exposing the vertebral artery. In addition, the costotransverse lamellae are resected. The spinal nerve lies posterior to the vertebral artery at the level of the foramen transversarium. The venous plexus, which accompanies the vertebral artery, is a common source of bleeding using this approach, and is best controlled with pressure packing. In fact this lateral approach is used only in cases of far-lateral pathology or if the vertebral artery requires exposure.

There are many decompressive and reconstructive procedures that can be performed on the cervical spine

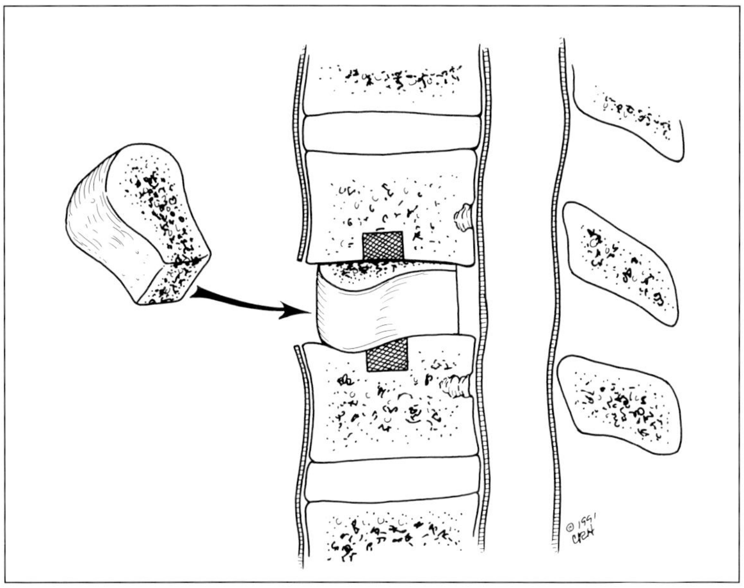

a

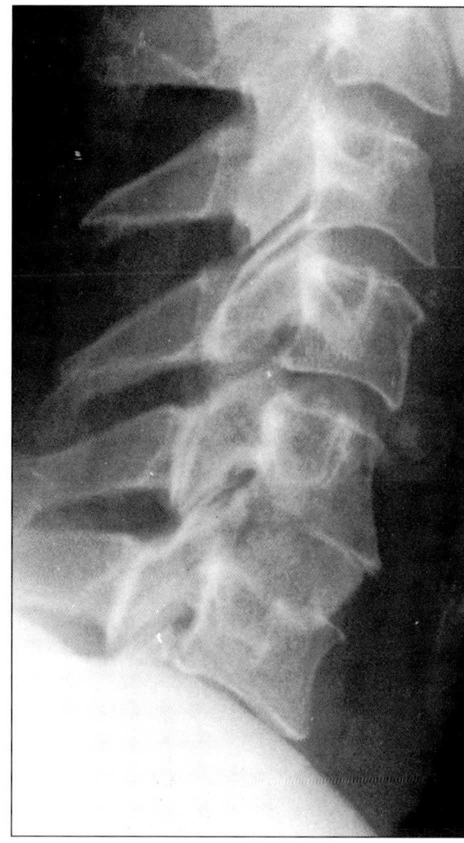

b

Figure 2.23
(a) A diagram of interbody fusion using a tricortical iliac crest graft. The graft should be countersunk about 2 mm, and should distract the interspace about 2 mm. (b) Lateral radiograph after Smith–Robinson type fusion, showing a good position of the graft

once the exposure is complete, including discectomy, vertebrectomy, interbody fusion, or strut grafting. Strict adherence to the sound surgical principles and techniques described in the rest of this book, together with knowledge of pertinent biomechanical features of the cervical spine, are imperative in the prevention of neurologic and structural complications.

Proper visualization of the operative field is a priority. Headlamp illumination and loupe magnification are a minimal requirement. An operating microscope, although not always required, is advised during resection of the posterior longitudinal ligament for removal of a sequestered disc fragment, and in spinal cord decompressive procedures.

Several techniques of anterior discectomy and fusion of the cervical spine are available, but the author favors the Smith–Robinson technique, because it is biomechanically superior to other procedures.[52,54] The height of the graft should be about 2 mm more than the degenerated disc space, but at least 5 mm to obtain maximal compressive strength and maximal enlargement of the neural foramina.[2] Distraction of the intervertebral space can be achieved by skull traction and/or laminar spreader. Traction with the head-halter device can also be effective. Graft extrusion can be avoided if the graft is countersunk 2 mm under the anterior cortical margin of the vertebral body (Fig. 2.23). Obviously, the graft should not be too deep, because impingement of the spinal cord must be avoided. Exact measurements of both the width and depth of the bone graft slot should be made using a caliper or ruler.

Simmons and Bhalla[43] have reported on the 'keystone' technique of anterior cervical grafting (Fig. 2.24). This technique involves the removal of the vertebral end-plate and exposure of cancellous bone for improved graft healing potential. However, there is a theoretical concern for inadequate maintenance of disc space distraction with this

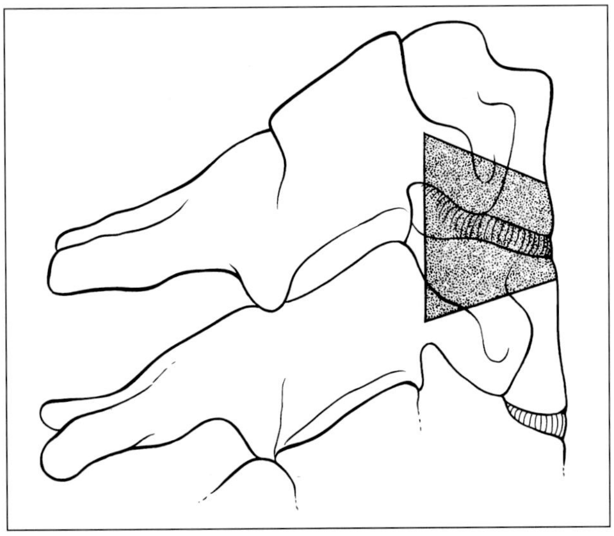

Figure 2.24
Simmons' keystone technique of anterior cervical fusion

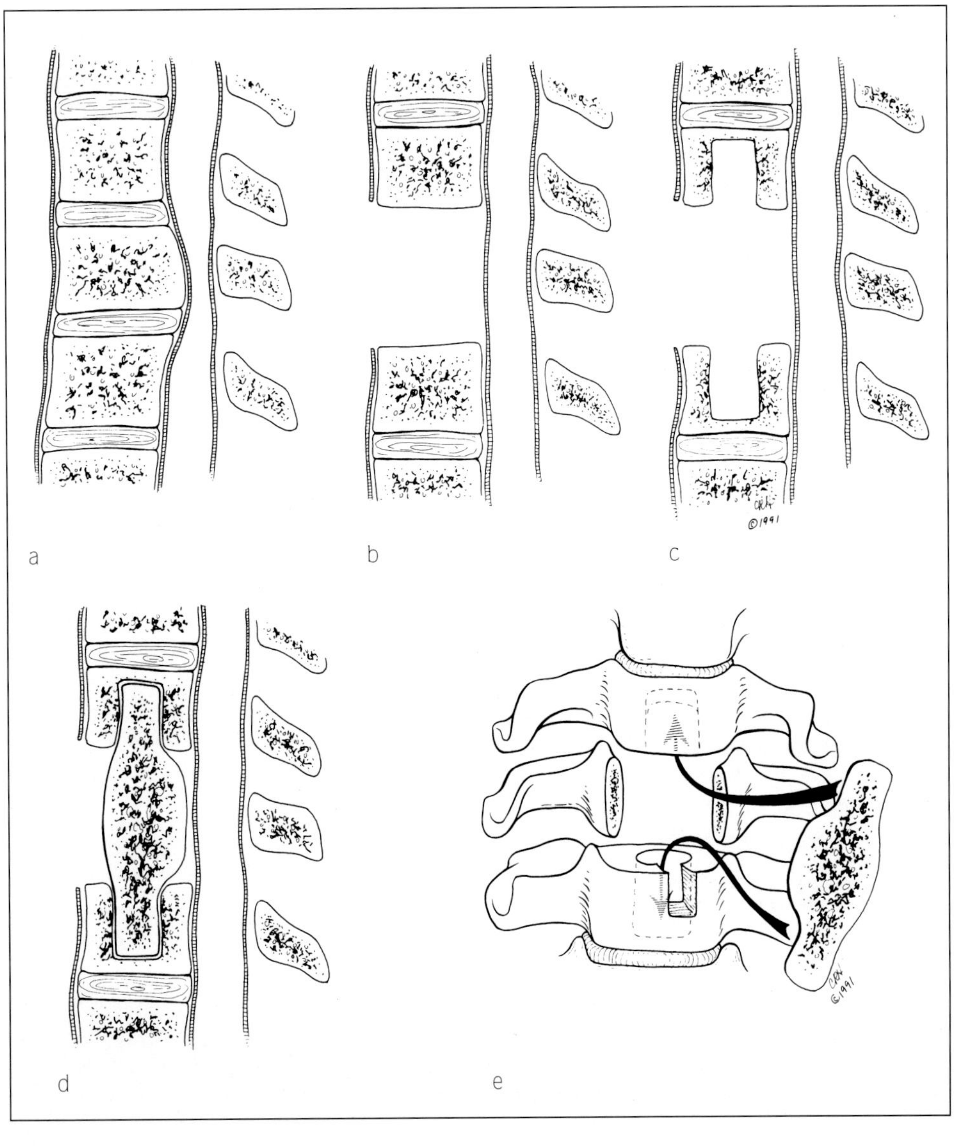

Figure 2.25
Vertebrectomy with strut grafting technique; (a) anterior spinal cord compression; (b) vertebrectomy and discectomy above and below the body; (c) slot preparation above and below the body; (d) strut graft countersunk against end-plates; (e) a window made inferiorly in order to insert the strut graft; and (f) lateral radiograph of healed anterior strut graft from C4 to C7

technique. The Cloward technique is mostly abandoned for reasons including inability to distract, poor biomechanical construct, and greater potential for technical mishaps.

Vertebrectomy with strut grafting is frequently done on patients with cervical spondylotic myelopathy, tumors, or burst fractures.[36,55] Again, several techniques have been reported in the literature. A tricortical iliac crest strut is adequate for reconstruction in most cases, but the fibula may be used if a vertebrectomy at three or more levels is carried out.[55] A power burr is used to take the vertebrectomy down to the posterior longitudinal ligament. Once the decompression is completed, the cervical spine must be reconstructed, and the strut graft countersunk to prevent graft dislodgement. The author has achieved satisfactory results with the slotted technique as shown in Fig. 2.25.[34] The bone graft is placed against the end-plates to achieve greater stability. Some surgeons prefer placement of the bone graft into the cancellous bone of the vertebral body (Fig. 2.26). If the graft is countersunk well inside the cortical margin of the vertebral body, this construct is also quite stable, although it can carry an increased risk of collapse and development of kyphosis (Fig. 2.27). If the strut graft is placed outside the cortical margin of the vertebral body, there is a potential for esophageal irritation as well as dislodgement of the graft. All these techniques are described in further detail in Chapter 9.

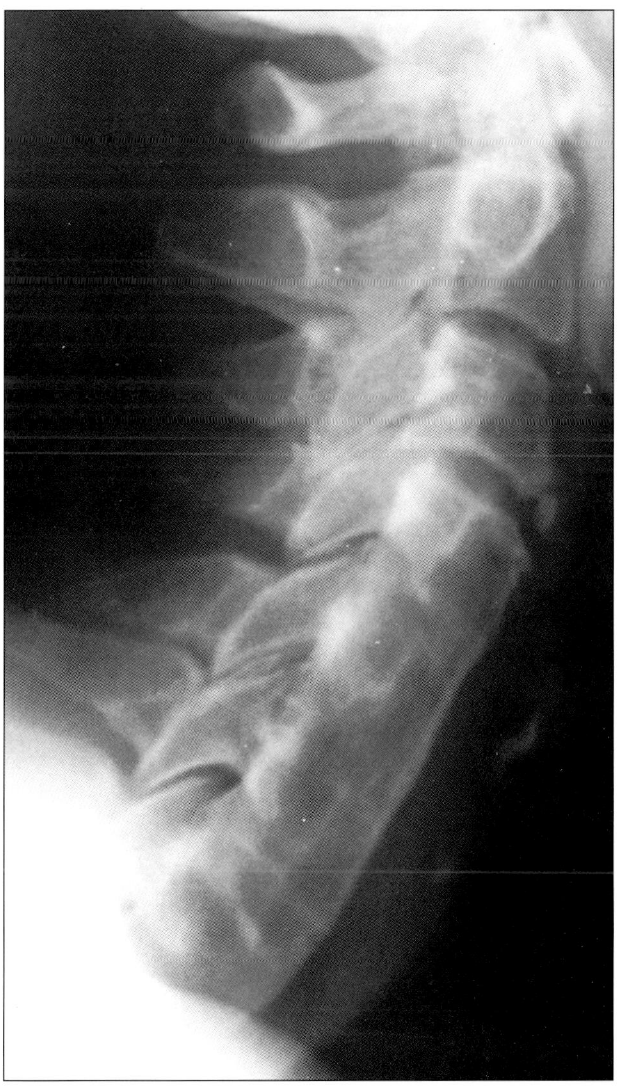

f

Potential complications associated with anterior operations of the upper and lower cervical spine can be numerous (Table 2.1). Proper positioning of the neck, fiberoptic, nasotracheal, conscious intubation and intraoperative monitoring of the spinal cord function are important measures to take in patients with myelopathy. As dissection is closely linked to vital neural, vascular, and visceral structures, thorough knowledge of the anatomy and experience are required to prevent injuries to these structures. Decompression of the spinal cord must be adequate, but not so far laterally as to endanger the vertebral arteries. After surgery, patients who have undergone a prolonged operation for decompression of the spinal cord should be intubated for 2–3 days until retropharyngeal edema subsides. Corticosteroids may decrease severe edema in the postoperative period. Airway obstruction and difficulty with swallowing as a result of retropharyngeal edema may require reintubation or tracheotomy.

The most devastating complication is neurologic deterioration.[16] Most spinal cord or nerve root injuries are associated with technical mishaps. Utmost care should be taken when removing osteophytes and disc material in the lateral corner close to the uncovertebral joint to avoid nerve root injury. If removal of the posterior longitudinal ligament or osteophytes is necessary because of perforating disc fragments or large osteophytes, an operating microscope should be used. Depth of the bone graft should be measured carefully. It is only necessary to use gentle tapping and stability should be maintained by compressive force on the graft. If neurologic complication is discovered after the operation, dexamethasone should be administered, and a lateral radiograph taken to determine the position of the bone graft. Computed tomography or magnetic resonance imaging may be valuable in ascertaining whether hematoma or cord contusion is present. If a hematoma or bone graft is suspected as the cause of postoperative myelopathy, expeditious re-exploration is required.

Dysphagia following anterior cervical surgery can result from postoperative edema, hemorrhage, denervation, or infection.[50] If persistent dysphagia is present, barium swallow or endoscopy should be considered. Esophageal perforation is a rare but serious complication of anterior cervical spine fusion,[56] occurring in about 1 of 500 procedures.[46] Sharp retractors must be avoided, and gentle

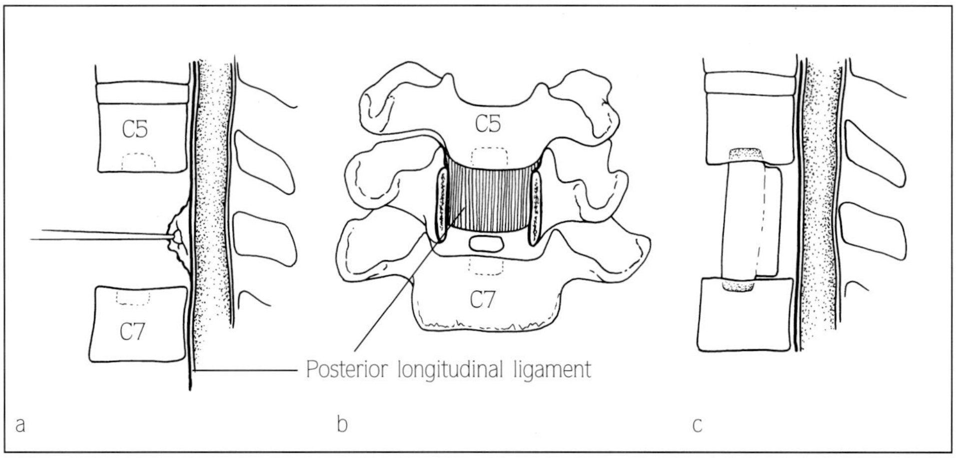

Figure 2.26
Vertebrectomy with strut graft technique: (a) removal of vertebral body and adjacent discs; (b) decompression performed to remove the posterior longitudinal ligament in myelopathic cases; and (c) a tricortical graft is countersunk

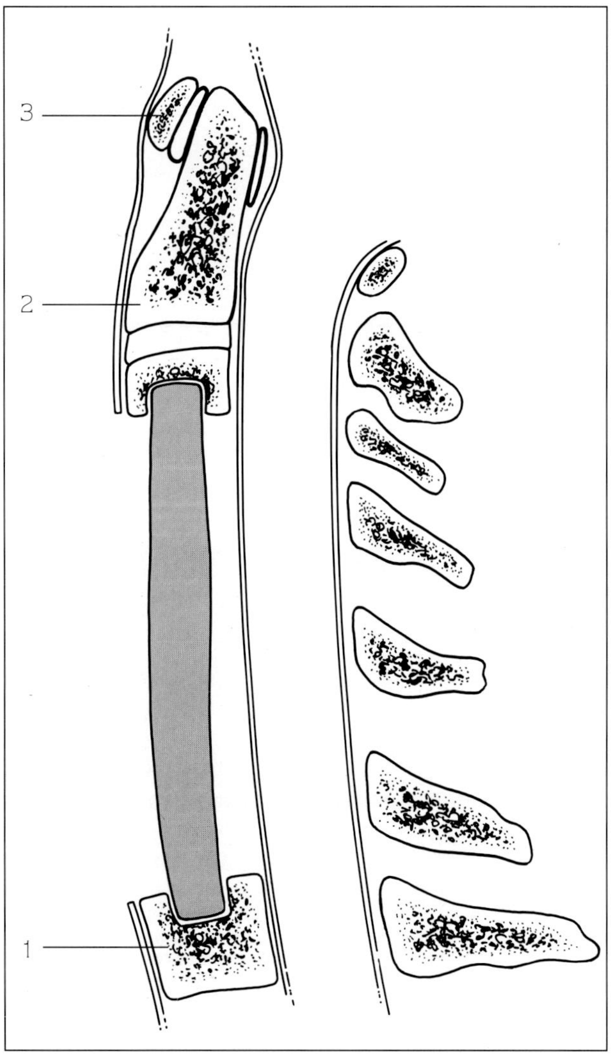

Table 2.1 Potential complications of anterior cervical fusion

Neural injury
Spinal cord injury
Nerve root damage
Dural tear
Vascular injury
Carotid artery
Internal jugular vein
Vertebral artery
Vocal fold damage (recurrent laryngeal nerve injury)
Esophageal perforation
Tracheal injury
Horner's syndrome
Thoracic duct injury
Pneumothorax
Bone graft complications
Extrusion
Collapse
Non-union
Donor site complications
Infection
Wound problems (hematoma, drainage, dehiscence)

Figure 2.27
A long strut fusion with a fibula

1 C7
2 C2
3 Anterior arch of atlas

handling of the medial soft tissue structures is mandatory. Use of a nasogastric tube may be helpful in identifying the esophagus during surgery and, if perforation is suspected, methylene blue can be injected for better visualization. Often, perforation is not recognized until the patient develops an abscess, tracheoesophageal fistula, or mediastinitis in the postoperative period. The usual treatment consists of intravenous antibiotics, nasogastric feeding, drainage, débridement, and repair. Early consultation with head and neck surgeons is recommended.

Minor hoarseness or sore throat after anterior cervical fusion may be the result of edema or endotracheal intubation, and occurs in nearly half the patients. However, recurrent laryngeal nerve palsy could be the cause of persistent hoarseness in a small number of patients, with an incidence of about 1%,[46] but possibly rising to 11%.[5,23] On the left side, the recurrent laryngeal nerve loops under the arch of the aorta, and is protected in the left tracheoesophageal groove. On the right side, it travels around the subclavian artery and passes from this to the right tracheoesophageal groove. The recurrent laryngeal nerve should be located when working down from C6 on the right. The nerve is in close proximity to the inferior thyroid artery as it enters the lower pole of the thyroid, and is protected by approaching the cervical spine from the left. If hoarseness persists for more than 6 weeks after anterior cervical surgery, laryngoscopy should be done to evaluate the vocal fold and laryngeal muscles. Treatment of inferior laryngeal nerve palsy should include a delay of at least 6 months to allow time for spontaneous recovery of function to occur. Further treatment or surgery by the otolaryngologist may be necessary in persistent cases.

Injury to the sympathetic chain may result in Horner's syndrome. The cervical sympathetic chain lies on the anterior surface of the longus colli muscles posterior to the carotid sheath, with subperiosteal dissection being important to prevent damage to the nerves. Horner's syndrome is usually temporary, although it can be permanent in some cases; the incidence of the latter is < 1%.[16] Ophthalmologic consultation may be needed for treatment of ptosis.

Fortunately, serious bleeding complications after anterior cervical surgery are rare. Wound hematomas are relatively uncommon, with an incidence of 9% in one series.[42] Hematomas may complicate wound healing, but are rarely responsible for airway obstruction or spinal cord compression.[41] The patient should have his or her head elevated in the immediate postoperative period, because the source of bleeding is frequently venous. Meticulous hemostasis and placement of a drain should be a routine part of the operative procedure to prevent these complications. Arterial bleeding from either the superior or inferior thyroid artery can be prevented by careful identification and ligation during surgery. Great care should be taken not to dissect too far laterally because the vertebral artery is in danger as well as the nerve roots. Tears on the vertebral artery should be repaired by direct exposure of the vessel in the foramen rather than by merely packing the bleeding site. Injuries to the carotid artery or internal jugular vein are exceedingly rare.

Airway obstruction after extubation may occur in the postoperative period.[13] Before extubation it must be ensured that the patient can exchange air. In cases requiring multiple vertebrectomy with retraction of soft tissues for a prolonged period of time, intubation should continue for a few days until retropharyngeal edema subsides. Corticosteroids may be used to decrease edema in these cases.

Complications associated with bone grafting and fusion are more common. Extrusion of graft usually occurs in an anterior direction away from the spinal cord, and it can be associated with dysphagia, tracheal obstruction, kyphotic deformity, or neurologic symptoms. The incidence is reported from 1% to 13%.[28] As mentioned before, meticulous surgical technique is the key to prevention of these problems. Treatment may simply include observation, or require reoperation, depending on the particular situation and symptoms produced. Graft collapse is another complication, which may or may not require active treatment. The incidence of graft collapse appears to be slightly higher for allografts than for autografts.[59] If graft collapse results in significant kyphosis, revision surgery may be required. The incidence of pseudoarthrosis after anterior cervical fusion has been reported as 0–26%. Failure of fusion is reported to be greater using the dowel technique, whereas the keystone method described by Simmons had no cases of non-union in one series.[43] Multi-level fusion has also been associated with a higher rate of non-union compared to single level fusion.[53,59] Many are asymptomatic despite radiographic evidence of non-union, and require no treatment.[25,42] Those with symptomatic non-unions may benefit from prolonged immobilization or revision surgery. Posterior foraminotomy is a good procedure following failed anterior cervical fusion for unilateral radiculopathy. Repeat anterior fusion may also be done in these cases with good success.

Cervicothoracic Junction

Anterior approaches to the upper thoracic vertebrae present a challenge to the spinal surgeon; anterior exposure may be accomplished through a low cervical approach, supraclavicular approach, sternum-splitting approach, or transthoracic approach. The low cervical approach is simply an extension of the anteromedial approach to the low cervical spine.[9,15] An oblique cervical incision starting 4 cm below the mastoid process and extending to the sternoclavicular joint, or a horizontal incision at the base of the neck, is made. After division of the platysma muscle, the

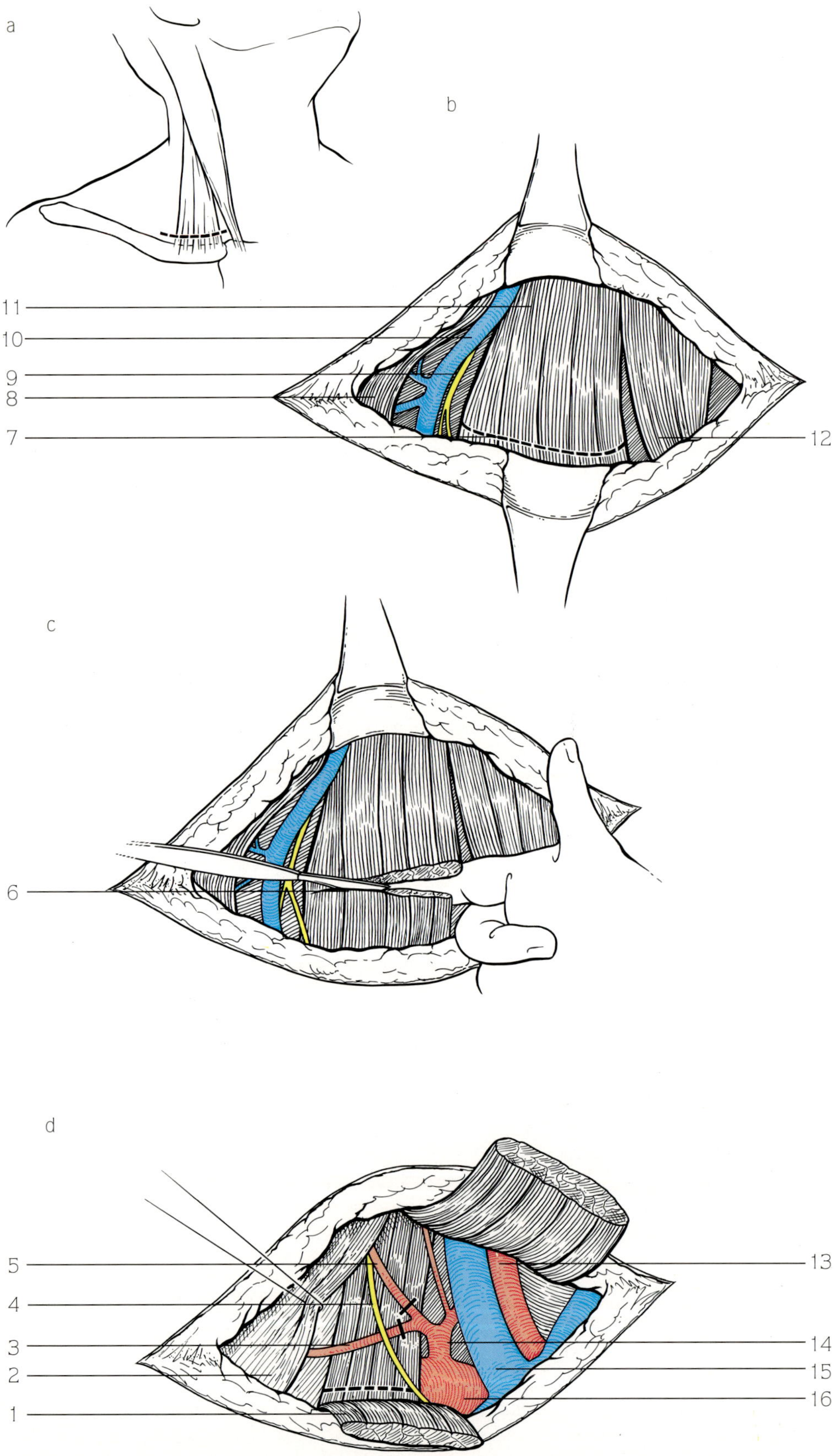

1 Sternomastoid m.
2 Omohyoid m.
3 Suprascapular a.
4 Phrenic n.
5 Transcervical a.
6 Division of clavicular head of sternocleidomastoid m.
7 Incision line
8 Platysma m.
9 Middle subscapular n.
10 External jugular
11 Clavicular head of sternocleidomastoid m.
12 Sternal head of sternocleidomastoid m.
13 Common carotid a.
14 Thyrocervical trunk
15 Internal jugular v.
16 Subclavian a.

Figure 2.28

(a) Supraclavicular approach entails a transverse incision above the clavicle. (b) Dissection posterior to the carotid sheath, followed by release of the clavicular head of the sternocleidomastoid. (c) The internal jugular and subclavian veins as well as the carotid artery must be protected from injury during division of the sternocleidomastoid muscle. (d) After division of the sternocleidomastoid muscle, the fascia beneath it is divided to release the omohyoid from its pulley. The subclavian artery and its branches, which include the thyrocervical trunk, suprascapular artery, and transcervical artery, must be identified. The suprascapular and transcervical arteries should be ligated as necessary. (e) The dome of the lung and the phrenic nerve are in close proximity to the scalenus anterior muscle. The phrenic nerve should be identified and retracted before division of the scalenus anterior muscle. The brachial plexus and supraclavicular nerves are more superficial at the lateral border of the scalenus anterior muscle, division of which exposes Sibson's fascia in the floor of the wound, which covers the dome of the lung. Sibson's fascia is divided transversely using scissors, and the visceral pleura and lung, retracted inferiorly. (f) The trachea, esophagus, and recurrent laryngeal nerve must be protected during medial retraction. The posterior thorax, stellate ganglion, and upper thoracic vertebral bodies are now visible looking down through the thoracic inlet. The recurrent laryngeal nerve should be identified and protected, and the inferior thyroid artery and vertebral artery identified

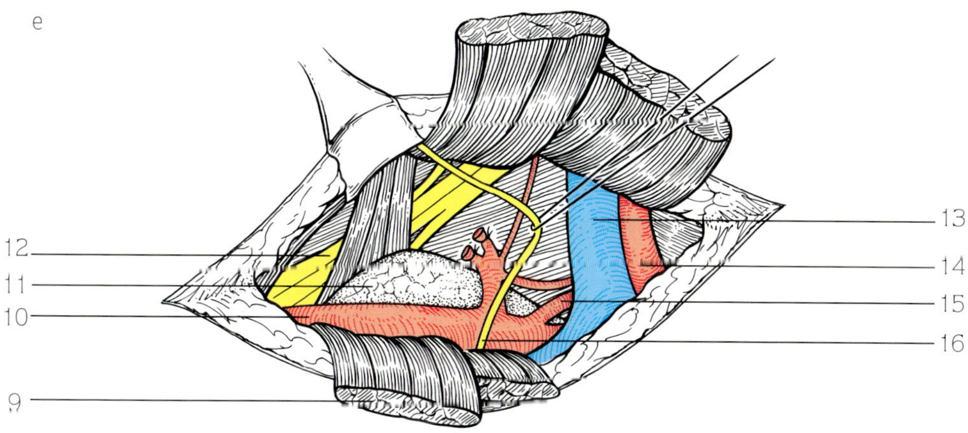

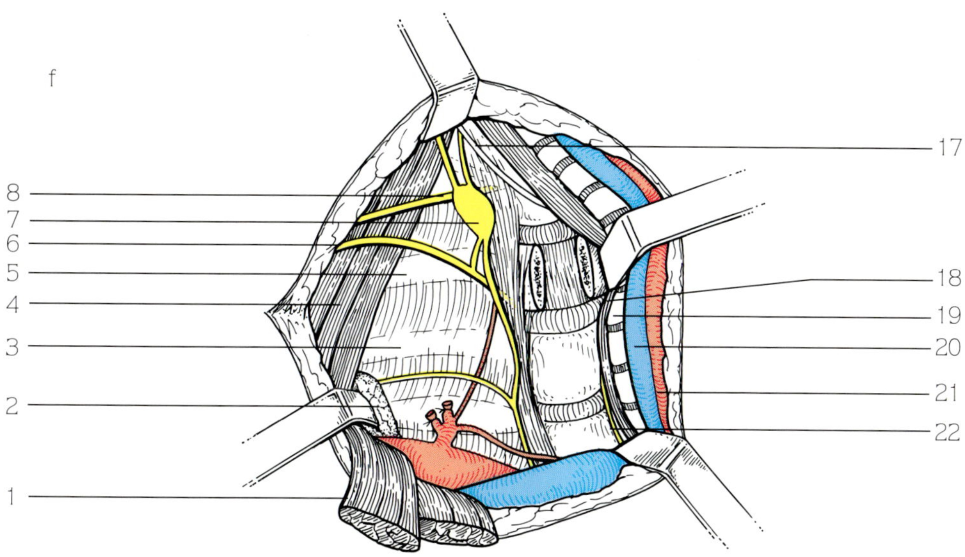

1 Anterior scalenus m.
2 Cupula of lung
3 Second rib
4 Scalenus medius m.
5 First rib
6 T1 root
7 Stellate ganglion
8 C8 root
9 Anterior scalenus m.
10 Subclavian a.
11 Cupula of lung
12 Brachial plexus
13 Internal jugular v
14 Common carotid a.
15 Vertebral a.
16 Phrenic n.
17 Phrenic a.
18 Esophagus
19 Trachea
20 Internal jugular v.
21 Common carotid a.
22 Recurrent laryngeal n.

dissection is taken between the sternocleidomastoid muscle laterally and the esophagus and trachea medially to reach the spine. The inferior thyroid artery and vein are ligated. The recurrent laryngeal nerve muscle must be identified from the right-sided approach, whereas the thoracic duct must be spared from the left-sided approach.

The supraclavicular approach uses a transverse incision above the clavicle and dissection posterior to the carotid sheath.[29] After incision of the platysma muscle, division of the clavicular head of the sternocleidomastoid is completed (Fig. 2.28). The internal jugular and subclavian veins as well as the carotid artery must be protected from injury during division of the sternocleidomastoid muscle. After division of the sternocleidomastoid muscle, the fascia beneath it is divided to release the omohyoid from its pulley. The subclavian artery and its branches, which include the thyrocervical trunk, suprascapular artery, and transcervical artery, must be identified and the last two ligated as necessary. The dome of the lung and the phrenic nerve are in close proximity to the scalenus anterior muscle; the former should be identified and retracted before division of the latter. The brachial plexus and supraclavicular nerves are more superficial at the lateral border of the scalenus anterior muscle, division of which exposes Sibson's fascia in the floor of the wound, which covers the dome of the lung. Sibson's fascia is divided transversely using scissors, and the visceral pleura and lung are retracted inferiorly. The trachea, esophagus, and recurrent laryngeal nerve must be protected during medial retraction. The posterior thorax, stellate ganglion, and upper thoracic vertebral bodies are now visible looking down through the thoracic inlet. The recurrent laryngeal nerve should be identified and protected, and the inferior thyroid artery and vertebral artery identified. The thoracic duct should be identified, if approached from the left, and, if damaged, it should be doubly ligated in both proximal and distal directions to prevent chylothorax.

The low cervical and supraclavicular approaches usually allow exposure of the lower cervical spine and the first and second thoracic vertebrae, but the distal extent of the exposure may be limited by the size and position of the anterior thorax. Additionally, obese or muscular patients with short necks are poor candidates for these approaches because of the limited distal extent of the exposure. Low cervical or supraclavicular approaches do not generally provide an extensile exposure of the upper thoracic spine, and all the complications discussed in the anteromedial approach to the low cervical spine apply to these approaches, particularly the injury to the recurrent laryngeal nerve, the thoracic duct, the lung, or the great vessels.

The upper thoracic vertebrae may also be approached through a standard thoracotomy which enters the chest through the bed of the third rib (Fig. 2.29). However,

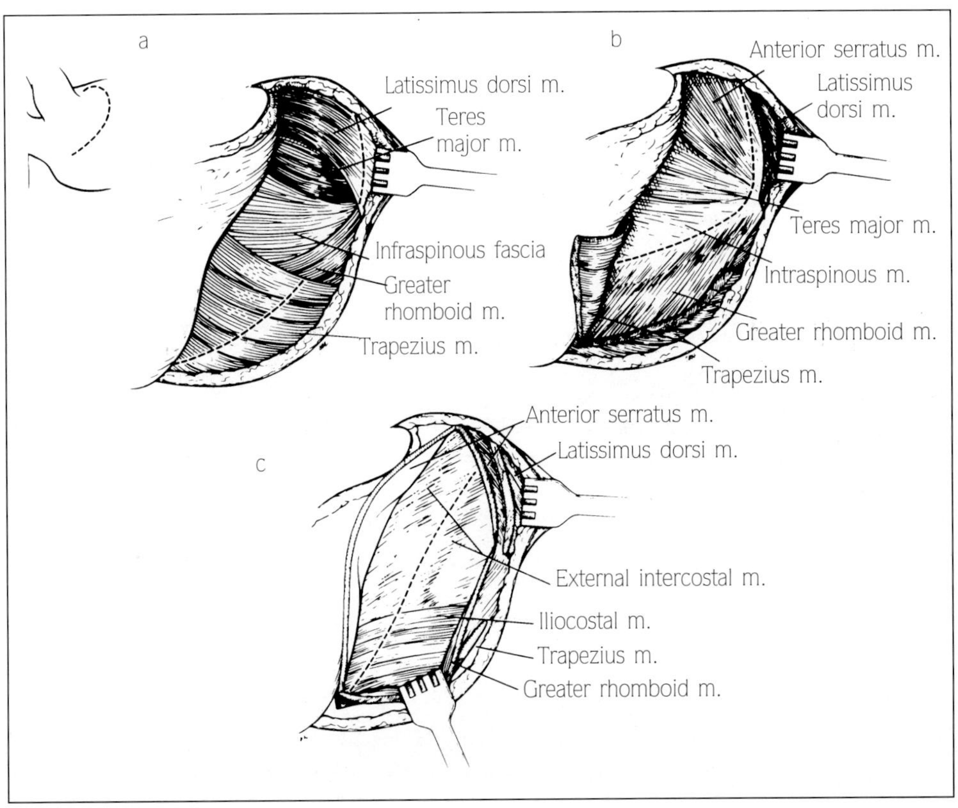

Figure 2.29
Transthoracic approach to the upper thoracic spine: (a) an incision around the scapula; (b) division of muscles; and (c) approach to the chest through the bed of the third rib

access to the lower cervical region through this approach is restricted by the scapula and remaining ribs.[31] Recently, Turner and Webb[47] have described a surgical approach to the upper thoracic spine from T1 to T3. The right-sided approach is preferred to the left, because the left subclavian artery is more curved than the right brachiocephalic artery. The incision for this approach is made medial and inferior to the scapula, which is retracted laterally by dividing the trapezius, latissimus dorsi, rhomboids, and levator scapulae muscles. The posterior 7–10 cm of each of the second, third, fourth and fifth ribs is removed. If T1 is involved, 2–3 cm of the first rib is also excised. Exposure of the vertebrae is made with an L-shaped incision in the pleura and intercostal muscles. Potential complications of this approach may be restriction of scapular movement and paralysis of intercostal muscles as a result of muscle-splitting aspects of this dissection. The authors recommend use of this approach only in older patients, and perhaps in those with malignant conditions.

The sternum-splitting approach provides better access to the cervicothoracic junction from C4 to T4, particularly in the obese patient (Fig. 2.30).[3,7] The skin incision is made anterior to the left sternocleidomastoid muscle, and then extended along the midsternal area down to the xiphoid process. After division of the platysma muscle and superficial cervical fascia, blunt dissection is done between the laterally situated neurovascular bundle and medial visceral structures. The retrosternal adipose and thymus tissues are retracted from the manubrium. Median sternotomy should be performed carefully to prevent injury to the pleura. Sternohyoid, sternothyroid, and omohyoid muscles are identified and transected as necessary. The inferior thyroid artery is ligated and transected. Blunt dissection is performed in a cranial-to-caudal direction, until the left brachiocephalic vein is exposed, which can be ligated and transected if necessary, although postoperative edema of the left upper extremity is often a problem. Great care should be taken to avoid injuries to the sympathetic nerves, the cupola of the pleura at the level of T1, the great vessels, and the thoracic duct, which passes into the left venous angle between the subclavian artery and the common carotid artery.

As there is a significant perioperative mortality associated with this sternum-splitting approach, Sudaresan and colleagues[44,45] perform a less aggressive T-shaped incision on the anterior chest wall (Fig. 2.31). Dissection is taken down to the level of the sternal body, manubrium, and clavicle, with ligation of the anterior jugular venous arch and medial supraclavicular nerves. The left-sided approach is preferred as the recurrent laryngeal nerve is less variable on the left and further from the midline. At the level of the manubrium and clavicle, the sternal and clavicular heads

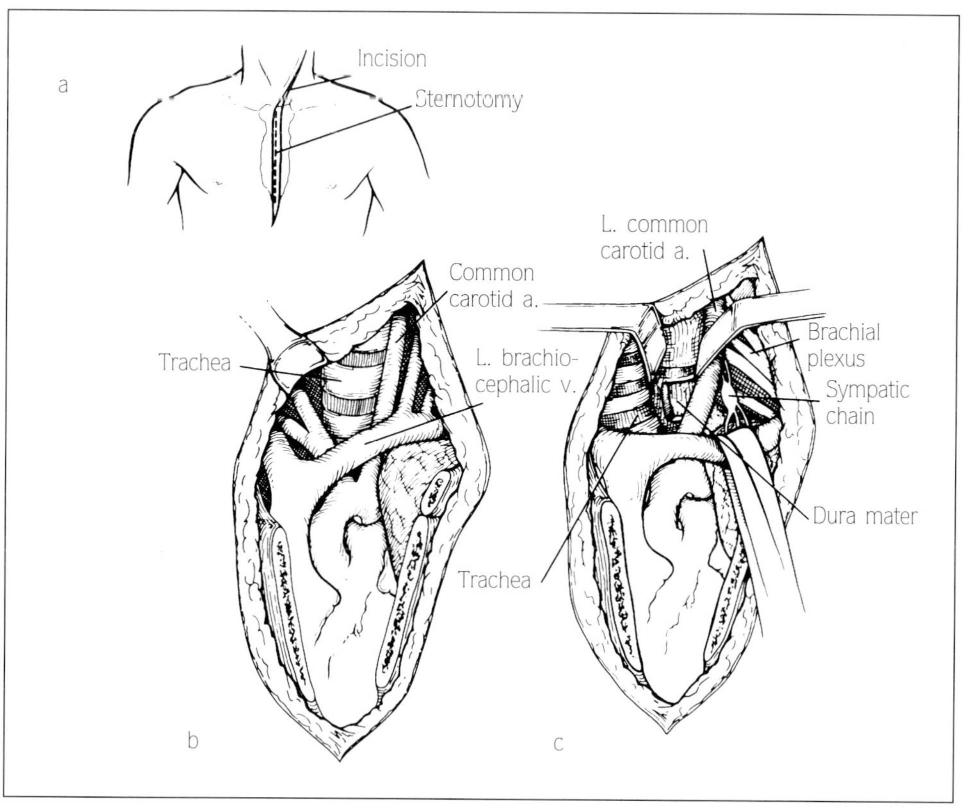

Figure 2.30
(a) Sternum-splitting approach through an incision anterior to the left sternocleidomastoid muscle and extended along the mid-sternal area down to the xiphoid process. (b) Blunt dissection between the carotid sheath and visceral structures proximally and a median sternotomy distally. (c) Following ligation and division of the inferior thyroid artery, the left common carotid artery and left brachiocephalic vein are retracted

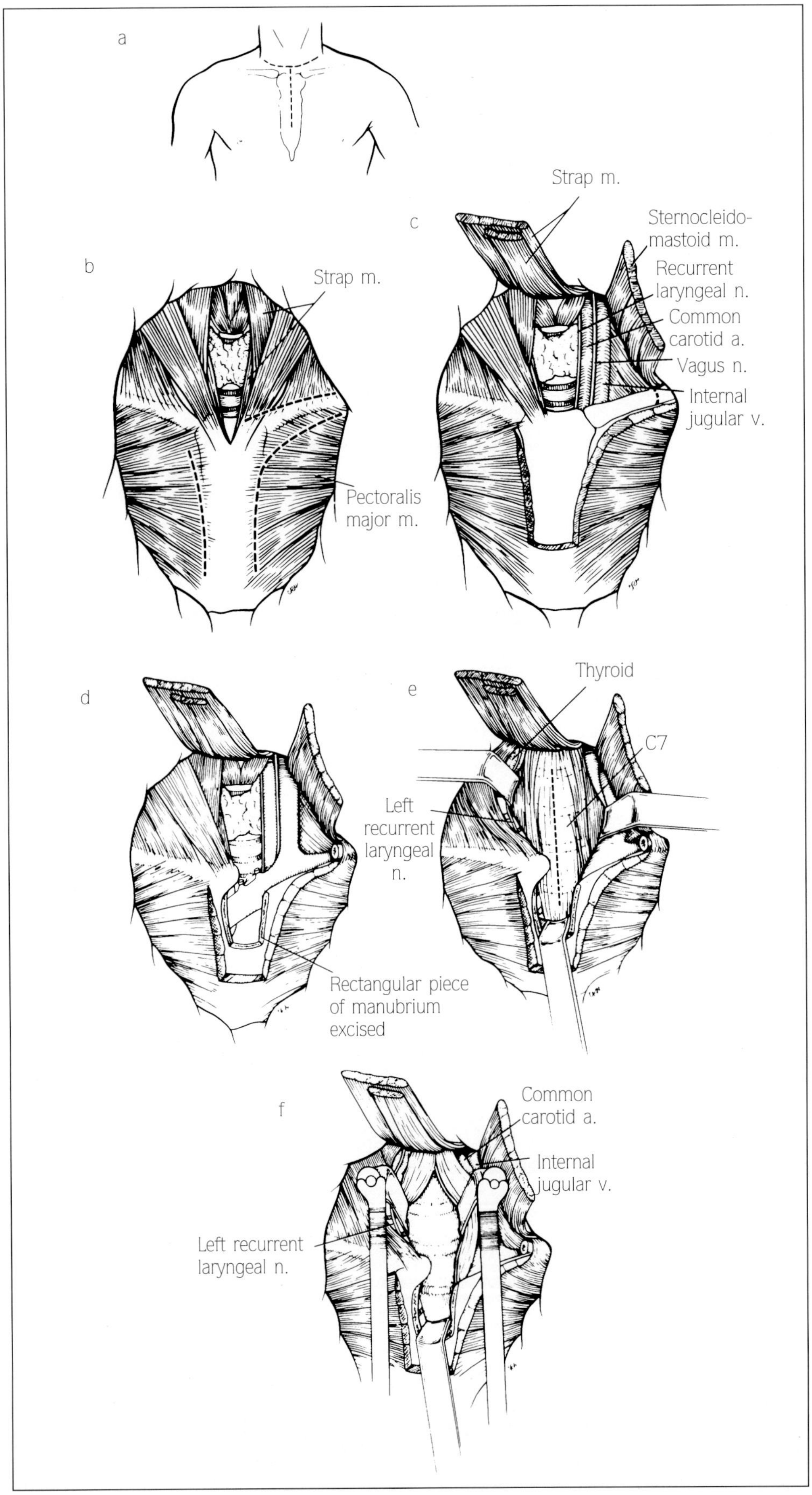

Figure 2.31
(a) T-shaped incision on the anterior chest wall. (b) Dissection is taken down to the level of the body manubrium and clavicle. (c) The sternal and clavicular heads of the sternocleidomastoid muscle are detached and retracted. The strap muscles on the ipsilateral side of approach are similarly detached and retracted. (d) The sternal origin of the pectoralis major is stripped laterally. The medial half of the clavicle is then stripped subperiosteally with removal of the medial third of the clavicle with a Gigli saw. A rectangular piece of the manubrium is removed along with its posterior periosteum. (e) Dissection between the left carotid artery on the left and the innominate artery, trachea, and esophagus on the right. (f) Self-retaining retractor in place

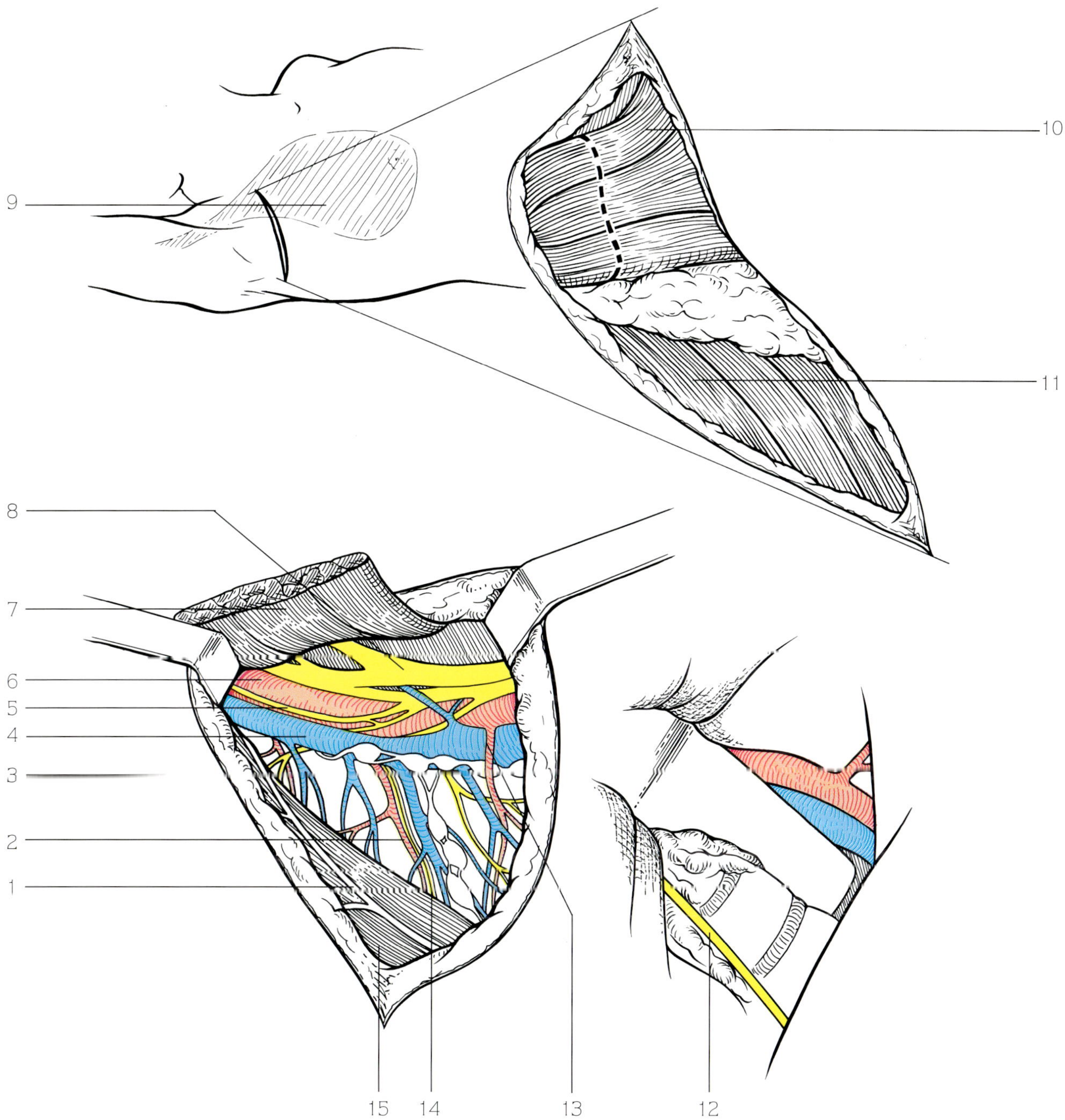

Figure 2.32
Axillary approach: (a) After placing the patient in a lateral decubitus position, a transverse incision is made at the base of the axillary hairline. (b) The pectoralis musculature is then divided. (c) Under the pectoralis muscle, neurovascular structures may be at risk such as the brachial plexus, axillary artery and vein, etc. (d) The chest wall is bluntly dissected by palpating the ribs. The sensory intercostobrachial nerve from the second intercostal space may have excision of a 4–5 cm peripheral segment. The third rib is excised and the parietal pleura is entered between the second and fourth ribs. Retraction and mobilization of the upper lobe of the lung exposes the upper segments of the thoracic vertebrae

1 Intercostal brachial n.
2 Thoracodorsal a.
3 Ulnar n.
4 Axillary v.
5 Medial cutaneous n.
6 Axillary a.
7 Pectoralis major m.
8 Brachial plexus
9 Pectoralis major m.
10 Pectoralis major m.
11 Latissimus dorsi m.
12 Intercostal brachial n.
13 Subscapularis a.
14 Thoracodorsal n.
15 Latissimus dorsi m.

of the sternocleidomastoid muscle are detached and retracted. The strap muscles on the ipsilateral side are similarly detached and retracted. After clearing the fatty and areolar tissues in the suprasternal space, the sternal origin of the pectoralis major is stripped laterally. The medial half of the clavicle is then stripped subperiosteally, and removal of the medial third of the clavicle completed with a Gigli saw. A rectangular piece of manubrium is removed along with its posterior periosteum and the exposed inferior thyroid vein, and if necessary the innominate vein, may be ligated.

Dissection is continued between the left carotid artery on the left, and the innominate artery, trachea, and esophagus on the right. Special attention must be given to protection of the thoracic duct and left recurrent laryngeal nerve. Sudaresan and associates[44] used this approach on seven patients with tumor involvement of the cervicothoracic junction. They noted one complication with a Steinmann pin migration in a patient stabilized with methylmethacrylate spacer. Charles[8] used this approach on ten patients with tuberculous or metastatic disease to the cervicothoracic junction. One death was noted in the perioperative period resulting from respiratory failure in a patient with previous chronic obstructive pulmonary disease. No ipsilateral shoulder problems to the side of clavicular resection were found, and all bone grafting matured to full fusion. One episode of early graft displacement without sequelae was recorded with an additional patient having temporary hoarseness.

Recently, Kurz and Herkowitz[32] presented a modified anterior approach to the cervicothoracic junction by removing the medial one-third of the clavicle. They reported no complications in four patients with tumors, except in one patient who had recurrence of the tumor. A combined low cervical and transthoracic approach has also been described to gain better access to the cervicothoracic junction in patients with severe kyphoscoliosis.[37]

Finally, a transaxillary approach to the upper thoracic spine is described (Fig. 2.32).[4] Either a right or left side approach can be made. After placing the patient in a lateral decubitus position, a transverse incision is made at the base of the axillary hairline; then the pectoralis musculature is divided. Underlying pectoralis muscle, neurovascular structures may be at risk such as the brachial plexus, axillary artery and vein etc. (Fig. 2.32c). The chest wall is bluntly dissected by palpating the ribs; a 4–5 cm peripheral segment of the sensory intercostobrachial nerve may be excised from the second intercostal space. The third rib is excised and the parietal pleura is entered between the second and fourth ribs. Retraction and mobilization of the upper lobe of the lung exposes the upper segments of the thoracic vertebrae.

This approach is rarely used because the highest upper vertebra exposed is T1 or C7, and exposure is more limited in obese patients or muscular males.

APPLICATION OF THE HALO VEST AND OTHER EXTERNAL CERVICAL ORTHOSES

The halo vest is significantly better than other orthoses in providing stabilization of the cervical spine in flexion–extension, rotation, and lateral bending. Distraction of the cervical spine is difficult to maintain, even with the halo vest. The surgeon should choose an appropriate orthotic device depending on the nature of the instability, the strength of the surgical construct, and the compliance of the patient. Unstable injuries of the upper cervical spine, such as odontoid fractures, Jefferson fractures, and hangman's fractures, are routinely treated with a halo vest. Occipitocervical and atlantoaxial arthrodesis with bone graft and wire should be followed by a postoperative halo vest for 3 months in most cases. Anterior strut graft without internal fixation is frequently supported with a halo vest, depending on the rigidity of the surgical construct.

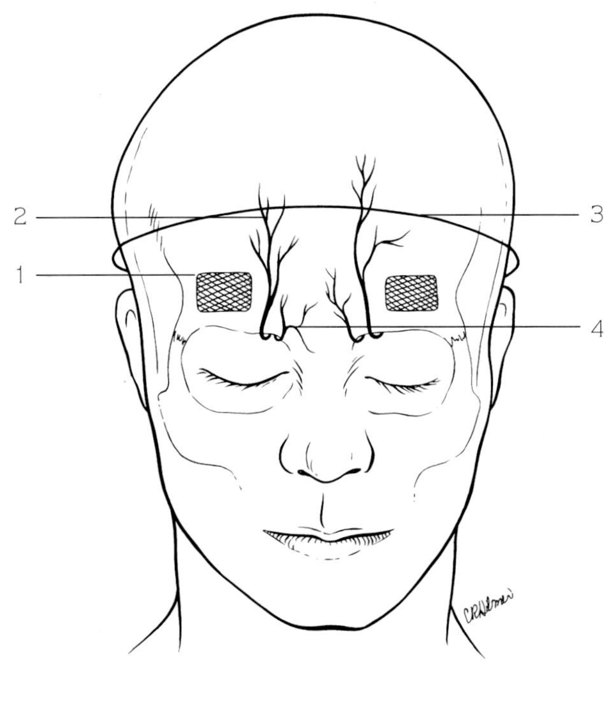

Figure 2.33
Halo pin sites: the anterolateral placement of the anterior pins avoids the thinner areas over the frontal sinus and the temporal fossae. The safe area for anterior pin placement is over the lateral eyebrow, avoiding the supraorbital nerve

1 Safe zone
2 Supraorbital n.
3 Equator
4 Supratrochlea n.

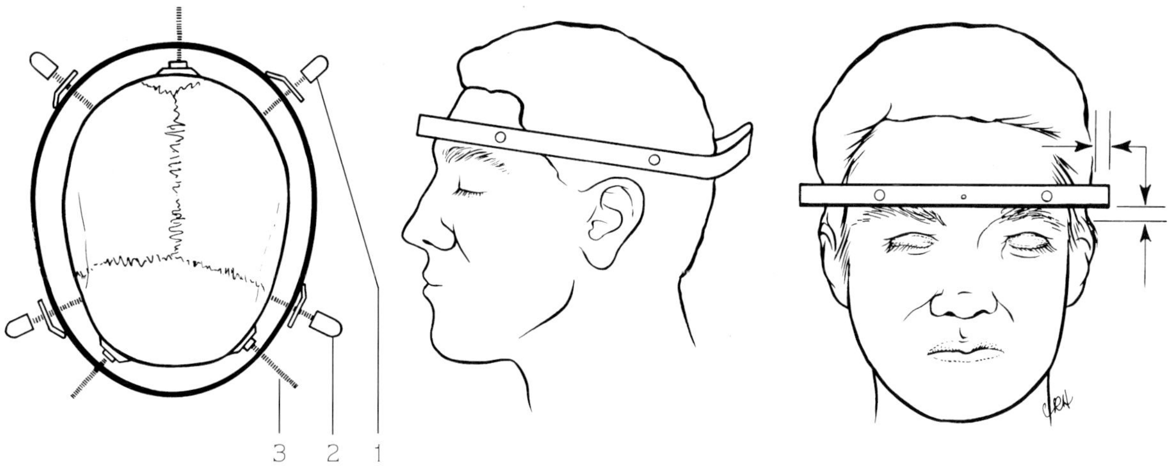

Figure 2.34
Halo application: the location for the posterolateral pins is anywhere behind the ears. The halo ring should be about 1 cm above the ears and 1 cm clearance around the skull

1 Posterior pins
2 Anterior pins
3 Positioning pins

The technique of halo application is simple, but complications of pin loosening, infection, and skin problems are common, and may result from improper halo vest application.[18] Although the halo vest is the most effective orthosis for cervical spine immobilization, loss of fracture reduction within the halo vest has been reported.

The application of a halo vest can be done in the patient's room, cast room, or in the operating room. The patient lies in the supine position with the head supported by an assistant or a narrow board. The head is usually extended, but the type of pathology or injury should dictate the exact position of the head. The circumference of the head should be measured, and an appropriate size halo ring selected. The halo ring should be positioned about 1 cm above the tip of the ears and 1 cm above the eyebrows. The halo ring is provisionally centered with positioning pins and base plates so that there is at least 1 cm of clearance between the skin and the ring circumferentially, and the ring should be positioned below the greater circumference of the skull to prevent cephalad slippage. The sites for pin insertion have been well defined by Garfin et al (Fig. 2.33).[18] The anterolateral placement of the anterior pins avoids the thinner areas over the frontal sinus and the temporal fossae. The safe area for anterior pin placement is over the lateral eyebrow, avoiding the supraorbital nerve. The location for the posterolateral pins is anywhere behind the ears. Once the sites are selected, the skin is prepared with antiseptic solution, followed by infiltration of local anesthetic without epinephrine. The needle is usually placed through the appropriate hole in the halo ring, and local anesthetic is injected down to the periosteum of the skull. The pins are

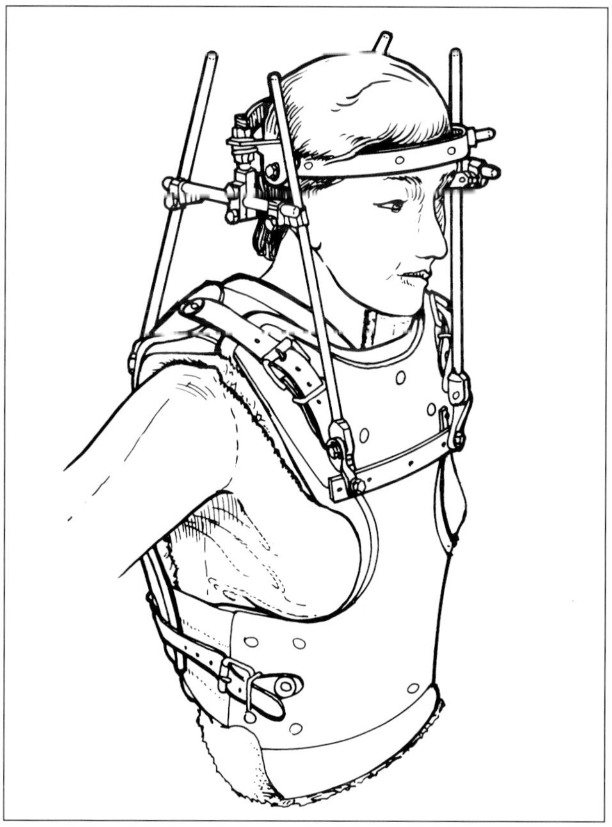

Figure 2.35
Halo-vest application: the posterior half of the vest is slid beneath the patient, followed by application of the anterior half of the vest; the connection between the vest and the halo ring is completed. The patient can be mobilized immediately

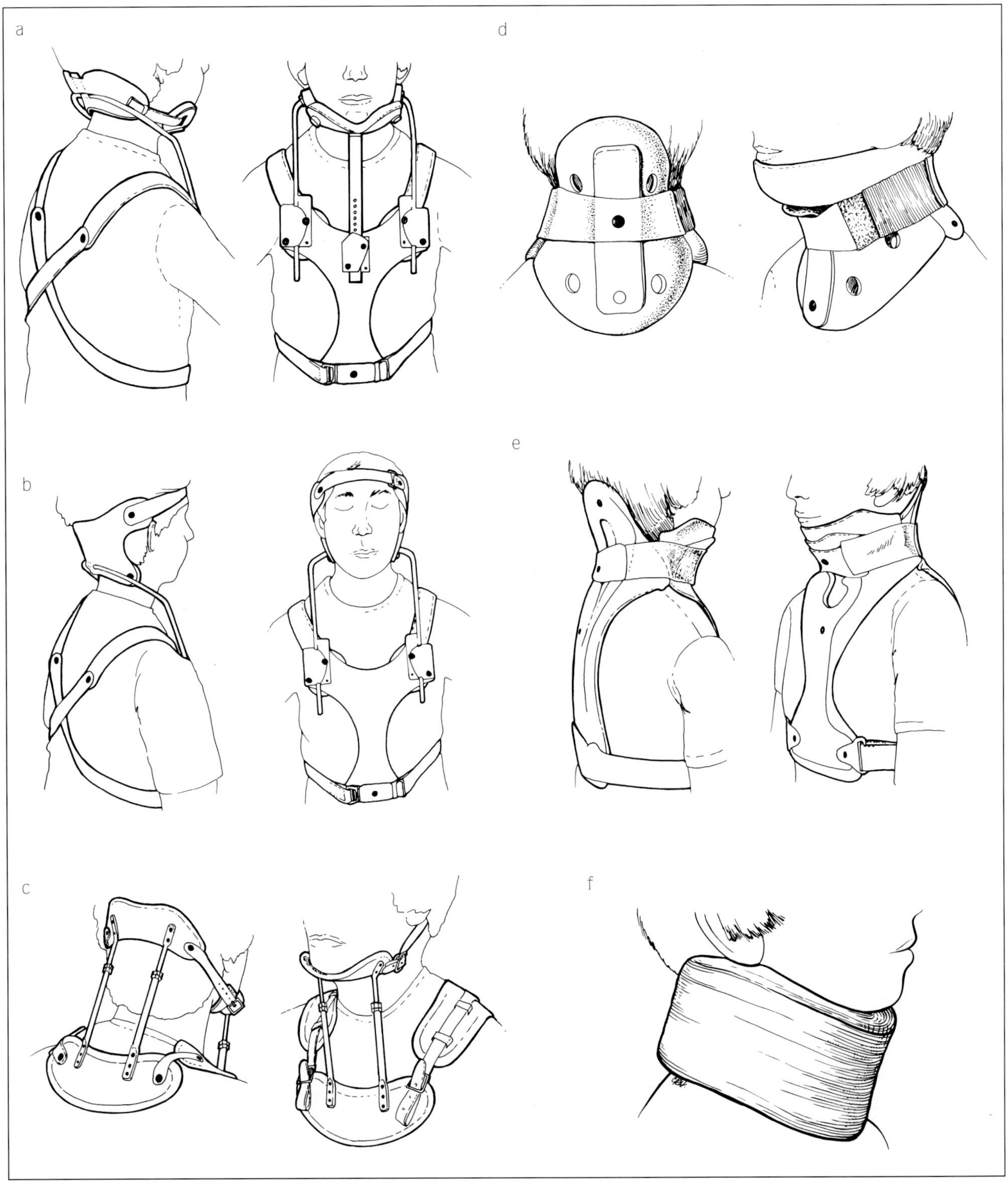

Figure 2.36
Cervical orthoses: (a) sternal occipital mandibular immobilizer (SOMI), which controls flexion better; (b) another SOMI-type brace with an optional strap to the head and greater support on the occiput to control more extension; (c) the four-poster brace; (d) the Philadelphia collar; (e) the extended Philadelphia collar; (f) the soft collar

then tightened so that the opposite pins are equally seated with finger pressure only (Fig. 2.34). At this time the positioning pins and the base plates are removed. Using a torque wrench, the pins are then tightened about 1 inch-pound of torque at a time until 6 inch-pounds of torque is reached. Then, the posterior half of the vest is slid beneath the patient, followed by application of the anterior half of the vest; connection between the vest and the halo ring is then completed (Fig. 2.35). The patient can be mobilized immediately. After 24 hours, the pins are retightened to 6 inch-pounds of torque, with no further tightening allowed. Skin care at the pin site and under the vest should be daily.

Other orthoses of the cervical spine include the Minerva brace, sternal occipital mandibular immobilizer (SOMI), the four-poster brace, Philadelphia collar, and soft collar (Fig. 2.36). Johnson et al[30] have contributed significantly to the understanding of the biomechanics of cervical orthoses. Basically, soft collars are used for patient comfort because they provide minimal counterforce against cervical spine motion. Philadelphia collars provide better external protection than soft collars, but are still inferior to other orthoses in controlling motion. The four-poster brace is an improvement over the Philadelphia collar in controlling flexion motion in the middle segments. Cervicothoracic braces which anchor more firmly to the trunk control flexion and extension motions better in the middle and lower cervical spine. The SOMI or Minerva brace controls flexion more effectively in the upper cervical spine. Nevertheless, these orthoses are still inferior to the halo vest in controlling all planes of motion, particularly in lateral bending and rotation. Plaster of Paris can be used to fabricate an orthosis of any type, and can be used in conjunction with a halo ring. A plaster of Paris orthosis is particularly useful in children.

SUMMARY

In summary, this chapter has reviewed surgical approaches to the cervical spine and use of orthoses. It should be remembered that in choosing a specific surgical approach, the patient's pathology, familiarity of the surgical approach, and complications associated with the approach should be considered. An appropriate orthosis should be chosen based on biomechanical stability provided by the device, and the degree of instability of the cervical spine.

REFERENCES

1 An HS, Gordin R, Renner K. Anatomic considerations for plate-screw fixation of the cervical spine. *Spine* **16**(10S): S548–S551, 1991.

2 An HS, Evanich C, Nowicki B, Haughton VM. Ideal thickness of Smith-Robinson anterior cervical fusion. *Spine* 18: 2043–2047, 1993..

3 Bauer R, Kerschbaumer F, Poisel S. *Operative Approaches in Orthopaedic Surgery and Traumatology,* 13–16. New York: Georg Thieme Verlag, 1987.

4 Breslau RC. Transaxillary approach to the upper dorsal spine. In Watkins RG (ed.) *Surgical Approaches to the Spine,* 58–63. New York: Springer Verlag, 1983.

5 Bulger RF, Rejowski JF, Beatty RA. Vocal cord paralysis associated with anterior cervical fusion: consideration for prevention and treatment. *J Neurosurg* **62**: 657–661, 1985.

6 Brooks AL, Jenkins EB. Atlanto-axial arthrodesis by the wedge compression method. *J Bone Joint Surg [Am]* **60**: 279–284, 1978.

7 Cauchoix J, Binet J. Anterior surgical approaches to the spine. *Ann R Coll Surg Engl* **27**: 237–243, 1957.

8 Charles R. Anterior approach to the upper thoracic vertebrae. *J Bone Joint Surg [Br]* **71**: 81–84, 1989.

9 Crenshaw AH. *Campbell's Operative Orthopaedics,* 7th ed., 3094–3095. St Louis: CV Mosby, 1987.

10 Crockard HA, Clader I, Ransford AO. One stage transoral decompression and posterior fixation in rheumatoid atlantoaxial subluxation: a technical note. *J Bone Joint Surg [Br]* **72**: 682–685, 1990.

11 Crockard HA. Anterior approaches to lesions of the upper cervical spine. *Clin Neurosurg* **34**: 389–416, 1988.

12 DeAndrade JR, MacNab I. Anterior occipitocervical fusion using an extra-pharyngeal exposure. *J Bone Joint Surg [Am]* **51**: 1621–1626, 1969.

13 Emery SE, Smith MD, Bohlman HH. Upper airway obstruction after multilevel cervical corpectomy for myelopathy. *J. Bone Joint Surg [Am]* **73**: 544–551, 1991.

14 Fang HSY, Ong GB. Direct anterior approach to the upper cervical spine. *J Bone Joint Surg* **44**: 1588, 1962.

15 Fielding JW, Stillwell WT. Anterior cervical approach to the upper thoracic spine. A case report. *Spine* **1**: 158–161, 1976.

16 Flynn TB. Neurologic complications of anterior cervical interbody fusion. *Spine* **7**: 536–539, 1982.

17 Gallie WE. Fractures and dislocations of the cervical spine. *Am J Surg* **46**: 495–499, 1939.

18 Garfin SR, Botte MJ, Waters RL, Nickel VL. Complications in the use of the halo fixation device. *J Bone Joint Surg [Am]* **68**: 320–325, 1986.

19 Grantham SA, Dick HM, Thompson RC, Stinchfield FE. Occipitocervical arthrodesis. *Clin Orthop* **65**: 118–129, 1969.

20 Griswold DM, Albright JA, Schiffman E, Johnson R, Southwick WO. Atlanto-axial fusion for instability. *J Bone Joint Surg [Am]* **60**: 285–292, 1978.

21 Hall JE, Denis F, Murray J. Exposure of the upper cervical spine for spinal decompression. *J Bone Joint Surg [Am]* **59**: 121–123, 1977.

22 Hamblen DL. Occipito-cervical fusion. *J Bone Joint Surg [Br]* **49**: 33–45, 1967.

23 Heeneman H. Vocal cord paralysis following approaches to the anterior cervical spine. *Laryngoscope* **83**: 17–21, 1973.

24 Henry AK. *Extensile Exposure,* 53. Baltimore: Williams & Wilkins, 1959.

25 Herkowitz HN. A comparison of anterior cervical fusion, cervical laminectomy, and cervical laminoplasty for the surgical

management of multiple level spondylotic radiculopathy. *Spine* **13**: 774–780, 1988.
26 Hirabayashi K, Miyakawa J, Satomi K, et al. Operative results and postoperative progression of ossification among patients with cervical posterior longitudinal ligament. *Spine* **6**: 354–364, 1981.
27 Hogson AR. An approach to the cervical spine (C3–7). *Clin Orthop* **39**: 129, 1965.
28 Horwitz NH, Rizzoli MV. *Postoperative Complications in Neurosurgery Practice, Recognition, Prevention, Management*, 30–98. Baltimore: Williams & Wilkins, 1988.
29 Johnson RM, Southwick WO. Surgical approaches to the spine. In Rothman RH, Simeone FA (eds) *The Spine*, 67–188. Philadelphia: WB Saunders, 1982.
30 Johnson RM, Hart DL, Simmons EF, et al. Cervical orthoses: a study comparing their effectiveness in restricting cervical motion in normal subjects. *J Bone Joint Surg [Am]* **59**: 332–339, 1977.
31 Kirkaldy-Willis WH, Allen PBR, Rostrup O, Willox GL. Surgical approaches to the anterior elements of the spine: indications and techniques. *Can J Surg* **9**: 294–308, 1966.
32 Kurz LT, Herkowitz HH. Modified anterior approach to the cervico-thoracic junction. *Spine* 5: 542–549, 1991.
33 Letts M, Slutsky D. Occipitocervical arthrodesis in children. *J Bone Joint Surg [Am]* **72**: 1166–1170, 1990.
34 Light TR, Wagner FC, Johnson RM, Southwick WO. Correction of spinal instability and recovery of neurologic loss following cervical vertebral body replacement. *Spine* **5**: 392–394, 1980.
35 McAfee PC, Bohlman HH, Riley LH, Robinson RA, Southwick WO, Nacholas NE. The anterior retropharyngeal approach to the upper part of the cervical spine. *J Bone Joint Surg [Am]* **69**: 1371–1383, 1987.
36 Meyer PR Jr. Surgical stabilization of the cervical spine. In Meyer PR (ed.) *Surgery of Spine Trauma.* New York: Churchill Livingstone, 1989.
37 Micheli JJ, Hood RW. Anterior exposure of the cervicothoracic spine using combined cervical and thoracic approach. *J Bone Joint Surg [Am]* **65:** 992–997, 1983.
38 Newman P, Sweetnam R. Occipito-cervical fusion. *J Bone Joint Surg [Br]* **51**: 423–431, 1969.
39 Riley LH Jr. Surgical approaches to the anterior structures of the cervical spine. *Clin Orthop* **91**: 16–20, 1973.
40 Robinson RA, Southwick WO. Surgical approaches to the cervical spine. In *American Academy of Orthopaedic Surgeons: Instructional Course Lectures.* Vol. XVII. St Louis, MI: CV Mosby, 1960.
41 Sang UH, Wilson CB. Postoperative epidural hematoma as a complication of anterior cervical discectomy. *J Neurosurg* **49**: 288–291, 1978.
42 Simeone FA, Rothman RH. Cervical disc disease. In Rothman RH, Simeone FA (eds) *The Spine*, 440–499. Philadelphia: WB Saunders, 1982.
43 Simmons EH, Bhalla SK. Anterior cervical discectomy and fusion. A clinical and biomechanical study with eight-year follow-up. *J Bone Joint Surg [Br]* **51**: 225–232, 1969.
44 Sundaresan N, Shah J, Feghali JG. A transternal approach to the upper thoracic vertebrae. *Am J Surg* **148**: 473–477, 1984.
45 Sundaresan N, Shah J, Foley KM, Rosen G. An anterior surgical approach to the upper thoracic vertebrae. *J Neurosurg* **61**: 686–690, 1984.
46 Tew JM Jr, Mayfield FH. Surgery of the anterior cervical spine: prevention of complications. In Dunsker SB (ed.), 191–208. *Cervical Spondylosis.* New York: Raven Press, 1981.
47 Turner PL, Webb JK. A surgical approach to the upper thoracic spine. *J Bone Joint Surg [Br]* **69**: 542–544, 1987.
48 Verbiest H. Antero-lateral operations for fractures and dislocations in the middle and lower parts of the cervical spine. *J Bone Joint Surg [Am]* **51**: 1489–1530, 1969.
49 Watkins RG. *Surgical Approaches to the Spine.* New York: Springer Verlag, 1983.
50 Welsh LW, Welsh JJ, Chinnici JC. Dysphagia due to cervical spine surgery. *Ann Otol Rhinol Laryngol* **96**: 112–115, 1987.
51 Wertheim SB, Bohlman HH. Occipitocervical fusion. *J Bone Joint Surg [Am]* **69**: 833–836, 1987.
52 White AA III, Panjabi MM. *Clinical Biomechanics of the Spine.* Philadelphia: JB Lipincott, 1991.
53 White AA III, Southwick WO, DePonte RJ, Gainar JW, Hardy R. Relief of pain by anterior cervical fusion for spondylosis – a report of sixty-five patients. *J Bone Joint Surg [Am]* **55**: 525–534, 1973.
54 White AA III, Jupiter J, Southwick WO, Panjabi MM. An experimental study of the immediate load bearing of three surgical constructions for anterior spine fusions. *Clin Orthop* **91**: 21–28, 1973.
55 Whitecloud TS, LaRocca H. Fibular strut graft in reconstructive surgery of the cervical spine. *Spine* **1**: 33–43, 1976.
56 Whitehill R, Sirna EC, Young DC, Cantrell RW. Late esophageal perforation from an autogenous bone graft. Report of a case. *J Bone Joint Surg [Am]* **67**: 644–645, 1985.
57 Whitesides TE Jr, Kelley RP. Lateral approach to the upper cervical spine for anterior fusion. *South Med J* **59**: 879–883, 1966.
58 Yasuoka S, Peterson HA, MacCarty CS. Incidence of spinal column deformity after multilevel laminectomy in children and adults. *J Neurosurg* **57**: 441–445, 1982.
59 Zdeblick TA, Ducker TB. The use of freeze-dried allograft bone for anterior cervical fusions. *Spine* **16**: 726–729, 1991.

3 Cervical spine biomechanics

Tom Reinsel and
Martin Krag

A thorough understanding of the biomechanics of the cervical spine is necessary to understand and intelligently treat cervical spine disorders. This chapter briefly reviews the anatomy of the cervical spine with a 'biomechanical slant'. Kinematics and instability of the cervical spine are also discussed. Finally, a biomechanical analysis of orthoses and surgical constructs is presented.

SPINAL COMPONENT BIOMECHANICS

Vertebrae

Upper Cervical

The occipito-atlantoaxial complex is one of the most complex articulations in the human body and functions as a transition zone between the head and spine. Several unique features in this transition zone afford a relatively large degree of motion to the head. One of the unique features, the absence of the C1 body, is a result of an elaborate embryological development[209] in which the C1 body is borrowed by C2 to form the dens. Another interesting aspect of this occiput–C1–C2 complex is the presence of only synovial articulations and the absence of any disc. This is the major reason for the selective occurrence of cervical spine problems in patients with rheumatoid arthritis in the upper cervical spine.

The occipital condyles are convex, directed slightly anterolaterally, and articulate with the concave C1 facets. The occipital condyles allow the weight of the skull to be directed over the large lateral masses of C1. The C1 structure, which has been well described elsewhere,[51,77,109] has three articulations with C2 – one facet over each C2 lateral mass and one between the C1 anterior arch and the dens. The two zygoapophyseal articulations are aligned in the transverse plane, which allows effective axial load transmission, but minimal anteroposterior stability which is, however, provided by the dens–C1 arch articulation. Although the other dimensions of this complex are surprisingly constant for various body sizes, the posterior prominence of the occiput is disproportionately large compared to the chest in children. As a result, the supine posture tends to produce cervical kyphosis, which can be harmful during the transportation of a child with a cervical spine injury.

Lower Cervical

The lower cervical vertebrae consist of C3–C7, although T1 and T2 are transitional in nature and share some lower cervical spine characteristics. Quantitative measurements have recently been carried out by Panjabi et al[174] and Liu[135]; relevant qualitative measurements have been performed as well[161]. The cervical vertebral body is roughly half the size of the lumbar, which reflects the lighter loads of the cervical spine. The concavity of the superior end-plate of the cervical body is effectively deepened by a ridge along each side of the superior end-plate. This uncinate process or neurocentral ridge, together with the convexity of the adjacent inferior end-plate, provides resistance to lateral shifting between adjacent pairs of vertebrae.[21] The area between the uncinate process and the adjacent inferior vertebral body is often referred to as the joint of Luschka. Although this is probably not a true synovial joint, debate on this topic continues.[63,104,166,178,222]

The pedicles connect the vertebral body to the posterior elements. The pedicles, in turn, form the upper and lower boundaries of the foramina, which are directed anterolaterally and inferiorly. Protruding anterolaterally from the pedicle is a rudimentary rib process whereas further posteriorly the transverse process projects posterolaterally from the pedicle. The transverse processes provide

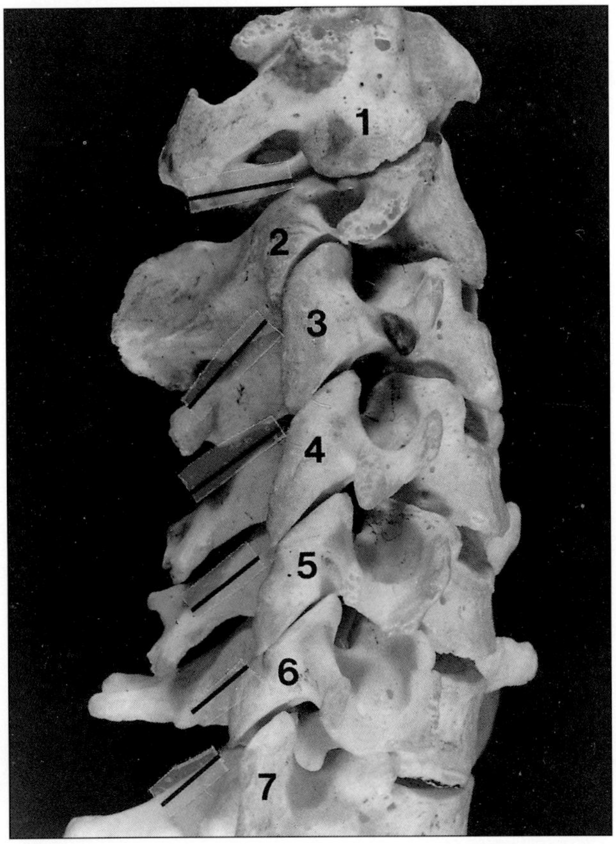

Figure 3.1
The facet orientation and its change at different anatomic levels

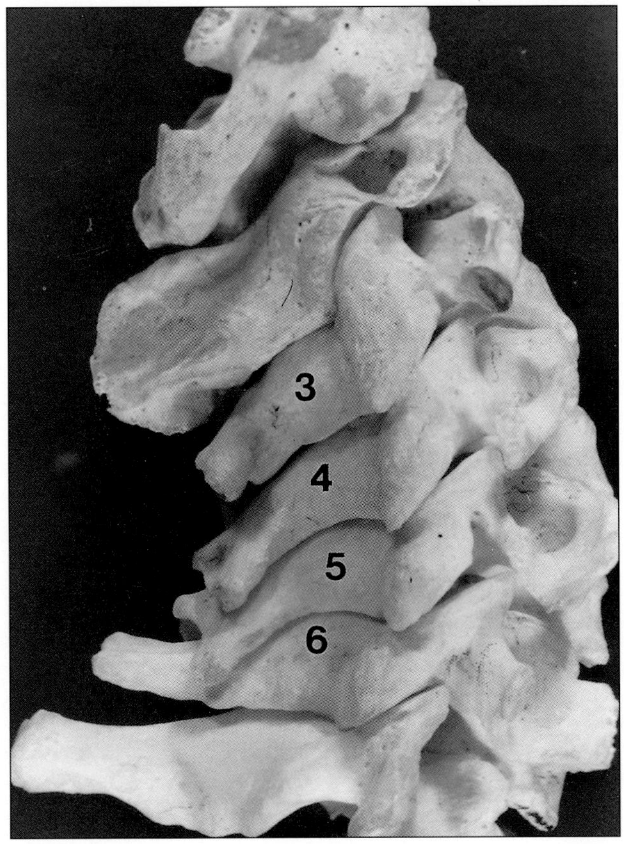

Figure 3.2
Spinous process length gradually increases caudally. Synovial joint orientation at C1–C2 is transverse while below this is oblique. Bifid spinous processes 'nest' together to allow extension without decrease in spinous process length

an important insertion site for various anterior and posterior neck muscles. The transverse process, together with the pedicle and rib process, form the foramen transversarium. The vertebral artery travels through this foramen transversarium except at C7 where the accessory vertebral vein usually travels.[103]

Connected posteriorly to the pedicles are the lateral masses, which include superior and inferior articular processes, each of which carries an articular facet. The facet joints appear to play some role in proprioception,[140] provide anteroposterior translation stability, and allow intervertebral motion.[71] The orientation of the facets (Fig. 3.1) changes from a nearly transverse orientation at C1–C2 to a 55–60° angle from C2–C3 to C7–T1 (measured with respect to the inferior end-plate).[21,43,111] The lateral masses which support the facets have become more surgically useful in recent years with the increased use of lateral mass screws and plates advocated by Magerl and others.[194]

Attached to the lateral masses by the lamina are the spinous processes, which increase in length from C3 to T1. Figuratively speaking they can be thought of as handles or levers for producing and controlling vertebral motion. The increase in spinous process length from C3 to T1 reflects the greater torque required to move the head as one moves caudally in the cervical spine. The spinous processes are bifid which allows them to nest (interdigitate) with one another and thus provide maximal extension without a decrease in spinous process length (Fig. 3.2).

The spinal canal is formed by the vertebral body, pedicles, lateral masses, and lamina. Spinal canal size and its relevance to cervical trauma has been thoroughly studied by Torg et al.[177,223] They found that a value of ≤ 0.80 for the ratio of the spinal canal to the vertebral body indicated canal stenosis and recommended against contact sports for athletes with a ratio < 0.5. This measurement has, however, been questioned in the case of professional football players whose vertebral bodies are unusually large in comparison to the spinal canal.

Discs

The six cervical discs (including C7–T1) are identical in nature and similar to thoracic and lumbar discs, consisting of an outer fibrous ring – the annulus fibrosus – and a semi-solid central core – the nucleus pulposus. This construct allows the transmission of compressive loads through a wide range of motion without producing excessive stress concentration. This is accomplished by the semi-solid nucleus pulposus which shifts posteriorly in flexion and anteriorly in extension, which probably produces a 'load-leveling' effect.[128] The discs are more closely contained than in the lumbar and thoracic area by the concave/convex arrangement of the vertebral body and by the 'joints' of Luschka. The weakest point of the annulus fibrosus, as in the lumbar spine,[241] is the posterolateral corner where the rate of curvature of the annulus fibrosus is greatest. The first cervical disc is between C2 and C3 because there are no discs between either occiput and C1 or C1 and C2.

Ligaments

Ligaments play an important role in the stability of the cervical spine. They may be considered in two groups: those that span multiple motion segments and those that link only one motion segment. The ligamentum nuchae is a dense, fibrous, posterior, midline band that runs from the C7 spinous process to the external occipital protuberance, and is the major ligament in the cervical spine which spans multiple motion segments. It is analogous to the lumbar spine's supraspinous ligament. In comparison to quadripeds, the ligamentum nuchae in humans is rather rudimentary, but it is generally agreed that it provides a major constraint to excessive cervical flexion, although others have found this is not always the case.[24,26,28,94,112] Intermediate attachments from C2 to C6 appear to be much weaker, perhaps explaining why a 'clay shoveler's' fracture most often occurs at C7.[201]

The ligaments that functionally span only one motion segment include the anterior longitudinal ligament (ALL), intertransverse process ligament, posterior longitudinal ligament (PLL), facet joint capsules, and ligamentum flavum. The ALL and PLL actually span multiple segments, but the firm attachments at each level effectively limit their action to single motion segments. The ligamentum flavum has a significant stabilizing effect on flexion because of its high elastic content, returning the neck to neutral position upon flexion.[176] More detailed anatomic descriptions as well as extensive biomechanical testing of ligament–bone constructs in the cervical spine have been reported elsewhere.[112,247]

The dens provides a solid post to which are anchored both the occiput and C1. Although the occiput has minimal attachments to C1 (limited to the facet capsules), the attachments to the dens are much sturdier and include the alar ligament and the less substantial apical and upper arm of the cruciform ligament. C1 attaches to the dens via the hefty transverse ligament and weaker accessory C1–C2 ligament and C1–C2 facets. The alar ligament is approximately half the strength of the transverse ligament as shown by Dvorak et al.[60]

Muscle

The muscles in the neck allow and provide for precise motion and control of the head. None of the passive elements (bone, disc, ligament, and joints) provides much resistance to flexion or lateral bending, and thus requires muscle action to prevent buckling collapse.[233] As in the axial skeleton there are gross-function and fine-function muscles distinguished primarily on the number of segments crossed.

Anteriorly the gross-function muscles include the longus capitis, longus collis, and scalenes. The fine-function muscles anteriorly are the intertransversarii. Posteriorly the muscle bulk is greater and is related to the fact that the head is usually positioned anterior to the center of gravity. This support includes the gross-function muscles such as splenius capitis, semispinalis cervices, longissimus cervices, and iliocostalis cervices. The fine-function muscles posteriorly are the interspinales, the intertransverarii, and the long and short rotatores. Quantitative detail of muscle site attachments as well as in vitro and in vivo muscle forces have been discussed elsewhere.[49,155,162]

Many of these muscles are oriented obliquely to the longitudinal axis of the spine. This allows rotation and shifting or translation of the head anteriorly, posteriorly, or laterally. For example, rotation of the head and neck to the left requires contraction of the left sternocleidomastoid and upper trapezius muscles in addition to the right splenius capitis and longissimus capitis muscles. In a recent review by Parke and Sherk,[176] the functional aspect of muscle structure is presented.

Cord, Dura, Nerve Roots

The biomechanics of the spinal cord is also an important topic that is often overlooked. Breig[24–29] has shown, using dynamic myelographic and cadaver studies, that the cord becomes longer and thinner with flexion, and shorter and thicker with extension. Excursion between the cord and vertebra of up to 18 mm occurred with motion; the neutral point – at which no relative motion occurs – is C5.[184] Magnetic resonance imaging (MRI) may be useful in documenting the extent of these motions.

This spinal cord motion generates tensile forces which are primarily borne by the dura and pia arachnoid. These forces are balanced by the nerve root dural sheaths and dentate ligaments. The effect of these mechanical changes on clinical findings and neurophysiological testing has been thoroughly investigated by Breig.[24–29] He noticed increased neurologic deficit with cervical flexion in some patients and felt that this was caused by increased contact pressure between the anterior aspect of the cord and posterior surface of the vertebral bodies. Applying this to the clinical situation, Breig recommended avoidance of flexion to prevent increased cord tension and abnormal intervertebral motion, both of which might worsen pre-existing neural damage.[29]

Spinal Cord Internal Stress/Strain

McVeigh[142] and later Omma[164] noted that axial compressibility was greater for the central gray matter than for the peripheral white matter. This is consistent with the observation that more tissue damage occurs centrally with external cord pressure.[34,146,202,203] A thorough analysis of spinal cord stress, both measured and calculated, is discussed by Panjabi and White.[167]

Experimental Cord Trauma

The ability to create cord trauma in vitro is important to the understanding and treatment of cord injuries. The Allen method (mass × drop distance) has seen many decades of use since first described in 1911, but new, more precise methods have allowed a more accurate study.[53,168,170,213] These methods have allowed Panjabi and Wrathall to correlate biomechanical input and functional outcome.[168]

SPINAL COMPOSITE BIOMECHANICS

The bony and soft-tissue components described above comprise the building blocks for the cervical spine. One important aspect of the interaction between these components is the motion or kinematics – that branch of mechanics that examines the motion of bodies without consideration of influencing forces.[110] Force considerations are not very useful clinically, because their direct measurement is not presently feasible.

A basic understanding of kinematics is important for the diagnosis and management of cervical spine pathology. As in the discussion of component biomechanics, the upper cervical (occiput–C1–C2) and lower cervical (C2–C7) kinematics will be discussed separately.

Upper Cervical

Flexion–extension motion, as demonstrated by radiographic measurement, occurs at both occiput–C1 and C1–C2. The average ranges of motion are 10° and 13.4° respectively.[9,10,25,110,179,234] This is consistent with predictions based upon anatomic considerations.

Axial rotation also occurs at both occiput–C1 and C1–C2. However, the deep fit of the convex occipital condyles in the concave facets of C1 somewhat restricts rotation at occiput–C1, as shown by several investigators.[39,50,59,245] Approximately half of the axial rotation of the entire cervical spine occurs at the C1–C2 level.[179,230,233,234] This large degree of motion can, however, cause kinking of the vertebral arteries at the occipital–C1 or C1–C2 joints.[14,208] Although symptom-free in most people, reported cases have been associated with hypermobility of the neck or with forceful manipulations.[110] The alar ligaments provide a check to rotation of both occiput–C1 and C1–C2: the left alar ligament limits rotation of the head to the right and vice versa.

Lateral bending occurs at the occiput–C1 probably to a small extent. Some controversy exists, however, as to the degree of motion. Werne[231] suggests that only 7.8° occur, whereas others[71] suggest up to 30–40°. Anatomic considerations prevent any appreciable lateral bending between C1 and C2.

It is usually agreed that translatory motion in occiput–C1 is < 1 mm. Worth,[245] however, noted translation of up to 5.5° in normal subjects. Translation does occur normally between C1 and C2. Radiographic studies by Jackson[108] demonstrated up to 2.5 mm in adults and 4 mm in children. Fielding,[73] based on cadaveric studies, feels that 3 mm is the upper limit of normal for C1–C2 translation and that any greater motion indicates transverse ligament rupture.

Lower Cervical

Here the range of motion can be approximated at roughly 10° each for flexion–extension, rotation, and lateral bending per motion segment.[73,137,233,234] The C5–C6 level is generally regarded as having the greatest range of motion, perhaps explaining the greater incidence of disc degeneration and herniation at this level.[11,57,137] The effect of motion on foraminal dimensions has been studied by Cailliet.[36] Yoo[248] et al found no significant increase with either flexion, extension, or rotation, but did find a significant decrease in foraminal size with extension.

The effects of age on range of motion have also been studied. Several studies have shown a decrease in range of motion with advancing age.[11,16,205] Recently, Dvorak et al[61] tested passive range of motion in asymptomatic volunteers using a three-dimensional electrogoniometric analyzer and found gender differences in range of motion as well as a general decrease with age, except for rotation at the atlantoaxial joint which increased or stayed the same. Other authors, however, have noted no decrease in the range of motion with age.[73,91,137,148]

Abnormal kinematics for cases in which there are no obvious fractures or dislocations have not been well defined. Amevo et al[4] found abnormal instantaneous axes of rotation in 46% of patients with chronic neck pain, but this correlated poorly with pain relief by facet blocks or with provocative discography. A 'stretch test' was developed by Schlicke et al[200] and applied to normal subjects. Application to individuals with neck pain to detect abnormal displacement under axial traction has not yet been studied.

INSTABILITY OR HYPERFLEXIBILITY

A large contributing factor to the confusion surrounding the term 'instability' is the lack of a generally agreed on or clear definition of its meaning. In a non-clinical context, instability may refer to unexpectedly large displacements in response to load, such as a canoe which tips to a surprising degree. Another meaning is that a system, after removal of some perturbation, does not tend to return to its initial state: beyond a certain point, further load to the edge of a canoe will cause it to continue to flip all the way over, even if the load is quickly removed.

In a clinical context, neither of these meanings of instability is very useful, mainly because controlled, gradually increasing loads cannot readily be applied to individual cervical vertebrae. Instead, the clinical term 'instability' usually refers to an anticipated unfavorable outcome in one way or another without a certain treatment, as indicated by actual or predicted hypermobility.

Given all these issues, the term 'mechanical insufficiency' seems to be a more appropriate term: it is usefully vague and does not suggest more than is presently understood.[124]

Despite the limitations of in vitro experiments, many contributions have been made to our understanding of spinal mechanical insufficiency ('instability') through cadaveric experiments. Cadaveric experiments have been performed by Panjabi et al[154,169,171,173] in attempts to quantify motion of the cervical spine. These authors have also studied the effects of sequential ligament transection on motion segment kinematics and found a 'pre-failure state' where cutting one more ligament would produce complete dislocation. Their criteria for 'instability', however, lack clinical correlation as discussed below. This biomechanical research forms the basis for one item on a 'checklist' used for defining 'clinical instability'.

Raynor et al[183] studied the effect of partial facetectomy on the kinematics of cervical spine cadaveric specimens. When 50% of each facet was excised, one-fifth failed under anterior shear load by articular process fracture. With excision of 70% of each facet, four-fifths failed with articular process fracture.

Although clinical recommendations have been made based on these studies, the relationship of these in vitro studies to in vivo kinematics is unclear for two reasons. First, the pattern of ligament disruption in vivo is probably different from sequential ligament transection; second, the force distribution in vivo is unknown and may be quite different from the in vitro forces used.

EXTERNAL SUPPORT

Orthosis Types

A discussion of the wide variety of orthoses is incomplete without a review of the nomenclature system.[96,113,115,243] Descriptions of orthoses are often dependent upon structural characteristics (e.g. halo vest) or place of origin (e.g. Philadelphia collar). These terms, however, often provide little descriptive information. Wolf and Johnson[243] patterned a nomenclature after orthoses named for the body part they immobilize, e.g. cervical, head–cervical, head–cervical–thoracic, and halo. This system has been modified slightly[124] (Table 3.1) because 'head' is fairly non-specific and 'halo' again names the device after a structural characteristic.

Unfortunately, reliance on biomechanical testing of these orthoses provides an incomplete picture for several reasons. First, the ultimate success of any orthosis should be based not on short-term mechanical testing, but on comparative study of patient outcomes: such studies remain to be done. Second, radiographic assessment of orthoses is limited by the fact that radiographs alone do not provide a full measure of the load distributions in the spine, which are ultimately what produce loss of reduction or undesirable motion. Finally, voluntarily produced neck motions in orthoses (by normal or patient volunteers) may be very different than those produced during daily activities. For example, soft foam neck collars can be easily

Table 3.1 Cervical orthoses

Category	*Example*
Cervical	Collar Collar and Chine piece Queen Anne Collar
Occipitomandibular–high thoracic	Philadelphia Four-poster
Occipitomandibular–low thoracic	Extended Philadelphia Sternal-occipital-mandibular immobilizer
Craniothoracic	Minerva Halo vest

deformed through a full range of motion[113] and yet patients wearing a collar usually move far less.

Cervical

These orthoses are usually referred to as neck collars and are usually composed of a soft (semi-compressible) material (Fig. 3.3). They provide little mechanical block to motion[3,42,113] and probably serve as a 'reminder' to restrict motion. Other cervical orthoses extend to the mandible with varying restriction of the occiput depending on the stiffness of the orthosis. Examples include the collar with a chin attachment or the Queen Anne collar.[42]

Occipital–mandibular–high thoracic

These orthoses, represented by the Philadelphia collar (Fig. 3.4a) and the 'four-poster' or Thomas collar (Fig. 3.4b), extend to the upper sternum and interscapular region.[113,189]

Occipital–mandibular–low thoracic

The extended Philadelphia collar (Fig. 3.5a), 'Yale brace' (Philadelphia collar with a rigid extension),[114] sternal occipital mandibular immobilizer (SOMI, shown in Fig. 3.5b) and 'cervicothoracic orthosis'[96,113] are examples of this type of orthosis which extends along the length of the sternum and thoracic spine.

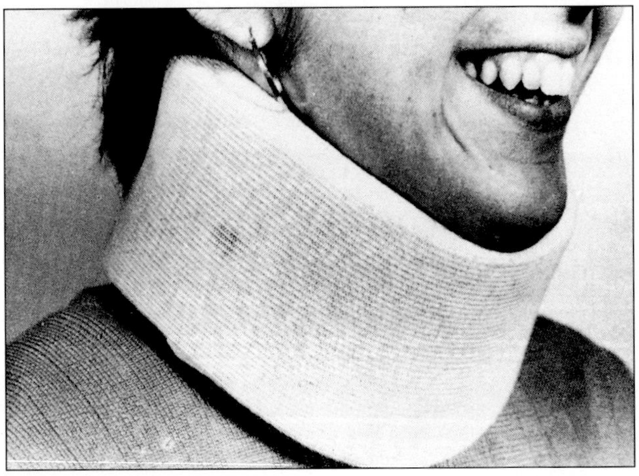

Figure 3.3
Cervical orthosis (soft collar)

Craniothoracic

A Minerva cast is one example of this, but the halo vest is much more commonly used – this attaches to the cranium via metal pins. The vest portion of the orthoses provides fixation to the trunk in varying degrees depending on the design.[15,125,149,159,181] The most recent design,[13,124,125,204] which incorporates four independently adjustable thoracic pads (Fig. 3.6), restricts neck motion to less than half that allowed by traditional vests.[22,126]

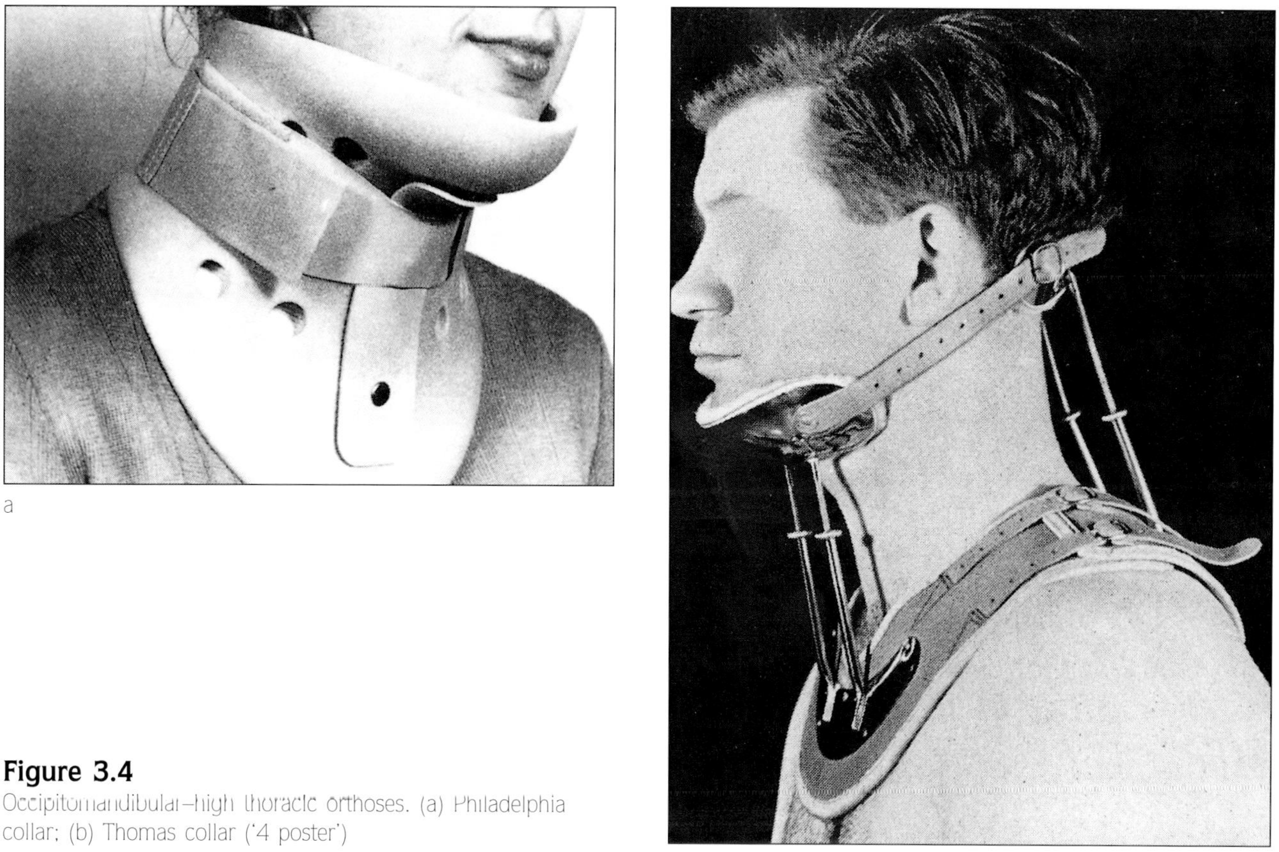

a

b

Figure 3.4
Occipitomandibular–high thoracic orthoses. (a) Philadelphia collar; (b) Thomas collar ('4 poster')

Orthosis Evaluation

As stated previously, clinical outcomes comparing different types of orthoses have not yet been done, although numerous studies have determined quantitatively motion restriction by orthoses. Early studies either used difficult-to-quantify cineradiography[97,116] or did not provide statistical analysis.[42] Fischer et al[75] used a standardized testing technique to examine motion in volunteers immobilized in a variety of orthoses (Philadelphia collar, four-poster, SOMI, and soft collar with chin and occipital pads). They found that:

1. For occiput–C2, 'paradoxical' motion occurred consisting of extension of the upper cervical spine with forward motion of the head and neck, and that this was greater with the Philadelphia and soft extended collar than with the other orthoses.
2. For C2–C3, all four designs restricted motion almost entirely.
3. For C3–C4 to C6–C7, the soft collar for extension and the Philadelphia collar for extension or flexion restricted motion to only two-thirds of normal, whereas the SOMI and four-poster design restricted motion down to one-third of normal.

Johnson et al,[113,114] in one of the most complete kinematic evaluations of orthoses, studied flexion–extension, lateral bend, and axial rotations voluntarily produced by seated subjects wearing each of the following: soft cervical collar, Philadelphia collar, Yale brace, SOMI, four-poster, cervicothoracic orthosis, and the halo vest. Their major findings were the following:

- the longer and stiffer devices generally provide greater immobilization;
- the non-halo devices restrict flexion and extension (13–74% of normal) and lateral bending (18–83%) to varying degrees, but provide little rotatory control (51–92%);

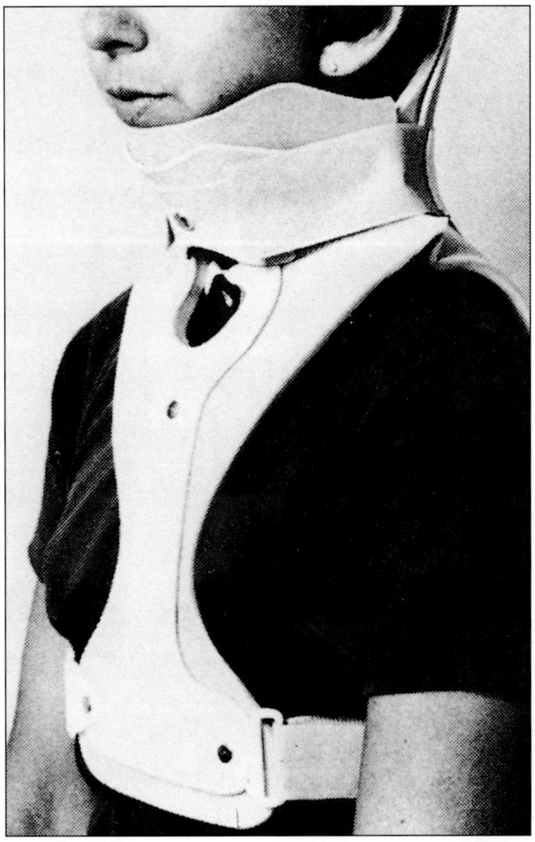

a

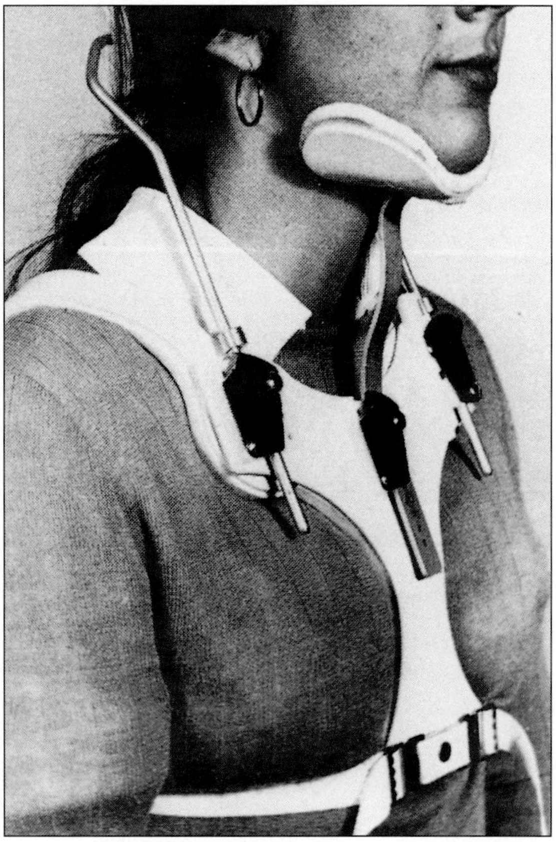

b

Figure 3.5
Occipitomandibular–low thoracic orthoses. (a) Extended Philadelphia collar; (b) Sternal–occipital–mandibular immobilizer (SOMI)

- the easily fabricated Yale brace functions much like the more complex 'cervicothoracic orthosis' or four-poster;
- the upper cervical spine is poorly immobilized by the non-halo devices;
- the halo vest allows motion in the lower cervical spine similar to some of the orthoses;
- the halo vest, although the best in the upper cervical spine, still allows roughly 20% of the flexion–extension motion at occiput–C1 and C1–C2, some of which is 'paradoxical' or 'snaking' motion (upper cervical extension and lower cervical flexion and produced by capital protraction, and the opposite produced by capital retraction). By controlling the motion between the orthosis and trunk, this snaking motion presumably can be controlled.

Benzel et al[15] found that a plastic Minerva orthosis provides better control of this motion compared to a standard type of halo vest.

Although popular and widely used, standard halo vests still have several problems.[13,81,125,240] Several authors have reported that a disturbingly large amount of motion occurs during activities of daily living – from 31% to 70% of the full normal range of motion.[6,122,133,134,229] It should be remembered that the 4% of normal flexion–extension range of motion reported by Johnson et al[113] was produced by subjects performing voluntary flexion–extension efforts in a seated posture, and not postural changes or activities of daily living.

Closely related to the large, undesired motion allowed by standard halo vests is the problem of large unintentional loads applied across the neck during their wear. Several authors

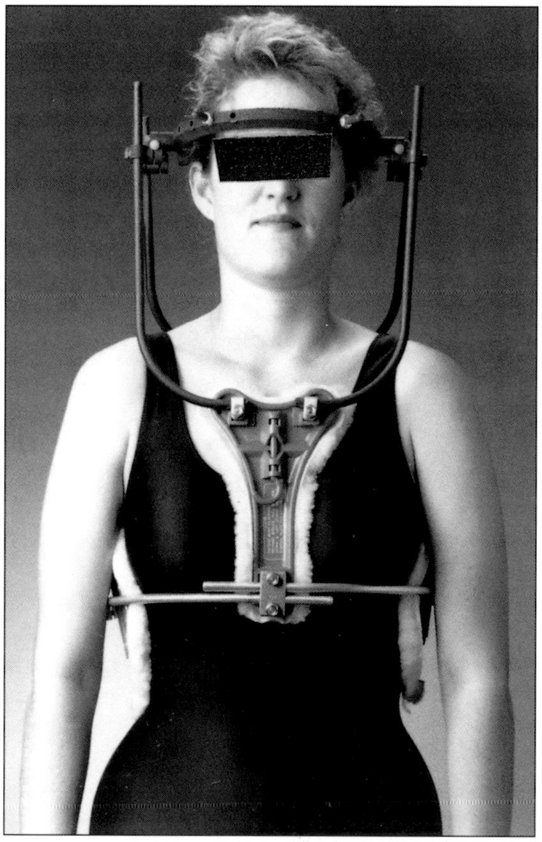

a

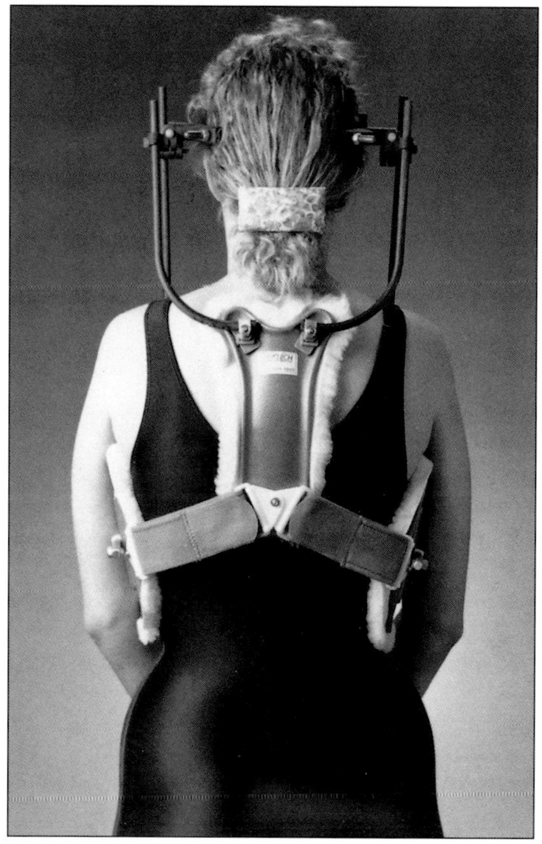

c

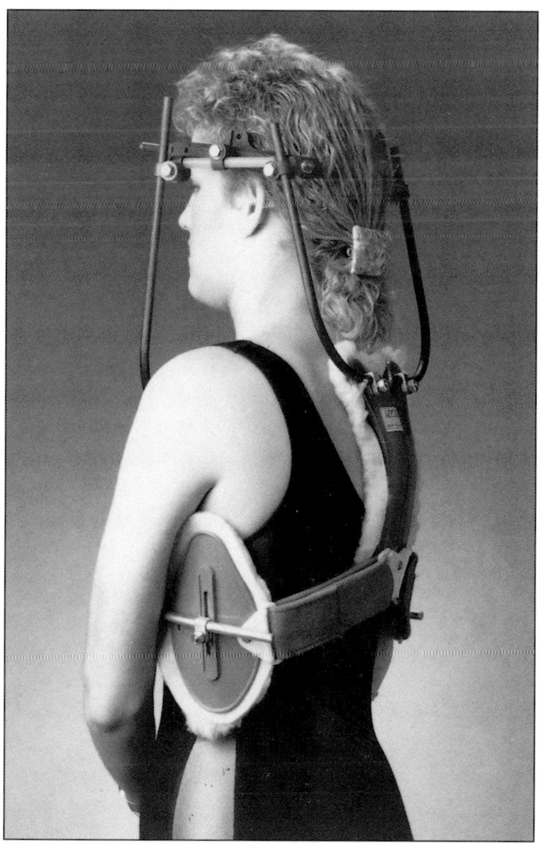

b

Figure 3.6
Levtech halo vest designed by Krag and Beynnon. The anterior sternal pad attaches to the side pads and contact fixation obtained anteriorly and laterally. Note the absence of shoulder straps; (b) lateral view of the pad system; (c) posterior view demonstration of the limited contact of the posterior pad to the interscapular area

have documented large distraction forces during shoulder shrug, coughing, and deep inspiration.[66,122,133,134] Others have shown high anteroposterior and mediolateral forces transmitted to the neck through the halo uprights.[228] These increased forces may lead to increased cranial pin loosening as well as, in the case of trauma patients, loss of intervertebral alignment.[33,64,98,118,122,125,132,159,180,226,228,237,244] Despite these problems, excellent results have been reported in the use of the halo with cervical spine trauma.[125,133,134]

Another group of problems with halo vests results from the covering by the vest of large areas of the thorax and upper abdomen (e.g. excessive warmth, sweating, and difficulty dressing). This also can contribute to the development of pressure sores under contact areas, particularly in insensate areas resulting from quadriplegia, as reviewed by Lind et al.[134]

In response to these problems, changes have been tried in halo-vest design. A halo fixed with screws to the clavicle was attempted,[8] but abandoned because of the uncontrolled movement between the clavicle, trunk, and the cervical spine. To decrease pin loosening, Garfin et al[81] designed and tested different pin tips as well as tightening torques. The forces exerted by the pins have been studied by Whitesides et al.[240] The effect of vest length was studied by Wang et al[229] who found that this did not affect intervertebral motion occurring above C4–C5. Paradoxically, at C6–C7 the longest vest worked least well. A fundamentally different halo-vest design and its initial biomechanical testing were reported by Krag and colleagues.[13,125,127] In that design, contact with the scapula and abdomen is completely avoided, and secure fitting of the vest to the thorax is made possible by means of four individually adjustable pads. Comparative biomechanical testing of this vest,[125] and clinical experience with it,[126,127,142] indicate that this vest provides a better grip of the thorax and thus allows less cervical motion to occur. In a recent clinical study of this halo vest,[126] allowed motion was only 43% of the motion allowed by standard vests. In the most recent and even larger clinical series,[221] the motion restriction is considerably more: down to 38% of that reported in standard vests.[122,133]

INTERNAL SUPPORT (FIXATION)

Surgically implanted devices designed for support of the cervical spine date back over a century, to when Hadra[92,93] used spinous process wires, initially to treat a cervical spine fracture–dislocation and later to treat Pott's disease. The use of internal support or fixation in the cervical spine has progressed and, in recent years, has developed rapidly. Along with internal fixation, the use of bone graft in promoting fusions has become widely used with the recognition that implant failure is likely unless solid fusion develops.[160] Indeed, in Hadra's first case, in which bone graft was not used, the spinous process wire loosened several weeks later and reoperation was necessary.

Despite the widespread use of bone graft with internal fixation, this certainly is not universal. Roy-Camille et al[194] did not use bone graft in a series of 221 posterior cervical fusions and Nielsen et al[160] found sufficient ligamentous healing without fusion, in their series of 30 patients with traumatic flexion injuries repaired by spinous process wiring alone.

Upper Cervical Spine (Occipital–C1–C2)

Wires or Hooks and Rods

Posterior wiring of C1–C2 is a standard procedure for immobilizing C1–C2; there are a variety of techniques. Mixter and Osgood,[151] in 1906, treated a chronic odontoid fracture by using 'stout braided silk ... passed about [the C1] posterior arch ... [and] firmly anchored by tying the silk band about the hooked spinous process of the axis ... '. Willard and Nicholson[242] described a technique widely attributed to Gallie – a loop passed around the C1 arch through which both ends were passed.

A high non-union rate with the above technique led to the use of an onlay bone graft held in place by the wire.[141] This accomplished two objectives: additional stability of the construct, and direct apposition and immobilization of the bone graft. Fusion rates of more than 90% were attained using two separate grafts on either side of the spinous process, under either one or two loops or wire.[32,88,215] Several modifications of this technique, first described by McGraw and Rusch, have been developed.[3,48,74,136,246] A disadvantage of the C1–C2 wiring is the limited ability to maintain a posteriorly directed force on C1, which is important, for example, in an anteriorly displaced odontoid fracture. With this in mind, Forsyth et al[76] described using a rib allograft anchored with sublaminar wires from C1 to C3.

An alternative method for achieving anteroposterior control of C1 is to immobilize the occiput–C1–C2 instead of C1–C3. However, with this immobilization there is also difficulty in achieving occiput–C2 anteroposterior control. In addition, there is greater mobility at occiput–C1 than at C2–C3, and there is difficulty and risk in achieving secure fixation to the occiput.

Many of the occiput–C1 fixation techniques[45,47,87,188,196] use internal fixation methods which are more secure than wire alone to overcome this relatively high level of occiput–C1 mobility. Wires have been used in combination with Luque rods[31,107,147,182] or Harrington rods.[157] Screws and plates have been used with no reconstruction plates,[59] Roy-Camille plates,[193] and others.[72,102] Other authors have suggested that internal fixation for occipitocervical fusion is unnecessary and increases the likelihood of surgical complications;[65] these authors have recently reported a fusion rate of 89% at an average of 12.8 weeks.

An alternative technique for C1–C2 fixation is the use of a hook and clamp system developed by Tucker in 1963 and named for Halifax, Nova Scotia where it was developed.[106,150,191,224] Although the absence of sublaminar wires and, as originally recommended, of bone graft initially made this technique appealing, complications of clamp loosening and increased pseudoarthrosis rates decreased its use.[46] Recently a report by Moskovich and Crockard reported an 80% C1–C2 fusion rate in which a Halifax clamp was used with the addition of an interposed bone graft. However, clamp loosening was still a problem in 20% of patients. A new clamp design (Codman and Shurtleff, Inc., Randolph, MA) is intended to lower the loosening rate.

Screws

In certain instances, for example with a hypoplastic, fractured, or surgically removed lamina, posterior wiring of C1 is not possible. In these cases posterior fixation with screws can be used, such a case first being described by Barbour,[12,58,211] who used two coronally oriented screws inserted from a bilateral approach to C1. Another method, described by Magerl,[144] uses a single posterior incision and, on each side, a screw which enters the C2 inferior articular process from below, angles up and anteriorly across the C1–C2 facet joint, and just penetrates the anterior cortex of the C1 lateral mass. This screw fixation is stronger and more rigid than wire fixation,[95] but is a technically exacting procedure with little margin for error and a large potential for neurologic and vascular damage. Magerl and Seeman,[144] however, have reported good results with this technique.

Screws can also be used anteriorly in the upper cervical region. The first use of odontoid screws for dens fractures is generally credited to both Nakanishi et al.,[158] Magerl,[144] and Bohler[18] who began using this type of fixation in 1978. Their reports,[144] as well as those of others,[1,22,67–69,84,121,131,152] have been sanguine in the use of this demanding technique. Biomechanical studies of odontoid screw fixation showed no significant difference between the use of one compared to two screws in oblique loading conditions in type II fractures.[197] There was a probable increase in torsional stability with two screws, but the authors questioned the clinical relevance of this increase. Another study examined the stability of single screw fixation in either type II or type III fractures.[52] They found that single screw fixation of either type II or III odontoid fracture provided approximately half of the strength provided by the intact dens. The screws failed by bending in type II fractures and cutting out in type III fractures.

Although attractive because this fixation preserves the almost 50% cervical rotation that occurs at the C1–C2 level, it is a very demanding technique, requiring meticulous set-up and biplanar fluoroscopy.

Anterior plates in the upper cervical spine have been reported, but clinical usefulness remains to be seen.[217–219]

Lower Cervical Spine

Spinous Process Wires

The first detailed description of posterior cervical wiring was by Ryerson and Christopher.[195] Their initial construct was without bone graft and involved wiring the middle of the C6 spinous process to the middle of the C7 spinous process. The former process broke after 9 weeks, prompting Ryerson and Christopher to reoperate using bone graft and positioning the wire around the C6 lamina and the whole of the C7 process.

The initial posterior cervical wiring, credited to Hadra[92,93] and performed in 1891, consisted of a figure-of-eight construct between the C6 and C7 spinous processes, which, however, required revision several weeks later. Gallie,[79,80] who was also an early pioneer in cervical wiring, gave no real description of his method, except that 'the spine of the two vertebrae involved [were fastened] together with fine steel wire'. Rogers[189,190] and later Forsyth et al.,[76] Bohlman,[20] and others[199,207] further modified the wiring techniques. However, differences in clinical outcome have not been documented between the different wiring techniques.[76,124]

Of these various wiring techniques, the Forsyth technique is a fairly simple procedure and includes the largest amount of spinous process within the wire loop. Because of the strength of spinous processes (indicated by the rarity of their fracturing after spinous process wiring), unless they are absent or fractured, the risk from placement of sublaminar wires in the lower cervical spine is probably unwarranted.[21,70]

Although no studies have documented any effect on clinical outcome by the type and diameter of wire used, these variables differ among authors. Two strands of 24- or 26-gauge wire twisted together[187,233] provide easy handling because of low flexural rigidity, and yet still have adequately high tensile strength. Multistrand cables, for example those developed by Songer et al,[214] are likewise attractive because of the even lower flexural rigidity without loss of adequate tensile strength. Multi-filament cables, however, are more difficult to secure: they require knotting or use of a special crimping fixation system.

Articular Process (Facet) Wires and Posterior Plates

When the lamina is not intact (e.g. fractured) or is absent (e.g. after laminectomy), several options are still available for performing a posterior arthrodesis. Robinson and Southwick[188] and others[37] described using wires passed through the inferior articular process. Recently these wires have been fixed to Harrington compression rods[82,157] which restricts cervical spine motion to 20% of normal.[86] Although the Harrington rod is probably less rigid than posterior plates, the graft bed is less obstructed and the risks associated with placement of lateral mass screws are avoided.

Articular process wiring is also useful in treating superior articular process fractures.[35] A wire is passed from the intact inferior articular process of the vertebrae above, obliquely down and around the spinous process of the fractured vertebrae. This wire applies a 'de-rotation force' which resists axial rotation and unilateral forward subluxation. This construct may be reinforced by spinous process wiring with a second wire.

Posterior plates have been used since the 1950s according to Roy-Camille and Saillant.[192] The plates, designed for use throughout the cervical spine, are flat, constructed of stainless steel and have holes placed 13 mm apart. Roy-Camille et al[194] describe placing the screw in the middle of the lateral mass at its most prominent point (the 'hillock') and directing it perpendicular to the longitudinal axis of the lateral mass and 10° laterally to avoid the vertebral artery. In their series of 221 patients, postoperative displacement of 5° or more occurred in only 6% of patients, and fusion occurred spontaneously without bone graft. Others also report good or excellent results with this method.[7,44,54,62,198]

An alternative to the posterior plate is the hook plate, which replaces the lower screw with a sublaminar hook attached just medial to the facet joint. Described by Magerl et al,[145] the hook plate produces less risk from lateral mass screw placement (because there is only one screw per plate) and yet still provides more rigid fixation than do wires.

Different screw placement methods for posterior plates have been studied.[5,99,153] One study showed that the longer screws allowed by an orientation anterolateral and parallel to the facet provide a stiffer construct than do the shorter screws resulting from the Roy-Camille technique, which tended to fail by screw pull-out.[5,99,153] However, questions still remain regarding the biomechanics of unicortical versus bicortical purchase, and regarding the trade-offs between the biomechanical and the safety of different methods of screw insertion.

Recently Grob et al[90,175,227] have developed an external fixator for diagnostic use in the cervical spine. Their external fixator, compared to one used in the lumbar spine, reduced flexion–extension by the same amount (approximately 50%), but was less effective in reducing lateral bending. Despite this, they stated that patients exhibited significant pain relief after temporary fixation and subsequent fusion, the performance of which was largely based upon the results from external fixator use.

Anterior Plates

Bohler[17] described the first use of plates anteriorly on the cervical spine in 1964, although the plates used by Bohler and others[30,168] were not specifically designed for this use. Later plates were designed specifically for the cervical spine.[19,129]

Bohler's work was advanced by Oroszco, Caspar, and others who promoted the clinical use of anterior plates.[30,38,78,100,129,163,219] A more detailed discussion of the early uses and testing of these plates is given elsewhere.[124] Plates in use today involve either bicortical or unicortical screws.[38,156] As reviewed elsewhere[124], the literature does not make a convincing case for the use of bicortical implantation to reduce screw loosening. This, plus the development by Lesoin et al[130] and later Morscher et al[156] of a unicortical screw with a locking set screw to prevent loosening, allows avoidance of the hazards involved in bicortical screw fixation in the cervical spine. The set screw expands one end of the screw which 'locks' the screw against either the plate[156] or the bone.[130] The Morscher screw and plate are titanium; the screws are either solid or hollow, fenestrated, and plasma sprayed. The latter allow bony ingrowth, but breakage of the hollow screws has recently been reported.[105]

The ease of implantation, the expected complete absence of graft extrusion, and the immediate stability of the anterior plate have led to increasing use of anterior plates in recent years.[2,83,185] Whether the benefits outweigh the risks remains an issue for further study. For multilevel arthrodeses this seems more likely to be true than for single-level ones, although even for the latter the use of plates may also be shown to be worth while.

Anterior Bone Grafts

Anterior interbody grafts, although not strictly implants, do function in a load-bearing capacity. First used by Bailey[9] and Badgley in 1952, this technique was later modified by Robinson and Smith[186] to include the use of a tricortical iliac 'horseshoe' graft. Variations of the interbody graft include the Cloward unicortical dowel-shaped graft,[40] a trapezoidal tricortical graft,[210] and fibular grafts,[235] as well as a double mortise and tenon graft.[142,216]

Mechanical testing of the interbody grafts showed that the tricortical graft was strongest primarily because the end-plates were left intact. Anterior dislodging of the graft can be a problem especially with longer grafts. One solution is the double mortise and tenon graft which 'locks' into place and prevents displacement.[142,216]

Mechanical Testing

There are several in vitro studies which compare different internal fixation devices for the cervical spine.[41,85,220,225] The most extensive of these reports[41] compared several different wiring techniques, and posterior and anterior plates. The major findings were that there were no significant differences between implants for most of the forces measured, and that the anterior plate alone was significantly weaker than the others for compression or flexion-induced strain.

Polymethylmethacrylate

The first application of polymethylmethacrylate in the spine was in 1959 by Knight[120] who used it for fusion in place of bone graft.[119] Although others have reported its use in place of bone graft in trauma patients,[23,117,212] its use in patients with a normal life expectancy remains controversial.55,138,239 Concern regarding the longevity of the polymethylmethacrylate construct and increased rates of infection, as well as results from animal studies[236,238] and mechanical testing,[170,172] have limited its use in patients with normal life expectancy.

However, in patients with a very short life expectancy polymethymethacrylate can provide very beneficial internal support. The typical patient will present with metastatic disease to the cervical spine and have either unrelenting pain or impending or actual neurologic compromise. These patients usually succumb to the disease before any long-term benefit from a bone graft is realized and before the bone resorption adjacent to the polymethylmethacrylate occurs. The morbidity of the bone graft harvest and the inconvenience of postoperative immobilization are thereby avoided.[56,123,165,206]

REFERENCES

1 Aebi M, Etter C, Coscia M. Fractures of the odontoid process: treatment with anterior screw fixation. *Spine* **14**: 1065–1070, 1989.

2 Aebi M, Zuber K, Marchesi D et al. Treatment of cervical spine injuries with anterior plating. Indications, techniques and results. *Spine* **16**: S38–S45, 1991.

3 Althoff B, Goldie F. Cervical collar in rheumatoid atlantoaxial subluxation: a radiographic comparison. *Ann Rheum Dis* **39**: 485–489, 1980.

4 Amevo B, Aprill C, Bogduk N. Abnormal instantaneous axes of rotation in patients with neck pain. *Spine* **17**: 748–756, 1992.

5 An HS, Gordin R, Renner K. Anatomic considerations for plate-screw fixation of the cervical spine. *Spine* **16**: S548–S551, 1991.

6 Anderson PA, Budorick TE, Easton KB et al. Failure of halo vest to prevent in vivo motion in patients with injured cervical spines. *Spine* **16**: S501–S505, 1991.

7 Anderson PA, Henley MB, Grady MS, et al. Posterior cervical arthrodesis with AO reconstruction plates and bone graft. *Spine* **16**: S72–9, 1991.

8 Appleby DM, Fu FH, Mears DC. Halo-clavicle traction. *J Trauma* **24**: 452–455, 1984.

9 Bailey RW, Badgley CE. Stabilization of the cervical spine by anterior fusion. *J Bone Joint Surg* **42**: 565–594, 1960.

10 Bailey RW, Sherk HH et al. (eds) *The Cervical Spine*, 2nd ed. Philadelphia: Lea & Febiger 1–881, 1989.

11 Ball J, Meijers KAE. On cervical mobility. *Ann Rheum Dis* **23**: 429, 1964.

12 Barbour JR. Screw fixation in fractures of the odontoid process. *South Austr Clin* **5**(1): 20–24, 1971.

13 Barr J Jr, Krag MH, Pierce DS. Cranial traction and the halo orthosis. In Bailey RW, Sherk HH, et al (eds) *The Cervical Spine*, 2nd ed., Chap. 6. Philadelphia: JB Lippincott; 299–311, 1989.

14 Barton JW, Margolis MT. Rotational obstruction of the vertebral artery at the atlantoaxial joint. *Neuroradiology* **9**: 117, 1975;

15 Benzel EC, Hadden TA, Saulsbery CM. A comparison of the Minerva and halo jackets for stabilization of the cervical spine. *J Neurosurg* **70**: 411–414, 1989.

16 Blanchard RS, Kottke FJ. The study of degenerative changes of the cervical spine in relation to age. *Bulletin of the University of Minnesota Hospital* **24**: 470, 1953.

17 Bohler J. Sofort- und Frühbehandlung traumatischer Querschnittlähmungen *Zeitschr Orthoäd Grenzgebiete* **103**: 512–528, 1967.

18 Böhler J. Anterior stabilization for acute fractures and non-unions of the dens. *J Bone Joint Surg* **64**: 18–27, 1982.

19 Böhler J, Gaudernak T. Anterior plate stabilization for fracture–dislocations of the lower cervical spine. *J Trauma* **20**: 203–205, 1980.

20 Bohlmann HH. Surgical management of cervical spine fractures and dislocations. *Am Acad Ortho Surg Instruct Course Lect* **34**: 163–186, 1985.

21 Braakman R, Penning L. *Injuries of the Cervical Spine*, 1–262. Amsterdam: Excerpta Medica, 1971.

22 Borne GM, Bedon GL, Pinaudeau M, et al. Odontoid process fracture osteosynthesis with a direct screw fixation technique in 9 consecutive cases. *J Neurosurg* **68**: 223–226, 1988.

23 Branch CL Jr, Kelly DL Jr. Failure of stabilization of the spine with methylmethacrylate. A retrospective analysis of twenty-four cases (letter). *J Bone Joint Surg* **69**: 1108–1110, 1987.

24 Breig A. *Biomechanics of the Central Nervous System. Some Basic Normal and Pathological Phenomena Concerning Spine, Discs and Cord.* Stockholm: Almqvist & Wiksell, 1960.

25 Breig A. Overstretching of a circumscribed pathological tension on the spinal cord–A basic cause of symptoms in cord disorders. *J Biomech* **3**: 7–9, 1970.

26 Breig A. The therapeutic possibilities of surgical bioengineering in incomplete spinal cord lesions. *Paraplegia* **9**: 173–182, 1972.

27 Breig A. Pathological stress in the pons-cord-tissue tract and its alleviation by neurosurgical means. *Clin Neurosurg* **20**: 85–94, 1973.

28 Breig A. *Adverse Mechanical Tension in the Central Nervous System.* Stockholm: Almqvist & Wiksell, 1978.

29 Breig A, El-Nadi AP. Biomechanics of the cervical spinal cord. Relief of contact pressure on and overstretching of the spinal cord. *Acta Radiol Diagn (Stockh)* **4**: 602–624, 1966.

30 Bremer AM, Nguyen TQ. Internal metal plate fixation combined with anterior interbody fusion in cases of cervical spine injury. *Neurosurgery* **12**: 649–653, 1983.

31 Bridwell KH. Treatment of a markedly displaced hangman's fracture with a Luque rectangle and a posterior fusion in a 71 year old man. Case report. *Spine* **11**: 49–52, 1986.

32 Brooks AL, Jenkins EB. Atlanto-axial arthrodesis by the wedge compression method. *J Bone Joint Surg* **60**: 279–284, 1978;

33 Bucci MN, Dauser RC, Maynard FA, et al. Management of post-traumatic cervical spine instability: operative fusion versus halo vest immobilization. Analysis of 49 cases. *J Trauma* **28**: 1001–1006, 1988.

34 Bucy PC, Heimburger RF, Oberhill HRO. Compression of the cervical spinal cord by herniated intervertebral discs. *J Neurosurg* **5**: 471–92, 1948.

35 Cahill DW, Bellesarrisue R, Ducker TB. Bilateral facet to spinous process fusion: a new technique for posterior spinal fusion after trauma. *Neurosurgery* **13**: 1–4, 1983.

36 Cailliet R (ed.). *Neck and Arm Pain.* Philadelphia: Davis Co., 1972.

37 Callahan RA, Johnson RM, Margolis RN, et al. Cervical facet fusion for control on instability following laminectomy. *J Bone Joint Surg* **59**: 991–1002, 1977.

38 Caspar W. Anterior stabilization with the trapezial osteosynthetic plate technique in cervical spine injuries. In: Kehr P, Weidner A (eds), *Cervical Spine I*, 198–204 New York: Springer-Verlag, 1987.

39 Clark CR, Goel VK, Galles K, et al. Kinematics of the occipito-atlanto-axial complex. *Transactions of the Cervical Spine Research Society*, 1986.

40 Cloward AB. The anterior approach for removal of ruptured cervical disks. *J Neurosurg* **15**: 602–617, 1958.

41 Coe JD, Warden KE, Sutterlin CE III, et al. Biomechanical evaluation of cervical spinal stabilization methods in a human cadaveric model. *Spine* **14**: 1122–1131, 1989.

42 Colachis SC Jr, Strohm BR, Ganter EL. Cervical spine motion in normal women: radiography study of effect of cervical collars. *Arch Phys Med Rehab* **54**: 161–169, 1973.

43 Condon BR, Hadley DM. Quantification of cord deformation and dynamics during flexion and extension of the cervical spine using MR imaging. *J Comput Assist Tomogr* **12**: 947–955, 1988.

44 Cooper PR, Cohen A, Rosiello A, et al. Posterior stabilization of cervical spine fractures and subluxations using plates and screws. *Neurosurgery* **23**: 300–306, 1988.

45 Crellin RQ, MacCabe JJ, Hamilton EBD. Severe subluxation of the cervical spine in rheumatoid arthritis. *J Bone Joint Surg* **52**: 244–251, 1970.

46 Cybulski GR, Stone JL, Crowell RM, et al. Use of Halifax interlaminar clamps for posterior C1–C2 arthrodesis. *Neurosurgery* **22**: 429–431, 1988.

47 de Groote W, Vercauteren M, Uyttendaele D. Occipitocervical fusion in rheumatoid arthritis. *Acta Orthop Belg* **47**: 685–698, 1981.

48 de los Reyes RA, Malik GM, Wu KK, et al. A new surgical approach to stabilizing C1–2 subluxation in rheumatoid arthritis. *Henry Ford Hospital Medical Journal* **29**: 127–130, 1981.

49 Deng YC, Goldsmith W. Response of a human head/neck/upper torso replica to dynamic loading. II. Analytical/numerical model. *J Biomech* **20**: 487–497, 1987.

50 Depreux R, Mestdagh H. Anatomic functionelle de l'articulation sous occipatale. *Lille Med* **19**: 122, 1974.

51 Doherty BJ, Heggeness MH. The quantitative anatomy of the atlas. *Proceedings of Cervical Spine Research Society*, 54–55, 1992;

52 Doherty BJ, Heggeness MH, Esses SI. A biomechanical study of odontoid fractures and fracture fixation. *Spine* **18**: 178–184, 1993.

53 Dohrmann GJ, Panjabi MM. 'Standardized' spinal cord trauma: biomechanical parameters and lesion volume. *Surg Neurol* **6**: 263–267, 1976.

54 Domenella G, Berlanda P, Bassi G. Posterior-approach osteosynthesis of the lower cervical spine by the Roy–Camille technique. (Indications and first results.) *Ital J Orthop Traumatol* **8**: 235–244, 1982.

55 Duff TA. Surgical stabilization of traumatic cervical spine dislocation using methylmethacrylate: long term results in 26 patients. *J Neurosurg* **64**: 39–44, 1986.

56 Dunn EJ. Role of methylmethacrylate in the stabilization and replacement of tumors of the cervical spine: a project of the Cervical Spine Research Society. *Spine* **2**: 15–24, 1977.

57 Dunsker SB, Colley DP, Mayfield FH. Kinematics of the cervical spine. *Clin Neurosurg* **25**: 174, 1977.

58 Dutoit G. Lateral atlantoaxial arthrodesis: a screw fixation technique. *South Afr J Surg* **14**: 9–12, 1976.

59 Dvorak J, Panjabi MM, Gerber M, et al. CT-functional diagnostics of the rotatory instability of the upper cervical spine. 1. An experimental study on cadavers. *Spine* **12**: 197–205, 1968.

60 Dvorak J, Schneider E, Saldinger P, et al. Biomechanics of the craniocervical region: the alar and transverse ligaments. *J Orthop Res* **6**: 452–461, 1988.

61 Dvorak J, Artinnes JA, Panjabi M, et al. Age and gender related normal motion of the cervical spine. *Spine* **17**: (10S): S393–S398, 1992.

62 Ebraheim NA, An HS, Jackson WT, et al. Internal fixation of the unstable cervical spine using posterior Roy–Camille plates: preliminary report. *J Orthop Traumatol* **3**: 23–28, 1989.

63 Ecklin U. *Die Alterveränderungen der Halswirbelsäule.* Berlin: Springer-Verlag, 1960.

64 Ekong CEV, Schwartz ML, Tator CH, et al. Odontoid fracture: management with early mobilization using the halo device. *Neurosurgery* **9**: 631–637, 1981.

65 Elia M, Mazzara JT, Fielding JW. Onlay technique for occipitocervical fusion. *Clin Orthop Rel Res* **280**: 170–174, 1992.

66 Ersmark H, Kalen R, Löwenhielm P. A methodical study of force measurements in three patients with odontoid fractures treated with a strain gauge-equipped halo-vest. *Spine* **13**: 433–455, 1988.

67 Esses SI, Bednar DA. Screw fixation of odontoid fractures and non-unions. *Spine* **16**: S483–S485, 1991.

68 Etter C, Coscia M, Ganz R, et al. Bone screw osteosynthesis of dens fractures. Technical surgical aspects and results. *Unfallchirurg* **92**: 220–226, 1989.

69 Etter C, Coscia M, Jaberg H. Direct anterior fixation of dens fractures with a cannulated screw system. *Spine* **16**: S25–S32, 1991.

70 Fairbank TJ. Spinal fusion after laminectomy for cervical myelopathy. *Proceed Soc Med* **64**: 634–636, 1971.

71 Fick R. *Handbuch der Anatomie und Mechanik der Gelenke unter Berücksichtigung der Bewegenden Muskeln*, 1904–1912. Jena: G Fischer.

72 Fidler MW. Posterior instrumentation of the spine: an experimental comparison of various possible techniques. *Spine* **11**: 367–372, 1988.

73 Fielding JW. Normal and selected abnormal motion of the cervical spine from the second cervical vertebra to the seventh cervical vertebra based on cineroentgenography. *J Bone Joint Surg [Am]* **46**: 1779, 1964.

74 Fielding JW, Hawkins RJ, Ratzan SA. Spine fusion for atlanto-axial instability. *J Bone Joint Surg* **58**: 400–407, 1976.

75 Fisher SV, Bowar JF, Awad FA, et al. Cervical orthoses effect on cervical spine motion: roentgenographic and goniometric method of study. *Arch Phys Med Rehab* **58**: 109–115, 1977.

76 Forsyth HF, Alexander EA, Davis CH, et al. Advantages of early spine fusion in the treatment of fracture-dislocations of the cervical spine. *J Bone Joint Surg* **41**: 17–36, 195.

77 *Francis (1952) quoted in CSRS p.55*

78 Fuentes JM, Blancourt J, Vlahovitch B, et al. Tear drop fractures. Contribution to the study of its mechanism and os osteo-disco-ligamentous lesions. *Neurochirurgie* **29**: 129–134, 1963;

79 Gallie WE. Skeletal traction in the treatment of fractures and dislocations of the cervical spine. *Ann Surg* **106**: 770–776, 1937.

80 Gallie WE. Fractures and dislocations of the cervical spine. *Am J Surg* **46**: 495–499, 1939.

81 Garfin SR, Lee TQ, Roux RD, et al. Structural behavior of the halo orthosis pin-bone interface: biomechanical evaluation of standard and newly designed stainless steel halo fixation pins. *Spine* **11**: 977–981, 1986.

82 Garfin SR, Moore MR, Marshall LF. A modified technique for cervical facet fusions. *Clin Orthop* **230**: 149–153, 1988.

83 Garvey RA, Eismont FJ, Roberti LJ. Anterior decompression, strut bone grafting, and caspar plate stabilization for unstable cervical spine fracture and or dislocation. *Spine* **17**: S431–S435, 1992.

84 Geisler FH, Cheng C, Poka A, et al. Anterior screw fixation of posteriorly displaced type II odontoid fracture. *Neurosurgery* **25**: 30–38, 1989.

85 Gill K, Paschal S, Corin J, et al. Posterior plating of the cervical spine: a biomechanical comparison of different posterior fusion techniques. *Spine* **13**: 813–816, 1988.

86 Goel VK, Clark CR, Harris KG, et al. Kinematics of the cervical spine: effects of multiple total laminectomy and facet wiring. *J Orthop Res* **6**: 611–619, 1988.

87 Grantham SA, Dick HM, Thompson RC Jr, et al. Occipitocervical arthrodesis, indications, technique and results. *Clin Orthop* **65**: 118–129, 1969.

88 Griswold DM, Albright JA, Schiffman E, et al. Atlanto-axial fusion for instability. *J Bone Joint Surg* **60**: 285–292, 1978;

89 Grob D, Dvorak J, Panjabi M, et al. Posterior occipitocervical fusion. A preliminary report of a new technique. *Spine* **16**: S17–S24, 1991.

90 *Grob* et al, *submitted Clin Orthop*

91 Hadley LH. Anatomicroradiographic studies: development and the cervical region. *The Spine*. Springfield IL: Charles C. Thomas, 1956.

92 Hadra BE. The classic: wiring of the vertebrae as a means of immobilization in fractures and Potts' disease. *Clin Orthop* **112**: 4–8, 1975.

93 Hadra BE. Wiring of the spinous process in injury and Potts' disease. *Trans Am Orthop Assoc* **4**: 206, 1981.

94 Halliday DR, Sullivan UR, Hollinshead WH, et al. Torn cervical ligaments: necropsy examination of normal cervical region. *J Trauma* **4**: 219–232, 1964.

95 Hanson P, Sharkey N, Montesano PX. Anatomic and biomechanical study of C1–C2 posterior arthrodesis techniques. *Proceedings of the Cervical Spine Research Society, 16th Annual Meeting*, 100–101, Key Biscayne FL, 1988.

96 Hart DL, Johnson RM, Simmons EF, et al. Review of cervical othoses. *Phys Ther* **58**: 857–860, 1978.

97 Hartman JT, Palumbo F, Hill BJ. Cineradiography of the braced normal cervical spine: a comparative study of five commonly used cervical orthoses. *Clin Orthop* **109**: 97–102, 1975.

98 Haw DW. Collapse of cervical spine treated by Down's Ace mark III halo assembly. *BMJ* **285**: 410, 1982.

99 Heller JG, Carlson GD, Abitbol JJ, et al. Anatomic consideration of the Roy–Camille and Magerl techniques for screw placement in the lower cervical spine. *Spine* **16**: S552–S557, 1991;

100 Hermann HD. Metal plate fixation after anterior fusion of unstable fracture dislocations of the cervical spine. *Acta Neurochir (Wien)* **32**: 101–111, 1975.

101 Herzenberg JE, Hensinger RN, Dedrick DK. Emergency transport and positioning of young children who have an injury of the cervical spine. *J Bone Joint Surg [Am]* **71**: 15–22, 1989;

102 Heywood AWB, Learmonth ID, Thomas M. Internal fixation for occipito-cervical fusion. *J Bone Joint Surg* **70**: 708–711, 1988;

103 Hollinshead HW (ed.) The neck. In *The Head and Neck*, 2nd ed; 501–603. MA: Harper & Row, 1968.

104 Hollinshead WH. The back. In *Anatomy for Surgeons*, Vol III: *The Back & Limbs*, 79–206. New York: Harper & Row, 1969.

105 Hollowell JP, Morgese V, Reinartz J, et al. Failure of synthes anterior cervical fixation device by fracture or Morscher screws. *Proceedings of the Cervical Spine Research Society* 185, 1992:

106 Holness RO, Huestis WS, Howes WJ, et al. Posterior stabilization with an interlaminar clamp in cervical injuries: technical notes and review of the long term experience with the method. *Neurosurgery* **14**: 318–322, 1984.

107 Itoh T, Tsuji H, Katoh Y, et al. Occipito-cervical fusion reinforced by Luque's segmental spinal instrumentation for rheumatoid disease. *Spine* **13**: 1234–1238, 1988.

108 Jackson H. The diagnosis of minimal atlanto-axial subluxation. *Br J Radiol* **23**: 672, 1950.

109 Jauregui N, Loncoln T, Mubarak S, et al. Surgically related upper cervical spine canal anatomy. *Proceedings of the Cervical Spinal Research Society*, 82–83, 1992.

110 Jofe MH, White AA, Panjabi MM. Clinically relevant kinematics of the cervical spine. In Sherk HH et al. (eds), *The Cervical Spine*; 57–69, Philadelphia: JB Lippincott, 1989.

111 Johnson RM, Southwick WO. Surgical approaches to the spine. In Rothman RH, Simeone FA, (eds), *The Spine*, 98–103 Philadelphia: WB Saunders, 1975:

112 Johnson RM, Crelin ES, White AA III, et al. Some new observations on the functional anatomy of the lower cervical spine. *Clin Orthop* **111**: 192–200, 1975.

113 Johnson RM, Hart DL, Simmons EF, et al. Cervical orthoses: a study comparing their effectiveness in restricting cervical motion in normal subjects. *J Bone Joint Surg* **59**: 332–339, 1977.

114 Johnson RM, Hart DL, Owen JR, et al. The Yale cervical orthosis: an evaluation of its effectiveness in restricting cervical motion in normal subjects and a comparison with other cervical orthoses. *Phys Ther* **48**: 865–871, 1978.

115 Johnson RM, Own JR, Hart DL, et al. Cervical orthoses: a guide to their selection and use. *Clin Orthop* **154**: 34–45, 1981.

116 Jones MD. Cineradiographic studies of the collar-immobilized cervical. *J Neurosurg* **17**: 633–637, 1960.

117 Kelly DL Jr, Alexander E Jr, Davis CH Jr, et al. Acrylic fixation of atlanto-axial dislocations. Technical note. *J Neurosurg* **36**: 366–371, 1972.

118 Kelly EG. Loss of reduction in cervical fracture–dislocations managed in the halo cast. *Proceed Am Ac Orthop Surg Ann Mtng*, 1981.

119 Knight G. Paraspinal acrylic inlays in treatment of cervical and lumbar spondylosis and other conditions. *Lancet* **ii**: 147–149, 1959;

120 Knight G. Acrylic inlay for instability of the cervical spine. *J Bone Joint Surg [Br]* **49**: 384, 1967.

121 Knöringer P. Double-threaded compression screws in osteosynthesis of acute fractures of the odontoid process. In Voth D, Glees O (eds) *Disease in the Cranio-Cervical Junction*, 217. New York: de Gruyter, 1987.

122 Koch RA, Nickel VL, The halo vest: an evaluation of motion and forces across the neck. *Spine* **3**: 103–107, 1978.

123 Kostuik JP, Errico TJ, Gleason TF, et al. Spinal stabilization of vertebral column tumors. *Spine* **13**: 250–256, 1988.

124 Krag MH. Biomechanics of the cervical spine, including bracing, surgical constructs, and orthoses. In Frymoyer JW, ed., *The Adult Spine: Principles and Practice* 929–965, 1991.

125 Krag MH, Beynnon BD. A new halo-vest: rationale, design and biomechanical comparison to standard halo-vest designs. *Spine* **13**: 228–235, 1988.

126 Krag MH, Longcope D. Improvement in cervical immobilization by halovest design change: four thoracic pads vs standard whole-torso vest. *Proceedings of the North American Spinal Society, 6th Annual Meeting*, Keystone, CO, 1991.

127 Krag MH, Beynnon BD, Gill K, et al. A new halovest: initial clinical experience and comparison to a 'standard' halovest. *Proceedings of the Cervical Spinal Research Society, 14th Annual Meeting*, Palm Beach, FL, 1986.

128 Krag MH, Seroussi RE, Wilder DG, et al. Internal displacement distribution from in vitro loading of human thoracic and lumbar spinal motion segment: experimental results and theoretical predictions. *Spine* **12**: 1001–1007, 1987.

129 Lesoin F, Cama A, Lozes G, et al. Anterior approach and plates in lower cervical posttraumatic lesions. *Surg Neurol* **21**: 581–587, 1982.

130 Lesoin F, Jomin M, Viaud C. Expanding bolt for anterior cervical spine osteosynthesis: technical note. *Neurosurgery* **12**: 458–459, 1983.

131 Lesoin F, Autricque A, Franz K, et al. Trancervical approach and screw fixation for upper cervical spine pathology. *Surg Neurol* **27**: 459–464, 1987.

132 Levine AM, Edwards CC. The management of traumatic spondylolisthesis of the axis. *J Bone Joint Surg* **67**: 217–226, 1985;.

133 Lind B, Sihlbom H, Nordwall A. Forces and motions across the neck in patients treated with halo vest. *Spine* **13**: 162–167, 1988;

134 Lind B, Sihlbom H, Nordwall A. Halovest treatment of unstable traumatic cervical spine injuries. *Spine* **13**: 425–432, 1988.

135 Liu YK, Clarke CL, Krieger KW. In: Sances A, Thomas DJ, Ewins CL et al. (eds) *Quantitative Geometry of Young Human Male Cervical Vertebrae. Mechanism of Head and Spine Trauma*, 417–431. New York, Goshen: Funterharnscheidt, 1986.

136 Louis R. *Surgery of the Spine: Surgical Anatomy and Operative Approaches.* New York: Springer-Verlag, 1983.

137 Lysell E. Motion in the cervical spine. *Acta Orthop Scand* **123**: 1–61, 1969.

138 McAfee PC, Bohlman HH, Ducker T, et al. Failure of stabilization of the spine with methylmethacrylate. *J Bone Joint Surg* **68**: 1145–1145, 1986.

139 McAfee PC, Cassidy JR, Davis RF, et al. Fusion of the occiput to the upper cervical spine. A review of 37 cases. *Spine* **16**: S490–S494, 1991.

140 McClain RF. Innervation of human cervical facets. *Proceedings of the Cervical Spine Research Society.* 49–50, 1992.

141 McGraw RW, Rusch RM. Atlanto-axial arthrodesis. *J Bone Joint Surg* **55**: 482–489, 1973;

142 McVeigh JF. Experimental cord crushes; with a special reference to the mechanical factors involved and subsequent changes in the areas of the cord affected. *Arch Surg* **7**: 573–600, 1923.

143 Magerl F. Sterilization of the lower thoracic and lumbar spine with external skeletal fixation. *Clin Orthop* **189**: 125–141, 1984;

144 Magerl F, Seeman P-S. Stable posterior fusion of the atlas and axis by transarticular screw fixation. In Kehr P, Weidner A (eds) *Cervical Spine I*, 322–327, New York: Springer-Verlag, 1987:

145 Magerl F, Grob D, Seemann P. Stable dorsal fusion of the cervical spine (C2–T1) using hook plates. In Kehr P, Weidner A (eds) *Cervical Spine I*, 217–221, New York: Springer-Verlag, 1987.

146 Mair WGP, Druckman R. The pathology of spinal cord lesions and their relation to the clinical features in protrusion of the cervical intervertebral discs. *Brain* **76**: 70–91, 1953.

147 Matsunaga S, Sakou T, Morizono Y, et al. Occipito-atlanto-axial fusion utilizing a rectangular rod. *Proceedings of the Cervical Spine Research Society, 16th Annual Meeting*, 106–107, Key Biscayne, FL, 1988.

148 Mayer T, Brady S. Tri-planar cervical spine motion assessment: methodology, normative data, age-related change and consistency of effort. *Proceedings of the Cervical Spine Research Society*, 138–139, 1992.

149 Millington PJ, Ellingsen JM, Hauswirth BE, et al. Thermoplastic Minerva body jacket. A practical alternative to the current methods of cervical spine stabilization. A clinical report. *Phys Ther* **67**: 223–225, 1987.

150 Mitsui H. A new operation for atlanto-axial arthrodesis. *J Bone Joint Surg* **66**: 442–445, 1984.

151 Mixter SJ, Osgood RB. Traumatic lesion of the atlas and axis. *Ann Surg* **51**: 193–207, 1910.

152 Montesano PX, Anderson PA, Schlehr F, et al. Odontoid fracture by anterior screw fixation. *Spine* **16**: S33–S37, 1991;

153 Montesano PX, Jauch E, Jonsson H Jr. Anatomic and biomechanical study of posterior cervical spine plate arthrodesis:

an evaluation of two different techniques of screw placement. *J Spin Dis* **5**: 301–305, 1993.
154 Moroney SP, Schultz AB, Miller JAA. Analysis and measurement of neck loads. *J Orthop Res* **6**: 713–720, 1988.
155 Moroney SP, Schultz AB, Miller JAA, et al. Load-displacement properties of lower cervical spine motion segments. *J Biomechan* **9**: 769–779, 1988.
156 Morscher E, Sutter F, Jenny H, et al. Die vordere Verplattung der Halswirbelsäule mit dem Hohlschrauben-Plattensystem aus Titanium. *Chirurg* **57**: 702–707, 1986.
157 Murphy MJ, Daniaux H, Southwick WO. Posterior cervical fusion with rigid internal fixation. *Orthop Clin North Am* **17**: 55–65, 1986.
158 Nakanishi T, Sasaki T, Tokita N, et al. Internal fixation for the odontoid fracture. *Orthop Trans* **6**: 176, 1982.
159 Nickel VH, Perry J, Garrett A, et al. The halo. A spinal skeleton traction fixation device. *J Bone Joint Surg* **50**: 1400–1409, 1968.
160 Nielsen FC, Annertz M, Persson L, et al. Posterior wiring without bony fusion in traumatic distractive flexion injuries of the mid to lower cervical spine. Long term follow-up in 30 patients. *Spine* **16**(4): 467–472, 1991.
161 Nissan M, Gilad I. The cervical and lumbar vertebrae: an anthropometric model. *Eng Med* **13**(3): 111–114, 1984.
162 Nolan JP Jr, Sherk HH. Biomechanical evaluation of the extensor musculature of the cervical spine. *Spine* **13**: 9–11, 1988.
163 Oliveira JC. Anterior plate fixation of traumatic lesions of the lower cervical spine. *Spine* **12**: 324–329, 1987.
164 Ommaya AK. Mechanical properties of tissues of the nervous system. *J Biomechan* **1**: 127–138, 1968.
165 Ono K, Tada K. Metal prosthesis of the cervical vertebra. *J Neurosurg* **42**: 562–566, 1975.
166 Orofino C, Sherman MS, Schechter D. Luschka's joint – A degenerative phenomenon. *J Bone Joint Surg* **42**: 853–858, 1960.
167 Panjabi M, White A III. Biomechanics of nonacute cervical spinal cord trauma. In Sherk HH et al (eds) *The Cervical Spine*, 2nd ed, 91–96, Philadelphia: JB Lippincott, 1989.
168 Panjabi MM, Wrathall JR. Biomechanical analysis of experimental spinal cord injury and functional loss. *Spine* **13**: 1365–1370, 1988.
169 Panjabi MM, White AA III, Johnson RM. Cervical spine biomechanics as a function of transection of components. *J Biomech* **8**: 327–336, 1975.
170 Panjabi MM, Dicker DB, Dohrmann GH. Biomechanical quantification of experimental spinal cord trauma. *J Biomech* **10**: 681–687, 1977.
171 Panjabi MM, White AA III, Keller D, et al. Stability of the cervical spine under tension. *J Biomech* **11**: 189–197, 1978.
172 Panjabi MM, Goel VK, Clark CR, et al. Biomechanical study of cervical spine stabilization with methylmethacrylate. *Spine* **10**: 198–203, 1985.
173 Panjabi MM, Summer DJ, Pelker RR, et al. Three-dimensional load-displacement curves due to forces on the cervical spine. *J Orthop Res* **4**: 152–161, 1986;
174 Panjabi MM, Duraceau J, Goel V, et al. Cervical human vertebrae quantitative three-dimensional anatomy of the middle and lower regions. *Spine* **16**: 861–869, 1991.
175 Panjabi MM, Lydon C, Vasavada D, et al. Biomechanical evaluation of diagnostic external fixation. *Proceedings of the Cervical Spine Research Society*, 59–60, 1992.
176 Parke WW, Sherk HH. Normal adult anatomy. In Sherk HH, et al (eds) *The Cervical Spine*, 2nd ed, 15–18, Philadelphia: JB Lippincott, 1989.
177 Pavlov H, Torg JS, Robie B, et al. Cervical spinal stenosis: determinations with vertebral body ratio method. *Radiology* **164**: 771–775, 1987.
178 Payne EE, Spillane JD. The cervical spine. An anatomico-pathological study of 70 specimens (using a special technique) with particular reference to the problem of cervical spondylosis. *Brain* **80**: 571–596, 1957.
179 Penning L, Wilmink JT. Rotation of the cervical spine: a CT study on normal subjects. *Spine* **12**: 732–738, 1987.
180 Perry J. Halo in spinal abnormalities – practical factors and avoidance of complications. *Orthop Clin North Am* **3**: 69–80, 1972;
181 Perry J, Nickel VL. Total cervical spine fusion for neck paralysis. *J Bone Joint Surg* **41**: 37–60, 1959.
182 Ransford AO, Crockard HA, Pozo JL, et al. Craniocervical instability treated by contoured loop fixation. *J Bone Joint Surg* **68**: 173–177, 1986.
183 Raynor RB, Push J, Shapiro I. Cervical facetectomy and its effect on spine strength. *J Neurosurg* **63**: 278–282, 1963.
184 Reid JD. Effects of flexion–extension movements of the head and spine upon the spinal cord and nerve roots. *J Neurol Neurosurg Psychiat* **23**: 214–221, 1960.
185 Ripa DR, Kowall MG, Meyer PR, et al. Series of ninety-two traumatic cervical spine injuries stabilized with anterior ASIF plate fusion technique. *Spine* **16**: S46–S55, 1991.
186 Robinson RA, Smith GW. Anterolateral cervical disc removal and interbody fusion for cervical disc syndrome. *Bull Johns Hopkins Hosp* **96**: 223–224, 1955.
187 Robinson RA, Southwick WO. Indications and techniques for early stabilization of the neck in some fracture–dislocations of the cervical spine. *South Med J* **53**: 565–579, 1960;
188 Robinson RA, Southwick WO. Surgical approaches to the cervical spine. *Am Acad Orthop Surg Instruct Course Lect* **27**: 299–316, 1960.
189 Rogers WA. Treatment of fracture–dislocation of the cervical spine. *J Bone Joint Surg* **24**: 245–258, 1942.
190 Rogers WA. Fractures and dislocations of the cervical spine. *J Bone Joint Surg* **39**: 341–376, 1957.
191 Roosen K, Travschel A, Grote W. Posterior atlanto-axial fusions: a new compression clamp for laminar osteosynthesis. *Arch Orthop Trauma Surg* **100**: 27–31, 1982.
192 Roy-Camille R, Saillant G. Chirurgie du rachis cervical, I, Généralités. Luxations pures des articulaires. *Nouv Presse Med* **1**(33): 2330–2332, 1972.
193 Roy-Camille R, Saillant G, Mazel C. Internal fixation of the unstable cervical spine by a posterior osteosynthesis with plates and screws. In Bailey RW, Sherk HH et al (eds) *The Cervical Spine*, 2nd ed, 390–403, Philadelphia: JB Lippincott, 1989.
194 Roy-Camille R, Saillant G, Laville C, et al. Treatment of lower cervical spine injuries. *Spine* **17**: S442–S446, 1992.
195 Ryerson EW, Christopher F. Dislocation of cervical vertebrae: operative correction. *JAMA* **108**: 468–470, 1937.
196 Sadeghpour E, Noer HR, Mahinpour S. Skull–C2 fusion in rheumatoid patients with atlanto-axial subluxation. *Orthopaedics* **4**: 1369–1374, 1981.

197 Sasso RC, Doherty BJ, Heggeness MH. Biomechanics of odontoid fracture fixation: a comparison on one and two screw techniques. *Proceedings of the Cervical Spine Research Society*, 61–62, 1992.
198 Savini R, Parisini P, Cevellati S. Surgical treatment of late instability of flexion rotation injuries in the lower cervical spine. *Spine* **12**: 178–182, 1987.
199 Schlicke LH, Schulak DJ. Wiring of the cervical spinous process. *Clin Orthop* **154**: 319–320, 1981.
200 Schlicke LH, White AA III, Panjabi MM, et al. A quantitative study of vertebral displacement and angulation in the normal cervical spine under axial load. *Clin Orthop* **140**: 47–49, 1979.
201 Schultz RJ. In Malabar FL, Krieger RE (eds) *The Language of Fractures*, 298–299. Baltimore: Williams & Wilkins, 1972.
202 Schneider RC, Kahn EA. Chronic neurologic sequelae of acute trauma to the spine and spinal cord. Part I. The significance of the acute-flexion or 'tear-drop' fracture–dislocation of the cervical spine. *J Bone Joint Surg* **38**: 985–997, 1956.
203 Schneider RC, Cheery G, Pantek H. Syndrome of acute central cervical spinal cord injury with special reference to the mechanism involved in hyperextension injuries of the cervical spine. *J Neurosurg* **11**: 546–577, 1954.
204 Schneiderman GA, Hambly M. Spinal orthoses. In Hockschuler SH, Cotler HB, et al (eds) *Rehabilitation of the Spine: Science and Practice*, Chap. 17; 213–222. St Louis: Mosby, 1993.
205 Schoening HA, Hannan V. Factors related to cervical spine mobility, part I. *Arch Phys Med Rehab* **45**: 602, 1964.
206 Scoville WB, Palmer AH, Samra K, et al. The use of acrylic plastic for vertebral replacement or fixation in metastatic disease of the spine: technical note. *J Neurosurg* **27**: 274–279, 1967.
207 Segal D, Whitelaw GP, Gumbs V, et al. Tension band fixation of acute cervical spine fractures. *Clin Orthop* **159**: 211–222, 1981.
208 Selecki BR. The effects of rotation of the atlas on the axis: experimental work. *Med J Aust* **1**: 1012, 1969.
209 Sherk HH, Parke WW. Developmental anatomy. In Bailey RW, Sherk HH, et al (eds) *The Cervical Spine*, 1–7, 2nd ed, Philadelphia: JB Lippincott, 1989.
210 Simmons EH, Bhalla SK. Anterior cervical discectomy and fusion. Clinical and biomechanical study with 8 year follow-up. *J Bone Joint Surg* **41**: 225–237, 1969.
211 Simmons EH, Dutoit G. Lateral atlanto-axial arthrodesis. *Orthop Clin North Am* **9**: 1101–1114, 1978.
212 Six E, Kelly DL Jr. Technique for C1, C2, and C3 fixation in cases of odontoid fracture. *Neurosurgery* **8**: 374–376, 1981.
213 Somerson SK, Stokes BT. Functional analysis of an electromechanical spinal cord injury device. *Expl Neurol* **96**: 82–96, 1987.
214 Songer MN, Specer DL, Meyer PR Jr, et al. The use of sublaminar cables to replace Luque wires. *Spine* **16**: S418–S421, 1991.
215 Sorenson KH, Husby J, Hein O. Interlaminar atlanto-axial fusion for instability. *Acta Orthop Scand* **49**: 341–349, 1978.
216 Stein A, Krag M, Hugus J. Anterior cervical interbody fusion: description of a new technique with clinical follow-up of the first 20 patients. *Proceedings of the Cervical Spine Research Society, 15th Annual Meeting*, Washington DC, 1987.
217 Streli R. Kompressionsosteosynthese bei Frakturen und Pseudarthrosen des Dens epistrophei. *Zeitschr Orthop* **119**: 675–676, 1981.
218 Streli R. Double hole plate fixation of the lower cervical spine. In Kehr A, Wiedner A (eds) *Cervical Spine I*, 175–179 New York: Springer-Verlag, 1987.
219 Streli R. Dens transfixation plate. In Kehr P, Weidner A (eds) *Cervical Spine I*, 239–243 New York: Springer-Verlag, 1987.
220 Sutterlin CE III, McAfee PC, Warden KE, et al. A biomechanical evaluation of cervical spine stabilization methods in a bovine model: static and cyclical loading. *Spine* **13**: 795–802, 1988.
221 Tomonaga T, Krag MH, Novotny J. 4-Pad halo-vest: clinical and X-ray experience. *Cerv Sp Res Soc*, 1993.
222 Töndury G. The cervical spine – its development and changes during life. *Acta Orthop Belg* **25**: 602–626, 1959.
223 Torg JS, Pavlov H, Genuario SE, et al. Neuropraxie of the cervical spinal cord with transient quadriplegia. *J Bone Joint Surg* **68**: 1354–1370, 1986.
224 Tucker HH. Technical report: method of fixation of subluxed or dislocated cervical spine below C1–C2. *Can J Neurol Sci* **2**: 381–382, 1975.
225 Ulrich C, Wörsdorfer O, Claes L, et al. Comparative study of the stability of anterior and posterior cervical spine fixation procedures. *Arch Orthop Trauma Surg* **106**: 226–231, 1987.
226 Van Peteghem PK, Schweigel JF. The fractured cervical spine rendered unstable by anterior cervical fusion. *J Trauma* **19**: 110–114, 1979.
227 Vasavada A, Lydon C, Grob D, et al. Diagnostic external fixation in the lower cervical spine: a biomechanical evaluation. *Trans Orthop Res Soc* **18**: 7, 1993.
228 Walker PS, Lamser D, Hussey RW, Rossier AB, et al. Forces in the halo-vest apparatus. *Spine* **9**: 773–777, 1984.
229 Wang GJ, Moskal JT, Pritts AT, et al. The effect of halo-vest length on stability of the cervical spine. *J Bone Joint Surg* **70**: 357–360, 1988.
230 Werne S. Studies in spontaneous atlas dislocation. *Acta Orthop Scand* **23**: 1–150, 1957.
231 Werne S. The possibilities of movements in the craniovertebral joints. *Acta Orthop Scand* **28**: 165, 1957.
232 White AA III. Clinical biomechanics of cervical spine implants. *Spine* **14**: 1040–1045, 1989.
233 White AA III, Panjabi MM. *Clinical Biomechanics of the Spine*. Philadelphia: JB Lippincott, 1978.
234 White AA III, Panjabi MM. The basic kinematics of the human spine. *Spine* **3**: 12–20, 1978.
235 Whitecloud TS III, La Rocca H. Fibula strut graft in reconstructive surgery of the cervical spine. *Spine* **1**: 33–43, 1976.
236 Whitehill R, Barry JC. The evolution of stability in cervical spinal constructs using either autogenous bone graft or methylmethacrylate cement: a follow-up report on a canine in vivo model. *Spine* **10**: 32–41, 1985.
237 Whitehill R, Richman JA, Glaser JA. Failure of immobilization of the cervical spine by the halo vest. A report of five cases. *J Bone Joint Surg* **68**: 326–332, 1986;
238 Whitehill R, Stowers SF, Fechner RE, et al. Posterior cervical fusions using cerclage wires, methylmethacrylate cement and autogenous bone graft: an experimental study of a canine model. *Spine* **12**: 12–22, 1987.

239 Whitehill R, Cicoria AD, Hooper WE, et al. Posterior cervical reconstruction with methylmethacrylate cement and wire: a clinical review. *J Neurosurg* **68**: 576–584, 1988.

240 Whitesides TE, Mehserle WL, Hutton WC. The force exerted by the halo pin. A study comparing different halo designs. *Spine* **17**(10S): S413–S417, 1992.

241 Wilder DG, Pope MH, Frymoyer JW. The biomechanics of lumbar disc herniation and the effect of overload and instability. *J Spin Dis* **1**(1): 16–32, 1988.

242 Willard D, Nicholson JT. Dislocation of the first cervical vertebra. *Ann Surg* **113**: 464–475, 1941.

243 Wolf JW Jr, Johnson RM. Cervical orthosis. In Bailey RW, Sherk HH, et al (eds) *The Cervical Spine*, 2nd ed, 97–105, Philadelphia: JB Lippincott, 1989.

244 Wolf JW, Jones HC. Comparison of immobilization of the cervical spine by halocasts versus plastic jackets. *Proceedings of the Cervical Spine Research Society Annual Meeting*, Palm Beach, FL, 1980.

245 Worth D. Kinematics of the cranio-vertebral joints. PhD Dissertation, Victoria Institute of Colleges, 1980.

246 Wu KK, Malik G, Guise ER. Atlanto-axial arthrodesis: a clinical analysis of 22 cases treated at Henry Ford Hospital. *Orthopaedics* **5**: 865–871, 1982.

247 Yoganandan N, Pintar F, Burlter J, et al. Dynamic response of human cervical spine ligaments. *Spine* **14**: 1102–1110, 1989.

248 Yoo JU, Zou D, Edwards WT, et al. Effect of cervical spine motion on the neuroforaminal dimensions of the human cervical spine. *Spine* **17**: 1131–1136, 1992.

4 Clinical evaluation of cervical spine disorders

J. Michael Simpson and Christopher P. Silveri

The cervical spine has been a source of great intellectual curiosity and marvel since the genesis of human anatomical study. Its configuration allows for an infinite array of fluid movement, often with tacit agility, yet it is prone to sudden and incapacitating pain and dysfunction. Rothman and Rashbaum stated, 'the price we pay for a mobile cervical spine, which allows us to focus our eyes and ears toward a stimulus, is early and almost universal attrition in that anatomic structure known as the cervical disc'.[35] The availability and sensitivity of such studies as magnetic resonance imaging and computed tomography have emphasized the ubiquitous nature of cervical spondylotic disease in the adult spine. What remains, however, is the discrepancy between the prevalence of such changes and their symptoms. The history and physical examination remain paramount in determining true pathologic changes from those of inevitable senescence.

The clinical evaluation of any disorder involves an appreciation of the patients' physical complaints as well as the emotional and social influences that contribute to their personality. With the numerous medicolegal and compensation issues facing the spine surgeon today, a dedication to the art of patient interviewing and examination is vital in the determination of appropriate management. The interview results in a tremendous exchange of information regarding the patient's condition, concerns, and anxieties, often more complex than the presenting complaint.

Whether cervical dysfunction is due to congenital, degenerative or traumatic pathology, the integrity of the cervical spine must be completely evaluated by a thorough history obtained from the patient, family members, or witnesses. Once the etiology is understood, the physician can then proceed with a thoughtful and directed physical examination.

Before starting an examination, the practitioner must appreciate whether the patients' symptoms involve only local neck discomfort or whether there is an associated radicular or myelopathic pattern to their complaints. The mechanism of injury and knowledge about the direction of forces are vital in the anticipation of various types of skeletal trauma or spinal instability as well as associated injuries.

HISTORY

Trauma

Emergency assessment always begins with a general evaluation of cardiorespiratory function. Forty-three percent of patients who experience blunt trauma involving the cervical spine have associated injury which may require urgent care.[12,20] It is the primary responsibility of the spine surgeon to oversee the activity of the other members of a trauma service as it pertains to the cervical spine, and to be in control of the neck during attempts at airway management, transferring, log rolling, etc.

All too often, perpetuation of a spinal cord injury results from an overly zealous or unorganized approach to such a trauma patient. Bohlman[4] showed that almost one-third of all cervical injuries were overlooked on initial evaluation. This critical diagnosis is frequently missed by simply not realizing its potential. Physical examination and evaluation of patients with potential cervical injury are often complicated by polytrauma, ethanol or drug intoxication, or head injury, resulting in an uncooperative or unresponsive patient. Although resuscitation efforts have vastly improved over the last 40 years, it had been estimated that almost 10% of neurologically intact patients develop deficits as a result of such measures.[33] Clinical suspicion and early diagnosis must therefore be emphasized. Of course life-sustaining activity takes precedence over spinal stabilization, although, in most instances, simultaneous management can be accomplished.

Inspection is critical in the initial management of the acutely injured patient. Although the patient may be unconscious, much can be derived from the general posture of the patient. The presence of maxillofacial trauma, lacerations, or other injury above the level of the clavicle, as well as ventilation difficulties, should lend suspicion to a cervical spine lesion.[28]

If the patient is unresponsive, a detailed history must then be obtained from family, friends, witnesses, the emergency medical systems (EMS), or police personnel. Reconstruction of the events leading up to the incident can provide the appropriate details needed to understand the forces involved and the mechanism of injury, both of which will allow the physicians to anticipate possible instability and jeopardy to the spinal cord.

Information gathered from the observations of the EMS at the scene also adds to the history. Position of the patient when found, level of consciousness, victim's initial complaints, and degree of motor function contribute to the history of the event. Occasionally a patient may have transient paraplegia or paralysis secondary to concussion of the spinal cord which recovers before arriving at the emergency room.[5]

If the patient is conscious, a detailed history of the incident should precede further evaluation. This should include type of injury, blunt versus a deceleration injury, level of consciousness, short- and long-term memory loss, dizziness, location of pain, numbness, paresthesia, or fasciculation at or since the time of the incident. If sudden flexion–extension forces were involved, the patient should also recount experience of acute sensory or motor symptoms in the extremities or an 'electric' shock sensation at the time of the incident.

Past medical history that is significant for pre-existing cervical spinal pathology is also important to note. Cervical spondylosis with congenital and rheumatologic causes of instability are important factors in predisposing the spinal cord to immediate injury with subsequent low tolerance for further motion as a result of the decreased space available for the cord.[3] With the space available for the cord already compromised, sudden angular or translational movements may cause cord contusion with varying neurologic sequelae.

Degenerative disorders

When the etiology of cervical dysfunction is degenerative or non-traumatic in origin, the history provides many clues as to the presence or absence of operative pathology. Frequently, just a detailed history and physical examination are sufficient to establish a probable diagnosis. With this information, the treating physician may then proceed with appropriate tests or treatment for the disorder. Initial evaluation begins the moment the patient enters the office. The patient's age, posture, attitude, degree of aggression or reservation, gait, body habits, general occupational status (laborer versus white collar), and, of course, obvious physical disability will flavor the entire interview. As the physician and patient initially interact, information regarding the patient's recreational interests, occupation, family situation, relationship to referring physician, frustration, and general temperament should be obtained and incorporated into the strategy of the interview. Once the patient–physician relationship has been explored, the patient usually begins to explain the reason for the visit.

Discussion usually starts with a description of the symptomatology. It is important to ascertain the location and nature of the symptom complex as it refers to neck pain, radiculopathy, or myelopathic disturbances. Cervical disc disease with associated neck or arm pain, whether acute or chronic, occurs in approximately 51% of adults at some time in their life.[17] Those patients who only develop neck pain are destined for conservative treatment. Those with a significant radicular component and predominant arm pain in addition tend to improve through various conservative measures. However, radicular arm pain which fails these measures, and with corresponding radiographic lesions, has shown excellent responses to surgical decompression.

Neck pain is a non-specific indicator of many different processes. The practitioner must be aware that, apart from spinal pathology, musculoskeletal, craniovertebral, shoulder, visceral, and cardiorespiratory ailments can refer pain to this region.[42] Neck pain of spinal origin can result from numerous mechanical processes such as disc degeneration, ligamentous strain, osteophyte impingement, ligamentum flavum hypertrophy, infection, and tumor. It is well known that chronic cervical disc degeneration is a long-term problem and not a brief, self-limiting disorder.[14,38]

Most practitioners evaluate patients who experience acute manifestations of chronic disease. These two processes differ primarily in the mode of presentation and acuity of the symptoms. In the acute setting, patients usually provide specific information, time of onset, and contributing factors, and often note a specific incident which instigated the current pain syndrome. Patients initially describe recent development of local symptoms of aching and stiffness often occurring at night, waking them up, and causing changes in neck position to maintain comfort. This discomfort results in further stiffness and the inevitable 'voluntary' immobilization. It is important to note the temporal relationship of the pain syndrome to sleep, position of neck, Valsalva maneuvers, and activity that exacerbates their symptoms. It is most important to elicit the positions of greatest discomfort from the history because this will undoubtedly aid in differentiating neck pain from multiple sources. Most often, in patients with cervical spondylosis, extension and rotation of the head toward the site of pain exacerbate the discomfort. It is important to note this because immobilization in certain cervical collars may promote extension and actually increase pain.[36] In patients with muscular strain or ligamentous instability, flexion of the head exacerbates the symptoms. Painful rotations with occipital headache may suggest C1–2 problems. Patients may reveal associated symptoms of headache in both occipital and temporal regions, retro-orbital pain, and, rarely, facial neuralgias. Bizarre symptoms related to esophageal, tracheal, or vertebral artery compression, as well as low back pain, may also be seen.[21,34]

Jackson specifically noted headaches frequently associated with cervical disc disease due to compression and irritation of nerve roots in the upper cervical segments.[18] Such pain is usually relieved with rest, although the supine position may exacerbate the neck pain because of the awkward neck position assumed during sleep. Such pain is also usually relieved with immobilization, and use of non-steroidal drugs.

The patient may also describe neck pain associated with a more indolent course of unusual symptoms and fluctuating degrees of impairment. Chronic disc degeneration causes overall failure and malfunction of the motor unit which leads to inefficient biomechanics and the development of primary and referred pain patterns secondary to the weakening of the unit structures. Patients may recount seemingly unusual symptoms such as dizziness, tinnitus, intermittent blurring of vision, and retro-ocular pain, all of which appear non-specific; however, they may be related to osteophyte formation in chronic cervical degenerative disease.[12,25]

If an osteophyte develops in close proximity to the neurocentral joints, the vertebral artery foramina may be compromised, producing a severe degree of vascular compression with the symptoms noted above as vertebral artery syndrome (Fig. 4.1). Progression of this pathology to complete occlusion of the artery will lead to Wallenberg's syndrome with sequelae of dysphagia, vocal fold paralysis, sensory loss to the fifth cranial nerve, Horner's syndrome, palatal weakness, cerebellar dysfunction, and potential death.[12,25] In such cases of advanced disease, dysphagia may also be the only aspect of neck pain noted by the patient, and at times is known to be related to large anterior vertebral osteophytes, compressing visceral structures in the anterior neck.[35]

Most patients, when describing pure axial pain about the neck, experience what Sypert referred to as myofascial syndrome.[42] Their symptoms consist of neck pain (at times related to mild trauma or whiplash syndrome) with diffuse non-specific shoulder, interscapular, and arm discomfort. These symptoms are not, however, associated with other findings such as numbness, paresthesiae, or weakness in a true radicular distribution. These myofascial syndromes may be a clinical manifestation of referred pain from the motion segment of the cervical spine.

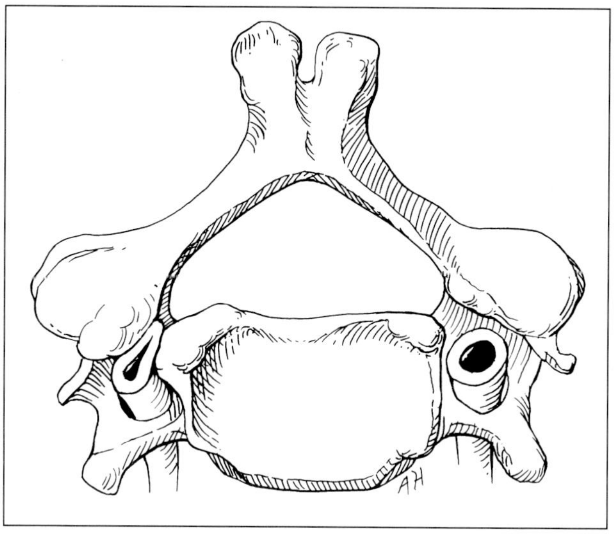

Figure 4.1
Compression of the vertebral artery occurring as a result of osteophyte impingement from both neurocentral and facet joints. Complete occlusion of the artery leads to Wallenberg's syndrome

When patients experience a true compressive neuropathy, their history moves away from a predominance of neck pain, and the physician elicits complaints of arm pain radiating from a cervical origin, often associated with non-specific symptoms of paresthesiae, dysesthesiae, and numbness along a similar distribution. The temporal relationship between neck and arm pain is often a classic reminder that compression without inflammation is not sufficient to produce radicular pain.[35] In a patient experiencing a soft disc herniation, on extrusion of the disc, the inflammatory process at the annular fibrosis subsides thereby diminishing the neck pain component. As the neural compression becomes the major remaining process, paresthesiae may develop from initial compression and, with subsequent inflammatory reaction, typical radicular pain ensues. Of course patients with a more chronic degenerative spine will not display such a classic presentation. Patients describe an increase in arm pain, typically with rotation and extension toward the side of the pathology. These maneuvers stretch the nerve roots and aggravate their impingement. Patients may note varying degrees of numbness and paresthesia, with or without muscle weakness. Often they do not realize initially the degree of weakness that is subsequently detected by their physician. Monoradicular symptoms of weakness usually progress slowly with the patient being able to compensate for the weakness with other muscles. Patients may have undergone diagnostic work-ups for carpal tunnel syndrome, shoulder and elbow pathology, or

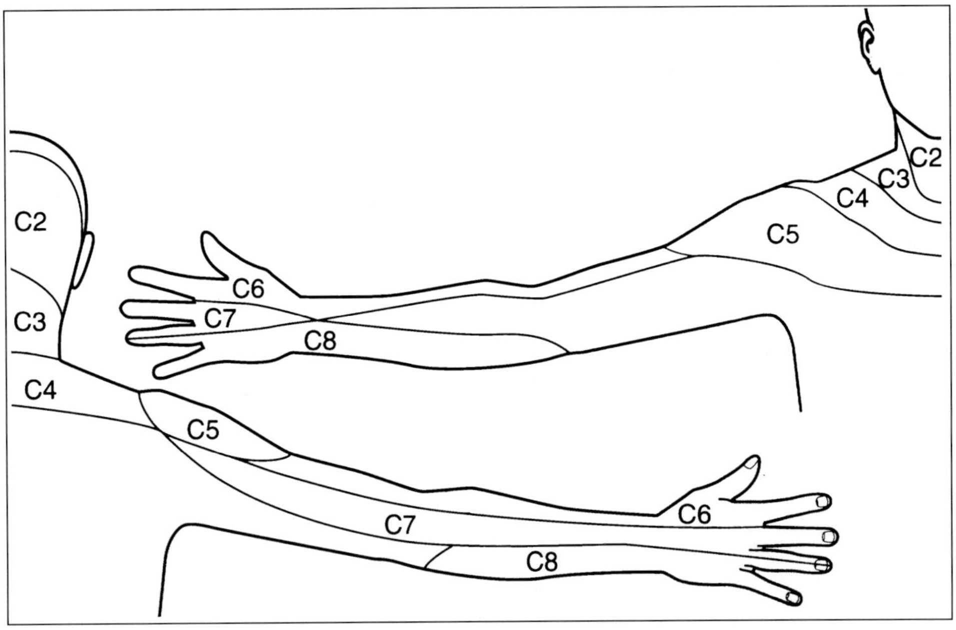

Figure 4.2
Dermotomes of the cervical nerve roots: compression of C2, C3, and C4 is uncommon and will only produce sensory discomfort about the posterior neck, occiput, trapezium, and chest wall. The lower cervical nerve roots are more commonly involved in cervical disc disease

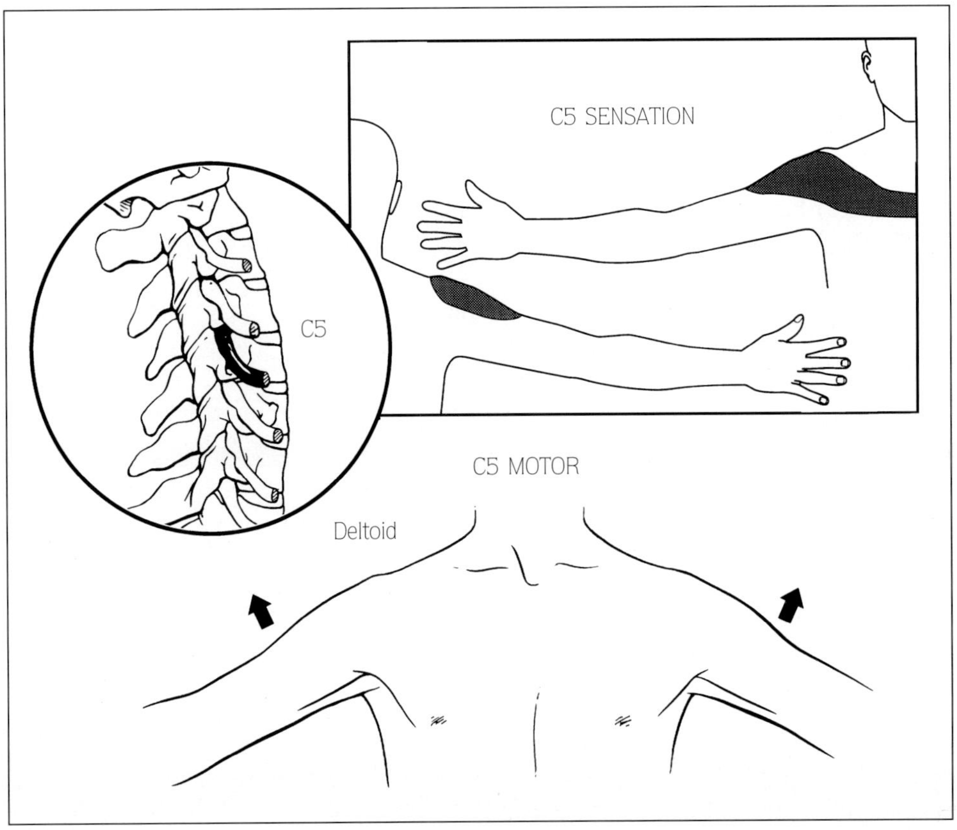

Figure 4.3
C5 radiculopathy: pain radiates over the shoulder and lateral aspect of the proximal arm. Weakness may be demonstrated in shoulder abduction as the deltoid and rotator cuff muscles are affected. The biceps reflex may also be diminished

tendinitis, etc., some patients actually having surgery without improvement due to misdiagnosis.[38]

Patients use several descriptions to explain their radicular discomfort. Typically, upper cervical segments exhibit radiculopathic pain syndromes which may be interpreted by the patient as tension or migraine headaches. C2 radiculopathy is rarely encountered; however, compression of C3 and C4 occur frequently and present clinically as sensory discomfort about the posterior neck, the occiput, and over the trapezium to the shoulder. Occasionally C4 may continue down the anterosuperior chest (Fig. 4.2).

A more classic presentation is with compression of the lower cervical nerve roots. Such radiculopathies are commonly described as sharp or lancinating, precipitated, or exacerbated by postural or Valsalva maneuvers.[26] Simeone[36] describes the C5 radiculopathy as the 'epaulet' pattern, which is highly specific, and radiates down over the shoulder to the lateral aspect of the proximal arm. Because the major motor innervation to the deltoid and rotator cuff arises from the C5 root, patients also complain of fatigue or frank weakness in shoulder abduction. The biceps muscle has dual innervation from both C5 and C6, whereas the deltoid is almost pure C5. The biceps reflex primarily indicates neurologic integrity of C5; however, the reflex also has a C6 component (Fig. 4.3). The C5 radiculopathy is often confused with shoulder problems, but meticulous physical examination of the neck and shoulder will usually distinguish these disorders.

Radiculopathy approximating the C6 distribution involves neck pain radiating across the biceps and anterior arm to the radial aspect of the forearm, and dorsum of the thumb and index finger. Weakness is described as that relating to biceps strength, although its extent is not appreciated by the patient. Wrist extensors are partially innervated by C6 and C7: specifically, extensor carpi radialis longus and brevis by C6, and extensor carpi ulnaris primarily by C7. Weakness in this general group could therefore reflect either C6 or C7 compressive pathology. The brachioradialis reflex is most directly affected by C6 compression. Subtle changes in the biceps reflex is suggestive of impairment given its dual innervation (Fig. 4.4).

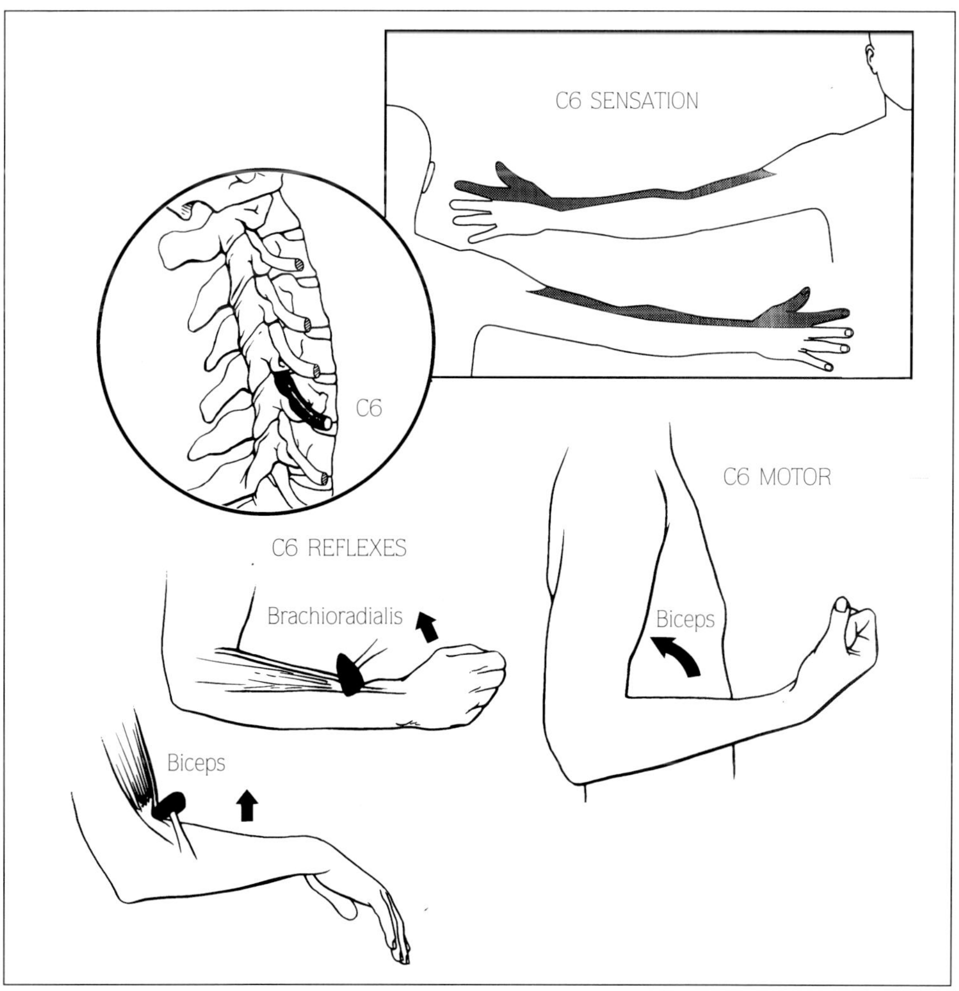

Figure 4.4
C6 radiculopathy: pain radiates from the neck along the biceps and anterior arm to the radial aspect of the forearm, and dorsum of the thumb and index finger. Weakness may be demonstrated in the biceps and wrist extensors. Reflex abnormalities may be seen in brachioradialis and biceps testing

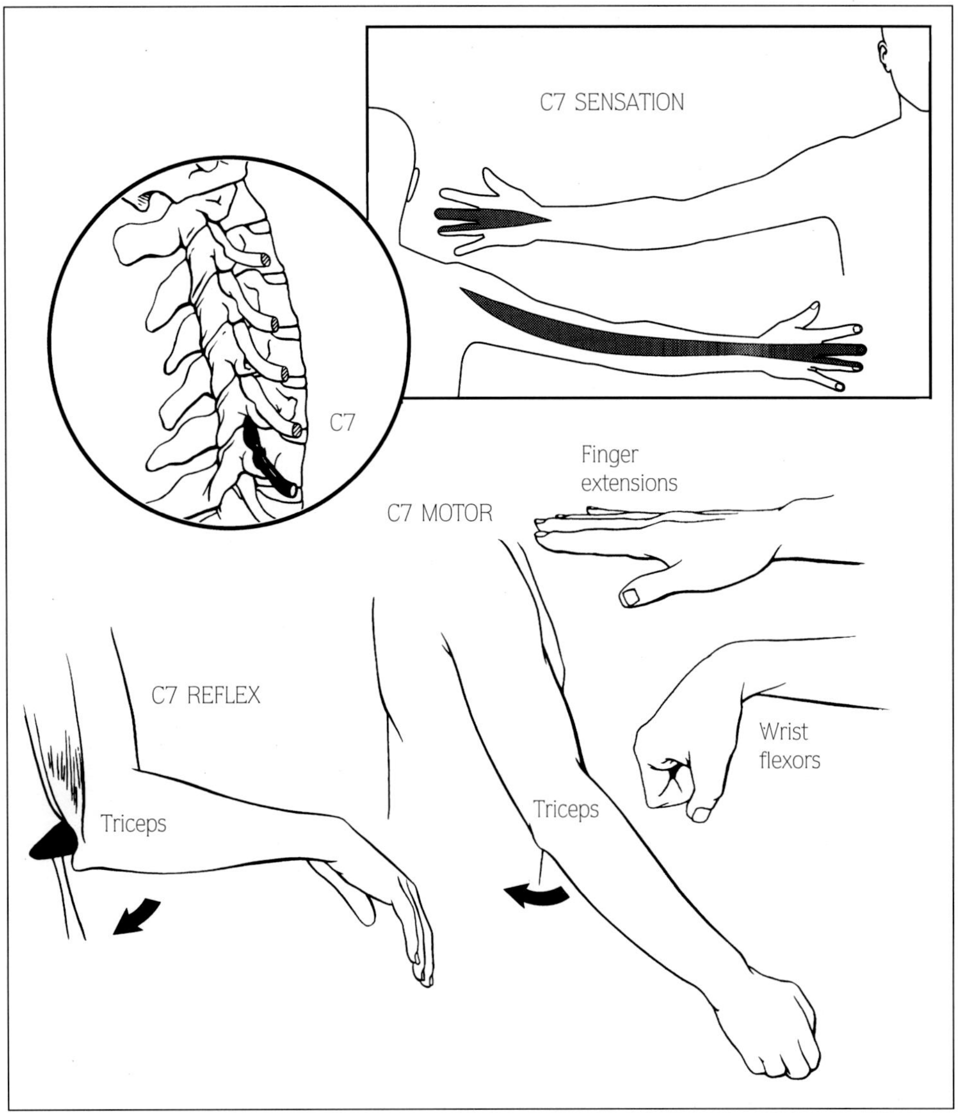

Figure 4.5
C7 radiculopathy: pain radiates along the posterior shoulder and arm – posterolateral aspect of the forearm to the middle finger. The triceps muscle is most commonly affected, resulting in weakness and diminished reflex. Weakness of finger extensors and wrist flexors may also be elicited on examination

Compressive pathology of the C7 nerve root presents with pain along the posterior shoulder and arm – the posterolateral aspect of the forearm to the middle finger. However, involvement of the index and ring fingers, as well as the first web space, can also be seen. The muscle most commonly affected is the triceps, resulting in weakness and diminished reflex, although weakness is rarely a patient complaint, unless in someone who is physically active (Fig. 4.5).

Radiculopathy associated with the C8 root is clearly the most characteristic feature. Patients describe a dermatomal distribution corresponding to the medial (ulnar) border of the arm and forearm to the fifth digit, and often the ulnar half of the fourth digit. Invariably, the symptoms are below the elbow with most dysfunction noted in numbness along the ulnar digits and a deficit in both abduction and adduction of the fingers as well as in finger flexion (Fig. 4.6).

The above patterns of pain distribution are classically described by those having a cervical compressive neuropathy; they are meant to be guidelines for the evaluation and diagnosis of such pathology. Of course, patients with a more chronic presentation will have less distinct findings. Many individuals with a long history of cervical dysfunction, and involvement at many levels, have pain of less severity, infrequently related to neck posture. They develop long-standing paresthesiae and occasionally undetected atrophy of the hand musculature with generalized weakness. The length of time the patient experiences these symptoms should be borne in mind, because those with long-standing compression tend to show less improvement in

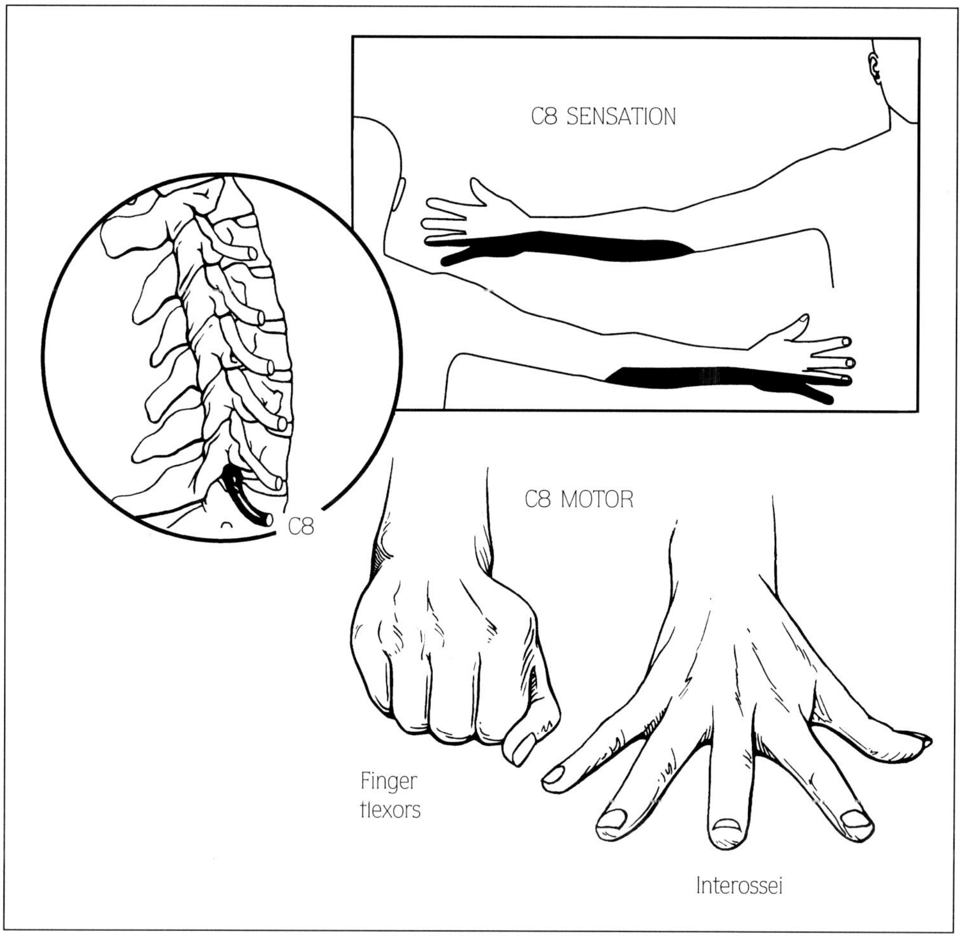

Figure 4.6
C8 radiculopathy: pain radiates from the lower ulnar border of the arm and forearm to the fifth digit and ulnar half of the fourth digit. Weakness can be demonstrated in finger abduction, adduction and flexion

function after definitive surgical care. In addition, physicians and their patients must not misinterpret paresthesiae and dysesthesiae as 'pain'. Decompressive procedures often resolve pain syndromes, but cannot be expected to relieve such sensory changes completely. More often they have residual paresthesiae after adequate surgical decompression as a result of the chronic nature of neural tissue damage, and the poor ability of the tissue to regenerate or repair such pathology. Simeone and Rothman[38] stated that most patients with failed disc surgery did not have convincing preoperative neurologic deficits.

It is also important for the physician to differentiate a history of peripheral nerve entrapment syndrome from cervical radiculopathy. Entrapment syndromes include carpal tunnel syndrome, anterior interosseous syndrome, pronator syndrome, cubital tunnel syndrome, Guyon's canal syndrome, radial tunnel syndrome and thoracic outlet syndrome. C6 radiculopathy is often confused with carpal tunnel syndrome, anterior interosseus syndrome or pronator syndrome, and C7 radiculopathy may present similarly to radial tunnel syndrome. Cubital tunnel syndrome, Guyon's canal syndrome and thoracic outlet syndrome should be ruled out in patients with a suspected C8 radiculopathy. Often peripheral nerve entrapment syndrome is present along with cervical radiculopathy, and this syndrome is known as the 'double crush' phenomenon.

Cervical spondylosis can further result in acute or chronic symptoms of myelopathy. Compression of the spinal cord can significantly alter the patient's ability to function, although most patients present with vague sensory and motor symptoms which have developed over a period of months or years. As this clinical syndrome is less characteristic than the more common radicular manifestations of cervical disc disease, the history and physical examination are critical in the diagnosis of such dysfunction.

Most often patients will present with a mixed picture, that is not discerned on initial evaluation.[11] The presence of both upper and lower motor neuron symptomatology, as well as the typically vague complaints given by these patients, can easily overwhelm the interviewing physician. Cervical spondylotic myelopathy has been stated as the most common cause of spinal cord dysfunction in patients aged over 55.[38] Less emphasis is placed on the degree of frustration experienced by the patients suffering from the sequelae. Unlike patients with nerve root compression, patients with evidence of myelopathy often have a difficult time pinpointing or describing their deficits. The elicitation of a history of specific patterns of dermatomal or motor deficits is not productive. In fact, in such circumstances the patient should be asked more general questions to provide more descriptive terms and examples which can help the practitioner translate the findings into clinical pathology.

Patients usually describe a long history of unusual difficulties in their upper and lower extremities. Manual dexterity is often affected, with a silent progression until patients are surprised at their lack of ability to complete activities of daily living, such as buttoning a shirt or writing. Descriptions of stumbling or generalized gait disturbances may also be apparent in the patient's history. The history is one of a slow, insidious onset of non-specific symptoms. Occasionally patients are only made aware of their habits by relatives or neighbors who note a shuffling gait or frequent falls, etc. The characteristic, stooped, wide-based gait of the elderly is a common end result.[7] Patients may also develop bowel and bladder complaints, although these usually coexist with other complaints and are unlikely to present on their own. With this in mind, a neurologic history should be ascertained, including frequency and changes in bowel/bladder habits. Emphasis should be placed on possible retention or incontinence, or on unusual patterns of frequency, dysuria and bladder discomfort.

It is generally agreed that lower extremity spasticity and dysfunction in gait will precede upper extremity symptoms in cervical spondylitic myelopathy.[15,24] Although the myelopathic hand syndrome noted by Ono[31] was associated with lower extremity symptoms, there are reports of purely upper extremity manifestations of this compressive pathology.[13,31] Surgeons must be aware that cervical lesions producing myelopathy can result in vague sensory or motor disturbances in one or both hands without significant lower extremity findings, and these must not be mistaken for peripheral compressive processes such as carpal tunnel syndrome, resulting in inappropriate surgery. Sensory dysfunction can be quite confusing because of the varied pathways that can be affected, with changes in touch, pain, and proprioception (temperature sensation). During history taking, each of these senses must be investigated in depth as to character and location.

The pain produced by cervical myelopathy is poorly characterized and almost unique.[6,34] Usually described as an ache, it can be associated with neck pain, nondescript, non-dermatomal arm or leg pain, or, as Rothman noted, with a bursting thermal quality. In certain provocative positions, the patient may experience a generalized electric shock sensation that involves upper and lower extremities as well as the trunk – this is known as Lhermitte's sign (Fig. 4.7).

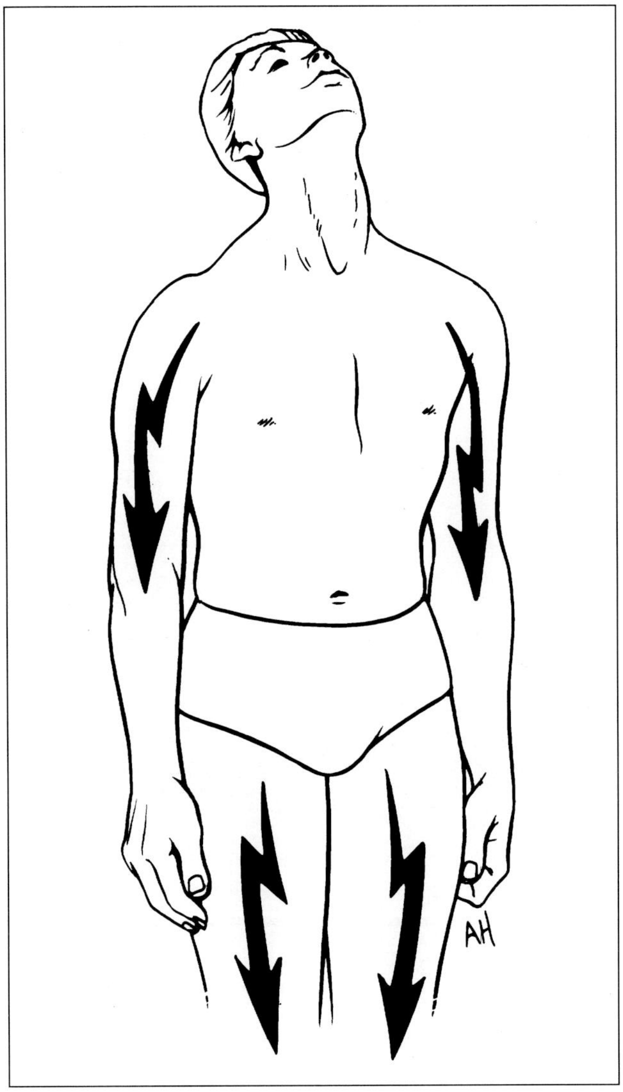

Figure 4.7
Lhermitte's sign: with certain provocative positions of the head and neck, the patient may produce an electric 'shock' sensation throughout the body when there is spinal cord compression

Combined myeloradicular symptoms may also be seen in these patients. The physician should not forget the potential for underlying myelopathic symptoms when there is presentation of monoradicular pain.[10]

As with any disease process, history taking would not be complete without a detailed account of the patient's past medical history. Underlying disorders can often present as cervical pathology, and vice versa. Such disorders include those that mimic cervical radiculopathy, for example, peripheral nerve neuropathies, carpal tunnel syndrome, inflammatory conditions, tendinitis, bursitis, thoracic outlet syndrome, infection, and tumor. Disease states such as diabetes mellitus, peripheral vascular disease, or central nervous system disorders may also disturb normal sensory or motor ability and so compromise adequate interpretation of the symptomatology, leading to a lesser potential for success through surgery.

A history of litigation, compensation, or drug dependence is also important in the prediction of successful outcome in the treatment of cervical spine disorders. An understanding of patients' psychosocial background, their expectations, their desire to return to work, their anger, and their present level of activity helps the surgeon to distinguish those individuals with surgically treatable lesions from those who are destined to have postoperative persistence of symptoms. Such emotional 'neuroses' place the patient in jeopardy of failure, and this is particularly true of drug addiction. Individuals with a self-induced or iatrogenic dependence on opiates for pain relief will inevitably develop a continued postoperative need for such relief. It is wise to investigate the dosage and frequency of such opiate use so that preoperative cessation by tapering can be addressed. If no attempt is made to diminish such dependence, a conditioned postoperative response of discomfort is almost inevitable whether similar to the preoperative syndrome or not. This then results in longer hospitalization and residual dysfunction. Perioperative management of such patients in pain clinics with concomitant detoxification is generally advised before any surgical intervention. Strict preoperative criteria for surgical indications are undoubtedly the most reliable predictor of success.

PHYSICAL EXAMINATION

Acute Evaluation of Cervical Spine Trauma

In the patient with cervical spine trauma, the physical examination is much more urgent and demanding than a routine office evaluation. Before the recent emphasis on increased awareness of cervical spine trauma by EMS and emergency room personnel, it was estimated that at least 10% of patients found to be neurologically intact on initial examination developed neurologic deficits after routine manipulation and resuscitation in the emergency room.[33] It is for this reason that prompt recognition of a potential spinal cord injury is mandatory and it is also mandatory that appropriate precautions are followed in the ensuing period of evaluation. Except for the immediately life-threatening emergencies, all aspects of the physical examination can and must be performed while maintaining stability of the cervical spine. In the ideal situation one individual, usually the orthopaedic or neurosurgical member of the trauma team, should be designated to oversee and scrutinize the handling of the spine during the resuscitation maneuvers. Iatrogenic injuries can be minimized with prior planning and education, as well as proper communication during these instances.

Initial patient assessment routinely begins with the well-known ABCs (airway, breathing, circulation), and is vital when dealing with cervical spine injuries because high lesions can quite easily depress or interrupt normal respiratory centers. Airway management becomes paramount in this setting, using the following indicators of respiratory distress: tachypnea, stridor, restlessness or combativeness, cyanosis or pallor, diaphragmatic breathing, use of accessory muscles, bradypnea, somnolence, and, finally, respiratory arrest. Inspection in this setting may reveal contusions, facial fractures or abrasions, swelling about the neck or head, blood in the nasopharynx or mouth, as well as rhinorrhea or otorrhagia. Presence of these injuries is highly suggestive of associated injury to the spinal cord. With such a degree of injury, a general inspection and palpitation may uncover other causes of respiratory distress, for example, fractured ribs or flail chest, with a potential hemo- or pneumothorax, abdominal pathology limiting diaphragmatic excursion, or occult penetrating injuries to the chest. Serial blood gas determinations are also crucial in diagnosing pulmonary insufficiency. Great care must be taken when establishing a means of ventilation, although protection of the cervical spine must not interfere with a successful resuscitation. It is best to obtain a lateral cervical spine radiograph before any manipulation of the airway; however, sometimes such delay is not possible because of the patient's respiratory condition. Endotracheal or nasotracheal intubation is often necessary and, if difficult, cricothyroidotomy can be carried out. If the patient is breathing, it is generally recommended that intubation is done through the nasal route, which requires the least amount of neck extension. Of course, even with oral intubation, the spine should remain as close to the neutral position as possible. In the apneic patient, laryngoscopy is mandatory and ventilatory support is managed through an oral airway.[39]

An assessment of the patient's circulatory status then follows, with a primary survey of sites of obvious hemorrhage and a secondary assessment of occult sources of blood loss. Injury to the spinal cord, however, may make interpretation of hemodynamic parameters quite difficult. With injuries above the midthoracic level (approximately T6), disruption of the sympathetic nervous system may result in loss of peripheral vascular tone and, more importantly, diminished ability of the heart to respond appropriately. As the vagal control over the heart is then unchecked[27] the characteristic hypotension is followed by bradycardia. Also, with loss of vascular tone, blood pools in the dilated peripheral vessels leading to hypothermia.[29]

Given these paradoxical cardiovascular responses, fluid resuscitation must be accomplished with great caution to avoid the development of congestive heart failure. Peripheral vasodilatation and bradycardia resulting, in a patient who is envolemic, from a neurologic insult will not respond to hydration as it would in one in hypovolemic shock. It is wise to consider vasoconstrictors such as dopamine for correction of spinal shock. Once the patient has been stabilized hemodynamically, a more critical look into the possibility of osseous and/or neural damage is can be made.

The physical examination of the cervical spine will be discussed in general in the next section; however, it is appropriate to consider certain aspects when dealing with the trauma patient. Part of the primary survey in the emergency room should include notation of certain neurologic criteria. The patient's level of consciousness is important to appreciate in the first instance because, with concomitant head and spinal injuries, there may be subtle deterioration in the patient. Alertness, orientation, patient cooperation, and ability to follow simple commands, as well as ability to communicate, are all descriptors that need to be noted. The Glasgow Coma Scale is also a standard by which the level of consciousness can be assessed (Table 4.1). At the same time, brain-stem function needs assessment, in addition to general motor function to determine the presence of any gross neurologic deficits. Pupil reaction, response to painful stimuli, posturing, flaccid extremities, signs of incontinence, and priapism need to be documented. The perianal neurologic examination is most important in the evaluation of such a trauma patient, and is important for determination of the existing level of injury, completeness of neurologic damage, and subsequent potential return of function. The presence of perianal sensation, proprioception, or motor function indicates an incomplete lesion with function below the level of injury. Continued neurologic recovery, although possible, can only be estimated. As Meyer[28] says, 'What may be stated more emphatically is that in the absence of perianal sensation, perianal voluntary motor function, and peripheral reflexes, in all likelihood, the neurologic injury is complete and recovery is not likely'. Contraction of the bulbocavernosus reflex itself has no prognostic value, except that it indicates the patient is out of spinal shock, and subsequent neurologic recovery is also unlikely. Palpation and manipulation of the cervical spine under traumatic conditions are contraindicated prior to plain radiographic assessment.

A careful neurologic examination in the emergency room is required. Additional confirmatory examinations should be performed by consulting services. The lowest functioning neurologic level must be documented, and any change or loss in neurologic function observed by other physicians or nursing staff reported immediately. The motor and sensory findings for each functional level of the cord are discussed later in this chapter.

Table 4.1 Glasgow Coma Scale

	Response	*Score*
Eyes open	Spontaneous	4
	To sound	3
	To pain	2
	Never	1
Best verbal response	Oriented	5
	Confused conversation	4
	Inappropriate words	3
	Incomprehensible words	2
	None	1
Best motor response	Obeys commands	6
	Localizes pain	5
	Flexion withdrawal	4
	Abnormal	3
	Extension	2
	None	1

Adapted with permission from Teasdale G, Jennett B. Assessment and prognosis of coma after head injury. *Acta Neurochirug* 34: 45, 1976.

General Evaluation of the Cervical Spine

As with any physical examination, the practitioner begins the assessment by inspection of the cervical spine and observation of the patient's gait, posture, and attitude. Loss of lordosis or presence of torticollis may indicate true spinal pathology which is also reflected in a cautious gait. A wide-based or unsteady gait may indicate a proprioceptive, sensory, or myelopathic process. Inspection of the neck includes appreciation of the overall symmetry of the head, neck and shoulder complex, muscle atrophy, hypertrophy, skin discoloration or skin lesions, as well as noting the overall relationship of the back musculature and scapulae with spinal alignment, rib prominence, thoracic rotation or curvature. The presence of scars, indicating previous surgery, skin lesions such as those from neurofibromatosis, and loss of normal skin creases are other important clues to note before the physical examination is started.

The practitioner is now ready to lay hands on the patient. In a gentle and systematic manner, palpation of the cervical spine is important to localize tenderness, changes in skin temperature, asymmetries or masses, and thorough evaluation of the soft tissues about the neck. Of equal importance is identification of the bony architecture of the anterior and posterior cervical region as well as assessment of those structures intimately associated with its function, namely the head occiput, shoulders, and thorax.

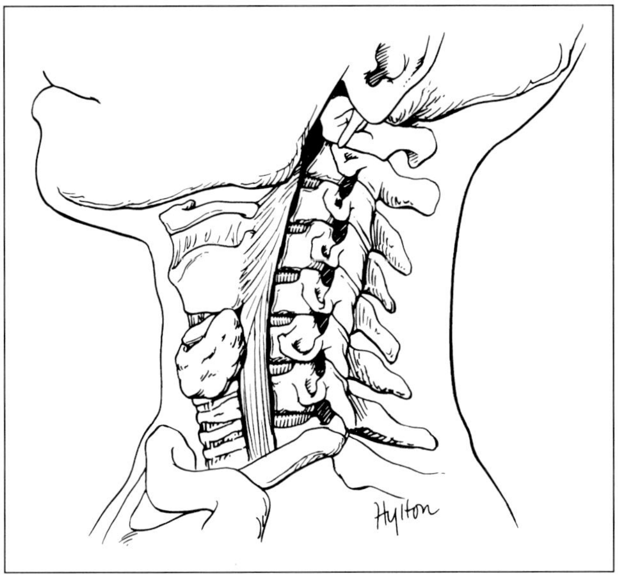

Figure 4.8
Anatomical landmarks of the neck as they relate to various levels of the cervical spine (see text for description)

Assessment of the head should include a general musculoskeletal palpation, noting areas of muscle tenderness or dermatomal areas of pain, such as those from an occipital neuroma. The occiput, inion, mastoid processes, superior nuchal line, and temporomandibular joints should all be evaluated before focusing on the neck. Bony palpation should then proceed to the anterior and posterior aspects of the neck. This is best done in both the erect and the supine position. Fig. 4.8 highlights the crucial anatomical landmarks as their position relates to the level of the spine.

In the anterior neck, the first cervical structures isolated are the lateral masses of the atlas, located just between the angle of the jaw and the styloid process. Moving in a caudal direction, the hyoid bone, located just above the thyroid cartilage, is palpable and can be felt to move upwards and then downwards with swallowing. This is a constant landmark approximating the level of the C3 vertebra. Next, the most easily palpable structure, the thyroid cartilage, is noted. It is posterior to this structure that the C4–C5 interval can be located. Below the obvious thyroid cartilage is the less distinguishable first cricoid ring. Not only is this an important site for emergent tracheotomies, but it is the landmark used in approximation of the level of C6. Lateral to this structure, in the interval between the sternocleidomastoid muscle belly and the tracheal airway, is the carotid tubercle or transverse process of C6. This is frequently used as an anterior landmark for the approach to the C5–C6 interspace, as well as identifying the planes of soft tissue dissection down to the anterior vertebral bodies. It is also commonly used as a site for injection of the stellate cervical ganglion.[16] The spinous processes, which are easily palpable, are posterior and should be assessed for rotational malalignment, degree of lordosis, and tenderness. Facet joint palpation is less distinct, lying deep to the trapezius and erector spinae musculature.

The soft tissue examination is equally important in evaluating the cervical spine and is accomplished together with palpation of the neck. The sternocleidomastoid muscle is best examined with the patient supine, and is palpated along its entire length, noting tenderness or spasm, asymmetry such as torticollic deformity, or swelling, such as that from hematoma formation or soft tissue masses. Anteromedial to this muscle belly lies the anterior lymph node chain. Enlargement of these nodes often indicates infection of the upper respiratory tract or ear, or nodal metastases of local tumors. The common carotid artery is best palpated in the same location most easily at the level of Chassaignac's tubercle (carotid tubercle). The magnitude of the pulsations, as well as the presence of bruits, should be noted. Palpation of both arteries together may precipitate bradycardia or syncope. Moving toward the midline, the thyroid gland is clearly palpable below the thyroid cartilage. The two main lobes as well as the isthmus, which gives it its characteristic 'H' shape, appear uniform and small, and are of concern only if asymmetry, nodules, or diffuse enlargement is noted. Similarly, the parotid gland, located laterally superficial to the angle of the mandible, is only detectable if enlargement is present, which may be indicative of acute obstruction, mumps, bacterial parotiditis, Sjögren's syndrome, or other inflammatory processes.[32] Finally, with respect to the anterior aspect of the neck, palpation should also include the supraclavicular areas, noting any fullness, pulsatile masses, presence of cervical ribs, or tenderness along the sternal notch, clavicle, or shoulder. On turning to the posterior aspect of the neck, the examination is best appreciated with the patient in the sitting position. Again, palpation of the head and occiput may locate areas of discomfort related to muscle spasm, occipital nerve inflammation, or musculoskeletal strain at the origin of the trapezius muscle or the superior nuchal ligament, as would occur after a flexion–extension injury. A chain of lymph nodes lies anterior to the lateral border of the trapezius muscle and these nodes may contribute to local pain or swelling.

Until now, the evaluation of the spine has been anatomic in nature. Such a complex construct allows for an almost infinite degree of freedom of motion, and allows the patient to focus or direct attention to a particular object at any given moment with great agility and swiftness. This complex mechanical fluidity is taken for granted unless suddenly limited by pain or dysfunction. The assessment of active range of motion in patients with cervical spine complaints begins with observation of the patient as he or she enters the room (Fig. 4.9). The clinical appreciation of cervical

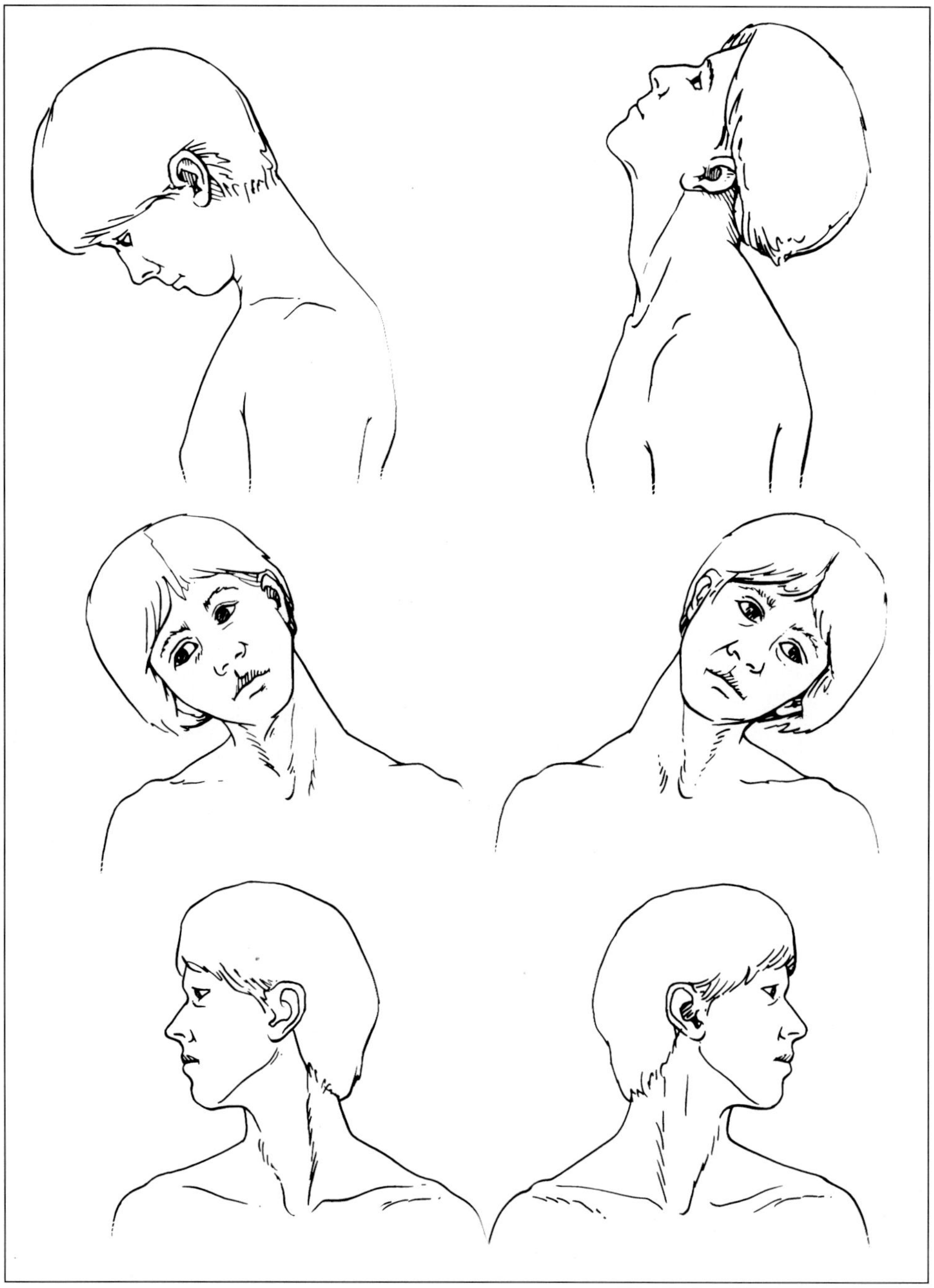

Figure 4.9
Cervical spine range of motion: flexion should almost bring the patient's chin to the chest wall, whereas extension should allow the patient to look directly upwards. Lateral bending should allow the ear to approximate the shoulder, whereas rotation puts the chin in line with the shoulder

movement is a compilation of flexion, extension, lateral bend, and rotation, as well as the degree of freedom afforded by the occiput–C1 and atlantoaxial articulations. Although biomechanical studies have documented individual ranges of motion for each level of the spine, the clinical evaluation is a more gross approximation of spinal mobility. Fig. 4.9 indicates the average ranges of flexion, extension, rotation, and lateral bend afforded between the occiput and thoracic spine, although it is helpful to remember simple guidelines. Normal flexion of the cervical spine should allow the patient to bring the chin down to the chest wall, and extension back to a level consistent with looking directly up at the ceiling. Rotational mobility should enable the normal individual to move the head so that the chin almost approximates a direct line with the shoulder. Functional loss of such mobility is easily noted by bilateral asymmetry. Finally, lateral bending should also be equal on both sides, with the patient able to bring the ear close to the ipsilateral shoulder.

Table 4.2 Clinical symptoms and findings of cervical nerve root involvement

Root	*Level*	*Sensory*	*Reflex*	*Motor*
C3	C2–3	Posterior neck to mastoid	None	Non-specific
C4	C3–4	Posterior neck to scapula and ± anterior chest	None	Non-specific
C5	C4–5	Lateral arm (axillary) to elbow	± Biceps	Deltoid ± biceps
C6	C5–6	Radial forearm to thumb	Biceps Brachioradialis	Biceps Wrist extensor
C7	C6–7	Midradial forearm to middle finger ± index/ring fingers	Triceps	Triceps Wrist flexor
C8	C7–T1	Ulnar forearm to little and ring fingers	None	Hand intrinsics Decreased grip strength Finger flexors
T1	T1–2	Medial upper arm	None	Hand intrinsics

Undoubtedly, the most important aspect of the cervical spine evaluation involves the neurologic examination. Nerve root or cord impingement by prolapsed nucleus pulposus, infection, tumor, or inflammatory tissue usually illicits characteristic neurologic deficits. There are eight cervical nerve roots, each of which exits through a foramen in relation to the corresponding vertebral body. The first seven exit above their corresponding vertebral body with only the eighth root exiting above the first thoracic vertebra. Given this structure of the cervical spine, accurate examination skills can often pinpoint the pathology to a specific level.

Motor examination of the uppermost cervical segments, C1–C4, is difficult to interpret. Diagnosis at these levels is usually aided by sensory deficits or a dermatomal distribution of pain. The intrinsic muscles of the neck are both innervated by cranial nerves and rami from the cervical roots. In the anterior neck, those strap muscles above the level of the hyoid bone are primarily innervated by the hypoglossal nerve. In the infrahyoid region, the ansa cervicalis contributes the nervous supply. The motor function of the trapezius and the sternocleidomastoid can be rather specifically isolated and represents the functioning of the spinal accessory nerve, or cranial nerve XI. The remaining cervical intrinsic muscles derive their motor input via the anterior primary rami off the cervical nerves and, except for electromyographic (EMG) studies, their individual function is difficult to ascertain during the physical examination.

The primary focus of the clinical evaluation involves the cervical contribution to the brachial plexus, namely C5–T1. The sensory and motor contributions of each root are outlined in Table 4.2. Although it has been shown that occasionally cross-over innervation or variations in root contribution to muscle groups exist, it is important to develop a standard operating criterion in the examination of patients for potential compromised nerve roots.[1]

Testing of motor function proceeds as indicated in Table 4.2. Involvement of the C5 root causes profound disability which is reflected in deltoid weakness. It is best to examine the strength of this muscle with both of the patient's arms held outstretched to each side. This removes any contribution of the long head of biceps to shoulder flexion, which is present when using the anterior portion of the deltoid to flex the arm. Patients are severely disabled with dysfunction of this particular root because it severely limits the ability to abduct the arm past the 90° position which is required for many activities of grooming and daily living. As the biceps has dual innervation by both C5 and C6, the deltoid is preferred for evaluating the fifth cervical root. Biceps testing is therefore an accurate predictor of competence of the C6 nerve root, as well as the wrist extensors (extensor carpi radialis brevis and longus), although there is also a small component of C7 reflected in its innervation of extensor carpi ulnaris. Along the same lines, there has been confusion in the literature concerning the appropriate use of the biceps reflex as an indicator of pathology. Although some authors state its use in evaluation of C5 function, the present authors feel that, as with motor strength, the primary innervation to the biceps, as well as the brachioradialis reflex, is C6. Depression of this reflex is most sensitive for C6 pathology.[2,16,20,23,37]

Moving to the seventh cervical root, the clinical picture becomes clear. The primary muscle group affected by an

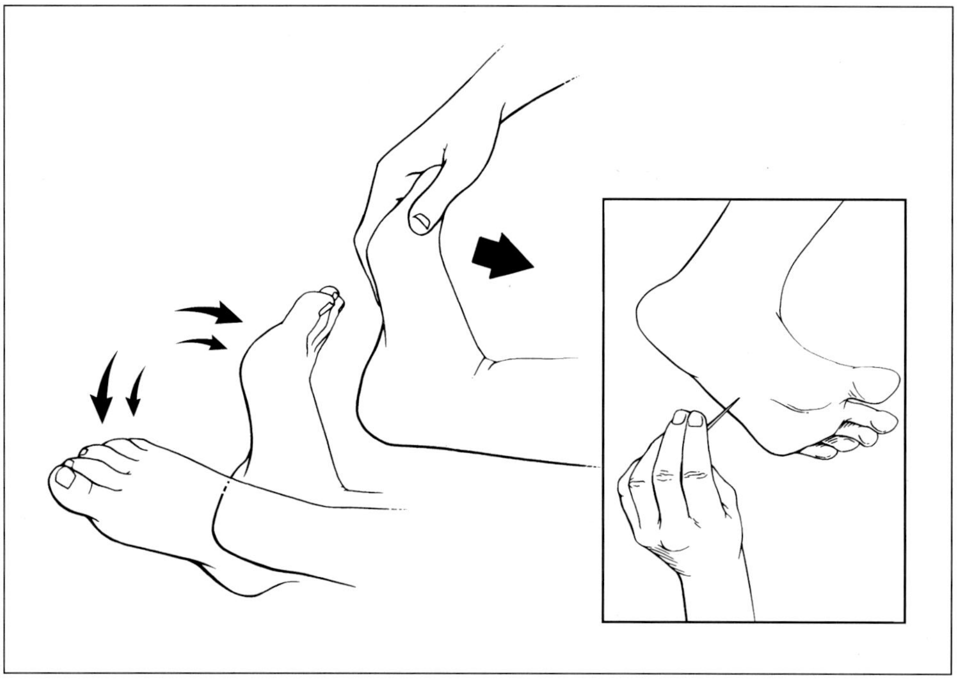

Figure 4.10
Babinski's extensor plantar response (Oppenheimer's test): extension of the great toe with light plantar stimulation is indicative of the upper motor neuron inhibition. Clonus is elicited by a quick, but lightly applied, thrust upward on the forefoot (box). Production of oscillating motion of the ankle joint is considered positive for spinal cord impingement

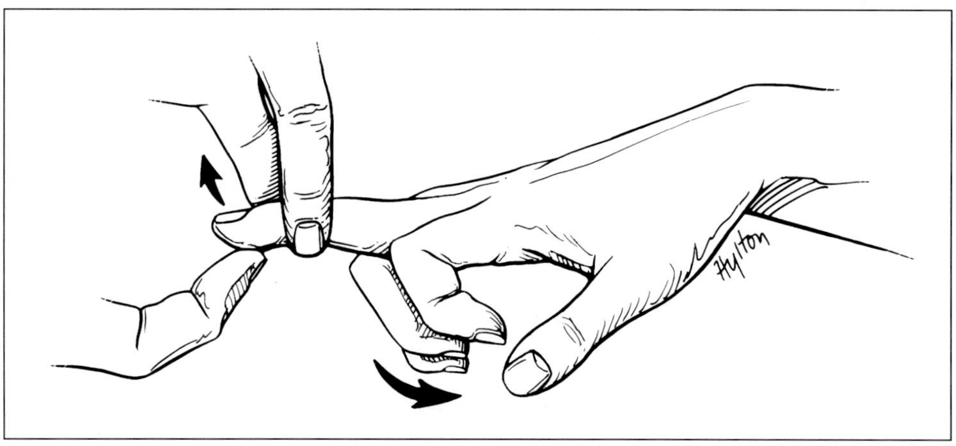

Figure 4.11
Hoffman's reflex is elicited by suddenly extending the middle finger distal interphalangeal joint. Production of reflex finger flexion, particularly when asymmetric, is indicative of spinal cord impingement

interruption in C7 function is the triceps mechanism. Equally, the triceps reflex is a sensitive means of further evaluation of this root. Also, for the sake of completion, the more powerful wrist flexor, flexor carpi radialis, is also innervated by the seventh cervical root. Although the flexor carpi radialis is assisted by the flexor carpi ulnaris (C8), weakness in the C7 distribution will markedly diminish wrist flexion clinically. Along these same lines, the finger extensors, extensor digitorum communis, extensor digiti indicis, and extensor digiti quinti, are also served mainly by the C7 root. The eighth cervical root is best tested by focusing on the muscle groups in the hand; the finger flexors obtain their function primarily via the C8 root. This will be reflected in a decreased grip strength, although at this level there is overlap with the innervation of the hand intrinsics by both C8 and T1. The C8 and T1 distributions both have no reflex abnormalities that need consideration. However, they have distinct sensory distributions, and it is generally agreed that hand intrinsics, namely interossei function, are innervated by T1, and grip function via the finger flexors represents primarily C8 contribution. Again, these are just guidelines, as there is considerable overlap at each level.

One final note on the motor examination involves various pathologic reflexes which must be tested, because they indicate the presence of a myelopathic process. The presence of lower extremity clonus, or Oppenheimer's or Babinski's extensor plantar response, indicates serious

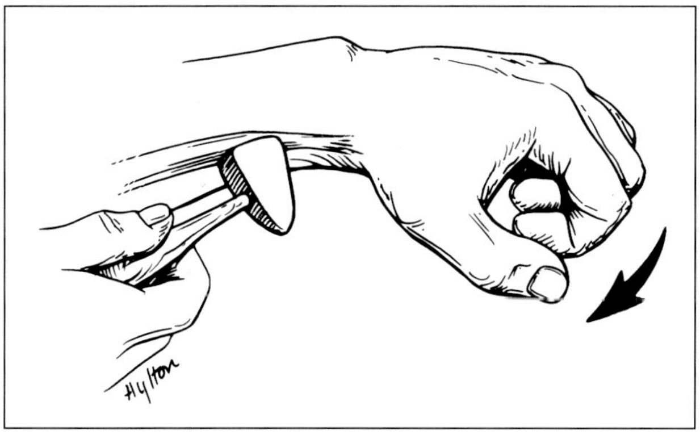

Figure 4.12
Inverted radial reflex: tapping of the distal brachioradialis tendon produces spastic contraction of the finger flexors

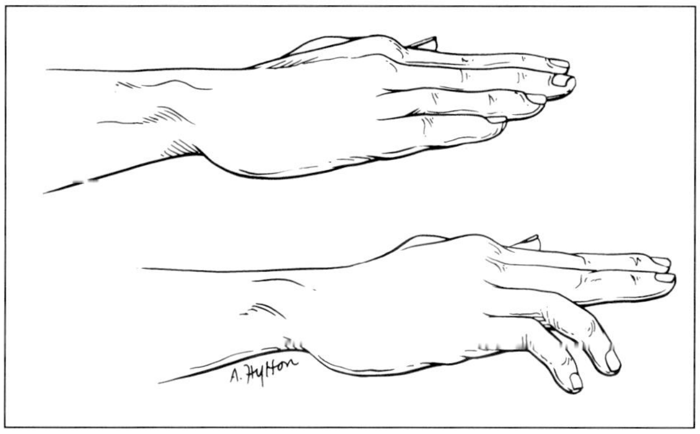

Figure 4.13
Finger escape sign: the patient is asked to hold all digits of the hand in an adducted and extended position. In cases of myelopathy, the two ulnar digits will fall into flexion and abduction, usually within 30 seconds

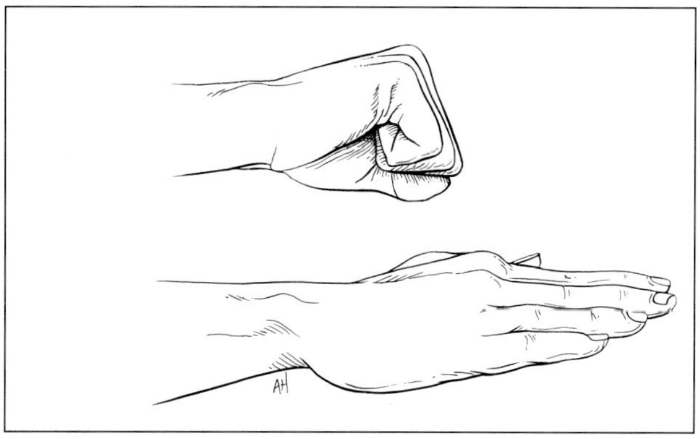

Figure 4.14
Grip and release test: the patient is asked to form a fist and then to release all digits into extension, rapidly repeating the sequence. A normal patient should be able to perform this motion 20 times within a 10-second period

disruption of the normal upper motor neuron inhibition, and should be noted (Fig. 4.10). Hoffman's reflex (reflex finger flexion with sudden middle finger distal interphalangeal joint extension), when present and especially when asymmetric, is strongly indicative of cervical cord impingement (Fig. 4.11). Also, patients with cervical cord impingement at C6 level may exhibit a paradoxical brachioradialis reflex where, by tapping the distal brachioradialis tendon, a diminished reflex is elicited with a reciprocal spastic contraction of the finger flexors; this is known as the inverted radial reflex (Fig. 4.12).[22,30,40] Finally, as discussed previously, patients may also describe sudden electric shock sensations throughout the trunk and extremities with neck flexion–extension. This can also, on occasion, be elicited on physical examination and is known as Lhermitte's sign, indicative of cervical myelopathy. Ono et al[31] have described the myelopathic hand syndrome. The finger adduction test and the grip and release test are helpful in delineating a myelopathic state. The finger escape sign is performed by asking the patient to hold all digits of the hand in an extended and adducted position (Fig. 4.13). With myelopathy, the ulnar digits will fall into abduction and some degree of flexion usually within 30 seconds. The grip and release test requires the patient first to form a fist and then to release all digits into extension, repeating the sequence rapidly. Under normal circumstances, a patient should be able to perform this maneuver 20 times within a 10-second period (Fig. 4.14).

The sensory examination and its relationship to nerve root dysfunction are given in Table 4.2 and illustrated in Fig. 4.2. As discussed in the previous section, the sensory evaluation begins with the history, and is largely subjective. Because of the varying patterns of innervation, the examination can be complicated and difficult to interpret or illicit. The most helpful aspect of the sensory examination involves the dermatomal nature of cervical radiculopathy. Patients will often note decreased sensation to light touch or pinprick across a specific radicular pattern. When correlated with the complete history and examination, this usually acts as confirmatory evidence that implicates a specific level of pathology. Myelopathic changes are, however, more diffuse, involving altered perception of pain and temperature as well as proprioception, vibratory and light touch appreciation. A compilation of these disturbances can lead

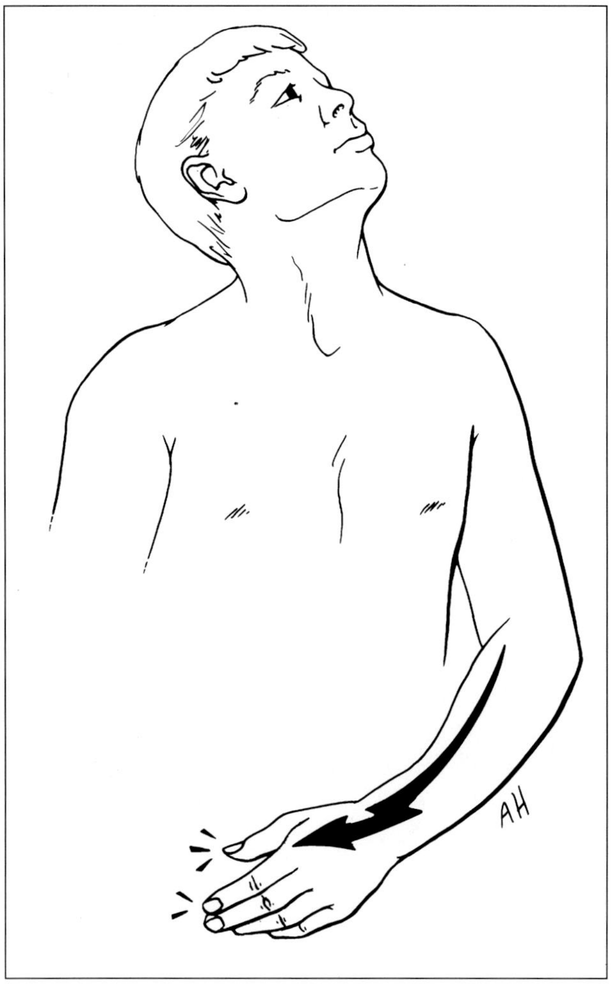

Figure 4.15
Spurling's sign: extension of the neck coupled with lateral rotation toward the affected arm will exacerbate cervical radiculopathy by further narrowing the neural foramina

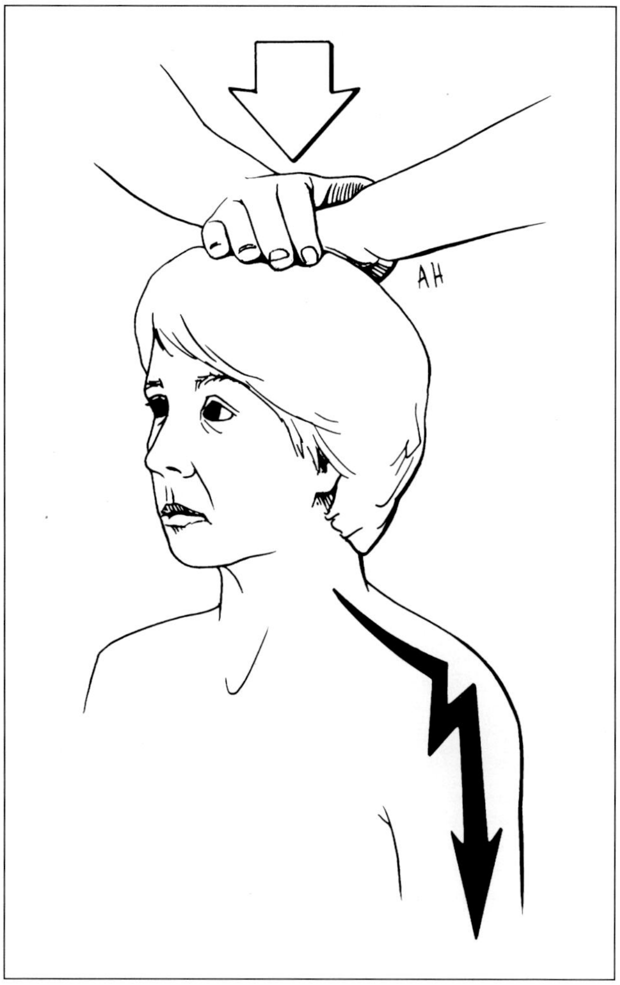

Figure 4.16
Axial cervical compression testing may also reproduce cervical radicular symptoms by narrowing the neuroforamina. Distractive forces may relieve root compression

to subtle or severe sensory deficits in both the upper and the lower extremities, and should be noted. Most importantly, the level at which normal function returns must be documented. This may be the only indication of spinal cord sparing in the trauma patient with severe motor paralysis.

To complete the physical examination, and to clarify the clinical suspicion of nerve root pathology, several provocative tests exist which are worth incorporating into the evaluation.[9,16] The Spurling sign produces arm pain with neck hyperextension and lateral cervical rotation toward the side of pathology[41] (Fig. 4.15). This causes further neural canal impingement and exacerbates the radiculopathy. In a similar fashion, an axial cervical compression test will elicit arm pain by narrowing the foramina, and distraction forces on the neck may relieve such nerve root compression (Fig. 4.16). Another provocative test is the Valsalva maneuver, which, through an increase in intra-abdominal pressure, simultaneously increases cerebrospinal pressure which, in turn, increases the pressure about the cervical roots.[16] The shoulder abduction test relieves arm pain by acting as a reverse tension sign (Fig. 4.17). This was shown to have a high correlation with extradural compression on the cervical nerve roots in the series of Davidson et al.[8] Finally, the swallowing test is a non-specific means of detecting irritation of the anterior neck structures by a

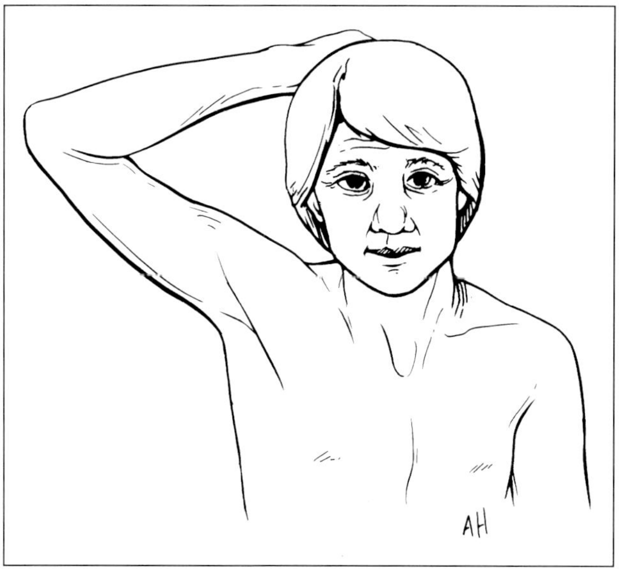

Figure 4.17
Shoulder abduction text: many patients with cervical radiculopathy will obtain relief in their arm pain with the shoulder held in an abducted position which alleviates tension

large anterior vertebral osteophyte, tumor, or inflammatory mass.[16,38]

To complete the history and physical examination, the physician needs to make a provisional diagnosis, which is later confirmed by appropriate testing. Development of a routine in history taking and examination, although seeming laborious, is necessary to prevent oversight or misdiagnosis. With the current advances in technology, the importance of these measures may be forgotten. However, if this happens, inappropriate testing and consultation can produce further undue anxieties and costs which complicate the practice of medicine.

REFERENCES

1 Benini A. Clinical features of cervical root compression C5-C8 and their variations. *Neurol Orthop* **4**: 74–88, 1987.
2 Boden SD, Weisel SW, Laws ER Jr, et al. *The Aging Spine: Essentials of Pathophysiology, Diagnosis, and Treatment*, 46. Philadelphia: W.B. Saunders, 1991.
3 Bohlman HH. Cervical spondylosis with moderate to severe myelopathy: A report of 17 cases treated by Robinson anterior cervical discectomy and fusion. *Spine* **2**: 151–162, 1977.
4 Bohlman HH. Acute fractures and dislocations of the cervical spine: An analysis of 300 hospitalized patients and review of the literature. *J Bone Joint Surg [Am]* **61**: 1119–1142, 1979.
5 Bohlman HH, Ducker TB. Spine Trauma in adults. Spine and spinal cord injuries. In Rothman RH, Simeone FA (eds) *The Spine*, 3rd ed, 973–1104. Philadelphia: WB Saunders, 1992.
6 Bradshaw P. Pain caused by cervical spondylosis. *Rheumatism* **17**: 2–7, 1961.
7 Clark CR. Cervical spondylitic myelopathy: History and physical findings. *Spinc* **13**: 847 849, 1988.
8 Davidson R, Dunn E, Metzmaker J. The shoulder abduction test in the diagnosis of radicular pain in cervical extradural compressive monoradiculopathies. *Spine* **6**: 441–446, 1981.
9 Dillin WH, Watkins RG. Cervical myelopathy and cervical radiculopathy. *Seminars in Spine Surgery* **1**(4): 200–208, 1989.
10 Epstein JA. Management of cervical spinal stenosis, spondylosis, and myeloradiculopathy. In Tindall GT (ed) *Contemporary Neurosurgery*, Vol 2, 1–6. Baltimore: Williams & Wilkins, 1985.
11 Ferguson RJC, Caplan LR. Cervical spondylitic myelopathy. *Neurol Clin North Am* **3**: 373–382, 1985.
12 Ford FR, Clark D. Thrombosis of the basilar artery with softenings in the cerebellum and brain stem due to manipulation of the neck. *Bull Johns Hopkins Hosp* **98**: 37–42, 1956.
13 Good D, Couch J, Wascaster L. 'Numb clumsy hands' and high cervical spondylosis. *Surg Neurol* **22**: 285–291, 1984.
14 Gore DR, Sepic SB, Gardner GM, Murray MP. Neck pain: A long term follow-up of 205 patients. *Spine* **12**: 1–5, 1987.
15 Gorter K. Influence of laminectomy on the course of cervical myelopathy. *Acta Neurochir* **33**: 265–281, 1976.
16 Hoppenfeld S. Physical examination of the cervical spine and temporomandibular joint. In *Physical Examination of the Spine and Extremities*, 105–132. Norwalk, CT: Appleton-Century-Crofts 1976.
17 Hult L. The Munkfors investigation. *Acta Orthop Scand Suppl* **16**: 1, 1959.
18 Jackson R. Headaches associated with disorders of the cervical spine. *Headache* **6**: 175–179, 1967.
19 Kraus JF, Franti CE, Riggins RS, et al. Incidence of traumatic spinal cord lesions. *J Chronic Dis* **28**: 471–492, 1975.
20 Kurz LT, Simeone FA, Dillin WH, et al. Cervical disc disease. In Rothman RH, Simeone FA (eds) *The Spine*, 3rd ed, 547–596. Philadelphia: WB Saunders 1992.
21 Langfitt T, Elliot F. Pain in the back and legs caused by cervical spinal cord compression. *JAMA* **200**: 112–116, 1967.
22 Lestini WF, Weisel SW. The pathogenesis of cervical spondylosis. *Clin Orthop* **239**: 69–84, 1989.
23 Liang MH, Katz JN. Clinical evaluation of patients with a suspected spine problem. In Frymoyer JW (ed) *The Adult Spine: Principles and Practice*, 223–239. New York: Raven Press 1991.
24 Lunsford LD, Bissonette D, Zorub D. Anterior surgery for cervical disc disease. Part 2. *J Neurosurg* **53**: 12–19, 1980.
25 MacNab I. Symptoms in cervical disc degeneration. In Sherk HH, Dunn EJ, Eismont FJ, et al (eds) *The Cervical Spine*, 2nd ed, 599–606. Cervical Spine Research Society, Philadelphia: JB Lippincott 1989.
26 McQueen DJ, Khan MI. Evaluation of patients with cervical spine lesions. In Sherk HH, Dunn EJ, Eismont FJ, et al (eds) *The Cervical Spine*, 2nd ed, 199–211. Cervical Spine Research Society, Philadelphia: JB Lippincott 1989.

27 Meyer GA, Berman IR, Doty DB. Hemodynamic responses to acute quadriplegia with or without chest trauma. *J Neurosurg* **34**: 168–177, 1971.

28 Meyer PR Jr. Acute injury retrieval and splinting techniques: On-site care. In Meyer PR Jr (ed) *Surgery of Spine Trauma*, 1–9. New York: Churchill Livingstone 1989.

29 Meyer PR Jr. Emergency room assessment: Management of spinal cord and associated injuries. In Meyer PR Jr (ed) *Surgery of Spine Trauma*, 23–60. New York: Churchill Livingstone 1989.

30 Montgomery DM, Brower RS. Cervical spondylitic myelopathy: Clinical syndrome and natural history. *Orthop Clin North Am* **23**: 487–493, 1992.

31 Ono K, Ebara S, Fiji T, et al. Myelopathic hand. *J Bone Joint Surg [Br]* **69**: 215–219, 1987.

32 Ray GC. Mumps. In Braunwald E, Isselbacher KJ, Petersdorf RG, et al (eds) *Harrison's Principles of Internal Medicine*, 11th ed, 709–711. New York: McGraw-Hill 1987.

33 Rogers WA. Fractures and dislocations of the cervical spine: An end result study. *J Bone Joint Surg [Am]* **39**: 341–376, 1957.

34 Rothman RH, Marvel JP Jr. The acute cervical disk. *Clin Orthop* **109**: 59–68, 1975.

35 Rothman RH, Rashbaum RF. Pathogenesis of signs and symptoms of cervical disc degeneration. In *American Academy of Orthopaedic Surgeons, Instructional Course Lectures*, Vol. XXVII, 203–215. St Louis: CV Mosby 1978.

36 Simeone FA. Cervical disc disease. Cervical disc disease with radiculopathy. In Rothman RH, Simeone FA, *The Spine*, 3rd ed, 553–560. Philadelphia: WB Saunders 1992.

37 Simeone FA, Dillin WH. Treatment of cervical disc disease. Selection of operative approach. *Contemp Neurosurg* 1–6, 1986.

38 Simeone FA, Rothman RH. Cervical disc disease. In Rothman RH, Simeone FA (eds) *The Spine*, 2nd ed, 440–497. Philadelphia: WB Saunders 1982.

39 Soderstrom CA, Brumback RJ. Early care of the patient with cervical spine injury. *Orthop Clin North Am* **17**(1): 3–13, 1986.

40 Spillane JD, Lloyd GH. The diagnosis of lesions of the spinal cord in association with 'osteoarthritic' disease of the cervical spine. *Brain* **75**: 177–186, 1952.

41 Spurling RG. *Lesions of the Cervical Intervertebral Disc.* Springfield, IL: Thomas, 1956.

42 Sypert GW. Neck pain and cervical syndromes: Part I – Evaluation. *Surgical Rounds for Orthopaedics*, 36–44, January 1990.

5 Radiology of the cervical spine

G. F. Carrera and
Howard S. An

Imaging studies influence the clinical care of patients with cervical spine disease throughout the diagnostic and therapeutic process. There are a wide variety of techniques and modalities available to image osseous structures and soft tissues of the cervical spine. Radioisotope scanning and magnetic resonance imaging (MRI) may demonstrate the physiologic activity of osseous structures and the intervertebral disc. To be efficient and cost-effective, it is necessary to have a good understanding of the specific types of information gained from each examination. Additionally, for some clinical entities, the correct sequencing of the various studies is imperative to maximize obtainable information and to improve cost-efficiency.

Correctly matching the information available from imaging studies to the clinical question at hand assures that crucial decisions are made rapidly and accurately. Imaging studies must be chosen with full attention to the diagnostic requirements of the clinical condition. Often, studies must be modified to answer specific questions. Complex cases require close communication between surgeon and imaging consultant to arrive at the best examination. As a general principle, abbreviated or incomplete examinations should be avoided unless necessary for patient safety. The savings in time, radiation, and money rarely compensate for inadequate diagnostic information. Advanced imaging modalities such as computed tomography, magnetic resonance imaging, and radioisotope techniques require both a sophisticated understanding of the technical requirements for adequate cervical spine studies, and commitment to the time and care needed to produce diagnostic studies.

Radiographic imaging of cervical spine disease is an extraordinarily complex subject, whose scope is well beyond the limits of this chapter. Many important subjects, such as evaluation of plain films or radiographs of cervical spine trauma, take up entire texts. The explosion of new imaging modalities has led to vast[32] changes in the way we evaluate the spine. A full understanding of the physical basis of these techniques is critical to grasp their use in cervical disease processes fully. A good, functional approach to imaging in cervical spine evaluation, however, can be grounded in a basic understanding of the major types of information each imaging modality provides. To some extent, appropriate imaging studies for each diagnostic entity will be reviewed in the ensuing chapters.

PLAIN RADIOGRAPHS

Plain radiographs of the cervical spine provide a rapid and accurate assessment of the anatomic relationship of bony structures, good definition of bone integrity, and a surprisingly effective screening examination for soft tissue structures surrounding the vertebrae. Examination of plain radiographs of the spine is widely available and applied as a screening modality and a diagnostic tool. Additionally, routine postoperative evaluation of many cervical spine disorders is also completed through radiography. Its use as a diagnostic study in such conditions as trauma, tumor, inflammatory disease, and degenerative disease of discs and joints has been extensively reviewed and is commonly understood. Fundamental radiographic principles of accurate, reproducible positioning, good exposure and processing, and complete examination (including special projections when clinically indicated), must be followed both to optimize diagnostic information and to minimize diagnostic failure resulting from inadequate or incomplete examination.[14,25,36,37,52]

Plain radiographs generally represent the first radiographic studies used to evaluate suspected cervical spine disease after clinical evaluation. In the acute trauma setting, initial evaluation should be performed while the patient remains protected by a rigid cervical collar. The radiographic examination should be limited first to those projections that can demonstrate lesions threatening neurologic status or life.

After examination of lateral projections (which should include the C7–T1 region of the spine unless the habitus or medical condition of the patient is prohibitive) for sagittal plane dislocations or displacements, fractures, or soft-tissue clues of osseous or discovertebral disruption, frontal and odontoid projections should be done to complete the acute examination. This series of views should reveal those lesions that are unstable or require treatment. If the patient remains symptomatic after initial treatment, or if there are clues to fracture on initial screening studies (especially disruptions in posterior elements), additional plain radiographs such as oblique projections, angled projections to demonstrate the lateral masses adequately, or flexion–extension radiographs may be performed. Such views may be required to solve problems, but are not generally required in the trauma-room setting.

Prevertebral soft-tissue swelling or small suspected fractures may indicate an unstable injury which can be shown with flexion–extension views. In the setting of acute trauma such projections should be performed with extreme care, because aggravation of an unstable injury with subsequent neurologic damage is a risk. Flexion–extension views of the spine in the patient suspected of acute fracture should be done under the supervision of the responsible clinician, and with the help of the patient in active positioning – never with forced or passive positioning.[1,15,23,27,28,54,66]

The plain lateral radiograph of the cervical spine remains the single most important imaging study for cervical spine trauma, and should first be evaluated with four imaginary lordotic lines which are formed by the anterior margins of the vertebral bodies, posterior vertebral margins, anterior cortical margins of the spinous process, and the tips of the spinous processes (Fig. 5.1). If there is any malalignment of a motion segment, the amount of translation and angulation should be measured as described by White and Panjabi.[67] Translations >3.5 mm and angulations >11° are regarded as unstable (Fig. 5.2). With unilateral facet dislocation, the articular facet of the vertebra above is perched or anteriorly dislocated on one side (Fig. 5.3). As a result of unilateral involvement, there is an associated rotatory deformity, and this can be appreciated on the anteroposterior view (Fig. 5.3c). The amount of anterior displacement is less than half the anteroposterior diameter of the vertebral body in unilateral facet dislocations. With bilateral facet dislocation, both articular facets of the vertebra above are perched or dislocated anterior to the superior articular facets of the vertebra below (Fig. 5.4), with the amount of anterior displacement more than half the anteroposterior diameter of the vertebral body. Such dislocations are more unstable injuries and have a higher incidence of associated spinal cord injury.

Vertebral bodies, facet joints, laminae, and spinous processes of the lower cervical spine must be carefully viewed to rule out fractures. An avulsion fracture of the spinous process is common in the lower cervical spine and is known as a clay shoveler's fracture. Compression or axial loading force may result in a compression wedge fracture or a more severe burst fracture with posterior cortex comminution. The 'tear drop' fracture refers to the avulsed triangular anteroinferior fragment of the vertebral body;[39] it is sustained by a flexion and axial loading mechanism of injury, and is usually associated with posterior ligamentous disruption and posterior displacement of the posterosuperior fragment into

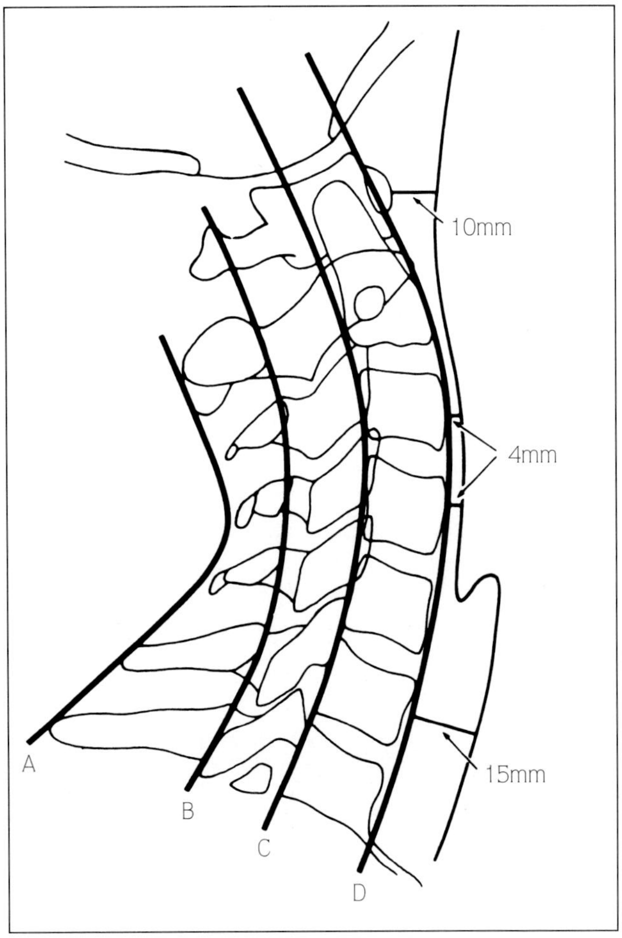

Figure 5.1
The lateral radiograph with four imaginary lordotic lines which are formed by the anterior margins of the vertebral bodies (a), posterior vertebral margins (b), anterior cortical margins of the spinous process (c), and the tips of the spinous processes (d). Normal width of retropharyngeal soft tissue is also shown. (From Meyer PR Jr, *Surgery of Spine Trauma*, New York: Churchill Livingstone, 1989, p.210)

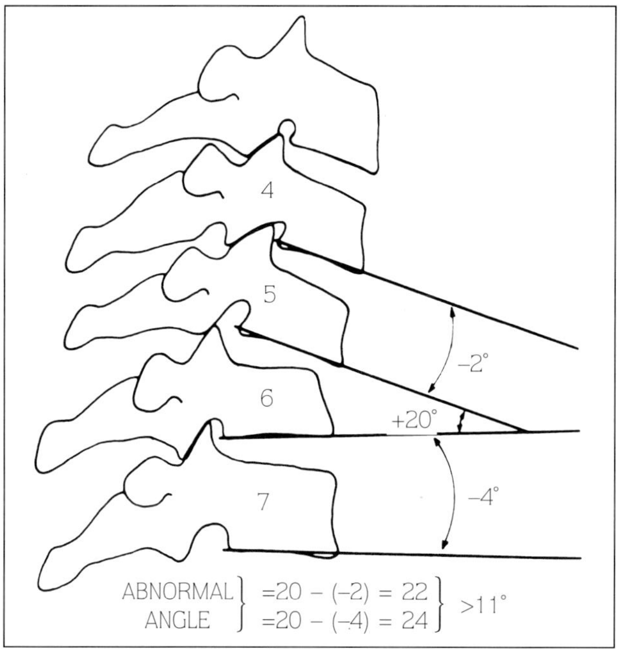

a

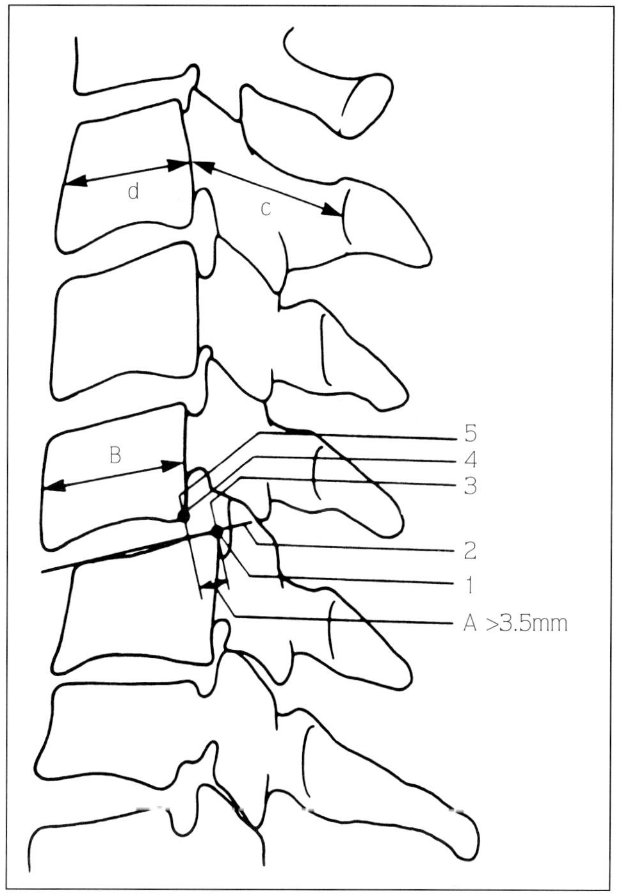

b

Figure 5.2
(a) The angulation between C5 and C6 is 20°, which is >11° more than at either adjacent interspace. (From White AA, Johnson RM, Panjabi MM, Southwick WO. Biomechanical analysis of clinical stability in the cervical spine. *Clin Orthop* 109: 85, 1975). (b) If the linear distance *A* is >3.5 mm, then it is considered to be unstable. If Pavlov's ratio (*c/d*) is <0.8, it is considered abnormal. (From White AA, Panjabi MM. *Clinical Biomechanics of the Spine*. Philadelphia, JB Lippincott, 1978, p.316)

the spinal canal (Fig. 5.5). Fracture of the superior articular facet may occur with a flexion force, and may cause nerve root dysfunction. An isolated fracture of the lamina may occur with a hyperextension injury, but most laminar fractures occur in association with burst fractures of the vertebral body.

Upper cervical spine injuries are also well demonstrated by the lateral radiograph. Occipitocervical dislocation is usually fatal, but patients may present with occipitocervical instability with subluxation and no neurologic deficit. Various methods are described to assess the instability of the occipitocervical spine. A line drawn from the clivus should intersect the odontoid process at the junction of its anterior and middle thirds. The posterior margin of the foramen magnum and the spinolaminar line of C1 should be in alignment. Power's ratio can also be calculated from the lateral radiograph to assess occipitocervical instability (Fig. 5.6). The distance between the clivus and the tip of the odontoid process should be 4–5 mm (Fig. 5.7). If the distance between the anterior arch of C1 and the odontoid process is >3 mm in adults, rupture of the transverse ligament is likely (Fig. 5.7). The space available for the spinal cord between the posterior margin of the odontoid process and the C1 ring should not be <13 mm (Fig. 5.7). The open-mouth anteroposterior view may also demonstrate asymmetry of the lateral mass of C1 in relationship to the odontoid process, suggestive of rotatory C1–C2 subluxation.

The ring disruption of the atlas or Jefferson's fracture is not easily demonstrated by the lateral radiograph. However, the anteroposterior view will show lateral displacement of the lateral masses of C1. If the combined lateral displacement of the lateral masses exceeds 6.9 mm,

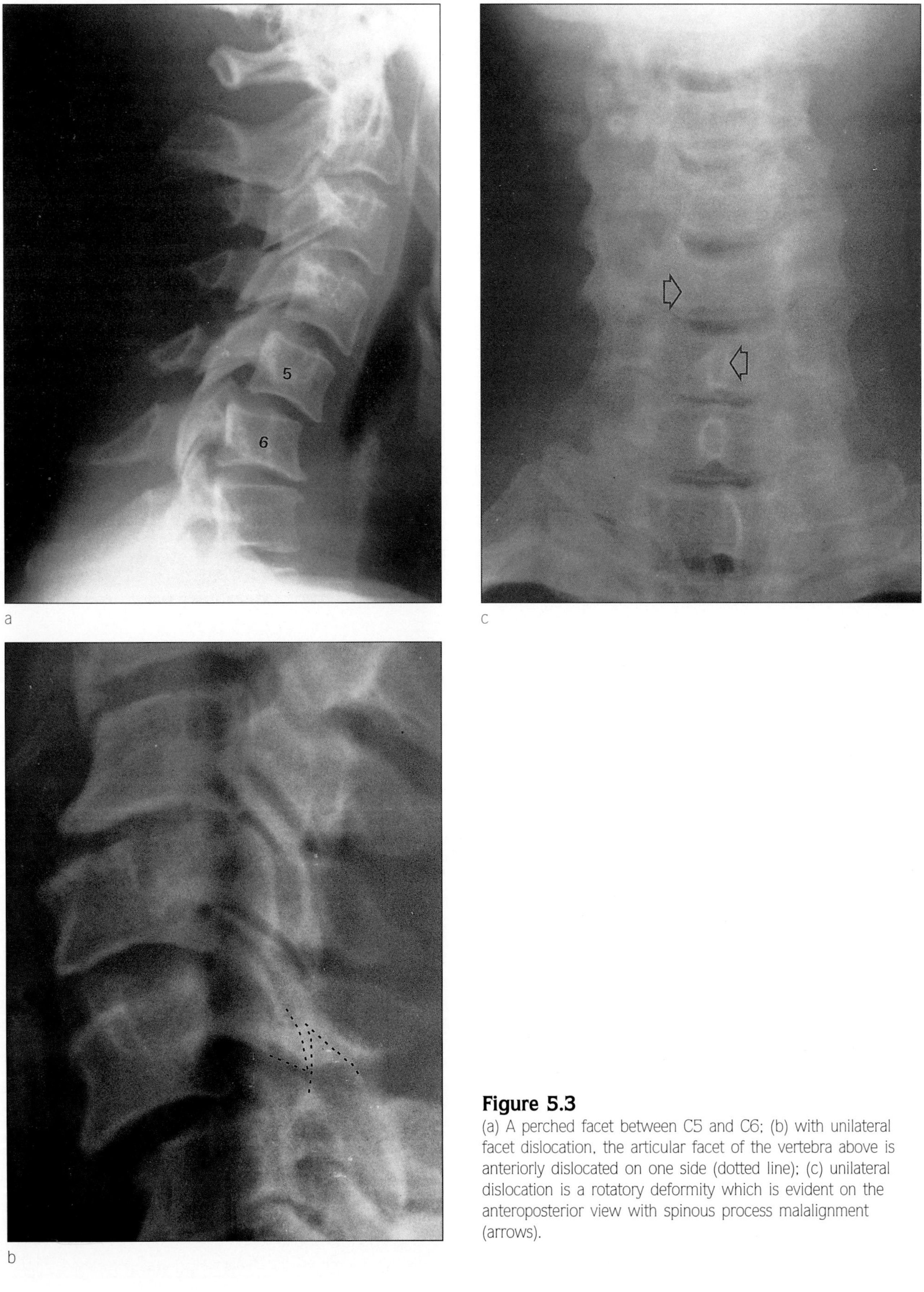

Figure 5.3
(a) A perched facet between C5 and C6; (b) with unilateral facet dislocation, the articular facet of the vertebra above is anteriorly dislocated on one side (dotted line); (c) unilateral dislocation is a rotatory deformity which is evident on the anteroposterior view with spinous process malalignment (arrows).

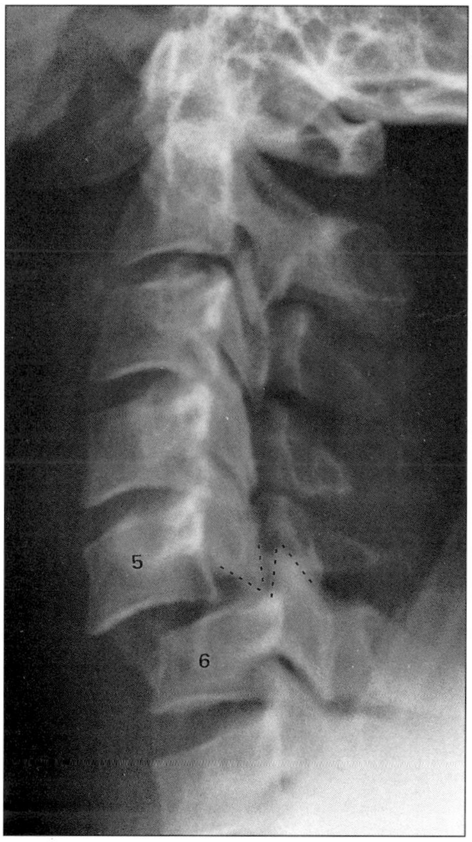

Figure 5.4
Bilateral dislocation of facet joints (dotted line) of C5 over C6 with >50% anterior displacement.

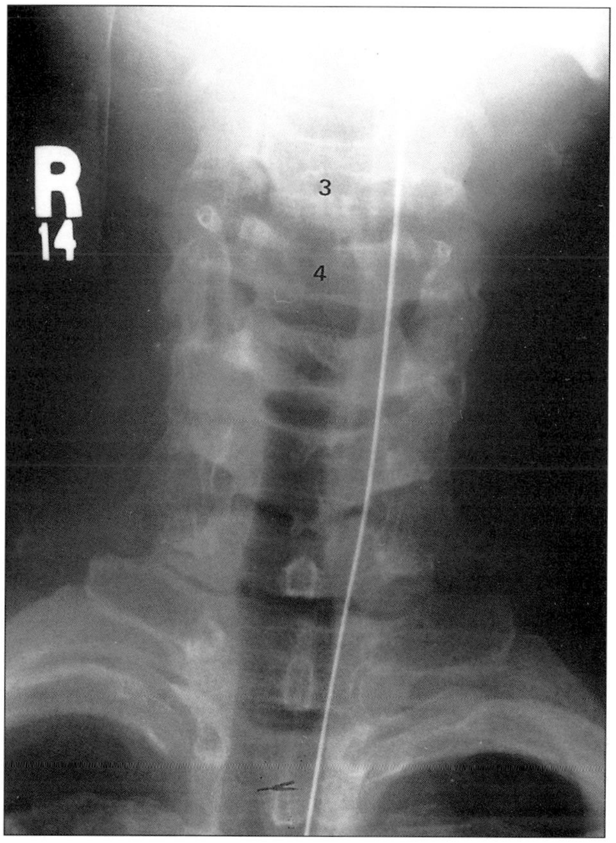

a

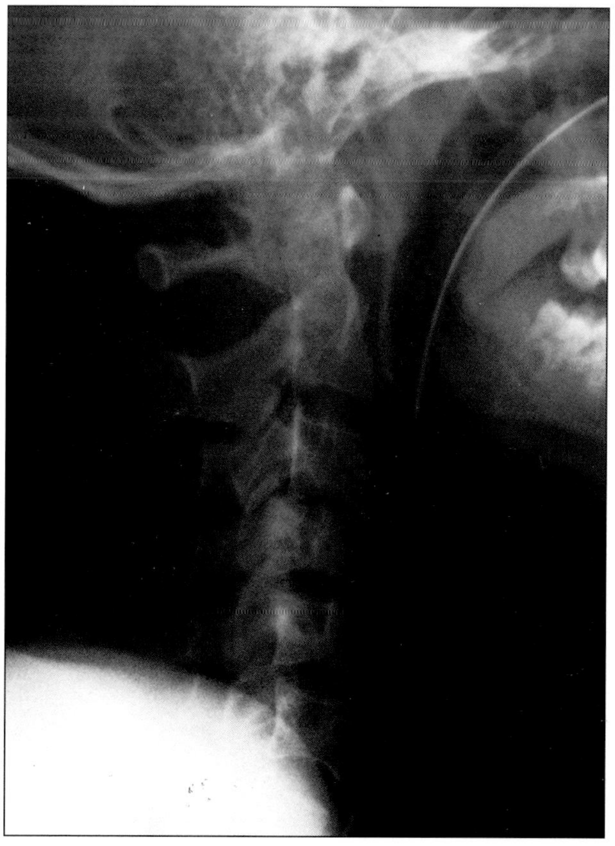

b

Figure 5.5
(a) Anteroposterior and (b) lateral radiographs following a motor vehicle accident show a flexion tear-drop fracture with bilateral facet subluxation at C3–C4. Anteroposterior radiographs show no fracture or malalignment, because the subluxation is bilateral. The nasogastric tube is deviated significantly to the left because of prevertebral hematoma. The lateral view is somewhat overexposed. Anterior subluxation of C3 on C4 with a flexion tear-drop fracture of the anterosuperior corner of C4 is apparent.

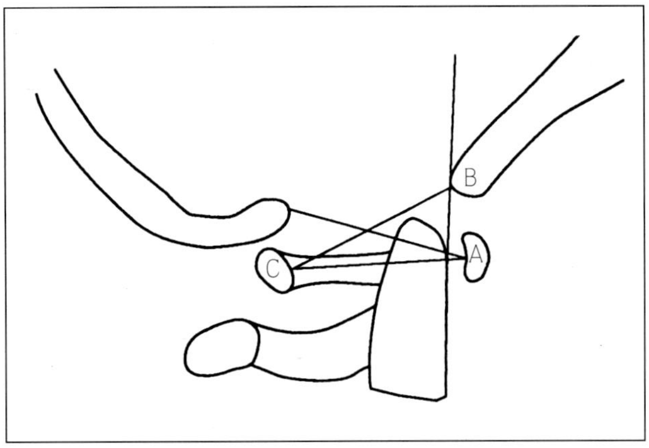

Figure 5.6
Power's ratio (BC/OA) >1 suggests anterior atlanto-occipital dislocation. The distance between the basion and the spinolaminar line of C1 is divided by the distance between the posterior margin of the foramen magnum (opisthion) and the posterior margin of the anterior arch of C1.

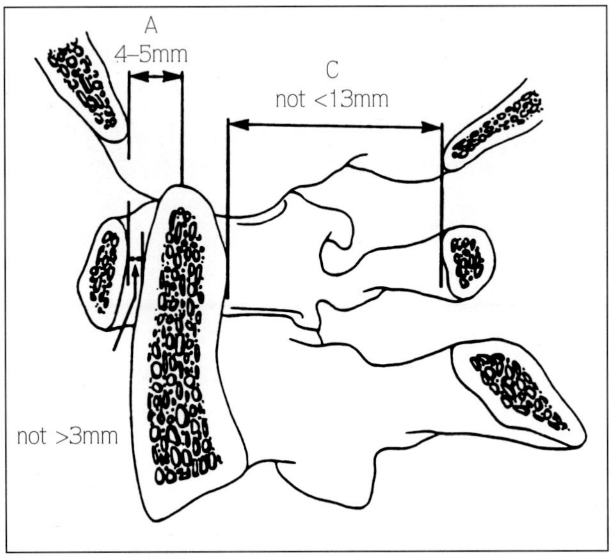

Figure 5.7
Critical measurements of the upper cervical spine. The distance between the clivus and the tip of the odontoid process should be about 4–5 mm. If the distance between the anterior arch of C1 and the odontoid process is >3 mm in adults, the rupture of the transverse ligament is likely. The space available for the spinal cord between the posterior margin of the odontoid process and the C1 ring should not be less than 13 mm.

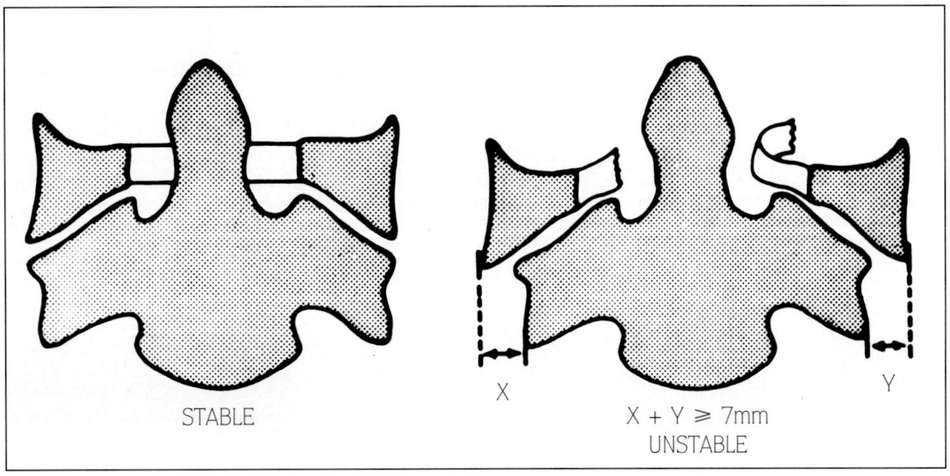

Figure 5.8
When the Jefferson fracture of C1 shows bilateral overhang of the lateral masses which totals 7 mm or more, a rupture of the transverse ligament is likely. (From White AA, Panjabi MM. *Clinical Biomechanics of the Spine.* Philadelphia, JB Lippincott, 1978, p.294)

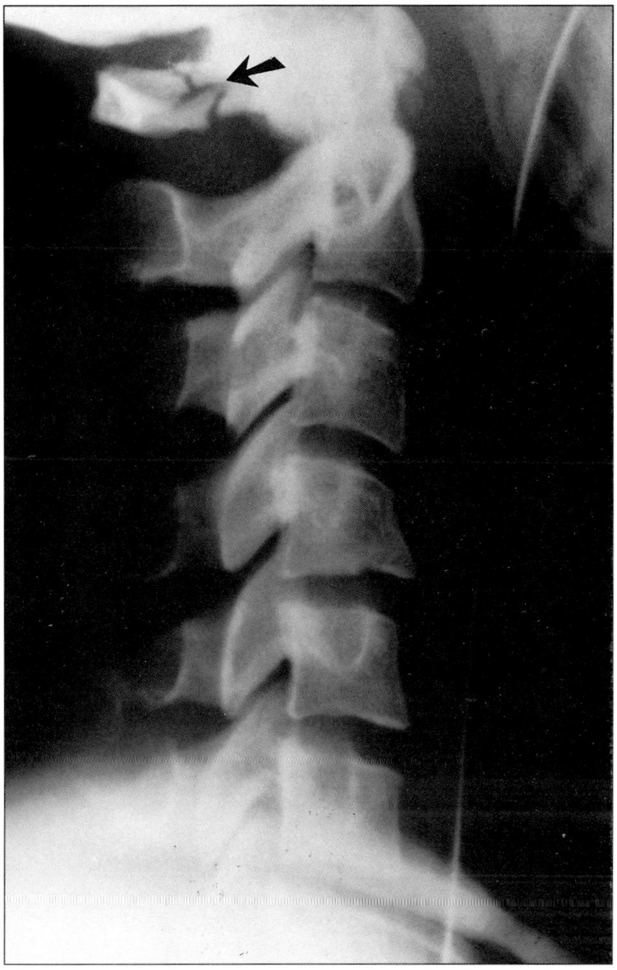

Figure 5.9
A fracture of the posterior arch demonstrated by the lateral radiograph (arrow). These fractures are a result of hyperextension injury as the posterior arch is compressed between the skull and the spinous process of C2.

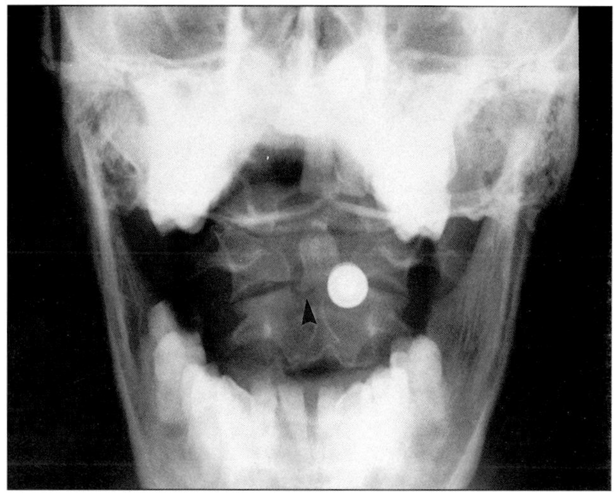

a

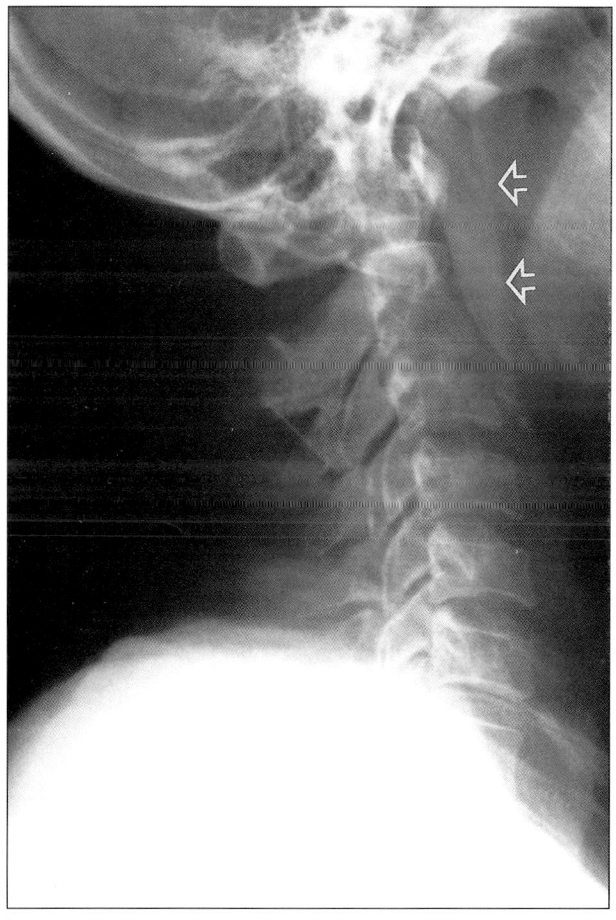

b

Figure 5.10
(a) Open-mouth anteroposterior and (b) lateral radiographs of the cervical spine after acute trauma show a type II odontoid fracture. The lateral view shows extensive anterior soft-tissue swelling (open arrows). Odontoid view shows the fracture line across the base of the odontoid (arrowhead). The importance of clearing overlying artifacts from critical areas is obvious.

the fracture is considered more unstable as the transverse ligament is most probably disrupted (Fig. 5.8).[24] Fracture of the posterior arch of the atlas is best demonstrated by the lateral radiograph (Fig. 5.9). These fractures are a result of a hyperextension injury as the posterior arch is compressed between the skull and the spinous process of C2. Fractures of the dens may result from a flexion injury with anterior displacement or an extension injury with posterior displacement. An open-mouth view will also demonstrate fractures of the dens (Fig. 5.10). Fracture patterns include an avulsion of the tip of the dens (type I), a transverse or oblique fracture through the base of the dens (type II), and a fracture that extends into the body of C2 (type III) (Fig. 5.11).[5] Fracture of the posterior arch of atlas is frequently seen with posteriorly displaced dens fractures. The fracture of the pars interarticularis of C2, commonly referred to as a hangman's fracture, is well demonstrated by the lateral radiograph (Fig. 5.12).[46] A classification of hangman's fracture is developed based on the amount of displacement (Fig. 5.13).

The width of the prevertebral soft tissue >10 mm at C1, >4–5 mm at C3–C4, and >15–20 mm at C6 is suggestive of soft-tissue swelling (see Fig. 5.1). Special views are sometimes necessary to detect subtle fractures. Oblique projections may demonstrate fractures of the pedicle, lamina, articular mass, and facet joint. A swimmer's view is indicated if the routine lateral radiograph with caudad traction of the shoulders fails to show the C7–T1 junction. The spinal canal should also be evaluated. Congenital or developmental narrowing of the canal may be evaluated using Torg's ratio[53]: with a ratio spinal canal/vertebral body of <0.8, the patient is thought to have an underlying cervical stenosis. Such findings may help explain neurologic deficiency without obvious abnormalities (see Fig. 5.2b).[60]

Patients being evaluated electively for cervical spine symptoms require a more extensive set of initial radiographs. Anteroposterior and lateral views, as well as an open-mouth odontoid projection and both oblique views, are necessary to visualize the entire cervical spine and the component articulations and foramina adequately. The 'screening lateral' view is to be decried as an adequate examination for symptomatic patients, because many lesions can be diagnosed only when orthogonal projections are examined. The responsibility of any examiner committing a patient to radiographic study is to provide an adequate examination for diagnosing all lesions demonstrable using that modality.

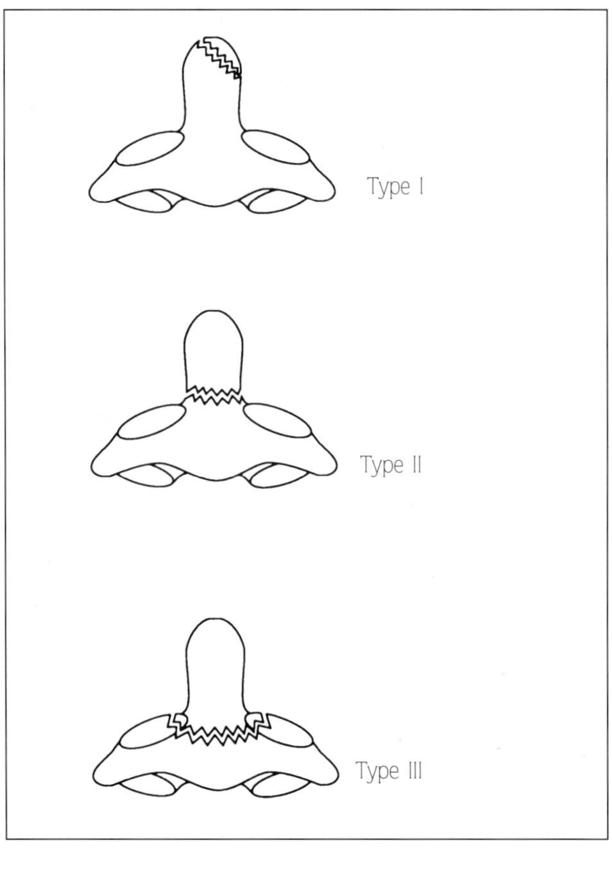

Figure 5.11
Fracture patterns include the tip of the dens (type I), the base of the dens (type II), and extension into the body of C2 (type III).

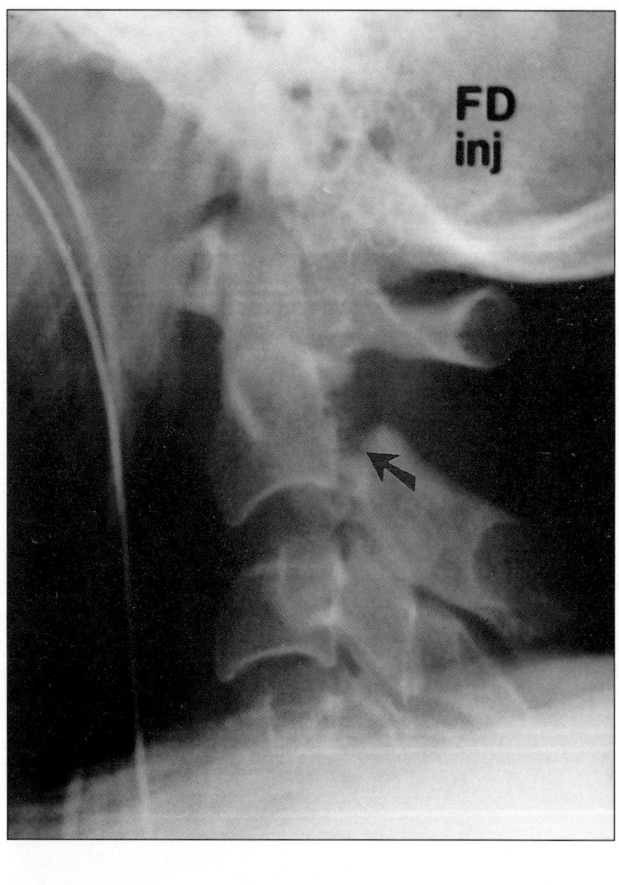

Figure 5.12
The fracture of the pars interarticularis of C2 or hangman's fracture is well demonstrated by the lateral radiograph (arrow).

The findings of neoplastic and inflammatory disease in the cervical spine are similar to those seen elsewhere in the skeleton. Osteolytic or osteosclerotic changes, frank destruction, and soft-tissue swelling or calcification are important clues to focal disease in the cervical spine (Fig. 5.14). Changes in the osseous structures resulting from intraspinal disorders such as tumors, cord expansion, or developmental anomalies of bone or neural structures are less common, but can present significant clues for diagnosis.

Degenerative disc disease and degenerative joint disease are common reasons for radiographic evaluation of the cervical spine (Fig. 5.15). Degenerative changes are very common in the symptom-free aging population, and are frequent sequelae to previous trauma. The importance of such changes as disc narrowing, vertebral osteophyte formation, and uncinate/foraminal osteophytes must be evaluated in light of the symptoms and findings on more specific examination of the soft tissues in and about the spinal canal. It must be emphasized that degenerative changes of the cervical spine as shown on plain radiographs may be very non-specific and require further correlative studies before specific treatment can be suggested. On the other hand, plain radiograph changes may serve to confirm the clinical suspicion of typical degenerative symptoms, and serve to reassure the clinician and patient alike that appropriate therapy is being followed and that a more sinister diagnosis is not warranted.

Postoperative plain radiograph evaluation of the cervical spine is important in following the integrity of complex procedures and their healing (Fig. 5.16). The critical element in the postoperative evaluation of the spine is reproducibility of the radiographs, so that subtle changes indicating complications can be diagnosed. If instrumentation has been applied it is crucial that the entire apparatus be imaged, and that similar projections are used on subsequent

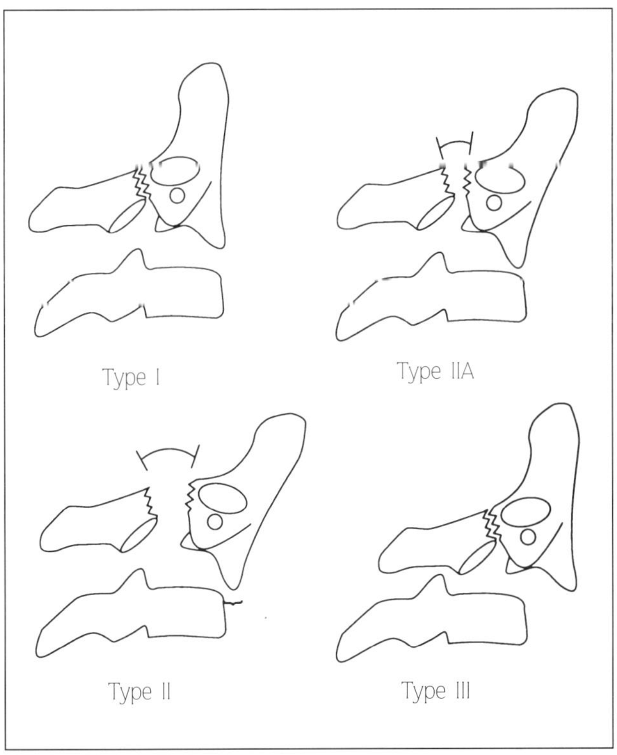

Figure 5.13
A classification of hangman's fracture based on the amount of displacement. Type I: minimal displacement (<3 mm); type II: >3 mm displacement and angulation; type IIa: severe angulation without significant translation; type III: associated facet dislocation of C2–C3.

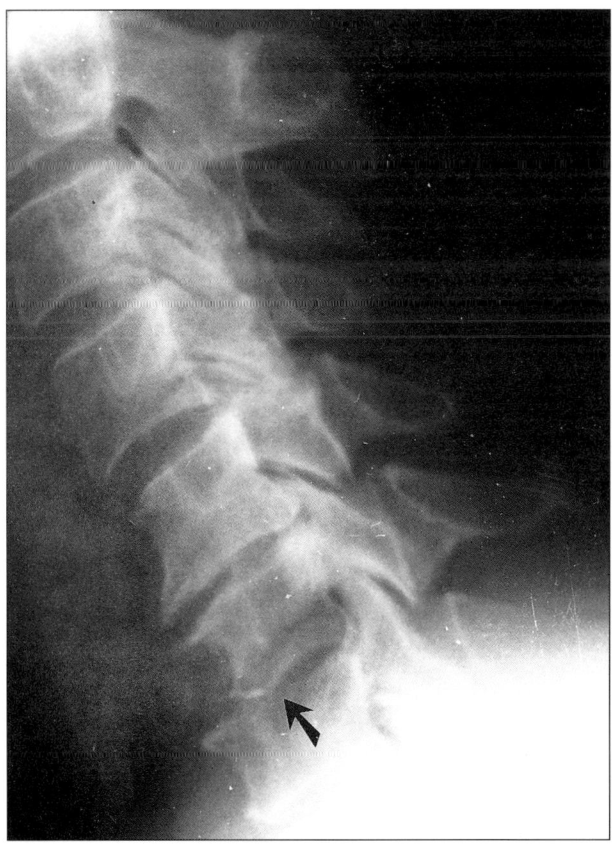

Figure 5.14
A lateral radiograph of a patient with osteomyelitis involving the C6–C7 region with disc collapse and osteolysis (arrow).

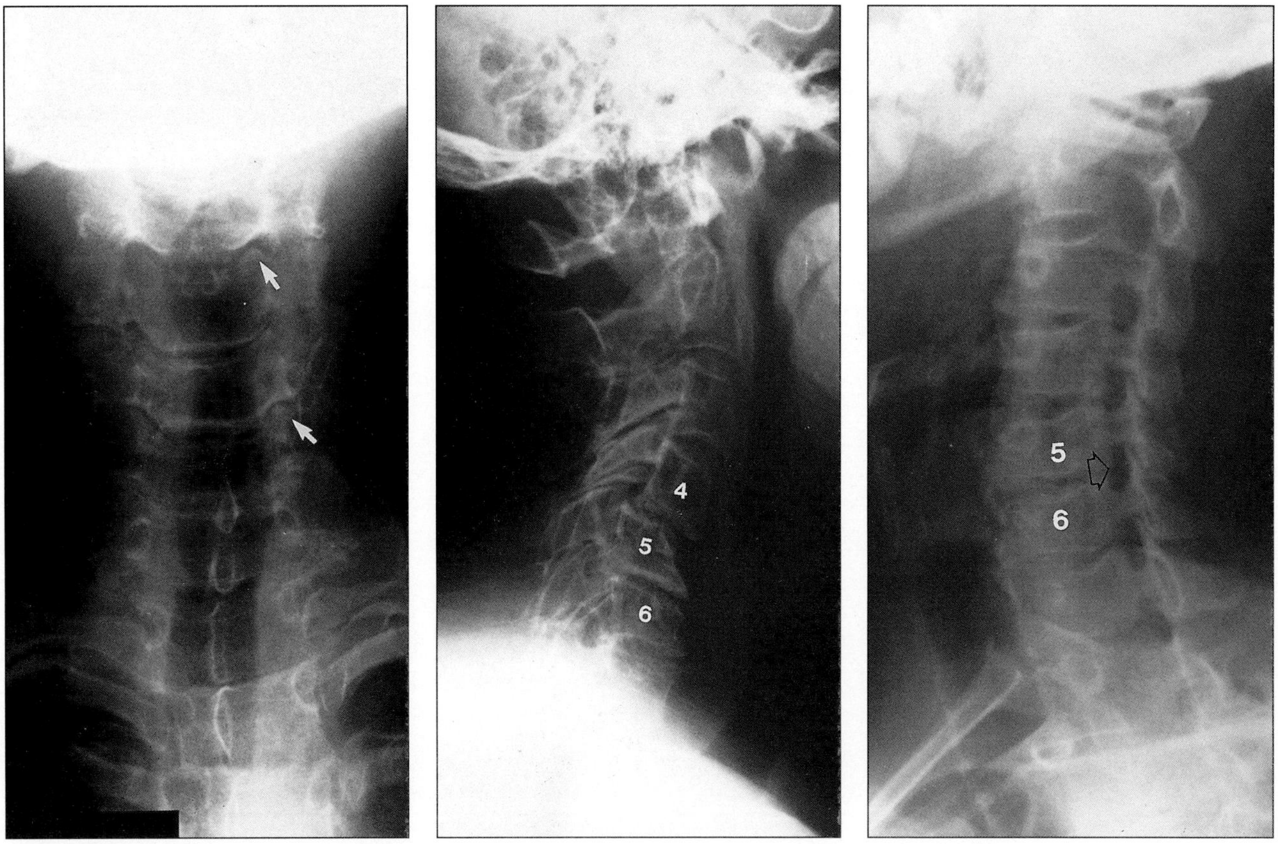

a b c

Figure 5.15
(a) Anteroposterior and (b) lateral radiographs of an elderly patient being evaluated for neck pain. Anteroposterior projection shows normal alignment. There are degenerative changes of the uncinate joints (arrows) including rounding and sclerosis. Lateral projection shows degenerative changes at multiple disc levels, and there is diffuse osteoporosis. There is spondylolisthesis at C4–C5 with reversal of the normal lordotic curve. Severe narrowing of all discs below C4 with end-plate sclerosis and irregularity are typical changes of degenerative disc disease, but are poorly correlated with specific symptoms. (c) An oblique radiograph of another patient showing very mild narrowing of right C5–C6 foramen (arrow).

studies. Changes in the relationship of hardware to osseous structures, altered alignment, lucencies around instrumentation, pseudarthrosis and fractures of instrumentation are all important findings in the evaluation for postoperative complication (Figs 5.17 and 5.18). Plain radiographs are limited, however, in the evaluation of bony structures in the postoperative spine. Additionally, symptomatic conditions such as arachnoiditis, recurrent herniated disc, foraminal stenosis, epidural infection and hematoma are not shown on plain radiographs and require different studies for definition. Stability of the postoperative, and particularly the post-fusion, spine can be evaluated with flexion–extension views. These studies are safer in the symptomatic postoperative patient than in the acutely injured, and may be performed in the radiology department under the supervision of the technician. All positioning, however, must be done by the patient, and passive flexion and extension must be avoided unless performed by the responsible surgeon (who should be prepared to handle any complications of the maneuver).

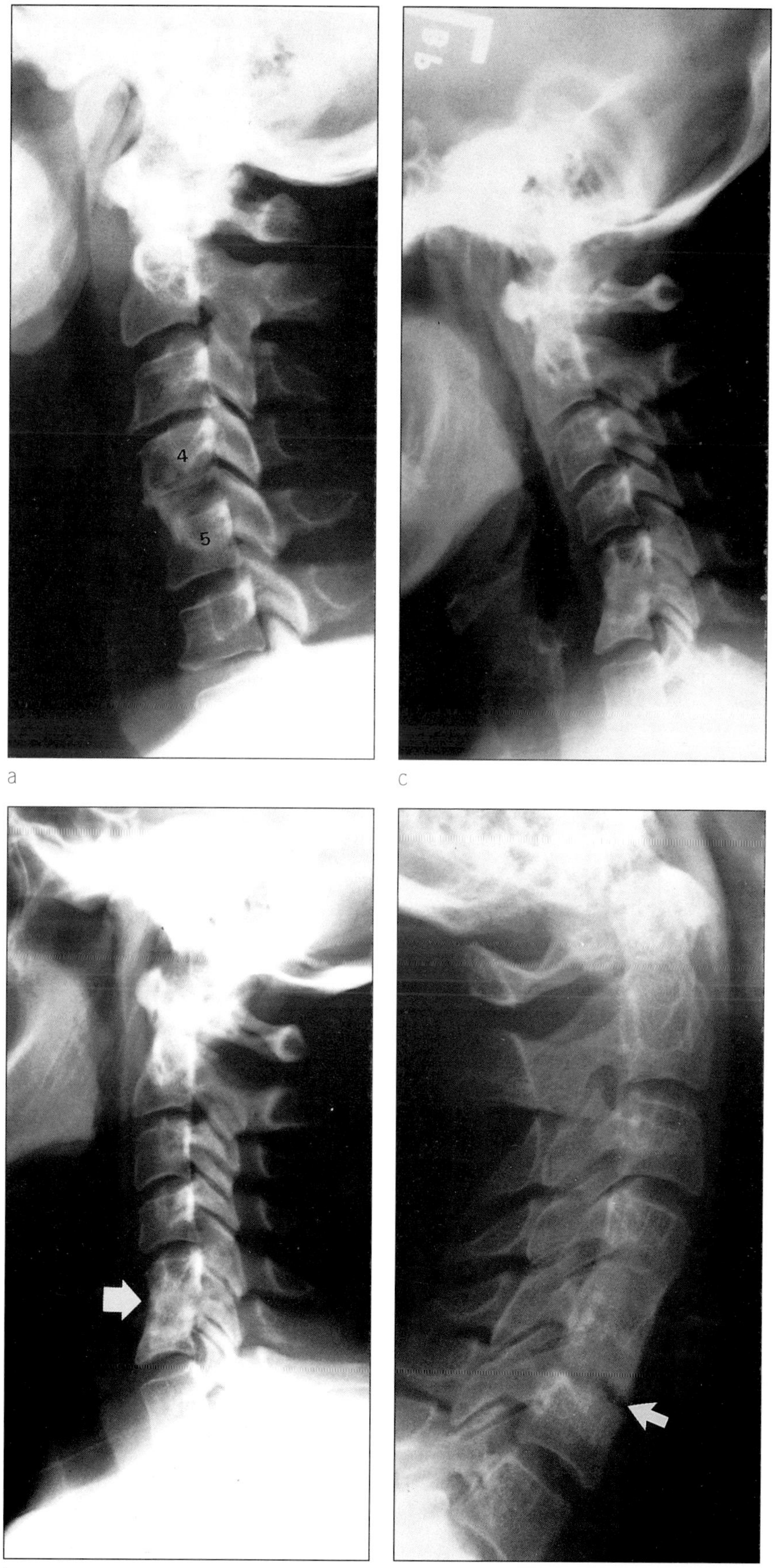

a c b d

Figure 5.16
(a) Lateral radiograph 6 months after operation shows a graft incorporation at C4–C5. The degenerative findings at C3–C4 are clearly evident. (b) Lateral radiographs of the cervical spine in a patient being evaluated for persistent discomfort 2 years after discectomy and interbody fusion at C5–C6. Healed interbody fusion of C5–C6 (arrow) is apparent. The cervical lordosis has been straightened. No complication is seen. (c) Lateral radiograph in flexion shows no change in the position of the fused vertebral segments. Motion with flexion occurs, as expected, at C4–C5, the segment above the fusion. Anterior displacement of 1–2 mm at C4–C5 is normal. (d) Lateral radiograph of a patient with recurrent neck and arm pain after anterior interbody fusion at C5–C6 and C6–C7. Pseudarthrosis at C6–C7 is evident (arrow).

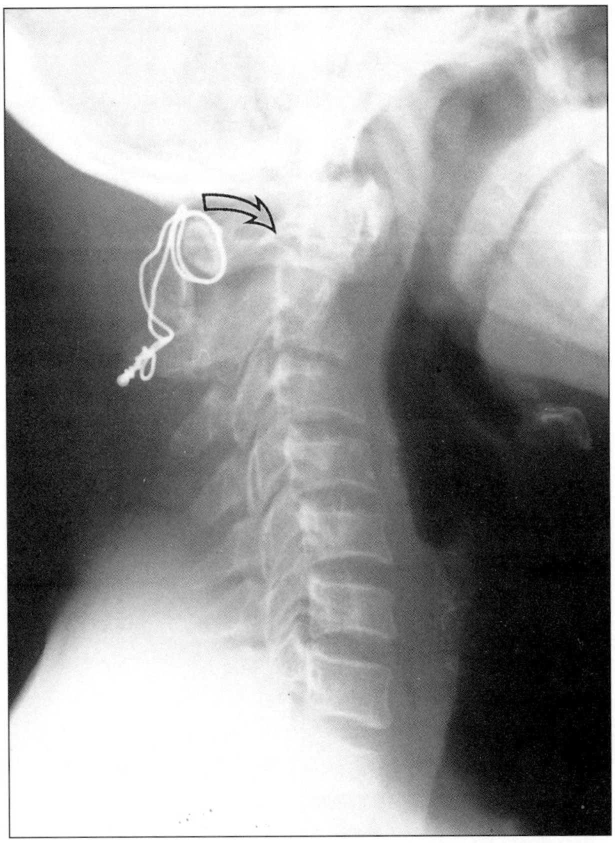

a

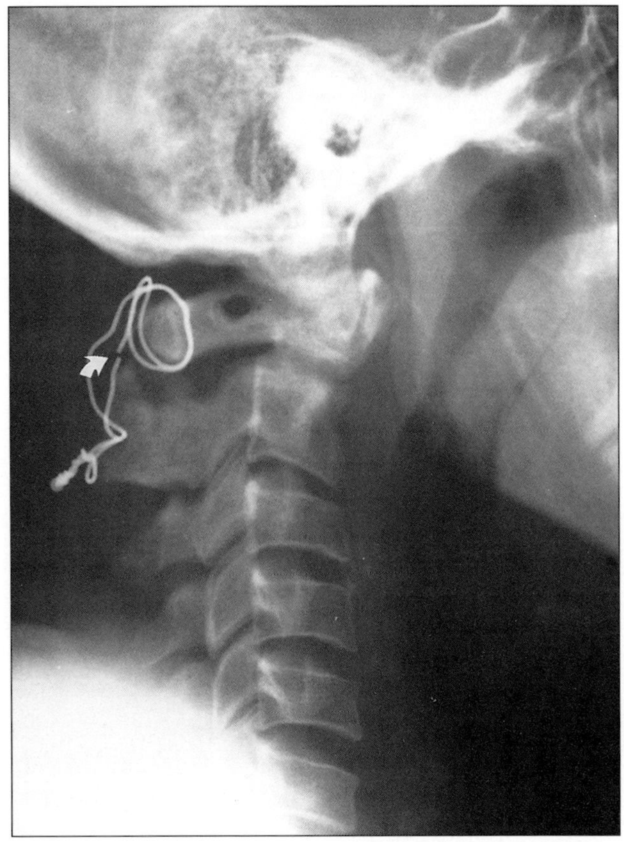

c

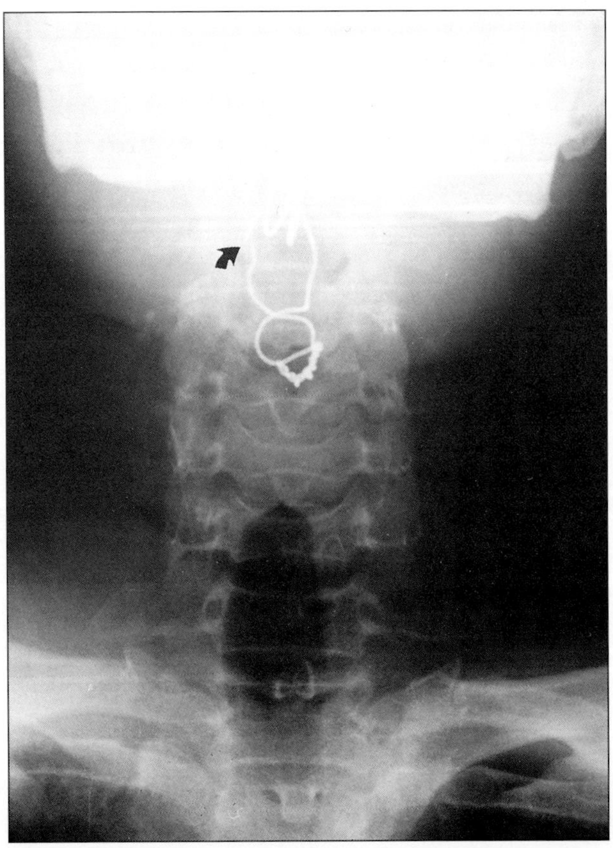

b

Figure 5.17
(a) Lateral radiograph 2 months after wire fixation shows progressive displacement of the fracture with deformity at the level of the odontoid (arrow). (b) Anteroposterior radiograph shows little change in the alignment or appearance of the cervical spine. The wire, however, is broken (arrow) confirming instability with motion at the fusion. (c) Lateral radiograph shows the broken wire more clearly with motion detected in flexion.

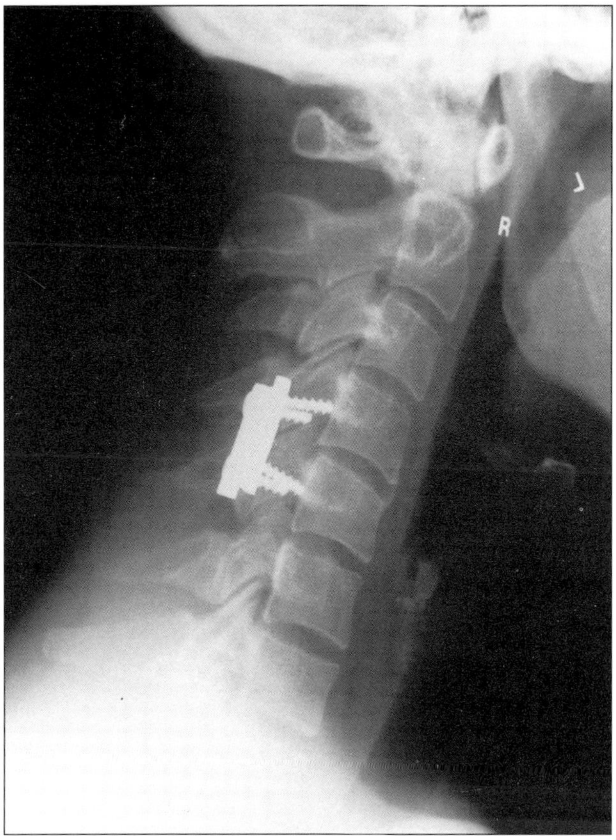

a

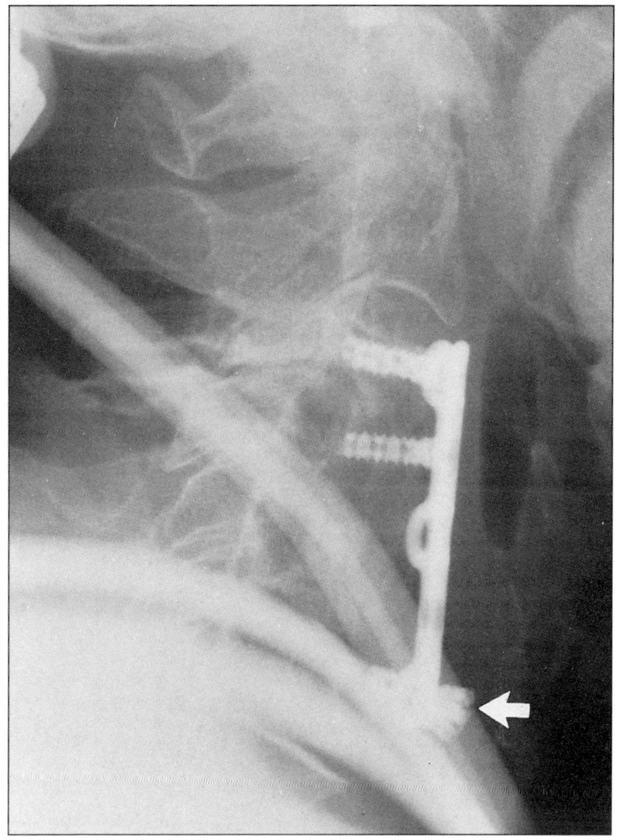

c

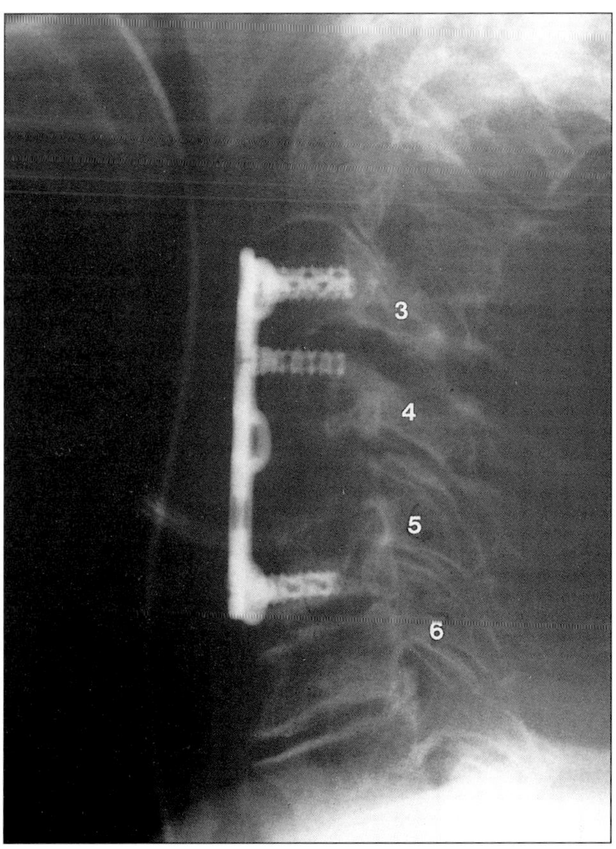

b

Figure 5.18

(a) Lateral radiograph showing a good alignment after posterior plate-screw fixation of C4–C5 in a patient with a facet dislocation. (b) Lateral radiograph after anterior vertebrectomy and fusion and plate-screw fixation in a patient with a neoplasm. (c) A follow-up radiograph showing a loosening and pull-out of the distal screws is noted in this patient (arrow).

CONVENTIONAL TOMOGRAPHY

Conventional tomography of the cervical spine, long a mainstay of problem-solving in the patient with negative or equivocal radiographs, has largely been supplanted by computed tomography and magnetic resonance imaging. The necessary equipment for conventional tomography, including special radiographic rooms, is becoming less widely distributed and enthusiasm for the technique is waning. The principle of conventional tomography is that of blurring all anatomy above and below a specific level in the plane of the radiographic table by moving the radiographic tube and film cassette. There are a variety of tube movement geometries (linear, circular, trispiral, hypocycloidal) which give different slice thicknesses, blur patterns, and exposure times. The nature of tomography allows improved resolution of bony structures in a thin plane which may be obscured by overlying anatomy in conventional radiographs, and subtle fractures or osseous destructive lesions can be shown to advantage. Computed tomography, however, with its superior resolving power and soft-tissue resolution has become widely recognized as a superior method for tomographic evaluation, and does not require the positioning maneuvers which characterize conventional tomography. Modern computed tomography is faster, more accurate, lower in radiation dose, and requires less patient cooperation than conventional tomography. As aqueous contrast media followed by plain radiography or computed tomography for myelography have supplanted gas myelography, which required conventional tomography, the requirement for plain tomographic evaluation has decreased dramatically.[57]

The use of conventional tomography today is basically limited to assessing certain fracture patterns and bone healing after injury or surgery (Figs 5.19 and 5.20). For example, the healing process of the base of dens may be better appreciated on conventional tomography than by computed tomography, particularly if an internal fixation was used in the patient.

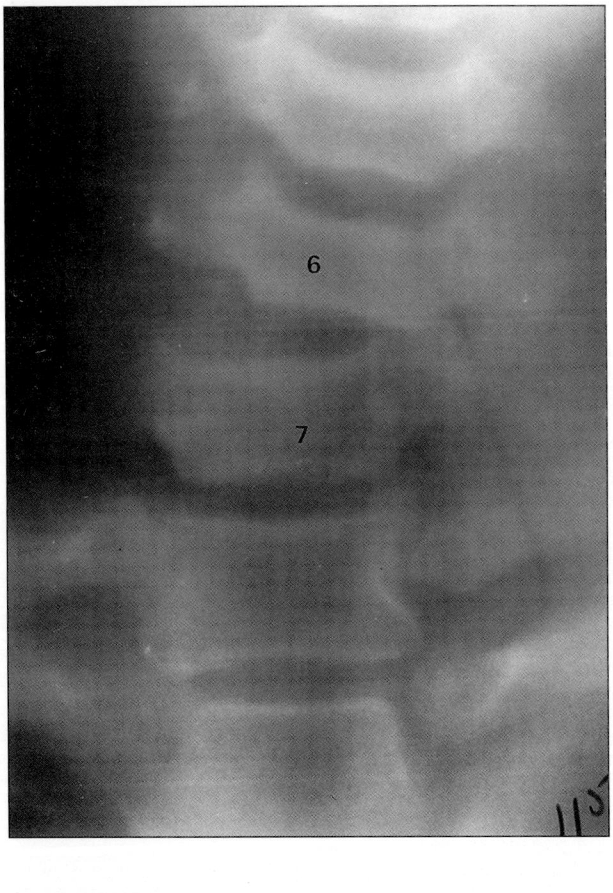

Figure 5.19
An anteroposterior tomogram showing an unusual lateral dislocation of C6–C7.

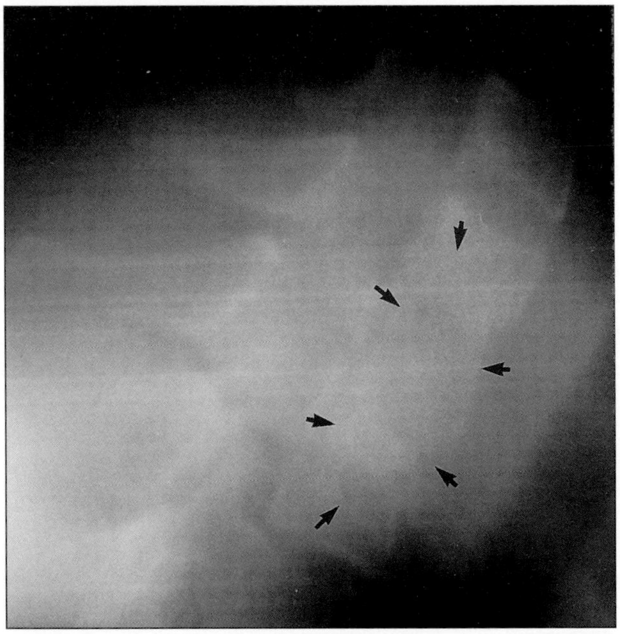

Figure 5.20
A lateral tomogram showing the proper placement of the anterior strut graft (arrow) between C6 and T1.

RADIOISOTOPE SCANNING

Intravenous injection of bone-seeking compounds, such as methylene diphosphonate, labeled with radioactive atoms such as technetium 99-m (^{99m}Tc), is followed by circulatory distribution of the radiolabel and accumulation in areas of osteoblastic activity. Regions with increased or accelerated bony repair, generally found in regions of response to mechanical, inflammatory, or adjacent neoplastic processes, lead to focal areas of increased radiolabel uptake. These regions can be detected by scanning with nuclear medicine cameras, and displayed as images representing the distribution of radiolabel and, therefore, of skeletal metabolic activity.

Modern, high-resolution γ cameras are capable of producing superb images of bone scans. Detection efficiency of relative radioactivity is excellent, and the total radiation dose from modern bone scans is very low (about 1.4 mGy/74 MBq or 140 mrad/20 mCi dose). Meticulous attention to radioisotope preparation and injection, calibration of equipment, and photography of the scans is necessary to allow maximum resolution of areas of increased uptake. Current practice in nuclear medicine includes obtaining spot views of regions of clinical concern using special, high-resolution collimators to discriminate adjacent anatomic structures.

The major application of radioisotope scanning in the cervical spine is in the diagnosis of neoplastic or infectious disease (Fig. 5.21). Bone scanning is much more sensitive to focal areas of reactive bone, found in both inflammatory and destructive processes, than conventional radiography. Although plain radiographs are often the first examination ordered in patients with spine symptoms, because of their universal availability and familiarity, bone scans become positive far earlier in the osteodestructive process than plain radiographs, and provide both prompt diagnosis and accurate direction for detailed anatomic study. Positive areas on bone scans are often the first indication of cervical spine involvement with metastatic disease, and occult primary lesions such as osteoid osteoma or osteoblastoma, which may be diagnosed after positive bone scans, are followed by tailored high-resolution imaging.

The role of bone scanning in degenerative disc disease is limited, but areas of increased uptake may be correlated with the changes on plain radiographs in patients with chronic neck pain (Fig. 5.22). The extent of active bone turnover, as shown on the isotope scan, is usually minimally increased in degenerative disorders as compared to neoplastic or infectious disorders. The role of bone scanning in cervical trauma is evolving. Patients with symptoms of persistent pain after major trauma despite

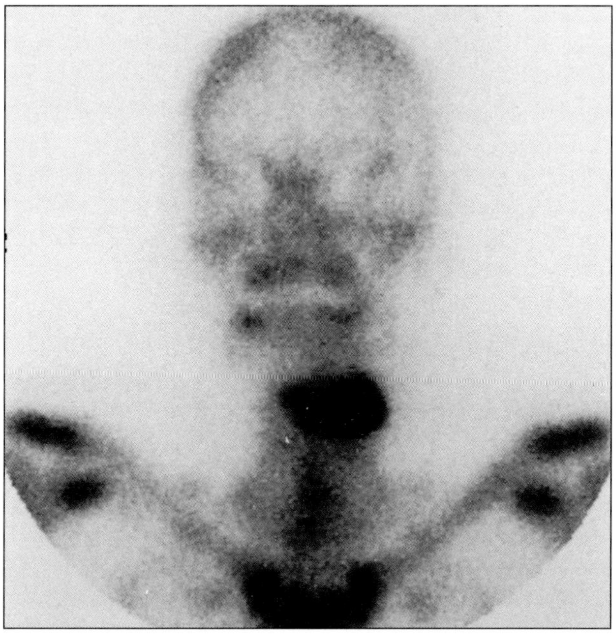

Figure 5.21
Static anteroposterior planar bone scan shows intense increased uptake in the neck extending somewhat asymmetrically to the left. This confirms extensive bone reaction, but is diagnostically non-specific. This patient had been involved in a motor vehicle accident, and had plain radiographs showing vertebral subluxation with an apparent surrounding mass and osteodestruction beyond that expected for simple compression fracture.

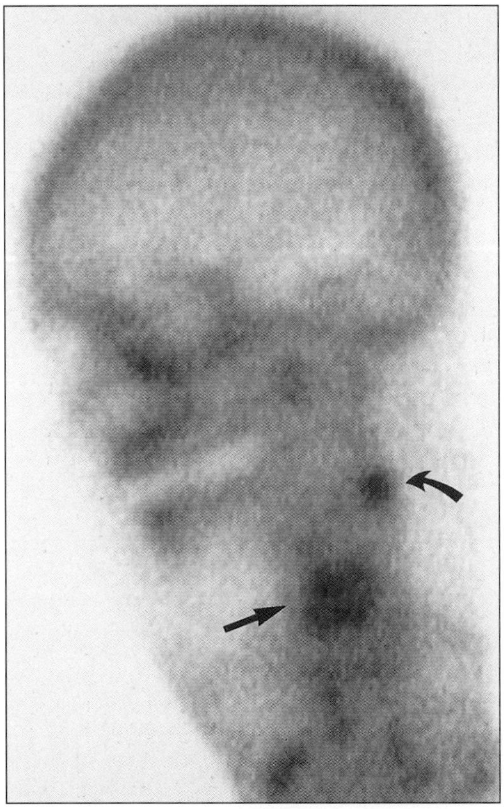

Figure 5.22
Oblique planar bone scan image shows area of increased uptake, indicating increased bone turnover and active metabolic activity, at the C4–C5 level posteriorly (curved arrow) and at C6–C7 (straight arrow) anteriorly. These findings correspond to abnormal areas on the radiograph. Note that the extent of radiographic abnormality is greater than the extent of active bone turnover as shown on the isotope scan.

normal conventional radiographs and equivocal clinical findings occasionally show unsuspected areas of osseous abnormality when studied with radioisotope scanning several days after the initial injury. Unsuspected fractures may be diagnosed using this technique, and often confirmed with carefully directed high-resolution anatomic studies such as thin-section computed tomography. Fracture healing is characterized by gradual return of positive areas to normal activity, but this process may take months to complete.[16,30,41,43,51,55,63]

Osteomyelitis and septic discitis produce areas of increased uptake on bone scans, much like the areas produced by traumatic or neoplastic disease. Although scan patterns may vary sufficiently to allow some differential interpretation, specific diagnosis usually requires further examination. Clinical status may clarify scan findings significantly, and must always command attention. Imaging with higher-resolution anatomic techniques may offer a more specific diagnosis, and almost always follows detection of abnormality with conventional scans. Radioisotope techniques other than that using ^{99m}Tc-labeled methylene diphosphonate (^{99m}Tc-MDP) have been developed for diagnosing infection, and are effective for this purpose. Combined ^{99m}Tc-MDP bone scanning and scanning using gallium-67 citrate or indium-111-labeled white blood cells is the currently accepted way of evaluating suspected infection using nuclear medicine techniques.[2,9,38,58,64,68]

In the postoperative spine special care must be taken to avoid overinterpretation of positive areas on bone scans. Operative manipulations such as instrumentation, osteotomies, and fusions lead to reactive bone and areas of increased uptake as a normal part of the postoperative healing response (Fig. 5.23). Suspected tumor or infection must be discriminated from normal healing, and this is often difficult using scans. The time course of abnormal activity, anatomic relation to the known operative procedure, and findings on other studies must be correlated for accurate diagnosis.

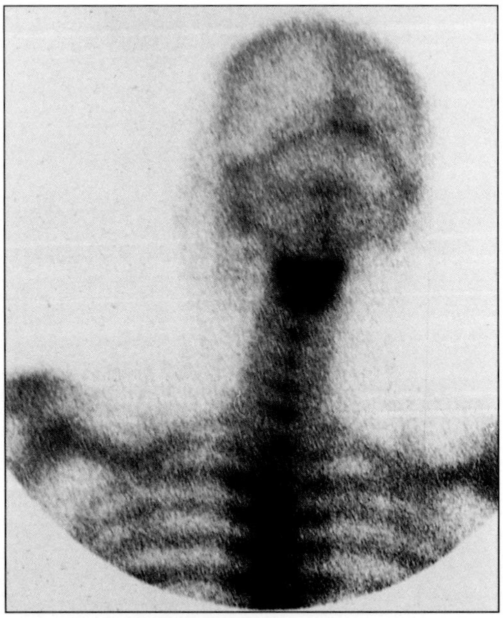

Figure 5.23
Radioisotope scan in anteroposterior projection 10 months after fusion, performed because of continued symptoms, shows dramatic increased uptake at the level of the fusion. Bone scan should show normalization of uptake by this interval after surgery.

MYELOGRAPHY

Until the development and refinement of magnetic resonance imaging (MRI), myelographic evaluation with water-soluble contrast media followed by plain radiography or computed tomography was necessary to evaluate the soft tissues of the spinal canal. Oil contrast agents such as iophendylate (Pantopaque), and gas (oxygen or air) contrast media have been replaced by modern water-soluble contrast media such as metrizamide or iohexol. Since the advent of MRI, the use of myelography has been limited to selected cases. Drawbacks of myelography are inadequate visualization distal to a complete block and invasiveness (Fig. 5.24). The complications of arachnoiditis, especially with iophendylate, and severe headache which followed removal of large amounts of cerebrospinal fluid during gas myelography have been significantly reduced with modern agents. Although complications of headache and nausea are relatively common with water-soluble agents, and more severe complications including seizures are reported, the margin of safety of these agents is significantly more favorable than that of previous media.

Myelography is, by nature, an indirect examination. The contrast column is visualized and displacements caused by extradural or intradural structures are used to diagnose lesions such as herniated disc, osteophytic encroachments, masses resulting from tumor or hematoma around the thecal structures, and intraspinal masses (Fig. 5.25). Cord atrophy, diastematomyelia, and other primary neural lesions demonstrate characteristic effects on the appearance of the opacified cerebrospinal fluid space shown at myelography. Myelography is extremely accurate for diagnosis of discogenic disease and other neurocompressive syndromes, and can serve as a major diagnostic step

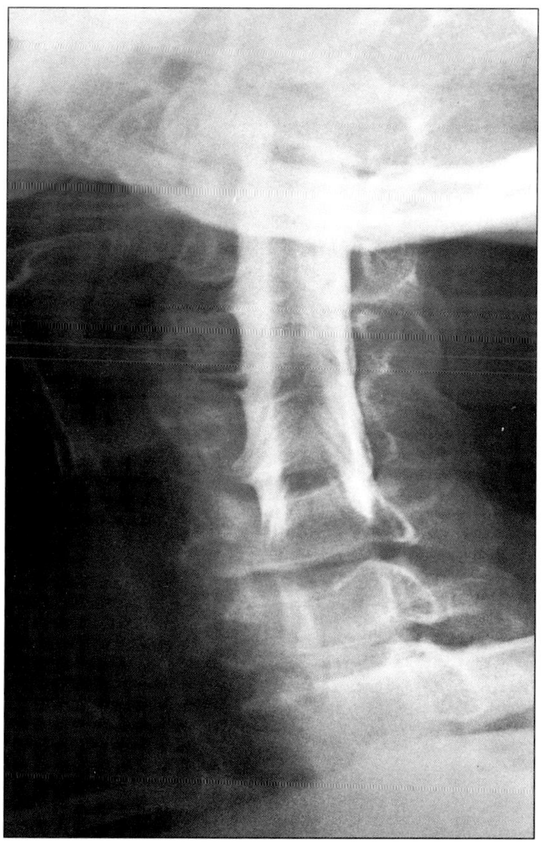

Figure 5.24
Oblique myelogram of the cervical spine by a C1–C2 puncture showing a complete block at C6 in a patient with cervical spondylosis. An additional puncture is needed to assess the distal extent of the lesion.

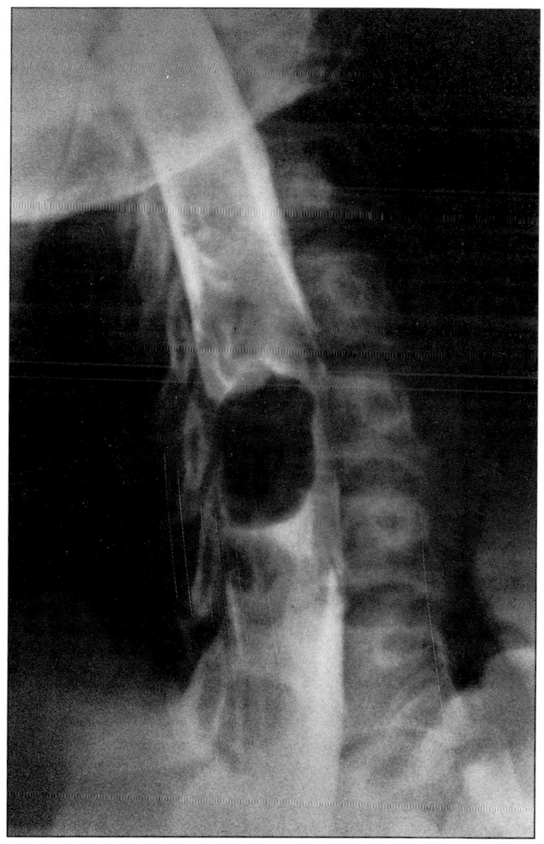

Figure 5.25
Cervical myelogram showing a smooth outline of the intradural lesion (neurofibroma).

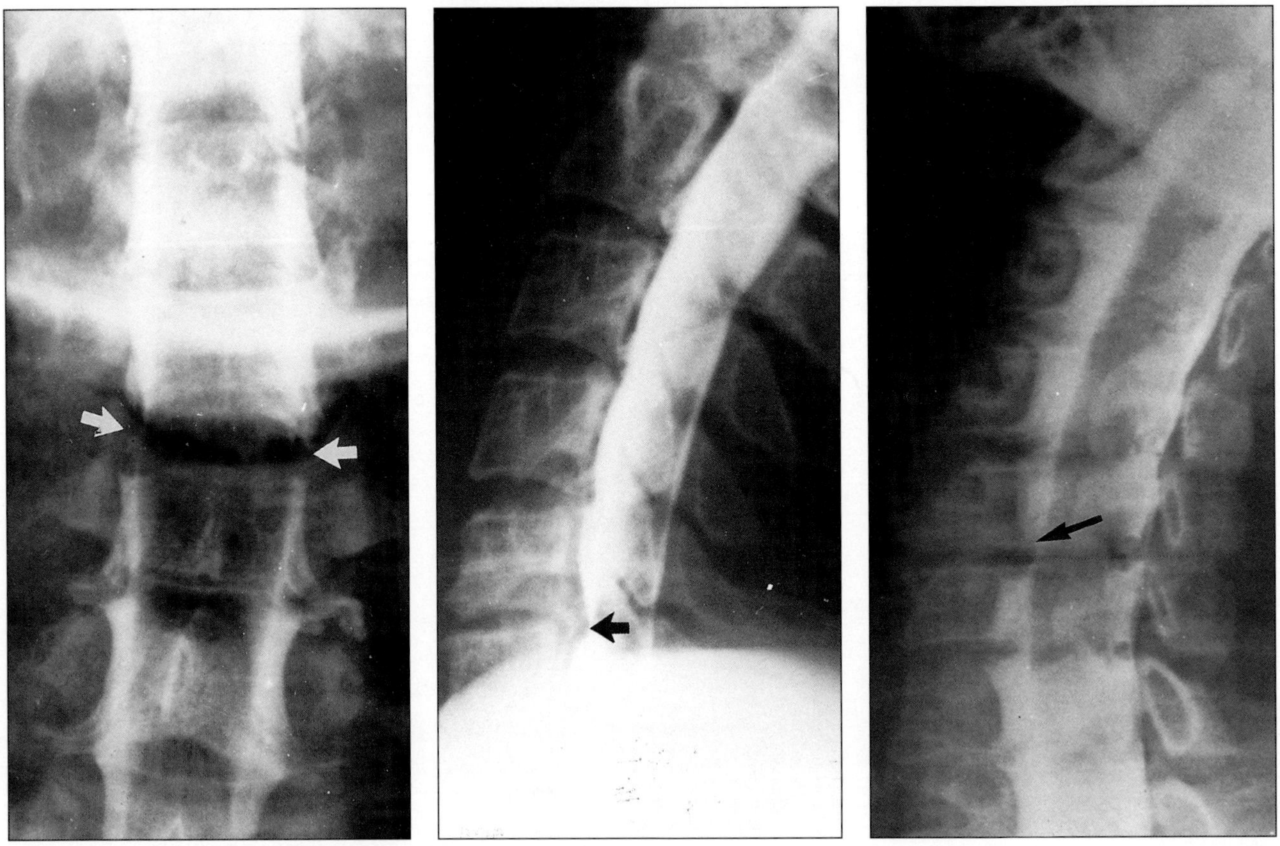

Figure 5.26
(a) Anteroposterior myelogram showing decreased filling of the C6 nerve roots bilaterally (arrows) in a patient with cervical spondylotic radiculopathy; (b) lateral view showing the indentation of the thecal sac at C5–C6 (arrow); (c) oblique views showing decreased filling of left C6 root (arrow).

in problem cases (Figs 5.26 and 5.27). The anteroposterior view will show exiting nerve roots to the level of the pedicle. A filling defect of myelographic dye on an oblique projection is a typical finding of nerve root compression. The spinal cord is well outlined by both anteroposterior and lateral views (Figs 5.26 and 5.27). The lateral view shows spinal cord compression by the disc or uncovertebral joint anteriorly and by the ligamentum flavum posteriorly (Fig. 5.28). Myelography is being applied as an outpatient procedure with increasing frequency because the complication rate using modest doses of water-soluble media is acceptable. Current practice includes computed tomography as a preferred method of imaging after myelographic injection of contrast, because the high-resolution and transaxial tomographic projection afforded by computed tomography provides an ideal way to evaluate the discovertebral complex and its relationship to intrathecal structures. Often, very low doses of myelographic contrast media, inadequate for myelography using plain radiographs, can serve to define these critical relationships adequately in cases of suspected herniated disc or foraminal stenosis.[54]

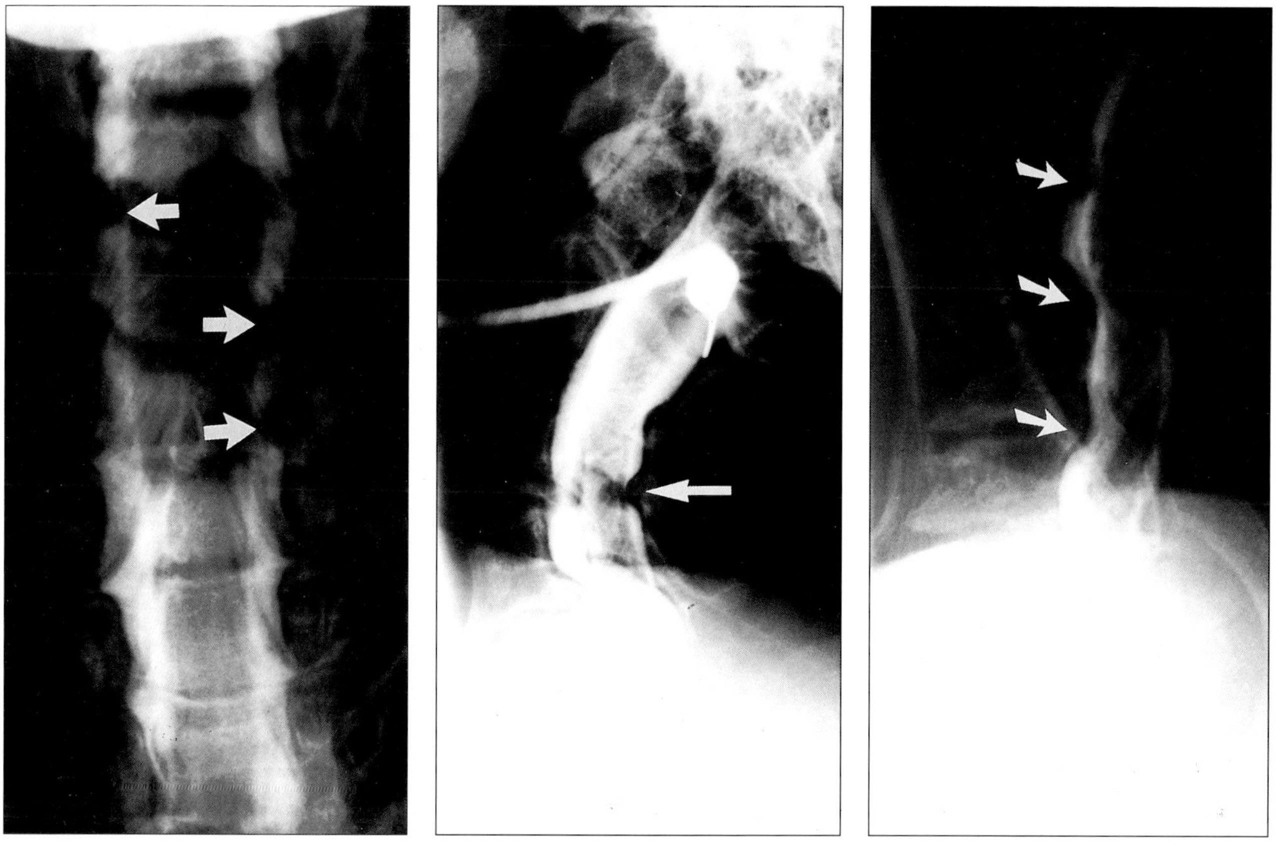

a b c

Figure 5.27
(a) Anteroposterior myelogram showing extradural defects on the right at C3–C4 and on the left at C4–C5 and C5–C6 (arrows), probably on the basis of uncinate hypertrophy. (b) Lateral view during injection showing posterior defect at C3–C4 (arrow) from hypertrophy of the ligamentum flavum. (c) Horizontal-beam, swimmer's lateral view showing anterior extradural defects from bridging discs and hypertrophied uncinate joints at C3–C4, C4–C5 and C5–C6 (arrows). There is evidence of mild cord compression with flattening at C5–C6.

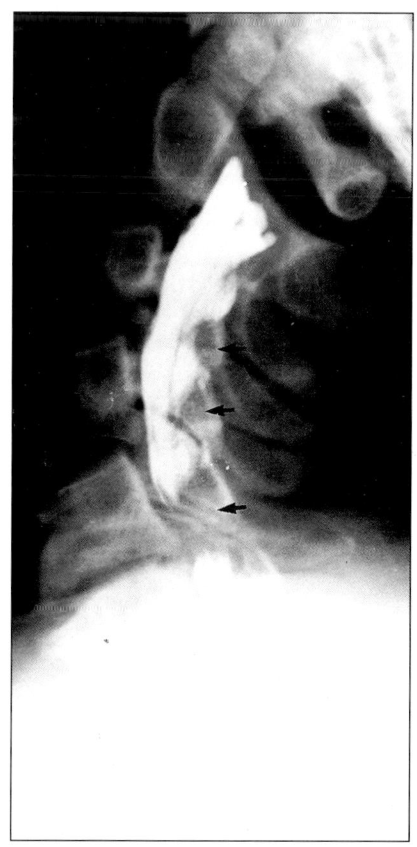

Figure 5.28
Lateral myelogram showing a large extradural defect at C5–C6 caused by disc herniation and posterior defects at C3–C4, C4–C5, and C5–C6, caused by ligamentum flavum hypertrophy or buckling (arrow).

COMPUTED TOMOGRAPHY

Application of the mathematics of Fourier transform analysis and filtered back projection using sufficiently robust computer systems and sensitive radiation detectors, which led to the development of computed tomography, created a revolution in diagnostic imaging. The same principles apply to nuclear medicine techniques (single photon emission computed tomography, SPECT) and magnetic resonance imaging, both essentially computed tomographic analysis using different energy signals from those of transmitted radiographic beams. Computed tomography has evolved over the last 20 years, with ever-improving detector systems, more powerful computer platforms which are capable of analyzing huge volumes of data, and advanced imaging algorithms which allow enhanced display characteristics for bony structures as well as multiplanar and three-dimensional displays. It is a radiographic modality, relying on computer analysis of radiographic density in a thin section of anatomy, displayed as a tomographic cut. Primary data acquisition in computed tomography always occurs in (or near) the plane perpendicular to the computed tomography table, whereas display in other planes requires reformation of the image (which means that resolution is, necessarily, lost in the process). Improvements in equipment have led to faster scans, thinner sections, and improved display characteristics for structures of high density such as bone. It is now sufficiently fast for even acutely ill patients to be rapidly and effectively studied while lying in protected positions with continuous monitoring.[33–35]

Only with improved computer technology has computed tomography been successfully applied to cervical spine disease. Accurate definition of subtle fractures and herniated discs in the cervical spine requires very thin sections and target reconstruction algorithms to correct for the small amount of soft-tissue surrounding the cervical vertebral column. Degenerative disc disease is challenging to evaluate effectively with computed tomography.[17] Contiguous thin sections (1.5 mm through the disc and neural foramina) are required and sections should be displayed at both bone and soft tissue settings to diagnose both soft-tissue lesions and osteophytes. The examination should cover the entire discovertebral apparatus at each level (from mid-body to mid-body), but contiguous 3-mm sections may be used on either side of the disc itself to save time and number of cuts. Osteophytes are clearly visible as irregular projections of bone or calcium density projecting from the bony structures into the spinal canal or foramen (Fig. 5.29). Deformity of the thecal sac or nerve roots indicates a neurocompressive lesion. Herniated discs are diagnosed as soft-tissue masses projecting into the spinal canal or foramen. The same effect on neural structures may be seen with calcified disc or osteophytes.

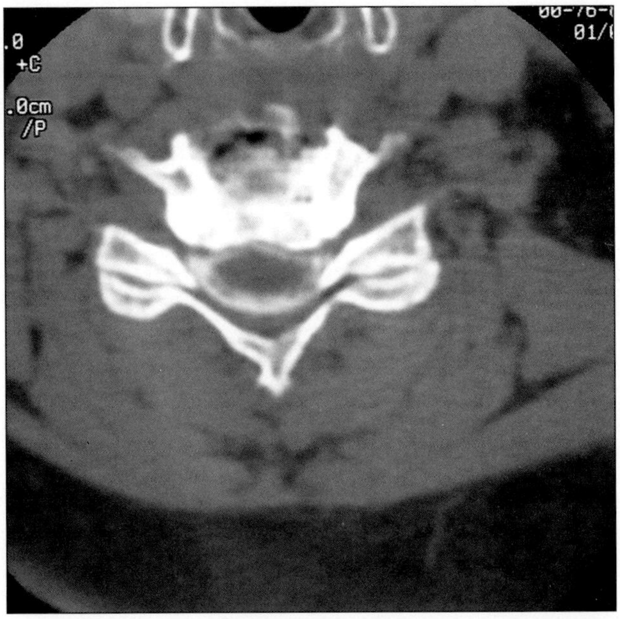

Figure 5.29
Computed tomographic myelogram in axial projection at C3–C4 revealing asymmetric uncinate hypertrophy with mild posterior cord displacement. The facet joints are essentially normal. Radio-opaque contrast in the thecal sac allows ready visualization of the spinal cord and dorsal nerve roots.

As cervical disc herniations may be small, and the amount of epidural fat surrounding the thecal sac is small, unenhanced computed tomography may not show significant lesions adequately. Computed tomography (CT) after enhancement of the cerebrospinal fluid with water-soluble contrast medium, either after conventional myelography or as part of a low-dose CT myelogram may be necessary to demonstrate subtle herniations and encroachments fully[33–35, 54, 55, 59] (Fig. 5.30).

Fractures are best studied with computed tomography. Disruptions of vertebral body, lamina, intracanal bone fragments, and facet joint alignment are clearly shown with or without reconstructed images (Figs 5.31 and 5.32). Multiplanar display, with reformation into sagittal or coronal projections, can greatly enhance demonstrations of fractures and other lesions that cover relatively long areas or are not optimally shown in the transaxial plane. Computed tomography remains the best imaging modality for evaluation of traumatic lesions of the cervical spine today. Tumors and infections are also adequately shown using contiguous 3-mm sections. Osteodestructive or sclerotic lesions and displacements are also usually well

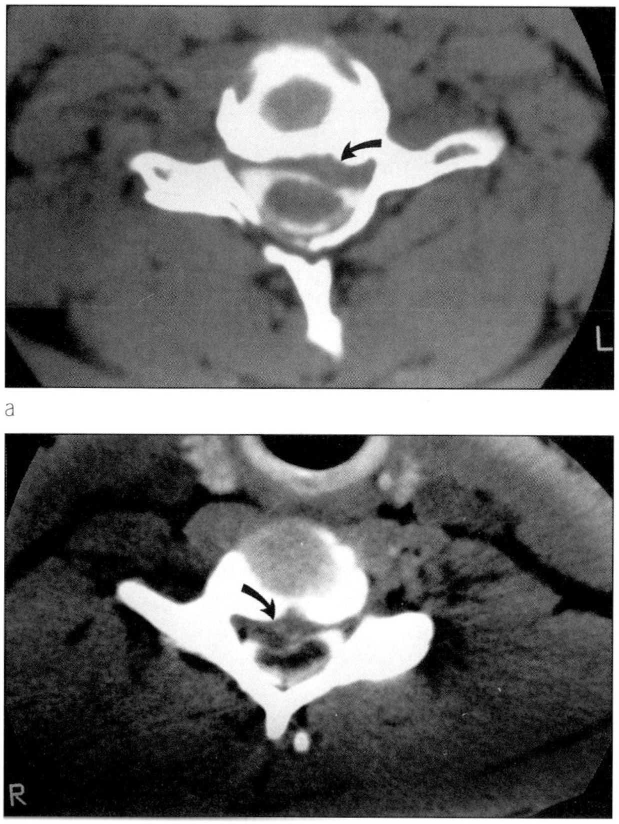

a

b

Figure 5.30
(a) Computed tomographic myelogram showing an intraforaminal herniation at C6–C7 with left C7 root impingement (arrow). (b) Computed tomographic myelogram showing a posterolateral herniated disc which compresses both the root and the spinal cord (arrow).

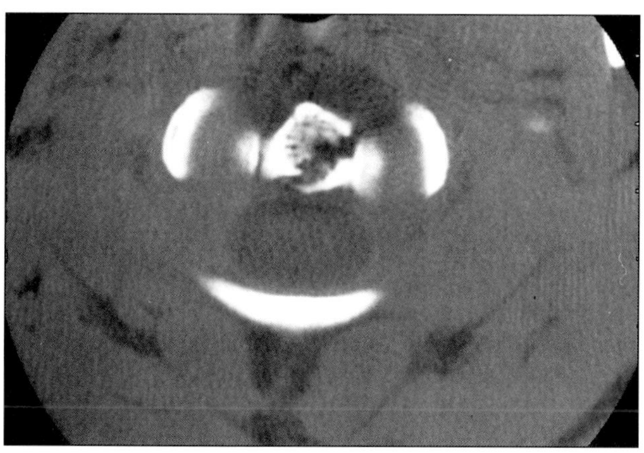

Figure 5.31
Unenhanced computed tomogram through the base of the odontoid confirming the fracture line. Although the image is taken at bone windows, the thecal sac and cord can be seen faintly.

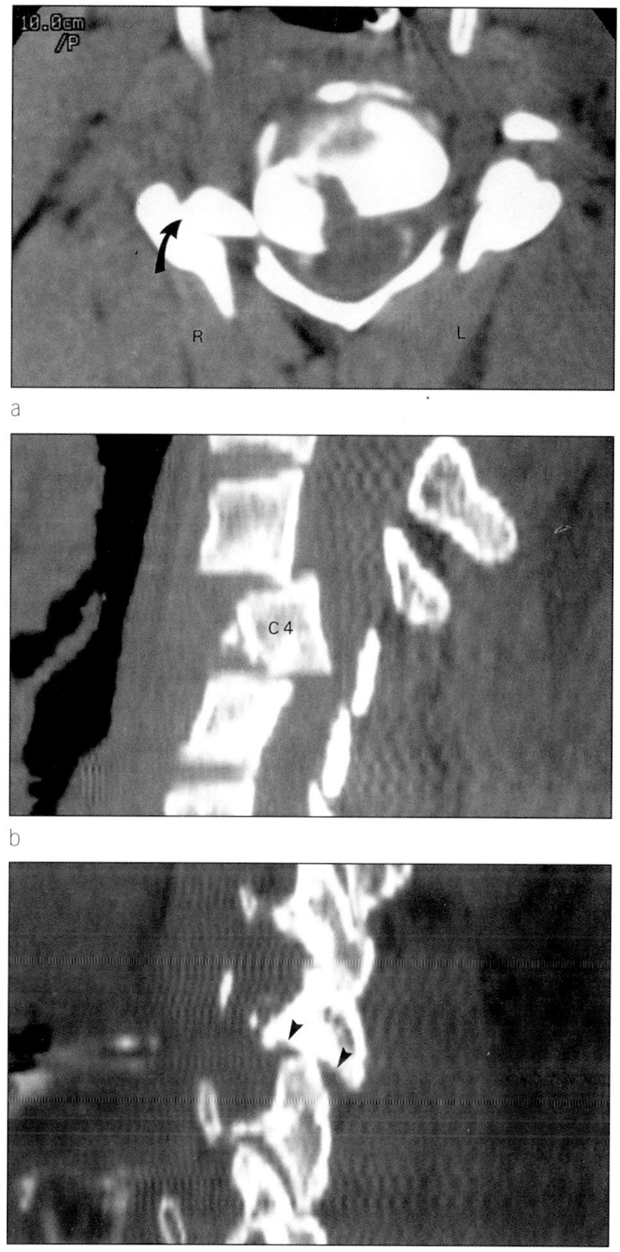

a

b

c

Figure 5.32
(a) Axial computed tomogram through the upper part of C4, after low-dose intrathecal contrast injection, displayed at soft-tissue windows, showing the severe fracture and effects on the cord. Posterior displacement of a large fracture fragment on the right deforms the cord. Facet subluxation (arrow) on the right is suboptimally shown at these display settings. (b) Sagittal reformatted computed tomograms in the midline. (c) Sagittal reformatted computed tomograms through the right facet joints. These scans show the extent of the fracture displacement and subluxation. Midline reformatted image shows the large retropulsed fragment of C4. Off-midline image shows that the right facet of C3 (arrowheads) is tilted and subluxed, but not perched or locked.

shown. Many lesions that are completely invisible on plain radiographs can be clearly demonstrated by computed tomography. Lesions that affect the neural structures, either by extrinsic encroachment or invasion, are well shown, but may require display on both bone and soft-tissue window settings.

Postoperative computed tomography studies may be significantly affected by instrumentation. Modern scanners provide a variety of methods for reducing the effect of a metallic artifact on the images, but hardware of any sort still introduces significant artifacts and may degrade computed tomograms. Complications of treatment including destructive lesions from infection and pseudoarthrosis from failed fusion are visualized well using appropriate high-resolution computed tomography.

MAGNETIC RESONANCE IMAGING

Magnetic resonance imaging (MRI) has followed on the heels of the computed tomography revolution in spinal imaging, and has become recognized as the best modality for examining the vertebral column and spinal contents.[12] Indeed, in many centers such techniques as conventional myelography and plain tomography are becoming rare or even non-existent as the extreme effectiveness of MRI in examining the spine becomes understood.

The technique is based on the fact that certain atomic nuclei, when exposed to a strong magnetic field, respond by aligning with (or against) the direction of the field.[11] Biologic atoms, such as hydrogen atoms in water and lipids, respond with sufficiently strong magnetization to allow imaging. When magnetized hydrogen atoms are exposed to a radiofrequency pulse of appropriate frequency the direction of the magnetic vector generated by these nuclei can be changed. MRI is accomplished by measuring the electromagnetic signal produced by these rotated nuclei, as they decay back to a resting state, in relation to the static magnetic field. A variety of decay properties can be detected and analyzed to produce images, allowing several biologic properties to be emphasized on the images. By selecting any of several rather complex parameters, including the energy and duration of the radiofrequency pulse, the time interval between pulses, the repetition rate of radiofrequency irradiation, and the time delay before signal detection, various image characteristics can be produced. In this way, fat or water ('free water' or fluid collections with high water content) can be displayed as 'bright' or 'high signal intensity' on MRI. Various biochemical conditions can influence local signal intensity, and thus influence image characteristics, in diagnostic ways (for example, the protein content of a fluid can affect signal intensity suggesting the nature of cyst contents). In addition, certain atoms and molecules perturb the local magnetic field in predictable ways ('paramagnetic effects'), allowing diagnosis of such lesions as hemorrhage, hematoma of various ages, iron deposition, etc[65]. Blood flow can be used to visualize vessels on MRI, and new techniques of reconstruction allow three-dimensional demonstration of blood vessels without using MRI contrast media.

In general, blood flow imaging and contrast media are not necessary for studies of the cervical spine. The overwhelming advantage enjoyed by MRI in this area is based on two facts: first, by their very nature, the image data acquired in MRI allow full-resolution display of images in any plane, unlike computed tomography which has full resolution only in the scan plane (axial or near-axial); this means that excellent images are available with MRI in the highly pertinent coronal and sagittal planes. Second, judicious use of pulse sequences allows the imager to emphasize marrow fat, which permits outstanding images of the vertebrae, or fluid, allowing enhancement of cerebrospinal fluid (pseudomyelogram effect); this, in turn, permits diagnosis of disc herniations and other neurocompressive lesions as readily as with contrast-enhanced computed tomography.

Current experience suggests that MRI is as accurate as, and far less invasive than, contrast myelography or computed tomographic myelography for diagnosing cervical disc disease. Conditions that affect osseous structures, such as tumors and infections, are shown with striking clarity using MRI because the neoplastic or septic pathologic process is often accompanied by local biochemical changes which produce areas of significantly altered signal behavior.

Excellent MRI requires a great deal of attention to detail; it is highly dependent on a carefully calibrated and meticulously maintained installation. Pulse sequences must be chosen to demonstrate the suspected pathology, and tailored sequences must often be added to imaging protocols to insure adequate examination[7]. Special imaging techniques such as application of local coils for signal detection ('surface coils'), gating of pulse and signal detection sequences to correct for the effects of the cardiac or respiratory cycle, and careful patient preparation to minimize the adverse effects of claustrophobia or prolonged imaging studies in an uncomfortable gantry, are critical for optimal examinations. The results of hasty or inexpert examinations extend beyond the failure to produce diagnostic quality examinations, because poorly conceived studies may generate images with misleading information.

Magnetic resonance imaging provides an effective diagnostic modality for patients with degenerative disc disease[18,19]. The clinician should be aware of the fact that many changes depicted on MRI have no symptoms, and, therefore, clinical correlation is extremely important. Computed tomography with intrathecal contrast has been considered the optimal examination for degenerative cervical disc disease, but MRI is becoming the first procedure of choice; it provides many advantages, including non-invasiveness, wide field of view, evaluation of intradural and extradural structures, and morphologic and pathophysiologic assessment of the intervertebral disc and marrow through different imaging planes, pulse sequences, and paramagnetic contrast enhancement. Despite these advantages, MRI does not demonstrate the cortical margins as well as a computed tomographic myelogram. If MRI findings are non-diagnostic in patients with cervical spondylosis, the latter may improve the diagnostic accuracy. Patients with contraindications to MRI (pacemaker, cochlear implants, intracranial ferromagnetic metallic clips) or claustrophobia, and patients with a metal implant in the cervical spine that will produce significant ferromagnetic artifacts should first have a computed tomographic myelogram.

For patients with degenerative disc disease plus radiculopathy or myelopathy, MRI techniques should include sagittal T1-weighted images, axial T1-weighted images, and sagittal T2-weighted images with spin echo, gradient echo, or fast spin echo technique. Gadolinium–^{99m}Tc-diethylenetriamine pentaacetic acid (Gd–DTPA) enhanced sagittal and axial T1-weighted MRI is used routinely in patients with suspected neoplasm, infection, or previous surgery. T1-weighted images provide the best images of the spinal anatomy. In sagittal T1 images, cortical bone of the vertebral body shows decreased signal intensity with higher signal intensity of fatty marrow in the cancellous vertebralbodies (Fig. 5.33). However, cortical margins seen in MRI are less distinct than on computed tomograms. The intervertebral disc shows low signal intensity with darker outer annular fibers, which merge with the posterior longitudinal ligaments. Spinal cord abnormalities such as cord atrophy, edema, and syringomyelia are also well demonstrated on sagittal T1-weighted images. Axial images may demonstrate a herniated disc, foraminal stenosis, or spinal cord abnormalities (Fig. 5.34).

Parasagittal images show low intensity nerve roots surrounded by high signal fat in the intervertebral foramen. Because of the oblique configuration of the cervical foramina, 45° oblique MRI can be done to demonstrate the foramina in selected cases (Fig. 5.35).[23] T2-weighted images give information about the hydration status of the intervertebral disc, the cerebrospinal fluid, and pathologic bone marrow changes. With the advent of gradient echo imaging or fast spin-echo techniques, the use of T2-weighted spin-echo studies has been decreased.

The use of MRI for the evaluation of intervertebral disc disease has been established as the first-line preferred imaging modality[48–50]. Central disc herniations are well detected on sagittal and axial views, and in addition the degree of spinal cord compression by the herniated disc can be assessed (Fig. 5.36). In cervical spondylotic myelopathy, MRI shows osteophyte protrusion in the spinal canal which indents the spinal subarachnoid space on both axial and sagittal views (Fig. 5.37). Posterior spinal cord compression by ligamentum flavum hypertrophy and facet disease is also well demonstrated with MRI (Fig. 5.38). T2-weighted sagittal images

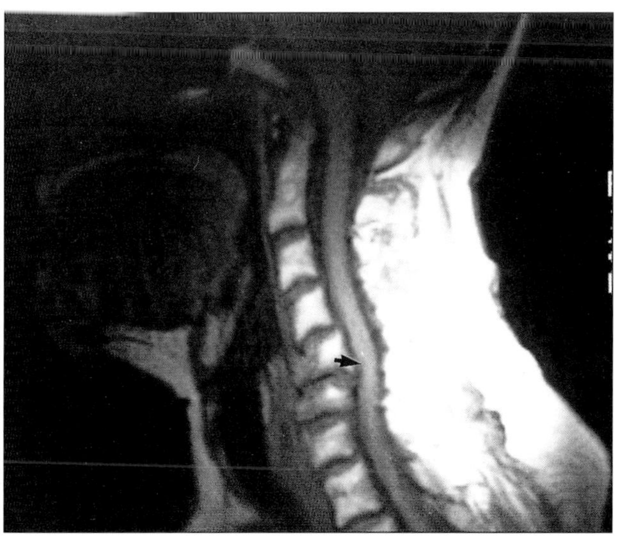

Figure 5.33
Sagittal T1-weighted MRI clearly shows the malaligned segments at C4–C5 and C5–C6. Posterior cord displacement (arrow) is apparent but there is no disc herniation.

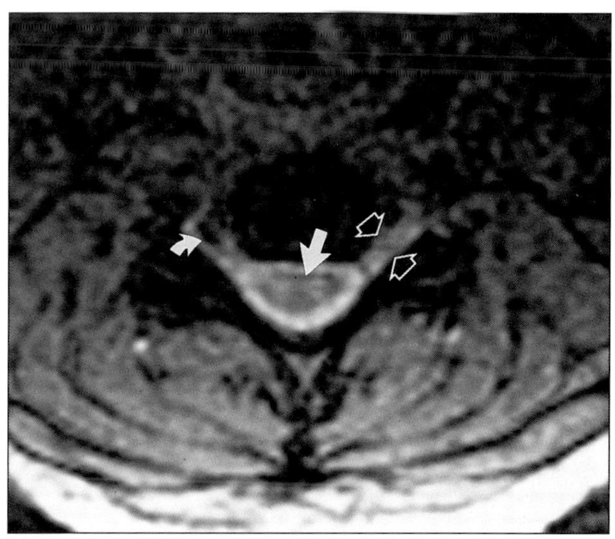

Figure 5.34
Axial T2-weighted MRI of a normal cervical spine. Spinal cord (large arrow), intervertebral foramen (open arrow), and nerve root (small arrow) are well outlined.

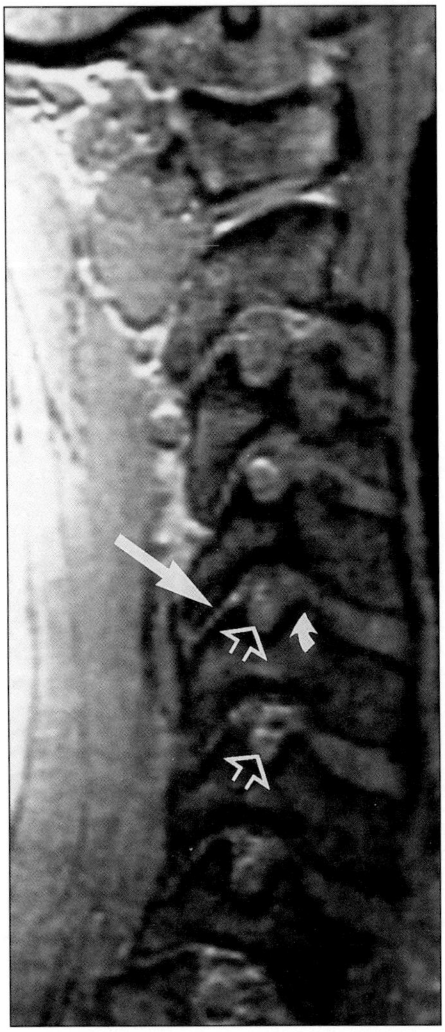

Figure 5.35
A 45° oblique MRI of a normal cervical spine demonstrating the foraminal anatomy better. Facet joint (large arrow), uncinate process (small arrow), and nerve root (open arrows) are clearly seen.

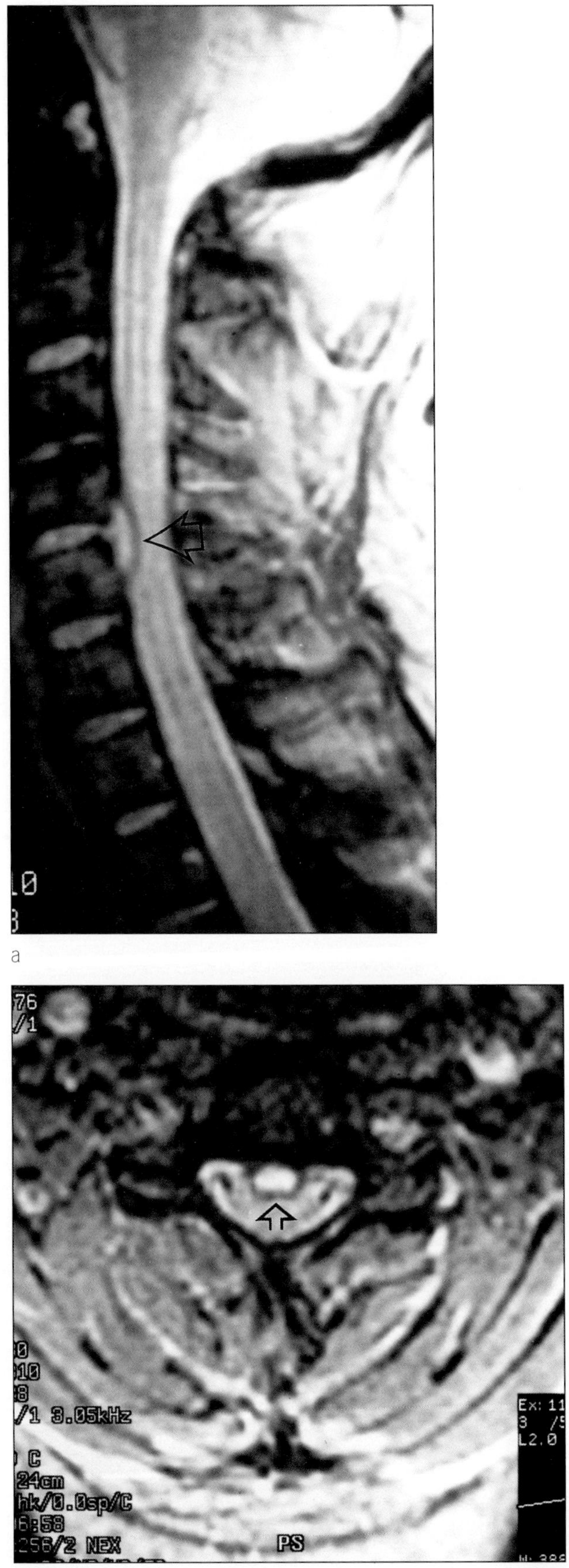

Figure 5.36
(a) Sagittal MR image using gradient-echo pulse sequence in a patient with neck and right arm pain shows a large herniated disc at C4–C5 (arrow). The herniation extends proximal and distal to the intervertebral space, but there is no separated fragment visualized. There is ventral cord compression. No other herniated discs are seen, but narrowing is noted at C3–C4. (b) Axial MR image through the C4–C5 disc showing the large, central, herniated disc compressing the ventral surface of the cord (arrow). On these pulse sequences the disc shows relatively high signal, clearly seen on both axial and sagittal images.

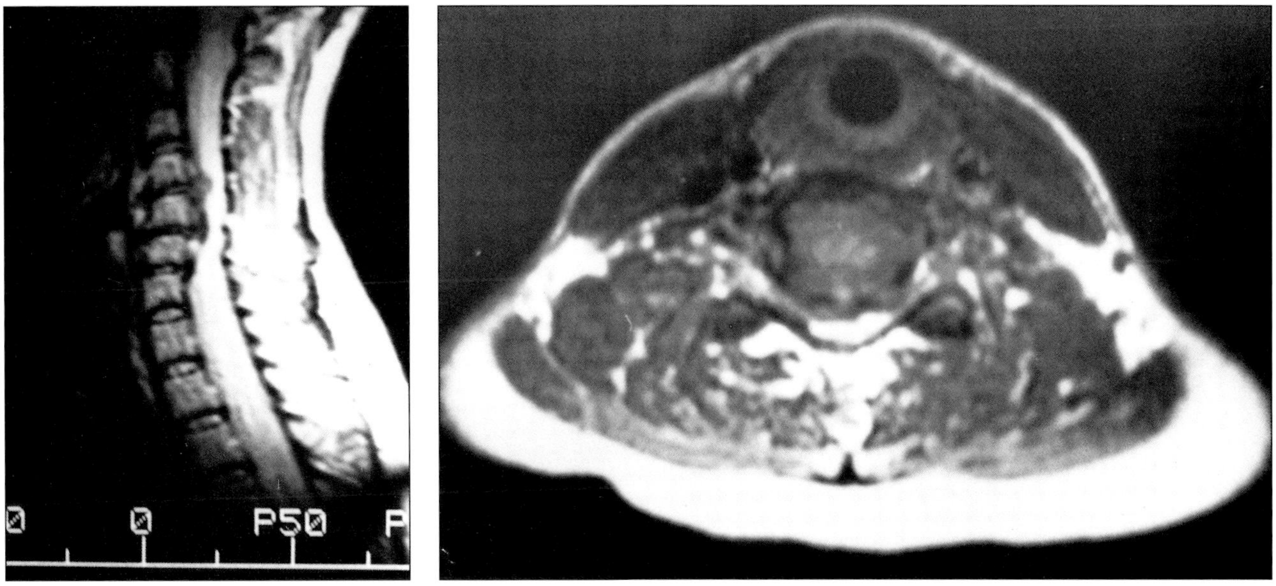

a b

Figure 5.37
(a) Sagittal T2-weighted MRI showing osteophyte protrusions in the spinal canal which indent the spinal subarachnoid space in a patient with cervical spondylotic myelopathy. (b) Axial view showing flattening of the spinal cord caused by disc and osteophyte protrusion.

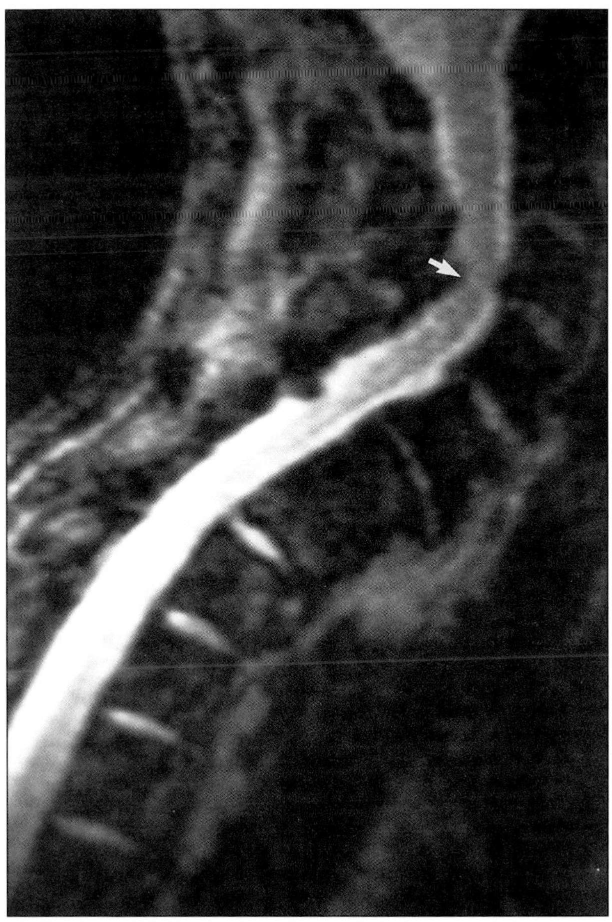

Figure 5.38
Sagittal T2-weighted MRI shows an impingement of the spinal cord from the posterior ligamentum flavum at C3–C4 (arrow) in a myelopathic patient with a hyperlordosis of the cervical spine. Incidentally, the patient had a previous anterior C6–C7 fusion.

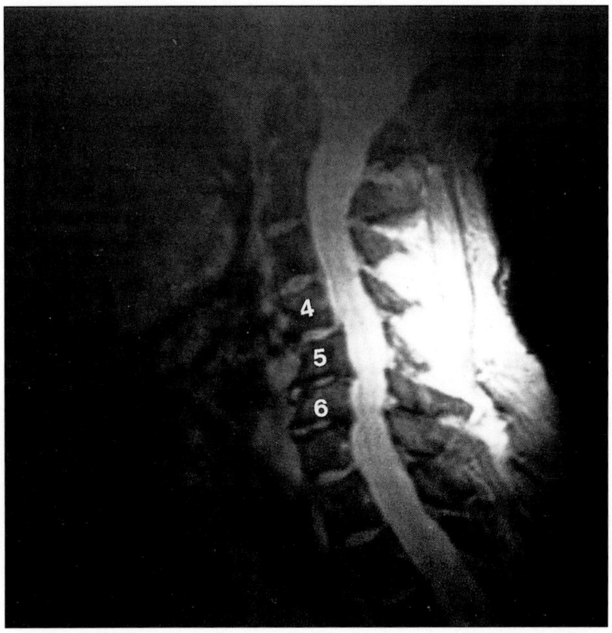

Figure 5.39
Sagittal MRI image using gradient-echo sequence clearly showing the malaligned segments at C4–C5 and C5–C6. Posterior cord displacement is apparent but there is no disc herniation.

demonstrate narrowing of the cross-sectional area of the spinal canal and a decrease or absence of subarachnoid cerebrospinal fluid signal at the stenotic levels (Figs. 5.36 5.37 and 5.39). Chronic spinal cord compression resulting from cervical spinal stenosis may lead to cord atrophy and edema within the cord which appears as high signal intensity changes on T2-weighted MRI. Lateral herniations are more subtle, and axial images demonstrate disc herniations in the posterolateral canal or in the foramen (Fig. 5.40). Foraminal stenosis by the hypertrophy of uncovertebral joints or the zygoapophyseal joints may also be demonstrated by MRI, although computed tomography is better for demonstrating bony margins.[69]

Magnetic resonance imaging has been used significantly in patients with cervical spine trauma.[10,26,40,44] Since the advent of MRI, the use of myelogram has reduced markedly in the evaluation of patients with spine trauma as in degenerative disc disease. Plain computed tomograms can complement MRI in the evaluation of bony abnormalities. Obvious advantages of MRI over plain computed tomography or computed tomographic myelogram are the lack of radiation, non-invasiveness, and the wide field of

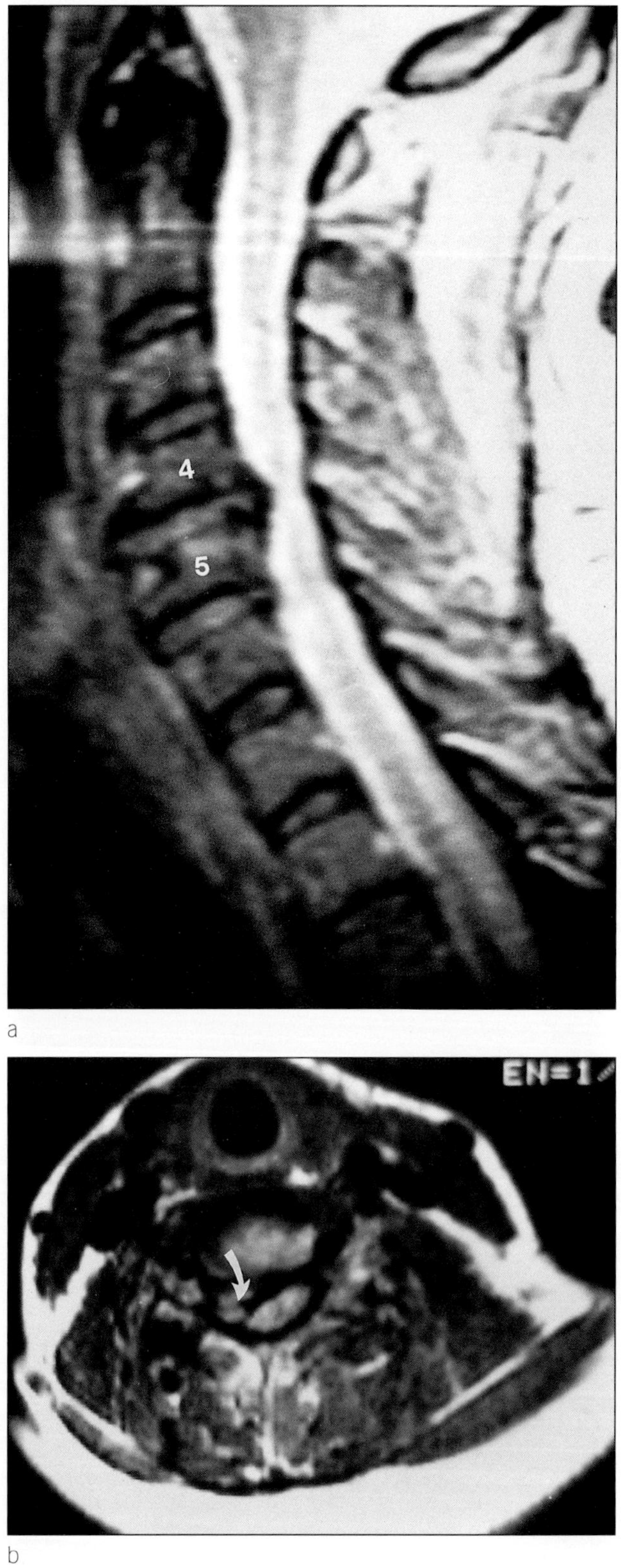

Figure 5.40
(a) Sagittal T2-weighted MRI shows a large herniated disc at C4–C5. (b) Axial T1-weighted MRI shows a large posterolateral herniated disc (arrow) impinging on the spinal cord.

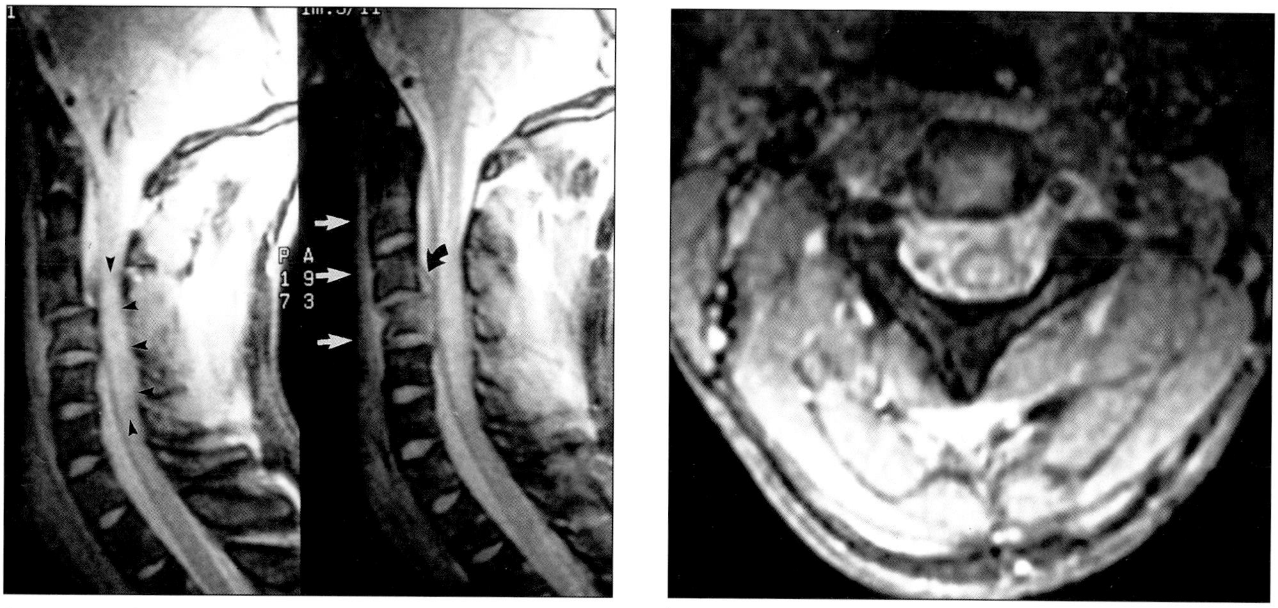

a b

Figure 5.41
(a) Sagittal T2-weighted MR image clearly shows the anterior displacement of C3, the retropulsed C4, and the impingement on the spinal cord at the level of the fracture. Increased signal ('bright signal') is seen in the cord (arrowheads) between C3 and C5, indicating cord edema. An anterior epidural hematoma (curved arrow) and prevertebral hematoma (straight arrows) are clearly shown. (b) Axial MR image using gradient echo sequence, at the level of C3, shows left and posterior displacement of the cord. This section is above the level of the fracture.

view. Other advantages include the ability to detect soft tissue and spinal cord abnormalities such as disc herniation, ligamentous disruption, hematoma, cord hemorrhage or edema, and syringomyelia. In patients requiring traction or orthoses, MRI-compatible cranial tongs or orthoses made with metals such as titanium must be used to minimize artifacts. MRI is usually indicated in patients with neurologic deficits and if plain radiographs and computed tomograms do not give enough information for definitive management.

Magnetic resonance imaging has recently been shown to provide some information on the prognosis of the spinal cord injury. Basically, hemorrhage of the spinal cord has a poor prognosis for neurologic recovery, whereas cord edema has a better prognosis.[10] Sagittal T2-weighted images are best for detection of cord hemorrhage or edema. Acute cord hemorrhages show decreased T2-weighted signal changes resulting from intracellular deoxyhemoglobin, but T2-weighted signal becomes hyperintense with time as a result of the T1-shortening effects of paramagnetic extracellular methemoglobin.[10,31] Acute cord edema is demonstrated by an area of hyperintense T2-weighted signal (Fig. 5.41a). Epidural compression of the spinal cord by bone fragment, disc, or hematoma is also well demonstrated by MRI (Fig. 5.41b), and it is particularly useful after reduction of facet dislocations to look for frequently associated herniated discs (Fig. 5.42). If the disc herniation impinges on the spinal cord, anterior discectomy and fusion should be considered in addition to posterior stabilization. Other soft tissue disruptions can also be demonstrated on MRI such as hematoma or disrupted posterior ligaments (Fig. 5.43). The disruption of the ligament shows a discontinuity in the normal low signal intensity of the ligament and increased signal on T2-weighted images resulting from edema and hemorrhage. It is important to assess the integrity of the posterior ligamentous complex, as a three-column injury is more unstable and may require both anterior and posterior stabilization procedures.

Magnetic resonance imaging is the procedure of choice in the evaluation of patients with suspected tumor or infection.[13,29,62] It is a non-invasive and non-ionizing method and provides direct sagittal, axial, and coronal images which can be obtained with a wide field of view. Any infiltrative process, such as tumor or infection which causes replacement of the normal fatty marrow with abnormal tissue

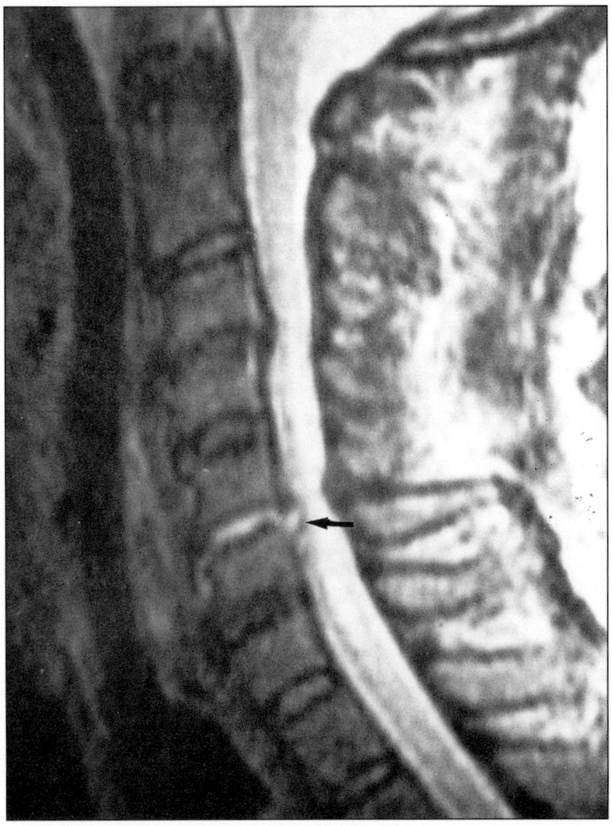

Figure 5.42
Sagittal T2-weighted MRI shows an associated herniated disc (arrow) at C5–C6 after reduction of facet dislocation.

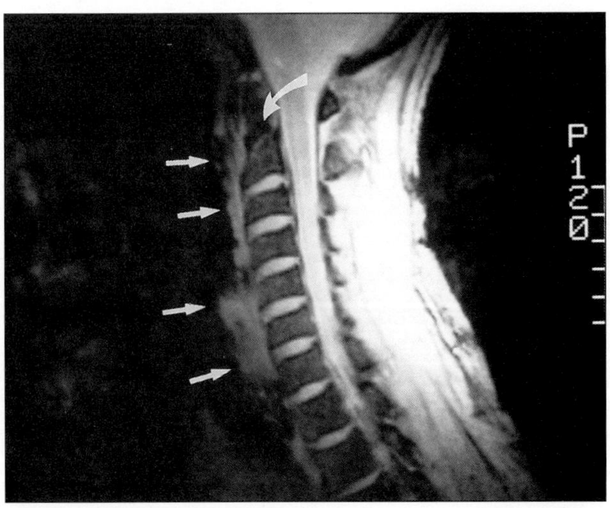

Figure 5.43
Sagittal gradient-echo MR image in the midline confirms the odontoid fracture (curved arrow). Minor disc bulges are seen at C2–C3 and C3–C4, but the cord is not displaced or deformed. Anterior hematoma (straight arrows) is well demonstrated.

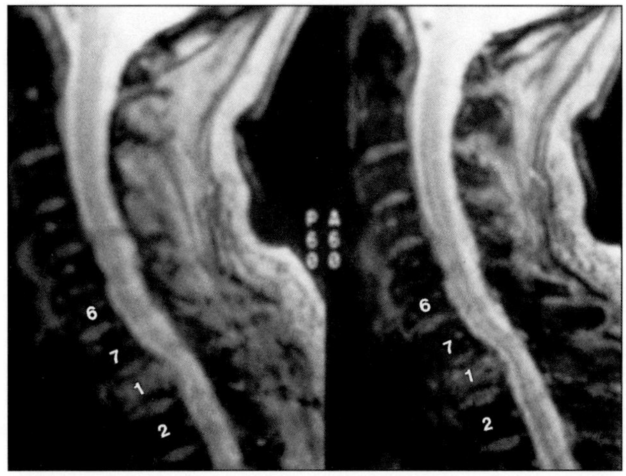

Figure 5.44
Sagittal T2-weighted MRI shows an increased signal intensity at T1 vertebral body with slight spinal cord impingement in a patient with metastatic prostate carcinoma. The adjacent intervertebral discs are normal.

associated with an increased water content and edema, will decrease the T1 intensity and increase the T2 signal. T2-weighted images allow the observer to differentiate among grades of inflammation. A focal area of high intensity on T2-weighted images usually represents a fluid collection, i.e. abscess, whereas a mild increase frequently indicates inflammation or early granulation tissue. Late granulation or fibrosis is dark on T2. More information can be gathered by the use of varied pulse sequences or the addition of intravenous gadolinium which enhances tissue contrast in cases of inflammation or scarring. With newer pulse sequences in use, such as STIR (short T1 inversion recovery technique), fatty marrow signal intensity is suppressed, thus highlighting the desired pathology. Gradient echo recall technique allows an increased rate of data acquision diminishing the image degradation caused by motion.

Abnormalities on MRI related to bone tumors and infections have been well described in the literature and are considered to be characteristic. MRI scanning allows the treating physician to detect the presence of infection or tumor early and to follow the patient's clinical course. Left untreated, spinal infections can progress to abscess formation, generalized sepsis, paraplegia, or even death. Donovan et al[21] noted the superiority of MR images over computed tomography and myelography in the diagnosis of discitis, osteomyelitis, and epidural abscess without concomitant meningitis. In cases of an associated meningitis, it is recommended that a high-resolution computed tomogram be obtained to differentiate an epidural abscess from the meningitis, due to the similarities of its signal

Figure 5.45
(a) Sagittal T1-weighted MR image shows kyphosis at the C3–C4 level with anterior destruction of the C3 and C4 vertebral bodies. An epidural mass severely displacing and flattening the cord at C3–C4 is noted, as is the caudal epidural extension of the tumor. Anterior tumor extension (arrows) is noted. The tumor shows high signal on T1 images because of intravenous gadolinium enhancement. (b) Sagittal MR image again demonstrates a huge, intermediate-to-high signal mass (arrows). Severe osseous destruction and effect on neural structures is clearly shown. (c) Transaxial T1-weighted images through the tumor done before and after intravenous gadolinium injection show effects of contrast enhancement. The large destructive lesion outlined on the pre-contrast scan (arrows) shows marked displacement of cord to the right. The signal enhancement on the post-contrast scan, in corresponding areas, shows the area of tumor involvement to better advantage.

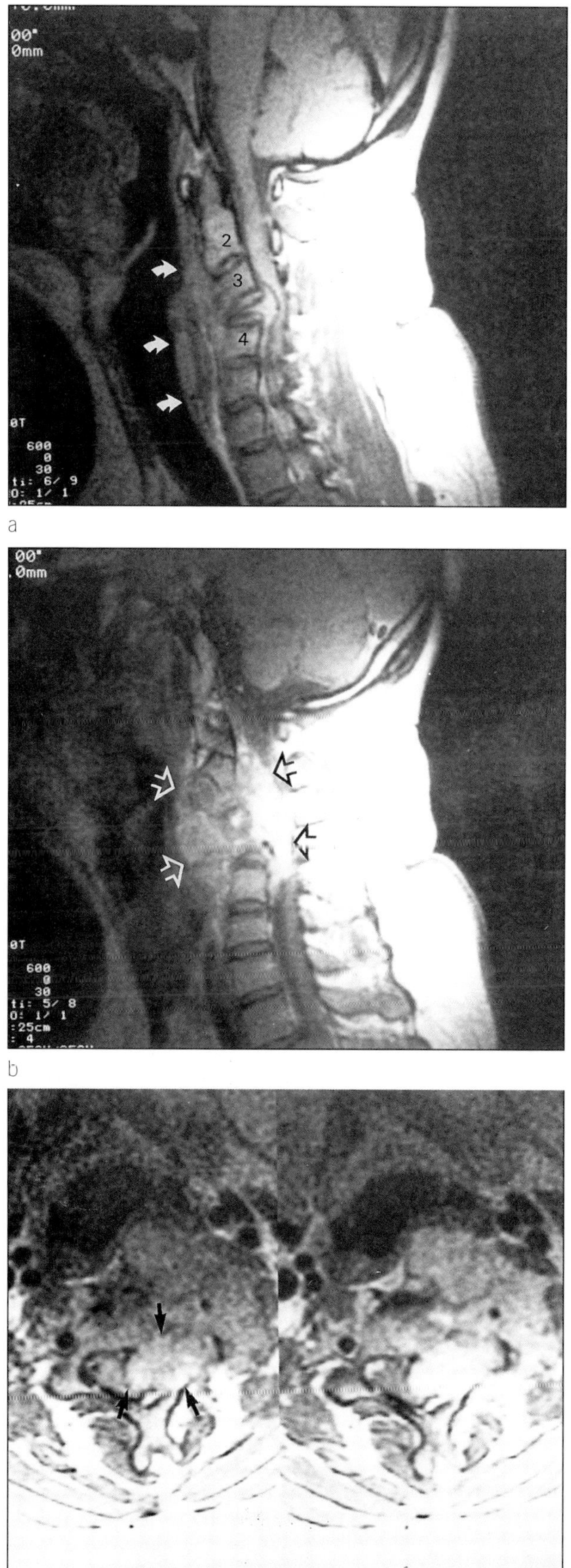

a
b
c

intensity with associated infected cerebrospinal fluid. Infections of the spine show decreased T1 signal intensity in the vertebral bodies and disc space, with with a corresponding increase in T2 signal. Contrast-enhanced MRI may increase the diagnostic accuracy of spinal infections, particularly early osteomyelitis and epidural abscess.[6] Magnetic resonance imaging has been used more frequently to assess tumors of the spine, and has even been found to have some merit in distinguishing benign from malignant processes, but it may be too sensitive in that non-neoplastic acute compression fractures may be falsely interpreted as metastatic disease. MRI has also been shown to distinguish tumors from infections of the spine reliably.[3,47,61] MRI characteristics of tumor include entire vertebral body destruction, with frequent pedicle and posterior element involvement. Primary neoplastic lesions usually have single body involvement with bony expansion and focal destruction whereas metastatic disease usually involves multiple vertebral levels with patchy vertebral involvement. Spinal infections usually reveal vertebral end-plate involvement located adjacent to the disc space with loss of vertebral end-plate definition and involvement of the contiguous vertebrae. Both neoplastic and infectious involvement of bone marrow will result in a decreased signal intensity on T1 and increased signal intensity on T2-weighted images. Neoplastic disease is differentiated from osteomyelitis by the lack of disc involvement with tumor (Fig. 5.44).

In addition to making the correct diagnosis of tumor or infection, MRI can demonstrate the extent of disease, soft-tissue involvement, and status of the spinal cord (Fig. 5.45).

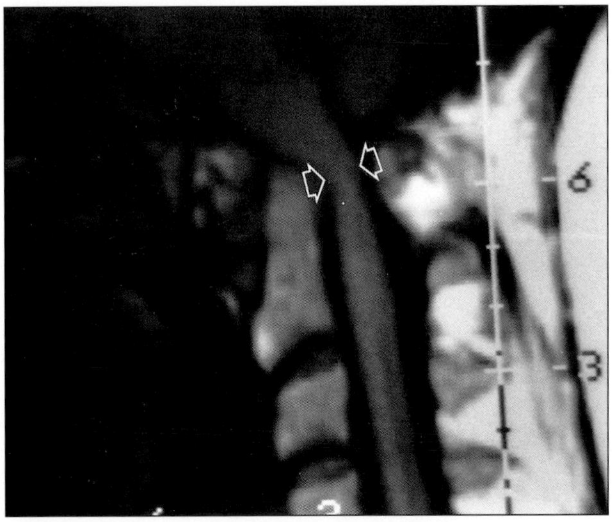

Figure 5.46
A sagittal T1-weighted MRI in flexion shows the impingement of the spinal cord (arrow) between the odontoid process and C1 ring in a rheumatoid arthritis patient with C1–C2 instability.

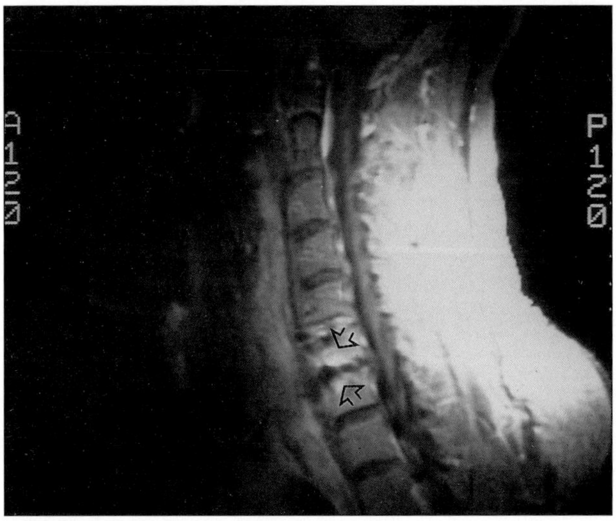

Figure 5.48
Sagittal T1-weighted MRI with gadolinium shows contrast enhancement (arrows) at C6–C7 suggesting a pseudoarthrosis process after 4 months after anterior discectomy and fusion of both C5–C6 and C6–C7. At C5–C6, a minimal contrast enhancement is noted suggesting a union process. This patient eventually had a non-union at C6–C7 and union at C5–C6.

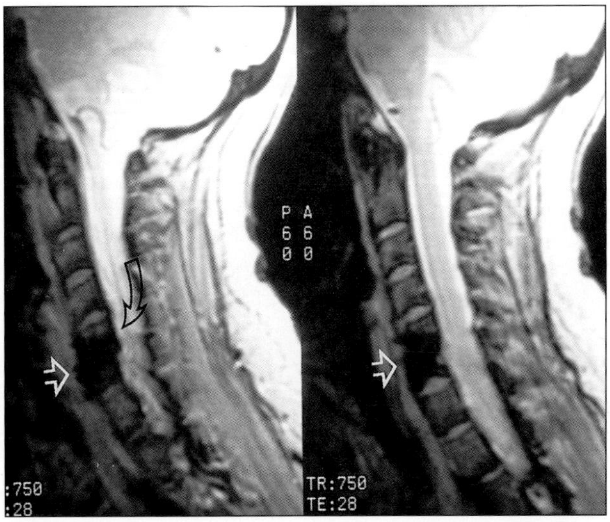

Figure 5.47
Sagittal MR image using gradient-echo sequence ('T2'-type image) renders cerebrospinal fluid bright (white) and spinal cord intermediate (gray) signal. Low signal in the fused segment from sclerotic bone is apparent (open arrows). The spinal canal is normal in the midline and shows minor deformity just off-center (curved arrow).

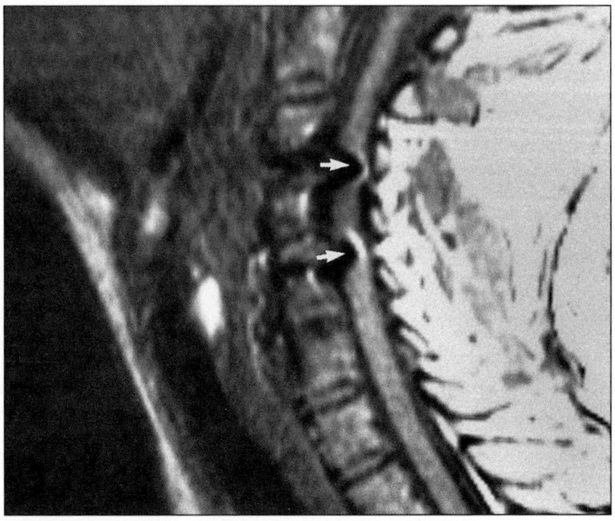

Figure 5.49
Postoperative T1-weighted MRI shows significant ferromagnetic artifacts at C3–C4 and C4–C5 (arrows) presumably resulting from small bits of metal in the disc space, which probably came from the use of a metal suction tip and power drill during surgery.

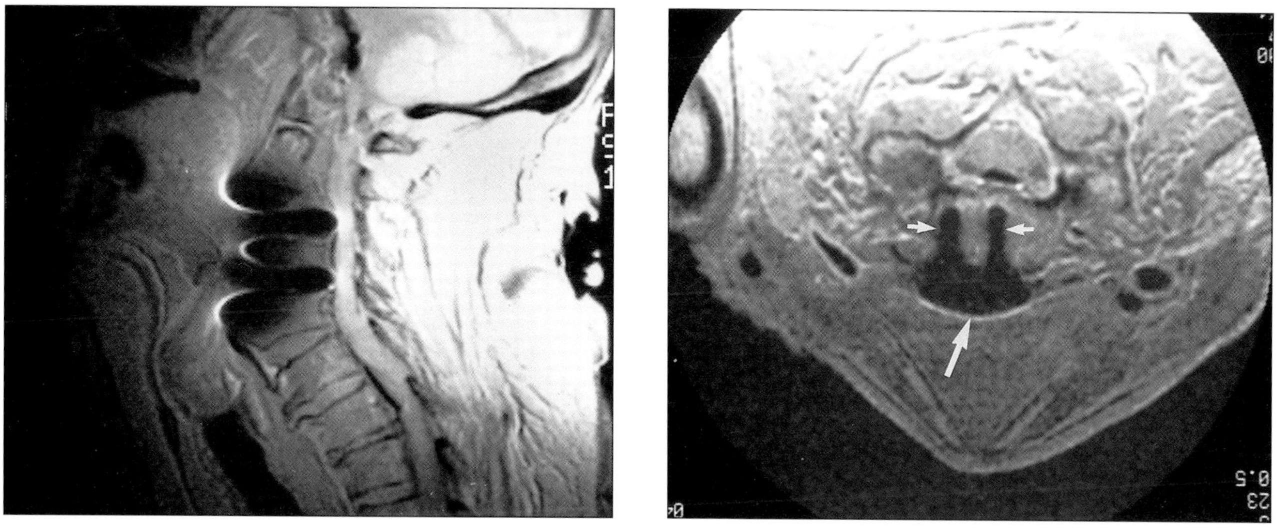

a b

Figure 5.50
(a) Sagittal MRI showing a significant ferromagnetic artifact produced by a stainless steel anterior plate-screw instrumentation. (b) Titanium plate (large arrow) and screws (small arrows) produce less ferromagnetic artifacts as shown in this axial MRI.

With or without administration of Gd-DTPA, MRI has been useful in evaluating patients with soft-tissue tumors, soft tissue abscesses, and intradural tumors. Dynamic MRI has been helpful in the assessment of spinal cord involvement associated with ankylosing spondylitis, rheumatoid arthritis, etc.[22] (Fig. 5.46).

In the postoperative period MRI may be helpful. It is valuable in demonstrating the position of an anterior graft, canal patency, spinal cord pathology, and bone healing. Fusion is usually evident if a homogeneous high signal is present from the vertebral body to the graft without visible space. However, low signal intensity does not necessarily indicate non-union, and may also indicate an artifact (Fig. 5.47).[56] Signal characteristics may change depending on the stage of healing. The authors' preliminary studies suggest that a low T1 signal and high T2 signal associated with contrast enhancement adjacent to the graft is usually predictive of non-union (Fig. 5.48). Postoperative evaluation with MRI may be limited because of ferromagnetic artifacts.[4] The authors' study has shown that after anterior discectomy and fusion MRI may be significantly distorted as a result of ferromagnetic artifact produced by small bits of metal, probably from the metal suction tip and power drill use during surgery (Fig. 5.49). Artifacts on MRI associated with metal implants can be reduced by using titanium instead of stainless steel (Fig. 5.50).[4,45]

Angiography of the Cervical Spine

Finally, selective angiography and embolization are occasionally necessary for certain spine tumors.[20,62] Spinal angiography is indicated for suspected known vascular tumors, such as hemangioma, aneurysmal bone cyst, or renal cell carcinoma, being considered for possible embolization, and also to evaluate the status of vertebral artery involvement by the tumor before surgery (Fig. 5.51). Arterial supplies to tumors may come from one or more of any neck arteries. Selective catheterization of all feeding arteries should be done to delineate the extent of tumor. Because of potential neurologic complications associated with spinal angiography, somatosensory evoked potentials should be used if possible.[8]

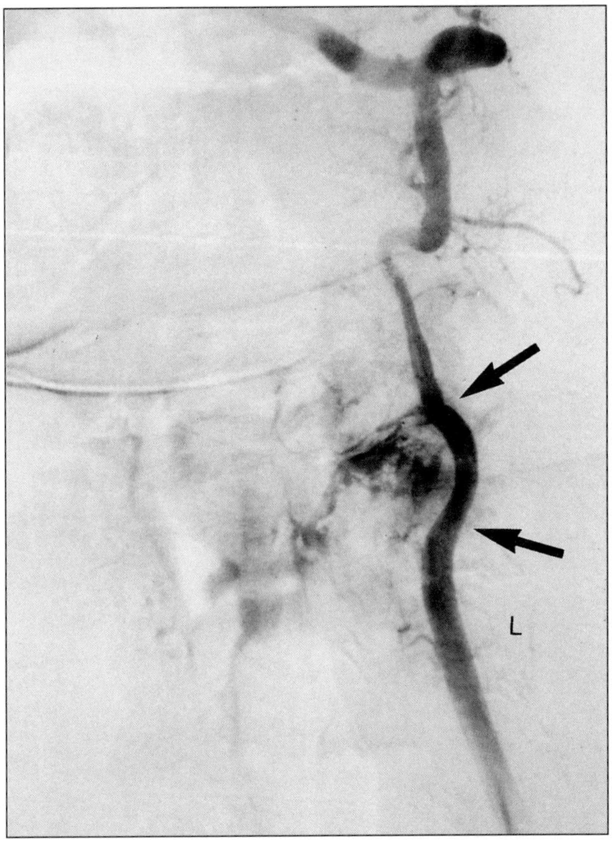

a

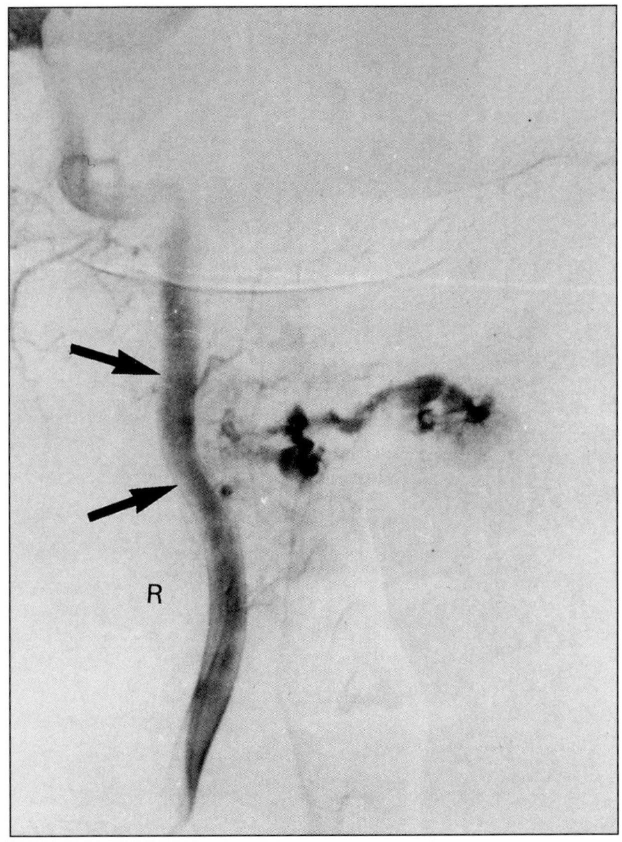

b

Figure 5.51
(a) Left and (b) right vertebral arteriograms with subtraction technique showing deviation of both vertebral arteries around the large central mass (arrows). Multiple small arteries feeding the tumor arise from each vertebral artery, but more arise from the left side.

SUMMARY

Many imaging options exist for diagnostic evaluation and therapeutic monitoring of patients with cervical spine disease. Screening examination with plain radiographs is universally accepted, and offers rapid and convenient evaluation of osseous structures as well as clues to soft-tissue disease. Often, major therapeutic decisions, particularly in the acutely injured patient, can be made on the basis of plain radiographs. Most larger practices and centers now use MRI as the primary diagnostic modality after initial screening for evaluating the spinal canal and discovertebral complex in the cervical spine. Lesions such as herniated discs, foraminal encroachments and stenosis, intrathecal lesions, and osseous lesions diagnosed with MRI often need no further evaluation with imaging. Nuclear medicine techniques fill a very important niche in the imaging sequence, because they are highly sensitive to significant osseous lesions in patients with confusing or multifocal clinical presentations, and are very useful in the longitudinal evaluation of postoperative patients. Complications associated with surgery and status of osseous healing can be efficiently evaluated with careful nuclear medicine studies, and allow for focusing of more specific anatomic studies. Computed tomography remains a major modality in the evaluation of the cervical spine. This is particularly true in instances where MRI is not available or when the patient cannot tolerate MRI, because of severe claustrophobia or complicating factors such as cardiac pacemakers or presence of ferromagnetic material. Some cases will need evaluation with both MRI and computed tomography to demonstrate complex lesions adequately or to clarify confusing situations. Myelography and computed tomography myelography, still widely applied because of broad clinical familiarity with the images, are rapidly becoming used as problem-solving techniques rather than primary diagnostic modalities.

REFERENCES

1 Abel MS (ed.) *Occult Traumatic Lesions of the Cervical Vertebrae.* St Louis, MO: Warren H. Green, 1970.
2 Al-Sheikh W, Sfakianakis GN, Mnaymneh W, et al. Sub-acute and chronic bone infections: Diagnosis using 111-In, 67-Ga, and 99m-Tc MDP bone scintigraphy and radiography. *Radiology* **155**: 501, 1985.
3 An HS, Vaccaro A, Dolinskas C, Balderston R, Cotler J. Distinction between spinal infection and spinal tumors by MRI. *Spine* **16**: S334–S338, 1991.
4 An HS, Thiel B, Nguyen C, Haughton V. Ferromagnetic artifacts associated with anterior cervical fusion and metal implants: a clinical and cadaveric study. Presented at the Cervical Spine Research Society, Palm Springs, CA, December, 1992.
5 Anderson LD, D'Alonzo RT. Fracture of the odontoid process of the axis. *J Bone Joint Surg [Am]* **56A**: 1633–1674, 1974.
6. Angtuaco EJ, McConnell Jr, Chadduck WM, Flanigan S. MR imaging of spinal epidural abscess. *ANJR* **8**: 879–883, 1987.
7 Axel L. Surface coil magnetic resonance imaging. *J Comput Assist Tomogr* **8**: 381, 1984.
8 Berenstein A, Young W, Ransohoff J, et al. Somatosensory evoked potentials during spinal angiography and therapeutic transvascular embolization. *J Neurosurg* **60**: 777–785, 1984.
9 Berkowitz ID, Wenzel W. 'Normal' technetium bone scans in patients with acute osteomyelitis. *Am J Dis Child* **134**: 828, 1980.
10 Bondurant FJ, Cotler HB, Kulkarni MV, McArdle CB, Harris JH Jr. Acute spinal cord injury: A study using physical examination and Magnetic Resonance Imaging. *Journal?* **15**: 161–168, 1990.
11 Bradley WG, Newton TH, Crooks L. Physical principles of nuclear magnetic resonance. In Newton TH, Potts DG (eds) *Advanced Imaging Techniques.* San Anselmo, Ca: Clavadel Press, 1983.
12 Bradley WG, Waluch V, Yadley RA, et al. Comparison of CT and MR in 400 patients with suspected disease of the brain and cervical spinal cord. *Radiology* **152**: 695–702, 1984.
13 Carmody RF, Yang PJ, Seely GW, et al. Spinal cord compression due to metastatic disease: diagnosis with MR imaging versus myelography. *Radiology* **173**: 225–229, 1989.
14 Cattell HS, Filtzer DL. Pseudosubluxation and other normal variations of the cervical spine in children. *J Bone Joint Surg [Am]* **47**: 1295, 1965.
15 Clark WM, Gehweiler JA, Laib R. Twelve significant signs of cervical spine trauma. *Skel Radiol* **3**: 201–205, 1979.
16 Collier BD, Johnson RP, Carrera GF, et al. Complementary use of radiography and single photon emission computed tomography in identifying painful sites of spondylolysis or spondylolisthesis. *Radiology* **149P**: 101, 1983.
17 Daniels DL, Grogan JP, Johansen JG, Meyer GA, Williams AL, Haughton VM. Cervical radiculopathy: Computed tomography and myelography compared. *Radiology* **151**: 109–113, 1984.
18 Daniels DL, Haughton VM, Naidich T (ed) *Cranial and Spinal Magnetic Resonance Imaging: An Atlas and Guide.* New York: Raven Press, 1987.
19 Daniels DL, Hyde JS, Kneeland JB, et al. The cervical nerves and foramina: Local-coil MR imaging. *Am J Neuroradiol* **7**: 129–133, 1986.
20 Djindjian R, Merland JJ. *Angiography of Spinal Column and Spinal Cord Tumors.* Stuttgart: Georg Thième Verlag, 1981.
21 Donovan JM, Quencer RM, Montalvo BM, Katz BH, Eismont FJ, Green BA. Spinal infection: Evaluation with MR imaging and intraoperative U.S. *Radiology* **169**: 765–771, 1988.
22 Dvorak J, Grob D, Baumgartner H, et al. Functional evaluation of the spinal cord by magnetic resonance imaging in patients with rheumatoid arthritis and instability of the upper cervical spine. *Spine* **14**: 1057–1064, 1989.
23 Edelman RR, Stark DD, Saini S, et al. Oblique planes of section in MR imaging. *Radiology* **159**: 807–810, 1986.
24 Effendi B, Roy B, Cornish B, et al. Fracture of the ring of the axis: a classification based on analysis of 131 cases. *J Bone Joint Surg [Am]* **63**: 319–327, 1981.
25 Fielding JW. Normal and selected abnormal motions of the cervical spine from the second cervical vertebra to the seventh cervical vertebra based on cineroentgenography. *J Bone Joint Surg [Am]* **46**: 1779, 1964.
26 Flanders AE, Schaefer DM, Doan HT, Mishkin MM, Gonzales CF, Northrup BE. Acute cervical spine trauma: Correlation of MR findings with degree of neurologic deficit. *Radiology* **177**: 25–33, 1990.
27 Gehweiler JA, Clark WM, Schaaf RE, Powers B, Miller MD. Cervical spine trauma: The common combined conditions. *Radiology* **130**: 77–86, 1979.
28 Gerlock AJ, Kischner SG, Heller RM, Kay JJ, (eds). *The Cervical Spine in Trauma.* Philadelphia: WB Saunders, 1978.
29 Godersky JC, Smoker WRK, Knutzon R. Use of magnetic resonance imaging in the evaluation of metastatic spinal disease. *Neurosurgery* **21**: 676–680, 1987.
30 Gumerman LW, Fogel SR, Goodman MA, et al. Experimental fracture healing: Evaluation using radionuclide bone imaging. *J Nucl Med* **19**: 1356, 1978.
31 Hackney DB, Asato R, Joseph P. Hemorrhage and edema in acute cervical cord compression: demonstration by MR imaging. *Radiology* **161**: 387–390, 1986.
32 Harris JH Jr (ed.). *The Radiology of Acute Cervical Spine Trauma.* Baltimore: Williams & Wilkins, 1978.

33 Haughton VM (ed.). *Computed Tomography of the Spine*. New York: Churchill Livingstone, 1983.
34 Haughton VM, Syvertsen A, Williams AL. Soft tissue anatomy within the spinal canal as seen on CT. *Radiology* **134**: 649–656, 1980.
35 Haughton VM, Williams AL (ed.). *Computed Tomography of the Spine*. St Louis, MO: CV Mosby, 1982.
36 Hinck VC, Hopkins CE. Measurement of the atlanto-dental interval in the adult. *Radiology* **84**: 945, 1964.
37 Hohl M. Normal motions in the upper portion of the cervical spine. *J Bone Joint Surg [Am]* **46**: 1777, 1964
38 Howie DW, Savage JP, Wilson TG, Paterson D. Technetium phosphate bone scan in diagnosis of osteomyelitis. *J Bone Joint Surg [Am]* **65**: 431, 1983.
39 Kim KS, Chen HH, Russell EJ, et al. Flexion teardrop fracture of the cervical spine: radiographic characteristics. *AJNR* **9**: 1221–1228, 1988.
40 Kulkarni MV, Bondurant FJ, Rose SL, Narayana PA. 1.5 tesla magnetic resonance imaging of acute spinal trauma. *RadioGraphics* **8**: 1059–1082, 1988.
41 Matin P. Appearance of bone scans following fractures, including immediate and long-term studies. *J Nucl Med* **20**: 1227, 1979.
42 Maurer AH, Chen DCP, Camargo EE, et al. Utility of three-phase skeletal scintigraphy in suspected osteomyelitis: Concise communication. *J Nucl Med* **22**: 941, 1981.
43 McMaster MJ, Merrick MV. Scintigraphic assessment of the scoliotic spine after fusion. *J Bone Joint Surg [Br]* **62**: 65, 1980.
44 Mirvis SE, Geisler FH, Jelinek JJ, et al. Acute cervical spine trauma: evaluation with 1.5 T MR imaging. *Radiology* **166**: 807–816, 1988.
45 Mirvis SE, Geisler FH, Joslyn JN, et al. Use of titanium wire in cervical spine fixation as a means to reduce MR artifacts. *AJNR* **9**: 1229–1231, 1988.
46 Mirvis SE, Young JWR, Lim C, et al. Hangman's fracture: radiographic assessment in 27 cases. *Radiology* **163**: 713–717, 1987.
47 Modic MT, Feiglin DH, Piraino DW, et al. Vertebral osteomyelitis: assessment using MR. *Radiology* **157**: 157–166, 1985.
48 Modic MT, Pavlicek W, Weinstein MA, et al. Magnetic resonance imaging of intervertebral disk disease. *Radiology* **152**: 103–111, 1984.
49 Modic MT, Weinstein MA, Pavlicek W, et al. Nuclear magnetic resonance imaging of the spine. *Radiology* **148**: 757–762, 1983.
50 Modic MT, Weinstein MA, Pavlicek W, et al. Magnetic resonance imaging of the cervical spine: Technical and clinical observations. *Am J Neuroradiol* **5**: 15–22, 1984.
51 O'Reilly RJ, Cook DJ, Gaffney RD, et al. Can serial scintigraphic studies detect delayed fracture union in man? *Clin Orthop* **160**: 227, 1981.
52 Paul LW, Moir WW. Non-pathologic variations in relationship of the upper cervical vertebrae. *Radiology* **62**: 519, 1949.
53 Pavlov H, Torg JS, Robie B, Jahre C. Cervical spine stenosis: determination with vertebral body ratio method. *Radiology* **164**: 771–775, 1987.
54 Pay NT, George AE, Benjamin MV, et al. Positive and negative contrast myelography in spinal trauma. *Radiology* **123**: 103, 1977.
55 Pech P, Daniels DL, Williams AL, Haughton VM. The cervical neural foramina: Correlation of microtomy and CT anatomy. *Radiology* **155**: 143–146, 1985.
54 Penning L. Prevertebral hematoma in cervical spine injury: Incidence and etiologic significance. *AJR Am J Roentgenol* **136**: 553–561, 1981.
55 Rosenthal L, Hill RO, Chuang S. Observations on the use of 99m-Tc phosphate imaging in peripheral bone trauma. *Radiology* **119**: 637, 1976.
56 Ross JS. Magnetic resonance assessment of the postoperative spine: degenerative disc disease. In Modic MT (ed.) Imaging of the spine. *Radiol Clin North Am* **29**: 793–808, 1991.
57 Russin LD, Guinto FC Jr. Multidirectional tomography in cervical spine injury. *J Neurosurg* **45**: 9, 1976.
58 Schauwecker DS, Park HM, Mock BH, et al. Evaluation of complicating osteomyelitis with 99m-Tc MDP, 111 indium granulocytes and 67 Ga citrate. *J Nucl Med* **25**: 849, 1984.
59 Tadmor R, Davis KR, Roberson GH, et al. Computed tomographic evaluation of traumatic spinal injuries. *Radiology* **127**: 825, 1978.
60 Torg JS, Pavlov H, Genuaria SE, et al. Neuropraxia of the cervical spinal cord with transient quadriplegia. *J Bone Joint Surg [Am]* **68**: 1354, 1986.
61 Unger E, Moldofsky P, Gatenby R, Hartz W, Broder G. Diagnosis of osteomyelitis by MR imaging. *Am J Roentgenol* **150**: 605–610, 1988.
62 Voegeli E, Fuchs W. Arteriography in bone tumors. *Br J Radiol* **49**: 407–415, 1976.
63 Wahner HW. Radionuclides in the diagnosis of fracture healing. *J Nucl Med* **19**: 1356, 1978.
64 Wald ER, Mirro R, Gartner JC. Pitfalls in the diagnosis of acute osteomyelitis by bone scan. *Clin Pediatr* **19**: 597, 1980.
65 Wehrli FW, MacFall Jr, Shutts D, Breger R, Herfkens RJ. Mechanisms of contrast in NMR imaging. *J Comput Assist Tomogr* **8**: 369–380, 1984.
66 Weir DC. Roentgenographic signs of cervical injury. *Clin Orthop* **109**: 9, 1975.
67 White AA III, Panjabi MM. *Clinical biomechanics of the spine*. Philadelphia: JB Lippincott, 1978.
68 Williamson BRJ, McLaughlin RE, Wang GJ, et al. Radionuclide bone imaging as a means of differentiating loosening and infection in patients with a painful total hip prosthesis. *Radiology* **133**: 723, 1979.
69 Youssem DM, Atlas SW, Goldberg HI, et al. Degenerative narrowing of the cervical spine neural foramina: evaluation with high-resolution 3DFT gradient-echo MR imaging. *AJNR* **12**: 229–36, 1991.

6 Non-surgical evaluation, treatment, and rehabilitation of cervical spine disorders

Steven M. Gnatz and J. Michael Simpson

The specialist in physical medicine and rehabilitation brings unique talents to the evaluation and treatment of the patient with cervical dysfunction and pain. Most of these patients will not require surgery.[29] Accurate identification of non-surgical etiologies for cervical dysfunction and timely conservative treatment will help assure the patient of a more favorable result. Electrodiagnostic studies are considered an extension of the history and physical examination by the physician. The electrodiagnostic consultation will assist the referring surgeon in determining the presence or absence of surgically correctable disease.

HISTORY AND DIFFERENTIAL DIAGNOSIS OF CERVICAL DYSFUNCTION

It is helpful, from a treatment and prognostic standpoint, to differentiate radicular from non-radicular causes of cervical dysfunction, and such a differential diagnosis is shown in Table 6.1. Regardless of the particular etiology, the most common cervical dysfunction noted clinically is that of musculoligamentous tightness and tenderness of the cervical soft tissues. Patients with such symptoms are not candidates for surgical procedures, and generally respond to conservative measures. Radicular causes of cervical dysfunction may also respond to conservative care, but in refractory cases are more likely to respond to decompressive types of surgical procedures. However, attention to rehabilitation after surgery remains an important means of ensuring against relapse.

Currently there are many sensitive and powerful tools to confirm or discard the diagnosis of cervical radiculopathy and other forms of nerve entrapment in the cervical region (magnetic resonance imaging (MRI), computed tomography, myelography, electromyography (EMG), etc.). However, our ability to diagnose non-radicular cervical pain remains dependent on the clinician's experience and the clinical picture presented by the patient.

In evaluation of the patient with cervical pain and dysfunction, the patient's history cannot be over-emphasized. In most cases, a provisional diagnosis can be made by history alone, with physical examination and ancillary tests used for confirmation. The onset and timing of the problem may offer clues as to the etiology. Was there a specific incident of trauma? If so, what was the specific mechanism of injury and how much force was involved? This information may be obtained from accident reports or, in the case of a motor vehicle accident, ascertained from how much damage was done to the car. Which anatomic structures were most probably damaged secondary to the proposed mechanism of injury? For example, an extension-type injury may result in symptoms in the anterior neck muscles (sternocleidomastoid and other strap muscles) and/or dysfunction of the posterior elements (facet joint, nerve root, etc.). It would be unlikely that this mechanism of injury alone would result in posterior neck muscle dysfunction, as these muscles would be relaxed during the accident. Unfortunately, the mechanism of injury is often unclear, particularly in motor vehicle accidents, where combined flexion, extension, lateral bending, and rotatory forces are often applied to the neck. This information also tends to be less useful as time elapses from the original incident. Patients' memories of the accident change, either magnifying or minimizing it. Anatomic structures initially injured may become secondary complaints, because the process of substitution and overuse of normal muscles and other supportive structures leads to development of new pain patterns. Nevertheless, the ability to correlate the known or suspected pathophysiologic mechanism of injury to the patient's reported symptoms may give the examiner an indication as to whether the distribution of pain makes sense physiologically, or if there is a significant psychological component to the patient's complaints.

Table 6.1 Classification of head and neck pain

I Intrinsic causes of musculoskeletal pain
- A Skeletal abnormalities
  - 1 Fracture
  - 2 Neoplasm, primary or metastatic
  - 3 Infection, osteomyelitis
  - 4 Paget's disease
  - 5 Osteoporosis
  - 6 Endocrinologic, hyperparathyroidism
  - 7 Arteriovenous malformations, aneurysms
  - 8. Hematologic, sickle cell, multiple myeloma
- B Joint abnormalities
  - 1 Synovitis, capsulitis, discitis
  - 2 Joint effusion, hemarthrosis
  - 3 Osteoarthritis
  - 4 Rheumatic disease, rheumatoid arthritis
  - 5 Disc derangements
  - 6 Joint instability, ligamentous laxity
  - 7 Biomechanical abnormalities
  - 8 Neoplasms, primary or metastatic
  - 9 Vasculitides
- C Ligaments
  - 1 Trauma, sprains, rupture
  - 2 Chronic laxity
  - 3 Contracture
  - 4 Neoplasms
  - 5 Infection
- D Muscles, tendons, fascia
  - 1 Myofascial pain, fibromyalgia
  - 2 Trauma, strains, tears, ruptures
  - 3 Inflammatory conditions, polymyositis
  - 4 Infectious conditions, trichinosis, etc.
  - 5 Polymyalgia rheumatica
  - 6 Vasculitides
  - 7 Metabolic, exercise induced, cramps
  - 8 Ischemic, claudication, compartment syndromes
  - 9 Neoplasms
  - 10 Contracture, biomechanical abnormalities
  - 11 Overuse syndromes
  - 12 Nutritional, avitaminosis
  - 13 Toxins, venom, etc.
- E Nerve structures
  - 1 Entrapment, compression
  - 2 Trauma, stretch, laceration
  - 3 Deafferentation, neuromas
  - 4 Reflex sympathetic dystrophy, causalgia
  - 5 Neuritis, neuralgia, tics
  - 6 Peripheral neuropathy, diabetes, toxins
  - 7 Ischemia, vasculitis
  - 8 Infection, herpes, AIDS
  - 9 Neoplasms

II Extrinsic causes of head and neck pain
- A Other organs referring pain to the musculoskeletal system
  - 1 Heart: myocardial infarction, angina
  - 2 Lungs: pleuritis, tumors (especially Pancoast's)
  - 3 Eyes: infection, strain
  - 4 Ears: infection, tumors
  - 5 Nose and sinus: infection, abscess, tumors
  - 6 Throat and teeth: infection, tumors
  - 7 Central nervous system: syringomyelia, Arnold–Chiari, spasmodic torticollis, tumors (especially acoustic neuromas, neurofibromas and other slow growing), infections, vascular abnormalities and accidents, and supratentorial

From: Referred pain syndromes of the head and neck. Gnatz SM. *Physical Medicine and Rehabilitation: State of the Art Reviews* 1991; 5: 585–596.

A history of pain, paresthesiae, and weakness of an extremity deserves special attention. These symptoms are often equated with nerve entrapment by both patients and physicians, although, this is not always the case. Other deep anatomic structures (most often muscles), which do not have direct somatosensory input to the sensory cortex, generate referred patterns of pain and numbness, and may result in a reflex-type weakness of the limb.[27] These referred pain patterns are not dermatomal or myotomal, and can be differentiated by careful history and physical examination. A muscular trigger point is the most common example of a referred pain syndrome in the neck and upper extremities.[68]

Certainly one of the most common deep somatic referred pain syndromes is myofascial pain as described by Travell and Simons.[69] Pain originates in the myofascial 'trigger point' and is referred in a pattern that is not dermatomal, myotomal, or sclerotomal, but instead follows one that is recognizable and reproducible. Studies with normal subjects show that local tenderness to palpation of muscle is common, and yet true trigger points with pain referred to another area are present in only 5–12% of normal individuals.[64] The most commonly involved muscles in the neck region are the cervical paraspinal muscles and the occipital or nuchal muscles. The trapezius, levator scapulae, infraspinatus, supraspinatus, and rhomboids may

Table 6.2 Comparison of fibromyalgia and myofascial pain

	Fibromyalgia	*Myofascial pain*
Sex (F:M)	2–4:1	Both males and females
Age	Young adults	Any age
Prevalence	Common	5–12%
Tenderness	>7 locations	1–5 locations
Trigger points	Possible	Yes
Somatic complaints	Common	Rare
Referred pain	Possibly, but not necessarily	Yes, in well-defined areas
Local twitch	Less likely	Yes
Etiology	Unknown, more probably a result of intrinsic factors	Unknown, may be due to trauma, overuse, biomechanics
Treatment	Multidisciplinary, general aerobic, reassurance, support	Local injections, stretch and spray, range of motion, motion

From: Referred pain syndromes of the head and neck. Gnatz SM. *Physical Medicine and Rehabilitation: State of the Art Reviews* 1991; 5: 585–596.

also be involved and can demonstrate referred pain patterns to the neck or proximal arms. The referred pain pattern can be associated with autonomic phenomena, such as piloerection, flushing, sweating, and skin temperature changes. Additionally, visceral symptoms, such as nausea and vomiting, may result from stimulation of the trigger area. Reflex weakness of the affected muscle can occur.

It may be helpful to distinguish myofascial pain syndromes from the more generalized fibromyalgia, although these two diagnoses may simply represent two ends of the same scale.[61] Fibromyalgia usually includes additional somatic symptoms, such as sleep disturbance, irritable bowel complaints, and multiple tender areas. Myofascial pain is usually more localized or regional, involves fewer muscles, may be induced by trauma, and responds better to local treatment (Table 6.2).

The pathophysiology of fibromyalgia and myofascial pain syndromes remains undetermined. Recent studies have demonstrated a reduction in high-energy phosphate levels in the myofascially involved muscle.[2] Similarly, decreased levels of high-energy phosphates and increased levels of low-energy phosphates have been demonstrated in the trapezius muscle of patients with fibromyalgia.[45] Whether these findings are the cause or effect of the myofascial process is unknown. Other suspected causative or perpetuating factors are stress, fatigue, poor posture, underlying medical problems, and dysfunctional habits such as smoking. Myofascial pain and fibromyalgia should be distinguished from myositis, because no inflammatory process involving muscle tissue has been identified. The lack of specific diagnostic testing for this syndrome has hindered the general acceptance of this common condition as a real entity. It has been suggested that MRI spectroscopy may be of potential value in the diagnosis of fibromyalgia.[41]

A history of progressive loss of a range of motion in the cervical region is often reported by the patient. This symptom suggests that a 'vicious cycle' has developed wherein the initial incident of cervical pain was followed by pain with motion of the spine. The patient subsequently moves the area less (a normal physiologic response to pain), but with this loss of movement, muscular stiffness and tightness follow. More pain is produced when the patient attempts to move again, restarting the cycle. It should be noted that, even if the original initiator of pain is gone, pain can continue because musculoligamentous tightness can produce its own pain when motion is pushed beyond certain tolerable limits. The only way to break this cycle is to identify the tight structures and bring them back to their normal length by physical rehabilitative methods.

A history of clicking, popping, and crepitation does not carry any specific pathophysiologic or prognostic value, because this symptom can be present in those with muscular tightness or underlying degenerative joint disease.

Radiographic evaluation of those suspected of having degenerative joint disease may be helpful. However, caution is advised when interpreting minimal-to-moderate degenerative changes in any given patient as the cause of the painful syndrome, because these changes are common in the normal population.[9]

Radiation of pain to the occipital region may suggest an entrapment of the greater occipital nerve as it passes through the upper cervical area.[31] Occasionally, a neuroma of this nerve can be palpated at the base of the skull with reproduction of the symptoms. If so, the neuroma may resolve after injection with steroid and local anesthetic.

A history of other head pain should be elicited. As many as 11% of patients with temporomandibular joint dysfunction present with neck pain as their chief complaint.[25] These patients may also complain of ear symptoms including tinnitus and loss of hearing. Pain behind the eye and sinus regions, and symptoms related to the jaw joint itself including clicking, popping, and locking may help differentiate the patient with temporomandibular joint dysfunction from the one with a primary cervical problem.[24] The former patient can also present with dysphagia, a symptom seen together with severe spondylosis of the cervical spine.[11] In addition, dizziness or vertigo may be reported in patients with either temporomandibular joint dysfunction[8] or cervical dysfunction and degenerative joint disease.[1] The symptoms of dizziness and vertigo are more often related to head position and can be reproduced by unusual head postures in the later group. Vertebrobasilar artery insufficiency should be ruled out in those patients with significant cervical spondylosis.[57] Evaluation of the vertebral basilar circulation by angiographic means or less invasive Doppler ultrasonography studies is advised in these cases.

A history of symptoms related to other joints of the body should be elicited. If any, for example, the knees, shoulders, hips, elbows, wrists, or small joints of the hands and feet, have become warm, erythematous, swollen, or tender, then a rheumatologic process may be present. In contrast to the temporomandibular joint, the cervical spine is one of the common regions to become involved in rheumatoid arthritis and may be symptomatic in 30–40% of such patients. The most dramatic manifestation of rheumatoid arthritis in the cervical region is atlantoaxial subluxation which may require arthrodesis, if unstable.[51]

In ankylosing spondylitis, the cervical region may become involved, but this generally occurs late in the course of the disease. Ankylosing spondylitis typically involves initially the lumbosacral spine, with development of characteristic rigidity and loss of lordosis. The remainder of the spine eventually becomes involved, extending to first the thoracic region and finally the cervical region. In severe cases, a chin-on-chest-type deformity can develop with significant disruption of normal visual fields.

Other rheumatologic and connective tissue diseases may affect articulations of the cervical spine, including systemic lupus erythematosus, Sjögren's syndrome and scleroderma. These syndromes can usually be identified by other characteristic findings. Involvement of the cervical spine generally follows the course of the disease process.

Retropharyngeal abscess, other hidden infectious processes, and malignant sources may be uncommon causes of neck and facial pain.[13] A history of night sweats or swelling of lymph glands may help identify an infectious or tumor process. These lesions may also cause cranial nerve abnormalities, prompting further investigation.

Torticollis is a condition that can usually be identified by patient history or an initial inspection by the examining physician. The etiology of torticollis is highly variable, but is generally classified as congenital or acquired. Acquired forms may be seen in post-traumatic conditions or may simply be idiopathic; occasionally they may be of a non-physiologic (functional) nature.[15] Patients may not realize they have a torticollis and may partially hide the muscle spasm by turning their body to compensate for the head tilt. Pain may be localized to the affected lateral, anterior, or posterior neck muscles or referred to the occiput or upper extremities.

Intrinsic shoulder pathology must also be considered. Shoulder pain from rotator cuff disease, impingement syndrome, bursitis, and tendinitis may present with localized pain or referred pain into the neck. Shoulder disorders may also refer pain into the arm; however, careful examination of the shoulder can easily differentiate these problems from underlying cervical pathology.[63]

Brachial neuritis, also known as neuralgic amyotrophy, classically presents as shoulder pain followed by weakness and muscular atrophy of the shoulder.[67] Occasionally this pain will be referred to the neck region. More commonly, however, as other muscle structures in the neck and shoulder region become overused, pain develops. Neuralgic amyotrophy can be identified by EMG testing.

Occasionally, patients with primary muscular diseases such as myotonic dystrophy, muscular dystrophies and inflammatory myopathies, will present with cervical and shoulder symptoms. Usually, these symptoms arise from muscular weakness and overuse of the remaining functioning muscular structures. These problems can be identified by their characteristic history and physical findings, EMG examination, and muscle biopsy.

Pain may be referred from other deep somatic structures to the neck and shoulder region. The most well-known example of this type of referred pain is angina pectoris, with cardiac ischemia producing referred symptoms into the left arm, neck, or jaw. Other visceral pain, such as that produced by cholecystitis or pneumonitis, may be referred to the shoulder region.[6]

Head and neck pain in an elderly patient is more probably the result of degenerative or possibly neoplastic processes. As such, many believe that a more aggressive diagnostic work-up is required to identify treatable pathology.[47]

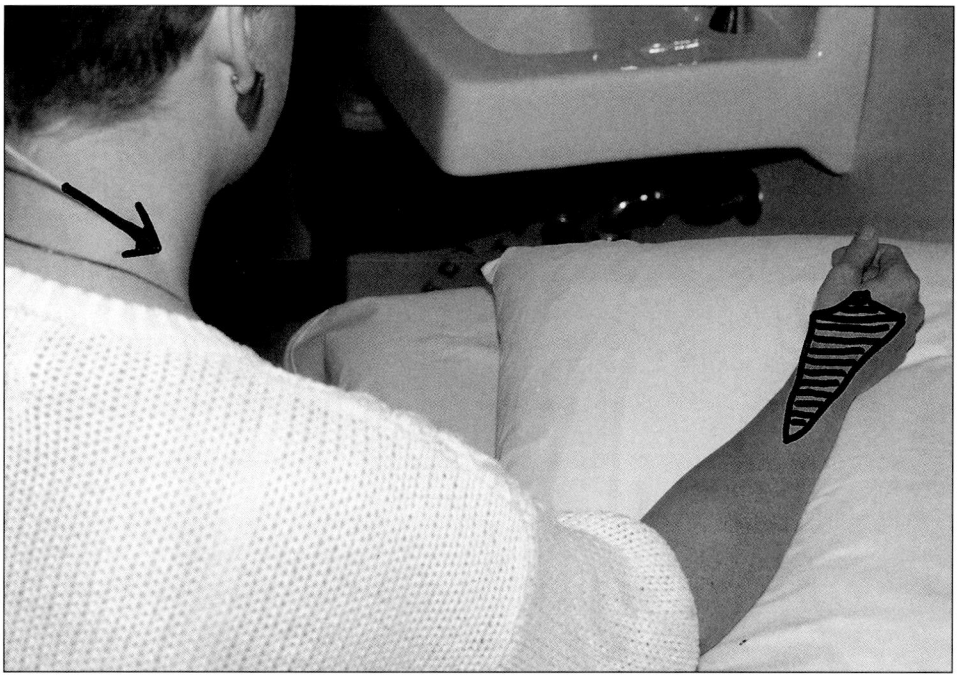

Figure 6.1
A myofascial trigger point identified by palpation; the referred pain zone is outlined

A history of pending litigation is an arguably poor prognostic sign for patients with cervical symptoms.[55] Many of these patients have been injured in motor vehicle accidents and have pending lawsuits, and yet, undoubtedly, many will recover with appropriate rehabilitation management. Many of these patients simply want assurance that no major medical problems or expenses will befall them in the future. The work-up in these cases will need to provide sufficient documentation and medical evidence to the physician and the patient of what, if any, future medical expenses will be incurred.

PHYSICAL EXAMINATION

Physical examination should include an evaluation of the static curvatures of the spine. Normal sagittal plane contours include a gentle cervical lordosis, thoracic kyphosis, and lumbar lordosis. The examiner is advised to evaluate the entire spine and posture, because abnormalities as remote as leg length discrepancy can have profound effects on cervicothoracic alignment. The identification of such sagittal or coronal plane deformities may point the examiner to a specific problem area.

Range of motion in the cervical region should first be evaluated with a request for active range of motion by the patient in the directions of flexion, extension, rotation, and lateral bending. These movements should be judged not only for their maximum limits, but also for fluidity and coordination of the individual spinal segments. Attention should be paid to the reproducibility of the maximum range of motion. If there is significant variation (>20%) in the maximum range of motion on repeated testing, a non-physiologic abnormality should be considered. Sophisticated electronic goniometric testing may be used to assist the examiner in evaluation and follow-up of the patient in treatment.[21]

Palpation of the muscular, ligamentous, bone, and joint structures of the cervical region may help to localize abnormalities. The paraspinal, scalene, and anterior strap muscles of the neck should be evaluated for tenderness or trigger points (Fig. 6.1). Muscles of the head, including occipital and masticatory muscles, and muscles of the anterior chest wall and scapular region should also be assessed. A trigger point, by definition, causes referred pain in a specific and reproducible pattern.[70] When identified, trigger points may be treated in several ways, as discussed later in the chapter. Tender areas of muscle without a referred pain zone should not be labeled as trigger points.[61] If multiple tender areas of muscle are discovered and accompanied by sleep disturbances and other associated somatic disturbances, such as irritable bowel syndrome, a diagnosis of fibromyalgia should be considered.[76]

The spinous processes are readily palpated and may help identify lesions of the vertebral body (e.g. metastatic

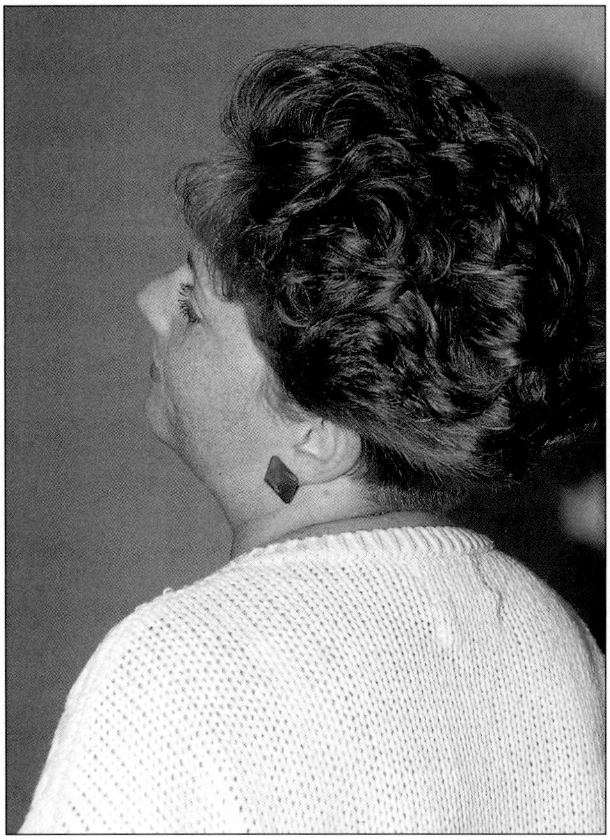

Figure 6.2
Demonstration of a combination of lateral bending, rotation, and extension placing stress on the posterior elements - including the facet joints. This position should increase pain of joint and nerve root origin but decrease muscular pain on the ipsilateral side

disease) or posterior elements. Palpation of the spinous process would not be expected to produce pain in muscular conditions. The vertical alignment of the cervical spinous processes should form a straight line. The interspinous ligament can be palpated and will be tender if damaged by a flexion injury. A combination of lateral bending and rotation of the head to the affected side should increase the pain of facet joint origin, but decrease muscular pain on that side, as these muscles are relaxed in this position (Fig. 6.2).

There are several other provocative maneuvers which can be used in evaluation of the cervical spine. Compression testing of the cervical spine is completed by placing the examiner's hand on the top of the patient's head and pressing downward. This maneuver may increase the pain of intervertebral disc origin, but is not specific.[33] Cervical distraction through manual cervical traction may be performed in an attempt to relieve radicular symptoms through volume expansion of the neuroforamina. Spurling's maneuver, in which the head is extended and rotated to the affected side, is a provocative maneuver which further narrows the neuroforamina, and may reproduce or exacerbate existing radicular symptoms. Axial compression may be applied during this maneuver, but is generally not required. Pain produced only in the neck region is not considered positive. The specificity of this test is questionable, as other referred pain patterns down the arm may be difficult to distinguish from radiculopathy. L'hermitte's sign is considered positive when an electric shock-like sensation down the back and into the legs is noted with extremes of flexion or extension of the neck. This test may be positive in cervical canal stenosis with myelopathy, but also in multiple sclerosis patients.[75]

Motor strength testing, sensory examination, and reflexes in the limbs are an important component of the examination. If dermatomal, myotomal, and reflex changes are found in a single nerve root distribution, a radiculopathy is suggested. Such findings are commonplace. Confirmatory electrophysiologic or radiographic testing is not required in the early treatment of these disorders as most improve over a short period of time with simple conservative measures. These tests are useful, however, in refractory cases where surgical decompression becomes a treatment option.

Other physical examination findings may be important in specific cases. The presence of a mass in the neck (thyroid, lymph nodes, etc.) must be addressed and worked up further. Cardiac examination and lung sounds may provide clues to other deep somatic structures which can refer pain to the neck region. Cranial nerve abnormalities may lead to suspicion of tumors or other space-occupying lesions. It may be helpful to listen for bruits over the cervical spine if arteriovenous malformations or vertebrobasilar artery insufficiency is suspected.

ELECTROMYOGRAPHY IN CERVICAL PAIN AND SUSPECTED RADICULOPATHY

Spinal nerve roots exit from the spinal column through the intervertebral foramina. Entrapment of the nerve root at the foramina may be the result of posterolateral disc herniation, osteophytes, tumor, arteriovenous malformations, or other space-occupying lesions.[53]

As the 31 pairs of spinal nerves (eight cervical, twelve thoracic, five lumbar, five sacral, and one coccygeal) leave the nerve root foramina they split into the anterior and posterior primary rami. The posterior primary rami segmentally innervate the deep paraspinal muscles, with some overlap. Anatomically, the vertebral level roughly corresponds to the level of posterior primary ramus innervation in the lumbar region. However, in the cervical region the paraspinal muscles fan out caudally. This anatomic disparity may lead to inaccurate interpretation of abnormal findings and complaints, if not considered by the treating physician.[34] The anterior primary ramus becomes a peripheral nerve through the cervical (brachial) and lumbar plexus, and directly innervates the anterolateral trunk musculature. Most muscles contain nerve elements from more than one root level.

The frequency of radiculopathy at the various root levels has been studied. Cervical radiculopathy accounts for between 5% and 36% of all patients with radiculopathy. C7 is by far the most frequently involved root level. C7 radiculopathy accounts for about 70%, C6 about 20–25%, C8 about 4–10%, and C5 about 2% of cervical radiculopathies.[49]

A compressive lesion producing radiculopathy can affect motor, sensory, and/or autonomic fibers of the nerve root. Many feel that the sensory and autonomic fibers are affected at least as often as the motor tracts. EMG and routine nerve conduction studies (NCS) test only the motor tracts in the case of radiculopathy.[32] Nerve root compression productive of a radiculopathy occurs proximal to the dorsal root (sensory) ganglion. Sensory nerve action potential (SNAP) abnormalities do not occur with radiculopathy, even in the presence of sensory loss, unless the dorsal root ganglion is somehow damaged as well. However, a unilateral SNAP abnormality can help differentiate radiculopathy from plexopathy. In brachial plexopathies, the nerves are affected distal to the sensory ganglion and, as such, the SNAP should be abnormal. Bilateral SNAP abnormalities are generally more consistent with a peripheral polyneuropathy.

The compound muscle action potential (CMAP) will show reduced amplitude in proportion to the amount of axonal degeneration that occurs after a compressive nerve root lesion.[38] The CMAP may be performed bilaterally, using the opposite side as a control. CMAP abnormalities may be even more marked when multiple roots are compressed, because compression of a single nerve root may have little effect on the total axon pool of a peripheral nerve. The loss of CMAP amplitude in peripheral nerves is most often seen in the situation of lumbar spinal stenosis, but is occasionally seen in severe spondylosis of the cervical region as well.

Nerve conduction velocity or latency should not be adversely affected by a focal proximal lesion such as radiculopathy. Nerve root stimulation techniques may be of more value than conventional NCS.[4] However, it should be noted that any form of this technique involves stimulation of the nerve distal to the site of compression. Abnormalities will be detected only if significant focal demyelination has occurred.

The H reflex is generally used in evaluation of an S1 radiculopathy.[7] The advantages are that the stimulation traverses the zone of injury using both sensory and motor pathways, and becomes abnormal soon after root compression. The H reflex may also be used in evaluation of C7, but if not obtained bilaterally does not indicate an abnormality.[18] Once affected, the H reflex tends to remain abnormal indefinitely, making it a less sensitive test in suspected radiculopathy. The H reflex will be affected by lesions anywhere along the pathway. It is not specific for a root lesion, even if unilateral. Lastly, it may be unaffected in proven radiculopathy, presumably because the large fibers that conduct the reflex are spared.

F waves represent a late motor response and can be obtained from more muscles than the H reflex, but have several disadvantages in the diagnosis of radiculopathy.[20] F waves represent only a motor response. They do not assess the sensory tracts which may play a significant role in radiculopathy. F waves evaluate the slowing or block to conduction through a few motor fibers at a time, along a long route, so as to dilute out any difference that might be seen from side to side. Similar to the H reflex, the F wave tests a peripheral nerve supplied by several roots, so that an abnormality of any one root may not result in a significant F wave abnormality.

Somatosensory evoked potentials (SSEPs) would appear to have some significant advantages over conventional NCS in the diagnosis of radiculopathy.[60] They cross the level of the lesion using sensory tracts, which are poorly evaluated by routine sensory studies. However, several technical problems have prevented more widespread use. SSEPs can be readily obtained from large mixed peripheral nerves such as the median nerve (Fig. 6.3). However, these nerves carry innervation from many root levels and therefore are less sensitive to compression from a single root level. Alternatively, individual cutaneous sensory nerves (e.g. radial sensory) can be stimulated and SSEPs recorded. This technique generally produces smaller and more variable potentials than large mixed nerve stimulation. These nerves also enter the central nervous system through several root levels, so the advantage of this technique is not clear at this time. Dermatomal SSEPs have been attempted in an effort to eliminate the problem of conduction of mixed nerve SSEPs at many root levels;[46] however, the potentials are difficult to obtain and the sensitivity for individual nerve root lesions has been unimpressive.

Certainly, the gold standard for electrodiagnosis of radiculopathy is needle EMG,[36] which assesses change in the muscle and thereby, indirectly, the motor nerve tracts. The focal demyelination of radiculopathy does not generally result in what would be considered hard evidence of radiculopathy (i.e. spontaneous motor activity), but rather

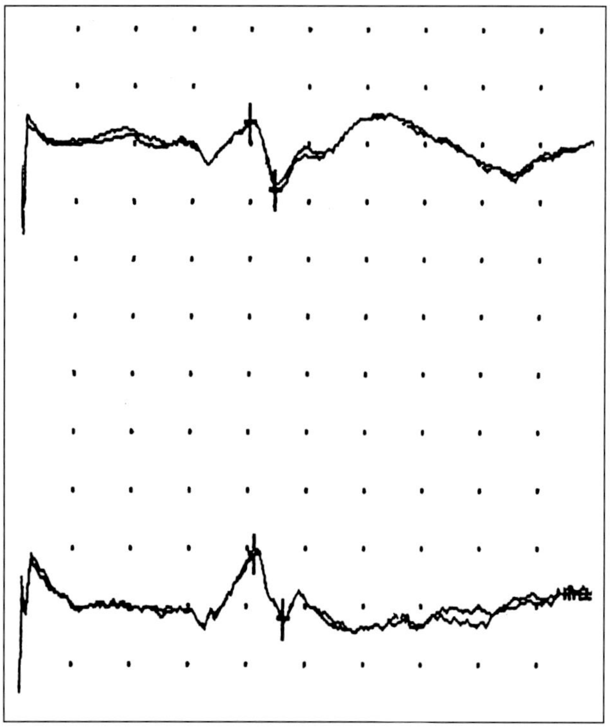

Figure 6.3
Somatosensory evoked potentials in the median nerve

a decrease in recruitment. It is only in the case of axonal degeneration of the motor fibers, with accompanying fibrillations and positive waves in a myotomal distribution, that lower motor neuron dysfunction consistent with radiculopathy can be inferred.

Electromyographic testing should include several muscles of the same nerve root innervation, both distal and proximal, mediated through different peripheral nerves. Muscles innervated by both the posterior primary ramus (paraspinals) and anterior primary ramus should be evaluated. It is quite common for muscle findings to be more pronounced in one particular muscle than another of the same root innervation, probably as a result of the anatomic positioning of the nerve fascicles at the root level.[36] However, without some abnormality in several muscles of the same myotome, a diagnosis of radiculopathy should be reserved. The sequence of electrophysiologic abnormalities seen in radiculopathy is shown in Table 6.3.

The earliest EMG finding in acute radiculopathy is a decrease in the number of motor unit potentials (MUPs) seen on recruitment. The recruitment frequency (the rate of firing of the first motor unit recruited at the moment the second motor unit appears) is increased early in radiculopathy. In other words, the initial motor unit recruited must fire faster before being able to recruit a second unit

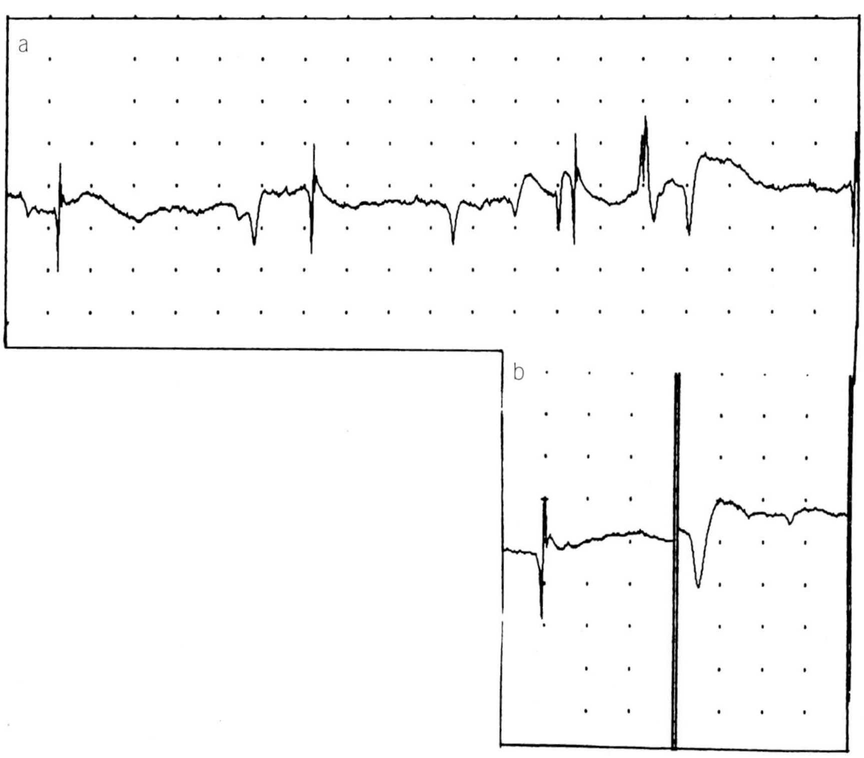

Figure 6.4
Spontaneous motor activity in a patient with cervical radiculopathy made up of fibrillations and positive waveforms firing in a relaxed muscle. (a) An isolated fibrillation potential; (b) an isolated positive wave

because there are fewer MUPs to recruit. This property is more readily appreciated by the audio signal of the EMG machine than on the oscilloscope of the MUPs. The frequency of the first MUP is heard to increase abnormally, before recruitment of a second one.

An early increase in the number of polyphasic potentials may be seen in radiculopathy. These have been postulated to occur, not on the basis of reinnervation, but rather as a result of ephaptic transmission, or neural cross-talk, between fibers through the zone of injury. These polyphasic potentials, if present, are generally smaller than those associated with reinnervation.

Spontaneous motor activity, fibrillations, and positive waves are the hallmark of acute radiculopathy when seen in a myotomal pattern (Fig. 6.4). They indicate abnormal muscle membrane irritability, not necessarily denervation. Fibrillations and positive waves are now thought to represent the same electrical events, viewed from a different distance and angle by the electrode. There is a delay in their appearance in the limb muscles as shown in Table 6.3. In general, fibrillation potentials and positive waves are larger initially and reduce in amplitude as time progresses.[40] They will ultimately disappear as reinnervation occurs, and muscle membrane irritability subsides.

Large, long duration, polyphasic potentials indicate reinnervation (Fig. 6.5). As the radiculopathy resolves, polyphasic potentials tend to reduce in number of phases, but the MUPs may remain larger and of longer duration than the normal MUPs of uninvolved muscles.

Electromyographic signs of chronic radiculopathy or ongoing root compression include complex repetitive discharges and fasciculations. These potentials are not limited to radiculopathy, however, so they should be interpreted cautiously.[17] One of the most common EMG signs of chronic radiculopathy with partial reinnervation is that of a reduced number of large, long duration (but not necessarily polyphasic) MUPs firing rapidly on attempted full recruitment.

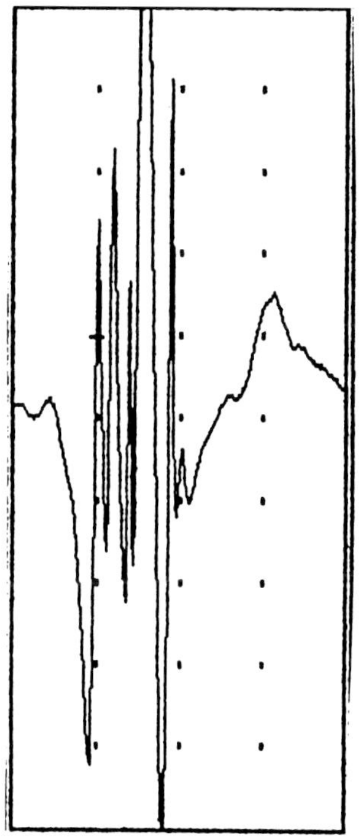

Figure 6.5
A polyphasic motor unit potential, indicating reinnervation

Table 6.3 Sequence of electrophysiologic abnormalities seen in radiculopathy

Days after onset	*Electrophysiologic findings*
0+	Reduced numbers of MUPs; reduced recruitment interval (increased recruitment frequency); increased proportion of polyphasic MUPs; fasciculation potentials may appear; prolonged H reflex latency in C7; reduced number of F waves in weak muscles
4+	CMAP amplitude will be reduced unilaterally if axonal degeneration is present
7+	Positive waves in posterior primary ramus innervated muscles (paraspinals)
12+	Positive waves in distal proximal limb muscles, fibrillations appear in paraspinals
15+	Positive waves in distal limb muscles and fibrillations in proximal limb muscles
18+	Fibrillation potentials occur in most affected muscles

Table adapted from Johnson EW. *Super EMG Syllabus*. Columbus, OH: Ohio State University, 1988.

Postoperative EMGs may present a diagnostic dilemma.[35] Spontaneous motor activity may be present in the paraspinal musculature for up to a year after surgery, as a result of disruption of the posterior primary ramus. This makes it sometimes impossible to obtain reliable information from muscles proximal to the suspected lesion. Additionally, the difference between poor recruitment, on the basis of new root compression, versus incomplete reinnervation may be possible only if the size and configuration of the remaining MUPs were familiar to the technician conducting the EMG from prior studies. Post-myelogram studies may show similar spontaneous motor activity in the paraspinal musculature, but usually for only 1–2 weeks.[74] If both a myelogram and EMG are required, it is ideal to obtain the EMG first. Diffuse abnormal spontaneous activity in the paraspinal muscles has been reported in diabetes[5] and occult malignancy.[73]

When interpreting EMG findings, it is important to bear in mind the limitations of EMG as a diagnostic tool for radiculopathy. First, EMG cannot 'rule out' a radiculopathy: a substantial portion of the time the motor tracts may not be involved. It is particularly important not to assume an etiology of nerve root compression, even when clear evidence of radiculopathy is present (i.e. pressure on the nerve root from a metastatic tumor looks the same on the EMG as a herniated nucleus pulposus).

Electromyography may be helpful in the identification of other cervical syndromes that involve the nerves or nerve roots. Cervical spinal stenosis clinically presents with a picture that can be easily confused with anterior motor horn cell disease.[65] In both diseases, there is generally a combination of upper and lower motor neuron signs and symptoms, including decreased reflexes in the arms and increased reflexes in the legs. Fasciculations and muscle atrophy may be present, especially in the hands. The EMG study will also appear similar in the affected muscles with fasciculations, fibrillations, and positive waves. Slightly low-to-normal CMAP amplitude, normal SNAP amplitude, and normal or near-normal conduction velocities are seen. However, the patient with cervical stenosis should have no EMG abnormalities above the level of the foramen magnum. If the tongue or facial muscles show significant EMG abnormalities, motor neuron disease should be suspected.

Nerve entrapment syndromes other than radiculopathy may cause or contribute to neck pain. Proximal shoulder and arm pain may be present in entrapment syndromes as far distal as median nerve entrapment at the wrist (carpal tunnel syndrome).[12] The combination of median neuropathy at the wrist and cervical radiculopathy (double crush syndrome) has been noted as a cause for this finding, but remains somewhat controversial.[50] Also, entrapment syndromes of the shoulder girdle muscles, such as the spinal accessory or suprascapular nerves, may cause pain in this area as a result of muscle weakness and splinting.[54]

CONSERVATIVE TREATMENT OF CERVICAL PAIN SYNDROMES

Acute cervical pain may be linked to a traumatic precipitating event. Other possible etiologies include: overuse syndromes, improper body mechanics (congenital or acquired), and other so-called 'micro-traumas'. Systemic or localized degenerative, inflammatory, infectious or malignant processes can be causes of and/or contributors to cervical pain syndromes.

In general, when prognosticating about the course of those patients with pain, it can be said that the longer the pain persists, the less likely a complete resolution becomes. This assumes that an adequate work-up for etiologic and contributing factors has been performed and that any perpetuating factors have been controlled as much as possible. Significant psychosocial overlay, lack of insight, or secondary gain motives do not bode well for recovery. Patients who are adaptable, educable, and show a willingness to take responsibility for aspects of the treatment within their control generally have a better outcome.[56] Education and supportive counselling along with lifestyle adjustment techniques may provide added effectiveness to the therapeutic plan. Psychological support may provide some help to the patient in coping with pain that cannot be controlled medically or surgically. It is also important to keep in mind that secondary gain, both monetary and emotional, can be persuasive and often totally subconscious motivating factors to continue pain behavior. Some patients need to have pain, and that secondary gain motive must be eliminated before they can hope to recover.

Treatment of acutely painful conditions differs from the treatment of chronic pain (Table 6.4).[66] In acute pain management, rest of the damaged structure is essential for recovery. This is in contrast to the management of chronic pain, where the patient usually requires a process of mobilization because of under-use of involved tissues. It is important to consider that contracture of collagenous structures, including tendon, ligament, and joint capsules, occurs rapidly in those patients experiencing a painful range of motion. Such patients require a range of gentle motion techniques that are active and passive to avoid the vicious cycle of pain, immobility, contracture, and increased pain. Similarly, atrophy of immobilized muscle should be avoided, if possible, through the use of isometric exercise.

The physical modalities of heat, cold, electricity, ultrasound, and hydrotherapy are used to accomplish goals of increased function while minimizing pain. Both heat and cold may provide analgesic effects.[42] The former is useful in management of both acute and chronic cervical pain, can provide analgesia and muscle relaxation, and lend some extensibility to collagen.[43] The latter may be more beneficial in acute pain for its ability to control edema. In fact, heat may exacerbate edema if present. The general guidelines of

Table 6.4 Characteristics of acute versus chronic pain

	Acute pain	*Chronic pain*
Time frame	Short (< 6 months)	Long (> 6 months)
Psychology	Few psychological factors	Many complex factors
Psychological profile	Pain + anxiety	Pain + depression
Value of pain	Represent tissue damage	Pain of no value
MD training	Focus of medical training	Few MDs experienced
Medications	Medicate 'prn'	Avoid addiction
Cure	Likely	Unlikely
Treatment	Rest	Mobilization

cold applied for the first 24–48 hours after an acute injury and heat thereafter are time tested.[58]

Many forms of heat are available including hot packs, short wave and microwave diathermy, and ultrasound. Hydrotherapy provides heat but is not very practical in the cervical region. Devices such as moist air cabinets and whirlpools may have some indication in cases of arthritic pain.

The depth of penetration of the various heating modalities varies. Hot packs provide superficial heat to the skin and subcutaneous tissue; microwave and short wave diathermy are capable of providing deeper heat, warming some muscle layers. Ultrasound is the only heating modality which can raise the intra-articular temperature of large joints significantly, because it works at the tissue/fluid interface.[44] Ultrasound may rarely exacerbate the pain of acute radiculopathy by a process not well understood.[26]

Contraindications to heat include heating of insensate areas where burns may occur, the presence of acute infection, inflammation or edema, and heating over areas of compromised vascular supply. Heat should not be used over either tumors or areas of unknown underlying pathology. Heat may exacerbate the weakness associated with multiple sclerosis and myasthenia gravis.

Transcutaneous neuronal electrical stimulation (TENS) is a modality which controls pain by means of electrical impulses applied to the skin.[59] There are two basic types of TENS: high-frequency, low-intensity TENS (conventional TENS) and low-frequency, high-intensity TENS (electro-acupuncture). Conventional TENS works by the 'gate' theory of pain.[72] Oversimplified, the 'gate' theory of pain states that there can be an inhibition of pain impulses carried by slow unmyelinated nerve fibers at the level of the dorsal column of the spinal cord by incoming cutaneous sensory and proprioceptive impulses carried through the larger myelinated fibers. These faster impulses arrive at the dorsal column first and in effect 'close the gate', not allowing propagation of the slower pain impulses.

The second type of TENS, high-voltage galvanic stimulation (HVGS) or electro-acupuncture, uses a more pronounced 'jolt' of electrical stimulation which has been shown to increase the endogenous opioid substances in the brain.[62] HVGSs are less useful in the treatment of some pain disorders because of the painful nature of the stimulus itself, and they tend to work better as a treatment modality with muscle tension, myofascial, and referred pain problems than with arthritic conditions.

There are few contraindications to TENS. it should not be placed over the anterolateral neck to avoid vagal stimulation; it may also, theoretically, cause malfunction of cardiac pacemakers, and hypersensitivity to the electrodes may be a contraindication; on occasion, skin irritation necessitates discontinuance, but can be minimized if hypoallergenic electrodes are tried. However, before stopping because no relief of pain is obtained, several different electrodes and stimulator settings should be tried; individual variation to TENS therapy is the rule.

TENS is non-invasive and may be highly effective in reducing or eliminating pain. Patients should be aware, however, that the unit only blocks pain; it is not a cure, and only works when the unit is on and the batteries charged.

Trigger point injections can be helpful if an isolated painful point in the muscle with a referred pain pattern (a trigger point) can be identified by palpation (Fig. 6.6);[69] 1–2 ml 0.5% procaine or 1% lidocaine (Xylocaine) without epinephrine (adrenaline) (which causes vasoconstriction) is used. Injection into and needling of the trigger point spreads out the offending muscle fibers and can provide relief for prolonged periods of time. The addition of corticosteroid

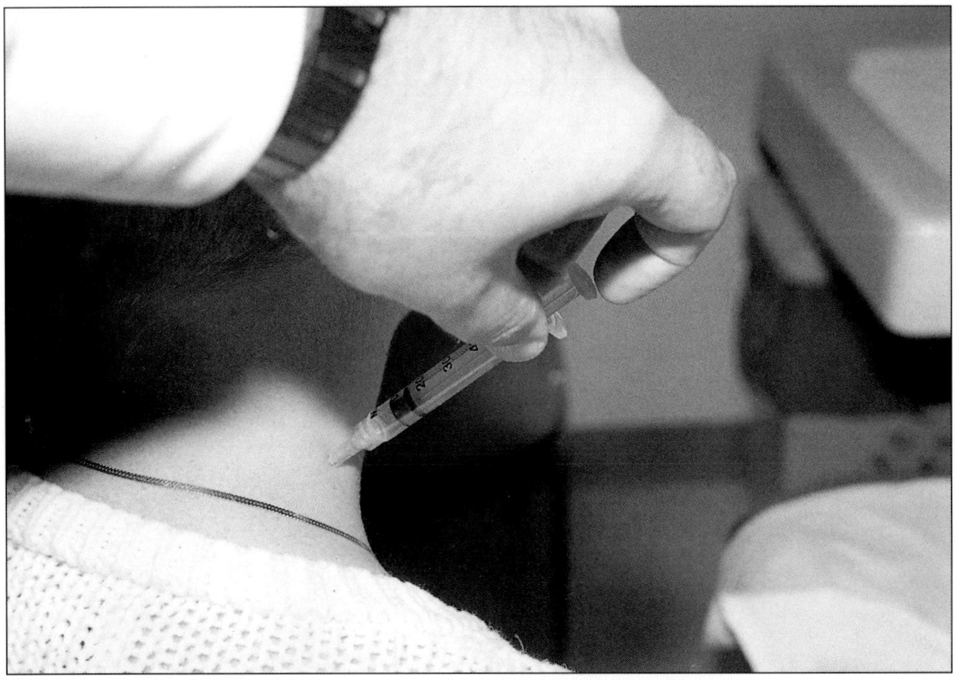

Figure 6.6
A trigger point injection technique to eliminate myofascial trigger areas using plain 1% lidocaine (Xylocaine). A fanning action with significant needling of the area is used. The injection is followed by application of ultrasound and stretch to the area

to the injected local anesthetic has not been shown to provide any additional effect.[30] In fact, a similar quantity of physiological saline may be as effective in spreading out the muscle fibers, but does not provide the immediate pain relief of the anesthetic agent.[23] Application of ultrasound to the injected area may provide longer lasting relief than injection alone. However, trigger points tend to recur unless a coordinated effort is made to eliminate the causative factors.

Spray and stretch technique using fluoromethane or a vapocoolant spray can also be effective if muscle tension of the trapezius or other large muscles is a problem.[68] This modality works using the counter-irritant effect that is similar to that of TENS and topical agents such as liniments.

Similarly, massage may be useful for short-term acute muscle tension. Massage is too labor intensive to be given on an ongoing basis in the physical therapy department. Many of the beneficial aspects of the therapy can be taught to the patient, or assisting family member, for use at home. Nevertheless, some patients may find it helpful to hire a massage therapist for intermittent or maintenance treatment, although the latter is not usually considered medically necessary by commercial insurance companies, making such treatment cost prohibitive.

The use of manipulation in the treatment of cervical pain disorders remains controversial.[19] There is some evidence in the literature that properly applied techniques may be useful in arthropathy of the cervical spine, especially facet joint arthropathy.[48] However, many unsubstantiated claims of cures and questionably trained providers make this a risky modality for most patients with pain. Chiropractors may also use other routine physical therapy modalities such as heat, ultrasound, and electrical stimulation, further clouding the effectiveness of manipulation itself as the therapeutic agent.

Cervical traction may be useful in the treatment of both radicular and non-radicular cervical pain. It has been shown that cervical traction in the range of 13 kg (30 pounds) of force can cause distraction of the cervical vertebrae.[14] In the case of cervical radiculopathy, this distraction force may provide relief of the impingement on the cervical nerve root. The traction force may be applied manually or through various mechanical devices. In the physical therapy department, both manual and mechanical traction may be performed. Generally, manual cervical traction is more likely to be helpful in patients with muscular symptoms in the cervical region or in those with a need for more careful attention to the amount and direction of the forces applied.[10] Mechanical devices can provide higher amounts of intermittent or constant force in one direction and are more useful with root impingement. At home, patients can use a device with a weight attached to a pulley over a door frame. Patients should be instructed that the proper angle of the neck during traction is about 20° of flexion. This means they have to face the door. If they face away from the door, extension combined with traction will tend to close the neural foramina, increasing pain.[16] The strap or halter should be carefully designed to avoid excessive force on the jaw and temporomandibular joint.[71]

Phonophoresis and iontophoresis are specialized modalities which cause the passage of drugs, particularly steroids, through the skin by the use of ultrasound and electrical current respectively. They may have beneficial effects under certain circumstances in conjunction with other therapeutic modalities but probably are less effective than direct injection.

Exercise is an important adjunctive therapy for patients with cervical pain. The ideal combination of rest and exercise is a difficult concept for patients and their physicians. When acute inflammation of the muscles or spinal joints is present, rest is necessary to allow healing to occur. However, muscle weakness and joint contracture can take place very rapidly when there is complete immobility. The key to proper management of the inflamed tissue is passive range of motion up to, but not past, the point of pain. The power required to range the joint may be provided by a therapist or by the patient after proper training. Production of pain during range of motion of the joint will only restart the vicious cycle of pain, immobility, contracture, and increased pain.

Isometric exercise may be initiated even in the face of acute joint inflammation. When combined with surface EMG biofeedback techniques, isometric contraction and relaxation of the muscle can easily be coordinated.

Therapeutic exercise of a subacute cervical spine problem begins with a gentle passive range of motion up to, but not past, the point of pain, after application of a suitable heating modality (usually hot pack and/or ultrasound). This will maximize range of motion and minimize pain. As inflammation subsides, the therapist allows the patient to become more active in the isotonic use of muscles around the spine, ultimately concentrating more on strengthening through resistive exercise. The timing of this program is highly variable depending on the tolerance of the patient and requires close follow-up by both the therapist and prescribing physiatrist.

The initiation of therapeutic exercise after surgery should be a decision made by both surgeon and physiatrist. After surgery, the tissues will require sufficient time for wound healing. This time varies, depending on the status of the tissue before surgery, the age of the patient, and many other factors pertaining directly to the type and extent of the surgery itself. Scar formation will occur during the healing phase and can lead to tissue tightness and weakness even more pronounced than before surgery. But if the tissues are not given sufficient time to heal, continued pain and unacceptable surgical results may occur. When an arthrodesis has been performed, time must be allowed before an aggressive range of motion is allowed. Isometric exercises can and should be instituted immediately. Even people in casts and other immobilizing devices can use isometric techniques to maintain some muscle strength and tone. Generally, performing a maximum voluntary contraction of the muscles without moving the joint, several times a day, is sufficient to maintain muscle strength while casted.[39] Once the cast or immobilizing device is removed, then more aggressive stretching and isotonic strengthening techniques may be employed.

It is a common misconception that patients with acute or subacute pain require strengthening exercises. It is difficult, if not impossible, to strengthen injured, painful muscles. To develop a muscle training response to exercise requires that force be applied to muscle and other tissues, which will not be tolerated by the patient in pain.

The three-stage treatment protocol of pain relief through modalities; range of motion and flexibility exercise to regain the normal resting length of the muscles and other tissues; and gradual strengthening to protect from further injury, will help assure a safe and successful recovery.

TREATMENT OF SPECIFIC CERVICAL DISORDERS

As mentioned previously, it is usually helpful to differentiate radicular from non-radicular causes of cervical dysfunction. The treatment of radicular neck pain initially involves rest and immobilization of the spine, and benefit may be felt from a soft cervical collar. Patients should be instructed on the proper orientation of the collar because, if placed backwards, the collar will put their neck into more extension, worsening their symptoms (Fig. 6.7). Additionally, the short-term use of opioid analgesics and muscle relaxants may be helpful, and manual cervical traction could be helpful in the acute stages. If beneficial, patients can be given a home traction unit, but should be instructed on proper usage necessary to avoid neck extension. If there is no improvement after a few weeks of appropriate rest, then further anatomic studies can be obtained to evaluate the extent of the lesion. There is no point in ordering EMG studies during the first week of symptoms. In fact, only limited information about the extent and localization of the lesion may be available at 3 weeks post-onset. Modalities other than superficial heat or cold should probably be reserved until after this initial rest period. Once the patient is up and around without significant pain, a more rigorous therapy program with stretching and flexibility can be initiated. However, only isometric exercises should be used until 6 weeks post-onset of true radiculopathy. After 6 weeks, if pain-free, further strengthening to protect the area is in order. If surgery is performed, then the post-surgical considerations as noted earlier apply.

Non-radicular forms of neck pain include a wide range of soft tissue, bone, and joint abnormalities. To a great

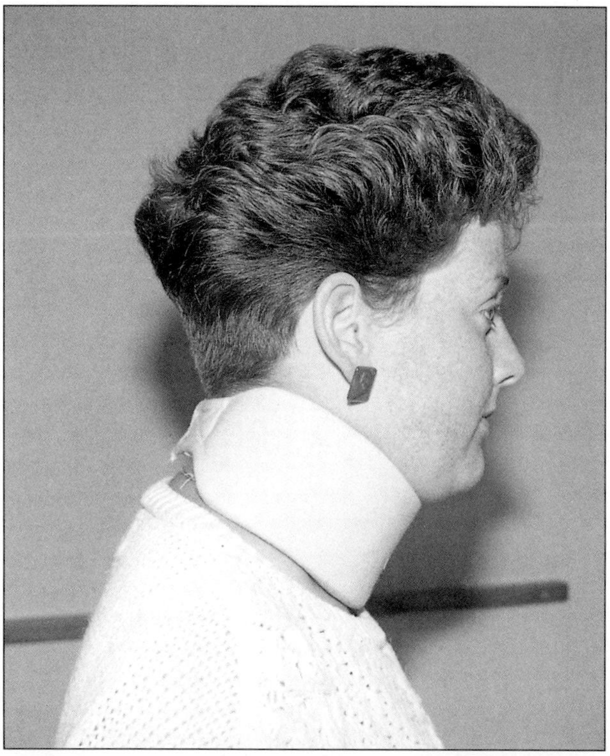

a

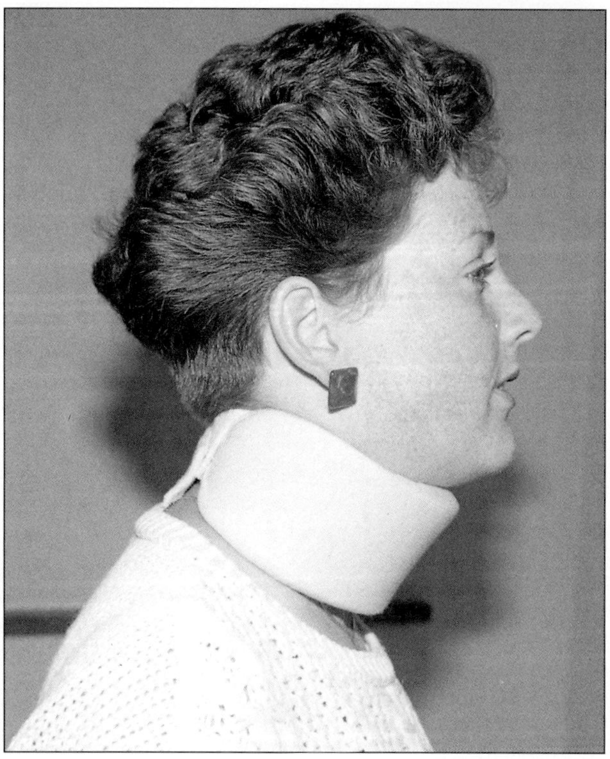

b

Figure 6.7
Proper (a) versus improper (b) soft cervical collar position for cervical radiculopathy. When extension results from the collar placement, worsening of the symptoms may result

extent, the treatment will depend on the underlying etiology of the pain. Despite thorough investigation, the cause of non-radicular neck pain may not always be clear. Nevertheless, in general, patients with non-radicular neck pain usually do better with a program of early mobilization. The use of heat and ultrasound modalities to loosen tight tissues followed by active and passive range of motion, and, finally, isotonic and isometric strengthening are advised. The one major exception to this protocol is the patient with significant underlying degenerative disease. In this case, the use of aggressive range of motion and isotonic strengthening may aggravate symptoms. This is opposite to the protocol used in muscular and myofascial pain syndromes of the neck. Unfortunately, both of these processes may present simultaneously in a patient and, under these circumstances, it is very difficult to incorporate sufficient mobilization and strengthening exercises to keep the muscles pain free, without aggravating the underlying joint disease. These patients often remain symptomatic despite treatment, simply because the treatments they require contradict one another.

For those patients with primarily muscular problems of the cervical region, treatment can be aimed at muscle relaxation, stretching, and gradual strengthening. Techniques such as surface EMG biofeedback and relaxation training may be helpful.[22] Attention to posture and ergonomic considerations may help eliminate the perpetuating factors. For those patients with fibromyalgia, a combination of reassurance, general non-traumatic aerobic conditioning exercise and medications, such as low-dose amitriptyline, for sleep and pain control may be helpful.[28] These patients require a well-coordinated education program regarding the benign, but cyclical, nature of their symptoms. Generally, they are taught to manage their muscular pain with non-opioid medications, self-massage, and aerobic conditioning.[52] These patients should not be placed on opioid analgesics or immobilized in devices such as cervical collars, because their problem will become chronic. Furthermore, employment of these types of interventions may be complicated by significant psychological or physical dependency issues.[3] Conversely, the older patient with significant degenerative disease may be prescribed a mild opioid analgesic, if non-steroidal anti-inflammatory medications are contraindicated or ineffective. Supportive devices, such as cervical collars, may increase their functional activities significantly. Although soft cervical collars do very little to immobilize the spine,[37] they do provide adequate support for some patients with degenerative joint disease. If a soft collar becomes less effective, a molded plastic collar can be fitted by the orthotist. These patients must be instructed in isometric strengthening exercises for the neck and must be made aware that some weakening of their cervical musculature may result.

Attention to posture and positioning considerations of the neck will help many patients. Elimination of habits such

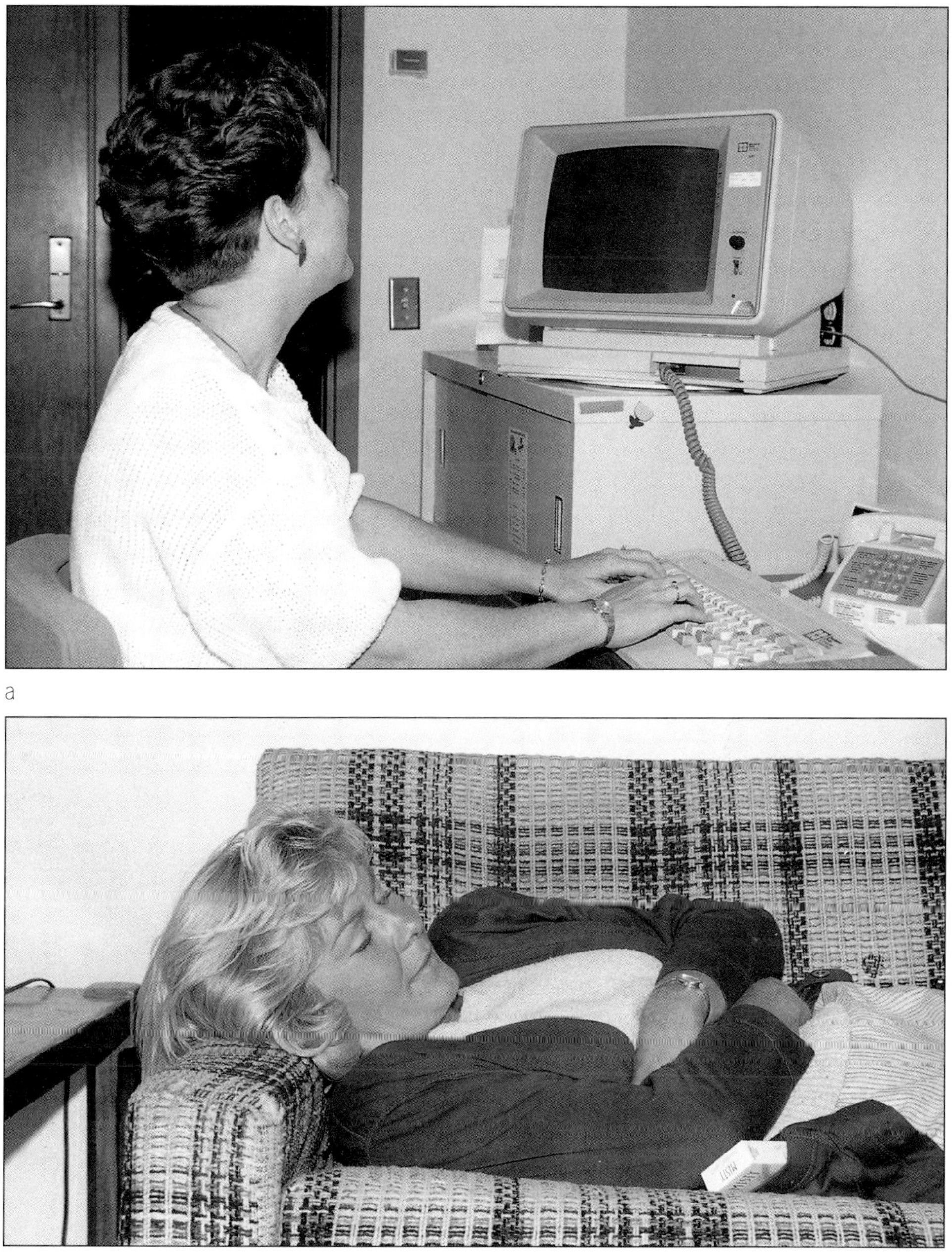

a

b

Figure 6.8
Neck postures to be avoided: (a) improper head position at the computer terminal; (b) prolonged neck flexion

as watching television while lying supine with the neck in a flexed position, and improper computer monitor and keyboard heights can make a major difference in neck symptoms (Fig. 6.8). Wearing soft-soled shoes and correction of mild leg length discrepancies may also assist the neck in maintaining normal posture. Some patients benefit from a more structured postural exercise program such as the Alexander technique or yoga.

Formal physical therapy should be discontinued when the patient has recovered adequately and been given a home program of exercise. Many patients will not be completely asymptomatic at the end of therapy, and some patients will need to learn to live with a certain degree of discomfort. The decision of when to discontinue formal therapy requires a re-evaluation by the physician to assess whether the goals of therapy have been obtained. There is no need for maintenance or ongoing therapy in most soft-tissue or degenerative cervical problems. Patients need to realize that they have the responsibility for the ongoing care of their musculoskeletal problem, but that, if they have a flare-up of symptoms, help is available.

CONSIDERATIONS IN THE SPINAL CORD-INJURED PATIENT

Management of patients sustaining spinal cord injury deserves special consideration. Our understanding of the potential associated medical complications has led to a significant decrease in patient morbidity and mortality, and increased life expectancy. The development of comprehensive spinal cord inury centers, which use a multidisciplinary approach to the management and rehabilitation of these patients, coupled with development of new technologies, has been responsible for improved survival and diminished complication.

In brief, the management protocols, restorative management, and rehabilitative processes will be reviewed.

Patient Management in the Acute Phase of Spinal Cord Injury

Although decisions are made concerning the need for surgical decompression and stabilization, therapeutic programs for maximization of physical function and avoidance of complication are structured and instituted to fit patient deficits. Neurologic assessment is the key in the evaluation process; chart documentation of sensory level function should be mapped and muscle grading is documented using a 0–5 scale, 5 being normal and 0 being absent. Results of rectal examination and bulbocavernosus reflex are recorded. The patient should also be assigned a motor index score, as developed by the American Spinal Injury Association (Table 6.5). In addition, the patient may be given a Frankel grade (Table 6.6). Serial examinations are required to recognize potential progressive neurologic loss.

There are essentially two types of spinal cord injury – complete and incomplete. With complete injuries, little or no neurologic return is expected. No injury may be considered complete until spinal shock has resolved. The bulbocavernosus reflex, which is elicited by genital stimulation and produces anal contraction, is used to determine the absence of spinal shock. If no motor or sensory function is present in the absence of spinal shock, the injury is considered complete. The determination of complete injury can usually be made within the first 24–72 hours after injury.

Incomplete spinal cord syndromes are characterized by the presence of some function below the level of injury. Classically, these have been divided into four syndromes: the anterior cord syndrome, central cord syndrome, posterior cord syndrome, and the Brown–Séquard syndrome (Table 6.7). Some patients will present with isolated nerve root dysfunction.

Table 6.5 Suggested spinal cord injury motor index score*

Grade on right	*Muscle*	*Grade on left*
5	C5	5
5	C6	5
5	C7	5
5	C8	5
5	T1	5
5	L2	5
5	L3	5
5	L4	5
5	L5	5
5		5
50		50
Total score 100		

This motor index score, when used accurately, provides a numerical grading system to document improvement or deterioration of motor function.
Motor grading system
0 absent – total paralysis
1 trace – palpable or visible contraction
2 poor – active movement through range of motion with gravity eliminated
3 fair – active movement through range of motion against gravity
4 good – active movement through range of motion against resistance
5 normal

	Present	*Absent*
Bladder function		
Bowel function		

* Motor index score adapted from scoring system by Lucas and Ducker.

Table 6.6 Frankel scale for spinal cord-injured patients

Frankel A	Complete paralysis
Frankel B	Sensory incomplete No voluntary motor function
Frankel C	Useless distal motor function
Frankel D	Useful distal motor function
Frankel E	Normal

Table 6.7 Classification of spinal cord injuries

Complete lesions
Posterior cord syndrome (crude sensation only)
Anterior cord syndrome
Central cord syndrome
Partial cord lesion, including Brown–Séquard type
Root syndrome

Above are the known and recognized spinal cord injury syndromes, including the syndromes of isolated nerve root compression.

Table 6.8 Incomplete spinal cord injuries

Syndrome	*Physical findings*	*Prognosis*
Anterior cord	Motor loss Pain and temperature loss	Poor
Central cord	Weakness in upper extremities, lower extremities Perianal sensation preserved	Variable return
Brown–Séquard	Ipsilateral paralysis Contralateral pain and temperature loss	Good
Posterior cord	Motor function usually preserved Sensory function lost	Unknown

The anterior cord syndrome is usually the result of compressive and/or flexion injuries to the spine. This syndrome is characterized by injury to the anterior horn cells opposite the area of spinal injury, and alteration of anterolateral, white-matter, column function controlling pain and temperature sensation. The posterior columns and posterior horn areas of the gray matter are variously spared, controlling deep pressure and posterior sensation. This syndrome carries the poorest prognosis, with return to motor function being rare.

The central cord syndrome is common, and involves an extension injury in an older patient with underlying spondylotic changes. A central hematomyelia results producing cord injury in the central gray matter where the motor horn cells for the upper extremities are housed. At this level, motor and sensory impulses in the sacral segments of the spinal cord are in the peripheral white matter, and may be preserved and provide sacral sensation. Upper extremity weakness is more pronounced than lower extremity weakness. Patients with this syndrome will experience variable return to function, but some degree of spasticity is likely.

The Brown–Séquard syndrome has the best prognosis of all incomplete syndromes. This syndrome is caused by transverse hemisection of the cord, and results in weakness; sensory loss is on the side of injury, with pain and temperature loss on the contralateral side. Stab wounds and other penetrating trauma are the most common cause. Brown–Séquard syndrome caused by blunt trauma has a favorable prognosis for neurologic recovery.

The posterior cord syndrome is rare. With this injury, the posterior columns sustain the brunt of the injury, preserving motor function, but there is associated loss of sensation below the injury level. Prognosis for this injury is uncertain (Table 6.8).

Restorative Management

Once the spine is appropriately stabilized, attention must be directed toward those functions that have suffered from loss of neurologic input.

Bladder Function

In the early stages of injury, bladder drainage is effectively accomplished by placement of an in-dwelling catheter. However, once the patient's medical status has stabilized, urinary tract management is best accomplished by intermittent catheterization. At first, this is completed every 4 hours, and later extended, depending on volumes of urine obtained. With return of reflex activity, a reflex bladder program may be instituted. With upper motor neuron lesions, the bladder reflex may be stimulated by stroking the inner thigh or tapping on the abdomen. The bladder subsequently contracts while the sphincter relaxes, emptying the bladder of its contents. Intermittent catheterization must be continued during the early phases of a bladder reflex program to ensure adequate voiding. The bladder should never be allowed to accumulate more than 400–500 ml of urine.

Infection is a common complication of a neurogenic bladder. This is generally the result of in-dwelling repetitive catheterization and can be minimized by sterile technique. With the bladder reflex technique, a reflex of urine may occur into the ureter and even into the kidney, potentially producing pyelonephritis. Intermittent catheterization is now the preferred method over an in-dwelling catheter, because the incidence is lessened. Prophylactic, suppressive, antibiotic coverage is no longer advised. When infection is suspected, cultures are obtained and appropriate antibiotics started once cultures are available. A voiding cystourethrogram can be obtained to exclude vesicourethral reflux.

Pulmonary Function

Pulmonary function is commonly compromised with cervical cord injury. With lesions at C3 or above, diaphragm function is lost and the patient is ventilator dependent. Patients with C4 level of function may initially require ventilator assistance, but with development of accessory muscle function they may become independent. Lesions below C5 do not usually require ventilatory support.

Secretion problems are commonplace and potentially life–threatening. Mucous plug formation and subsequent airway obstruction may necessitate emergent resuscitative measures. Atelectasis may develop secondary to recumbency. These airway complications are best averted with routine chest therapy inclusive of postural drainage, chest percussion, incentive spirometry, bronchodilators, and frequent suctioning of bronchial secretions. Bronchoscopy is indicated for examination and removal of any mucous plug responsible for segmental lung collapse.

Aspiration of varying degrees is probably common, but not always productive of pneumonia. Aspiration probably results from uncoordination of the oropharynx and larynx during swallowing. There is no good preventive measure, although tracheobronchial suctioning after oral feeding may be helpful. If aspiration pneumonia is suspected, broad-spectrum aerobic and anaerobic antibiotics should be instituted before culture results are received.

Pulmonary embolism may or may not be preceded by deep venous thrombosis of the lower extremity. It is one of the most common causes of sudden death. All spinal cord-injured patients should be given prophylactic heparin, 5000 units subcutaneously every 8 hours. Sequential compression stockings are also used regularly. The incidence of deep venous thrombosis has been estimated to affect 25–30% of patients clinically.

Bowel Function

As in bladder function, sphincter control of the bowel is lost with spinal cord injury. In a similar fashion, the sphincter can be relaxed through reflex stimulation. The bowel reflex is stimulated by stretching the external anal sphincter, which then relaxes the reflex-controlled internal anal sphincter and bowel contraction occurs, allowing the bowel to empty.

The goal of a bowel program is to create a regulated program inclusive of proper fluid intake, high fiber diet, and exercise. Routine use of laxatives or enemas is discouraged because it is eventually ineffective.

Skin Management

Skin ulcers may develop as a result of prolonged and excessive pressure on insensitive areas. Early prevention is centered around patient turning and appropriate padding of bony prominences. Frequent turning of the patient on a Stryker frame or Clinitron bed is also an effective means of shifting body weight.

In the subacute setting, the goal of any skin program is to maintain skin integrity, increase skin tolerance to pressure, and education of patients and daily caretakers in skin maintenance.

Cardiovascular Considerations

In the acute phase of cervical spinal cord injury, spinal shock is common; in such injury hypotension develops secondary to bradycardia, peripheral vasodilatation, and a diminished venous return for the lower extremities. However, the systolic pressure, rarely falls below 90 mmHg unless there is concomitant loss of blood. If excessive intravenous fluid or blood replacement is given, fluid overload and/or congestive heart failure may occur. This is especially true 3–4 days post-injury, when sympathetic tone begins to return, potentially causing overload of the cardiovascular system and producing diuresis. During this time, diuretic agents and cardiotrophic drugs may be required.

As the parasympathetic supply of the heart is derived from the vagus nerve and sympathetic supply from the upper thoracic spinal cord, bradycardia or even sinus arrest may occur. Administration of atropine intravenously or subcutaneously will usually result in an appropriate response.

When the patient is mobilized, postural hypotension is commonly seen. This is a manifestation of persistent peripheral vasodilatation, decreased venous return, and malfunction of normal carotid baroceptor reflexes. For refractory symptomatic cases, elastic and/or abdominal binder may be helpful. Additionally, ephedrine, taken just before mobilization, will help prevent postural hypotension.

Autonomic dysreflexia is clinically manifested by diaphoresis above the injury level, flushing of the face, headache, severe hypertension, and bradycardia. This disorder is usually the result of bladder distension or constipation which then produces a reflex vasoconstriction and increase in blood pressure. An increased blood pressure is sensed by baroreceptors secondarily producing bradycardia. Nifedipine (10 mg under the tongue) is very effective in treating the acute hypertensive phase; however, treatment of the underlying source of the autonomic dysreflexia is imperative (i.e. catheterization of bladder).

Musculoskeletal Considerations

Daily range of motion and stretching must be completed to prevent contractures. In the upper extremities, the shoulders are particularly prone to becoming tight and require passive motion two to three times per day. Flexion contractures of the foot and ankle are also common, and best treated with early stretching and bracing.

Heterotopic ossification may occur within 3 months of injury and most frequently affects the hip. Extensive ossification can severely limit motion and ability to sit in the upright position. During the bone formation phase, the patient may be mistakenly thought to have deep venous thrombosis. Heterotopic ossification occurs in 20–30% of spinal cord-injured patients.

Treatment for heterotopic ossification has been less than satisfactory. Disodium etidronate, which may prevent deposition of calcium around the affected joint, is the only currently available treatment. In more severe cases, surgical excision of the heterotopic bone is often necessary. Timing of excision is, however, important. It cannot be done in the acute phase, only when the alkaline phosphate level has returned to normal, bone scan is normal, and the plan radiographic appearance of the mass is one of maturity. After excision, disodium etidronate is given for one year.

Fractures are seen even with minor trauma in these patients secondary to developing osteoporosis. The most common sites of fracture include the femoral neck, supracondylar region of the femur, and tibia. Operative stabilization is preferred, but sometimes allows continued mobilization without the risks associated with external mobilization or prolonged bedrest.

SUMMARY

Through a well-coordinated approach to the diagnosis and treatment of cervical problems, most patients can enjoy a more pain-free and productive lifestyle. Careful history taking, detailed physical examination, and timely use of radiographic and electrodiagnostic testing will maximize the physician's ability to delineate the source of musculoskeletal pain about the head and neck, and subsequently allow for efficient treatment and return to function. The spinal cord-injured patient represents a special challenge to the team of physicians. With an integrated approach to management, the physical and emotional complications of spinal cord injury can be effectively dealt with and the return to function maximized.

REFERENCES

1 Beisinger E. Vertigo caused by disorders of the cervical vertebral column. *Adv Otorhinolaryngol* **39**: 44–51, 1988.
2 Bengtsson A, Henriksson KG, Larsson J. Reduced high-energy phosphate levels in painful muscle in patients with primary fibromyalgia. *Arthrit Rheumat* **29**: 817–821, 1986.
3 Bennett RM. The fibrositis-fibromyalgia syndrome. In Schumacher HR (ed), *Primer on Rheumatic Diseases*, 9th ed., 227–299. Atlanta, GA: Arthritis Foundation, 1988.
4 Berger AR, Busis NA, Logigian EL, et al. Cervical root stimulation in the diagnosis of cervical radiculopathy. *Neurology* **37**: 329–332, 1987.
5 Bicknell JM, Johnson SF. Widespread electromyographic abnormalities in spinal muscles in cancer, disc disease and diabetes. *University of Michigan Medical Center Journal* **42**: 124–127, 1976.
6 Bonica JJ (ed), *The Management of Pain*. Philadelphia: Lea & Febiger, 1954.
7 Braddom RL, Johnson EW. H reflex: Review and classification with suggested clinical uses. *Arch Phys Med Rehab* **55**: 412–417, 1975.
8 Brandenberg G, Leibrock LG. Dysphagia and dysphonia secondary to anterior cervical osteophytes. *Neurosurgery* **18**: 90–93, 1986.
9 Cailliet R. *Neck and Arm Pain*, 2nd ed., 103 Philadelphia: FA Davis, 1981.
10 Cailliet R. *Neck and Arm Pain*, 2nd ed., 128–129. Philadelphia: FA Davis, 1981.
11 Campbell CD, Loft GH, Davis H, et al. TMJ symptoms and referred pain patterns. *J Prosth Dent* **47**: 430–433, 1982.
12 Cherington M. Proximal pain in carpal tunnel syndrome. *Arch Surg* **108**: 69, 1974.
13 Cohen SG, Quinn PD. Facial trismus and myofascial pain associated with infections and malignant disease *Oral Surg Oral Med Oral Pathol* **65**: 538–544, 1988.
14 Colachis SC, Strohm BR. A study of tractive forces and angle of pull on vertebral interspaces in the cervical spine. *Arch Phys Med Rehab* **46**: 820–830, 1965.
15 Colbassani HJ, Wood JH. Management of spasmodic torticollis. *Surg Neurol* **25**: 153–158, 1986.
16 Crue BL. Importance of flexion in cervical traction for radiculitis. *US Air Force Med J* **8**: 374–380, 1957.
17 Daube J. *AAEM Minimonograph No.11: Needle Exam in Clinical EMG*. Rochester, Minnesota: American Association of Electrodiagnostic Medicine, 1979.
18 Deschuytere J, Rosselle N, DeKeyser C. Monosynaptic reflexes in the superficial forearm flexors in man and their clinical significance. *J Neurol Neurosurg Psychiat* **39**: 555–565, 1976.
19 Dixon GW. The current status of the scientific basis for manipulation. *Current Concepts Rehab Med* **2**: 3–5, 1985.
20 Eisen A, Schomer D, Melmed C, et al. The application of F-wave measurements in the differentiation of proximal and distal upper limb entrapments. *Neurology* **27**: 662–668, 1977.
21 Engelberg AL. *Guides to the Evaluation of Permanent Impairment*, 3rd ed., 79–83. Chicago: American Medical Association, 1988.
22 Ferraccioli G, Ghirelli L, Scita F, et al. EMG biofeedback training in fibromyalgia syndrome. *J Rheumatol* **14**: 820–825, 1987.
23 Frost FA, Jessen B, Siggard-Andersen J. A controlled, double blind comparison of mepivacaine injection versus saline injection for myofascial pain. *Lancet* **i**: 499–500, 1980.
24 Gelb H. Present day concepts in diagnosis and treatment of craniomandibular disorders. *NY Dent J* **51**: 266–271, 1985.
25 Gelb H, Bernstein I. Clinical evaluation of two hundred patients with temporomandibular joint syndrome. *J Prosth Dent* **49**: 234–243, 1983.

26 Gnatz SM. Increased radicular pain due to therapeutic ultrasound applied to the back. *Arch Phys Med Rehab* **70**: 493–494, 1989.

27 Gnatz SM. Referred pain syndromes of the head and neck. *Phys Med Rehabil State of the Art Reviews* **5**: 585–596, 1991.

28 Goldenberg DL. Fibromyalgia syndrome: an emerging but controversial condition. *JAMA* **257**: 2782–2787, 1987.

29 Gore DR, Sepic SB, Gardner GM, et al. Neck pain: A long-term follow-up of 205 patients. *Spine* **12**: 1–5, 1987.

30 Gottlieb NL, Riskin WG. Complications of local corticosteroid injections. *JAMA* **243**: 1547–1548, 1980.

31 Hammond DR, Danta S. Occipital neuralgia. *Clin Exp Neurol* **15**: 258–270, 1978.

32 Hong CZ, Lee S. Cervical radiculopathy – clinical, radiographic and EMG findings. *Orthop Rev* **15**: 31–37, 1986.

33 Hoppenfeld S. *Physical Examination of the Spine and Extremities*, 126–127. Norwalk, CT: Appleton-Century-Crofts, 1976.

34 Johnson EW. *Super EMG Course Syllabus*. Columbus, OH: Ohio State University, 1988.

35 Johnson EW, Burkhart JA, Earl WC, et al. EMG in post laminectomy patients. *Arch Phys Med Rehab* **53**: 407–409, 1972.

36 Johnson EW, Melvin JL. The value of electromyography in lumbar radiculopathy. *Arch Phys Med Rehab* **52**: 239–243, 1971.

37 Johnson RM, Hart DL, Simmons EF, et al. Cervical orthoses: A study comparing their effectiveness in restricting cervical motion in normal subjects. *J Bone Joint Surg [Am]* **59**: 332–339, 1977.

38 Kimura J. *Electrodiagnosis in Diseases of Nerve and Muscle: Principles and Practice*, 85–86. Philadelphia: FA Davis, 1989.

39 Kottke FJ. The effects of limitation of activity upon the human body. *JAMA* **196**: 117–122, 1966.

40 Kraft GH. Fibrillation potential amplitude and muscle atrophy following peripheral nerve injury. *Muscle Nerve* **13**: 814–821, 1990.

41 Kushmerick MJ. Muscle energy metabolism, nuclear magnetic resonance spectroscopy and their potential in the study of fibromyalgia. *J Rheumatol* **16**(supp19): 40–46, 1989.

42 Lehmann JF (ed). *Therapeutic Heat and Cold*, 3rd ed. Baltimore: Williams & Wilkins, 1982.

43 Lehmann JF, Masock AJ, Warren CG, et al. Effects of therapeutic temperatures on tendon extensibility. *Arch Phys Med Rehab* **51**: 481–487, 1970.

44 Lehmann JF, McMillan JA, Brunner GD, et al. Comparative study of the efficiency of short-wave, microwave and ultrasonic diathermy in heating the hip joint. *Arch Phys Med Rehab* **40**: 510–512, 1959.

45 Lund N, Bengtsson A, Thorborg P. Muscle oxygen pressure in primary fibromyalgia. *Scand J Rheumatol* **15**: 165–173, 1986.

46 Machida M, Asai T, Sato K, et al. New approach for diagnosis in herniated lumbar discs: Dermatomal somatosensory evoked potentials (DSSEPs). *Spine* **11**: 380–384, 1986.

47 MacRae D. Head and neck pain in the elderly. *J Otolaryngol* **15**: 224–227, 1986.

48 Maigne R. Manipulation of the spine. In Basmajian JV (ed) *Manipulation, Traction and Massage*, 3rd ed, 77–78. Baltimore: Williams & Wilkins, 1985.

49 Marinacci AA. A correlation between operative findings in cervical herniated disc with the electromyograms and opaque myelograms. *Electromyography* **6**: 5–20, 1966.

50 Massey EW. Coexistent carpal tunnel syndrome and cervical radiculopathy (double crush syndrome). *South Med J* **74**: 957–959, 1981.

51 Mathews JA. Atlanto-axial subluxation in rheumatoid arthritis. *Ann Rheumat Dis* **28**: 260–266, 1969.

52 McCain GA. Role of physical fitness training in fibrositis/fibromyalgia syndrome. *Am J Med* **81**(supp 3A): 73–77, 1986.

53 Mixter WJ, Barr JS. Rupture of the intervertebral disc with involvement of the spinal canal. *N Engl J Med* **211**: 210–215, 1934.

54 Norden A. Peripheral injuries to the spinal accessory nerve. *Acta Chir Scand* **94**: 515–532, 1946.

55 Norris SH, Watt I. The prognosis of neck injuries resulting from rear-end collisions. *J Bone Joint Surg [Br]* **65**: 608–611, 1983.

56 Pilowski I, Chapman CR, Bonica JJ. Pain, depression and illness behavior in a pain clinic population. *Pain* **4**: 183–192, 1977.

57 Ryan GMS, Cope S. Cervical vertigo. *Lancet* **ii**: 1355–1358, 1955.

58 Schmidt KL, Oh VR, Rocher G, et al. Heat, cold and inflammation. *Rheumatology* **38**: 391–404, 1979.

59 Shafer N, Kitay G. Transcutaneous electrical nerve stimulation and pain relief: An overview. *Am J Electromed* **2**: 9–13, 1987.

60 Siivola J, Sulg I, Heiskari M. Somatosensory evoked potentials in diagnostics of cervical spondylosis and herniated disc. *Electroencephal Clin Neurophysiol* **52**: 276–282, 1981.

61 Simons DG. Myofascial pain syndromes: Where are we? Where are we going? *Arch Phys Med Rehab* **69**: 207–212, 1988.

62 Sjolund BH, Terenius L, Erickson MBE. Increased cerebrospinal fluid levels of endorphin after electro–acupuncture. *Acta Physiol Scand* **100**: 382–384, 1977.

63 Sola AE. Evaluation of the patient presenting with upper extremity pain. In Wall PD, Melzack R (eds) *Textbook of Pain*, 2nd ed., 354–367. London, Churchill Livingstone, 1989.

64 Sola AE, Rodenberger ML, Gettys BB. Incidence of hypersensitive areas in the posterior shoulder muscles: A survey of two hundred young adults. *Am J Phys Med* **34**: 585–590, 1956.

65 Stark RJ, Kennard C, Swash M. Hand wasting in spondylotic high cord compression: An electromyographic study. *Ann Neurol* **9**: 58–62, 1981.

66 Sternbach RA. Acute vs chronic pain. In Wall PD, Melzack R (eds) *Textbook of Pain*. Edinburgh: Churchill Livingstone, 1984.

67 Subramony SH. Neuralgic amyotrophy (acute brachial neuropathy). *Muscle Nerve* **11**: 39–44, 1988.

68 Travell J. Myofascial trigger points: Clinical view. In Bonica JJ, Albe-Fessardi D (eds) *Advances in Pain Research and Therapy*, Vol. 1, 919–926. New York: Raven Press, 1976.

69 Travell JG, Simons DG. *Myofascial Pain and Dysfunction*, 12. Baltimore: Williams & Wilkins, 1983.

70 Travell JG, Simons DG. *Myofascial Pain and Dysfunction*, 59–63. Baltimore: Williams & Wilkins, 1983.

71 Walker GL. Goodley polyaxial traction – a new approach to a traditional treatment, *Phys Therapy* **66**: 1255–1259, 1986.

72 Wall PD. The gate control theory of pain mechanisms. A re-examination and re-statement. *Brain* **101**: 1–18, 1978.

73 Watson R, Waylonis G. Widespread paraspinal EMG abnormalities as a predictor of occult carcinoma. *Arch Phys Med Rehab* **56**: 216–220, 1975.

74 Weber WJ, Weingarden SI. Electromyographic abnormalities following myelography. *Arch Neurol* **36**: 588–589, 1979.

75 Weisberg LA. *Essentials of Clinical Neurology*, 98–100. Baltimore: University Park Press, 1983.

76 Yunus MB. Diagnosis, etiology, and management of fibromyalgia syndrome: An update. *Comprehensive Therapy* **14**: 8–20, 1988.

7 Congenital abnormalities of the cervical spine

Peter D. Pizzutillo and John B. Catalano

Congenital abnormalities of the cervical spine, although relatively uncommon, pose a challenge for the spine surgeon. Although the medical literature reports on the more frequent problems of traumatic, infectious, neoplastic and degenerative disorders of the spine, congenital malformations of the spine are of concern because of the potential for neural compromise, severe disability or restriction of activities in a much younger age group. Understanding of the etiology, natural history, neurologic risk, and surgical and non-surgical management of each abnormality is essential; a review of the etiology, clinical presentation, natural history, neurologic risk, and treatment options will be presented for each of the specific cervical spine anomalies.

BASILAR IMPRESSION

Basilar impression, the protrusion of the tip of the odontoid into the foramen magnum, is the most common congenital anomaly at the atlanto-occipital region. The odontoid may encroach on neural structures or embarrass vascular or cerebral spinal fluid flow. The etiology of primary basilar impression is a developmental defect in the occipitocervical junction although secondary forms are associated with disease processes such as rickets, osteogenesis imperfecta, Paget's disease, or rheumatoid arthritis. Primary basilar impression is associated with vertebral defects such as Klippel–Feil syndrome or anomalies of the odontoid or atlas. There is also a significant correlation with the Arnold–Chiari malformation.[3]

Basilar impression may present with long tract signs, weakness, or sensory changes in any or all four extremities. Cerebellar ataxia, lower cranial nerve compromise, nystagmus, or vertebral artery insufficiency syndromes have been associated with basilar impression. If posterior encroachment predominates, the presenting symptoms may be those of increased intracranial pressure or hydrocephalus. The clinical appearance of these patients include a short neck (78%), asymmetry of the facial skull (68%), or torticollis.[3] These findings are shared with other vertebral anomalies and are not pathognomonic for this syndrome.

Although basilar impression is congenital, patients who become symptomatic usually develop symptoms later in life, typically in the fourth decade. Three theories have been proposed to explain this. The first proposes a delayed myelopathy secondary to ligamentous laxity which progresses to instability with increased physical demands. The second theory suggests that the symptoms result from the development of degenerative arthritis. The third and most accepted theory suggests that the young central nervous system is resilient and more tolerant of compression, whereas the aging brain becomes more susceptible to direct and indirect insults. The presentation of symptoms later in life may confuse the diagnosis of basilar invagination with other conditions such as amyotrophic lateral sclerosis, trauma, tumor, or multiple sclerosis.

The radiographic evaluation of basilar impression may be difficult. Many methods of evaluating the relationship of the odontoid to the foramen magnum have been described including those of Chamberlain,[5] MacGregor,[23] McRae[26] (Fig. 7.1), and Fischgold and Metzger (Fig. 7.2).[10]

Chamberlain's line extends from the posterior lip of the foramen magnum to the dorsal margin of the hard palate (Fig. 7.2). Any projection of the odontoid above this line is an indication of basilar invagination. It is not always possible to use this method, because the posterior lip of the foramen magnum may be difficult to identify and, in some patients with basilar invagination, the posterior lip of the foramen may actually be invaginated.

MacGregor's line extends from the upper surface of the hard palate to the most caudal portion of the occiput which is readily identified. The distance between the tip of the odontoid and MacGregor's line is measured. A distance

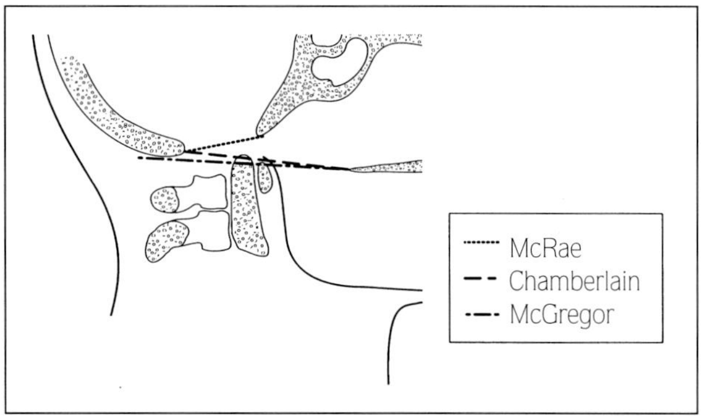

Figure 7.1
Lateral representation of (····) McRae's, (– –) Chamberlain's, and (–·–·–) McGregor's line in the evaluation of basilar impression

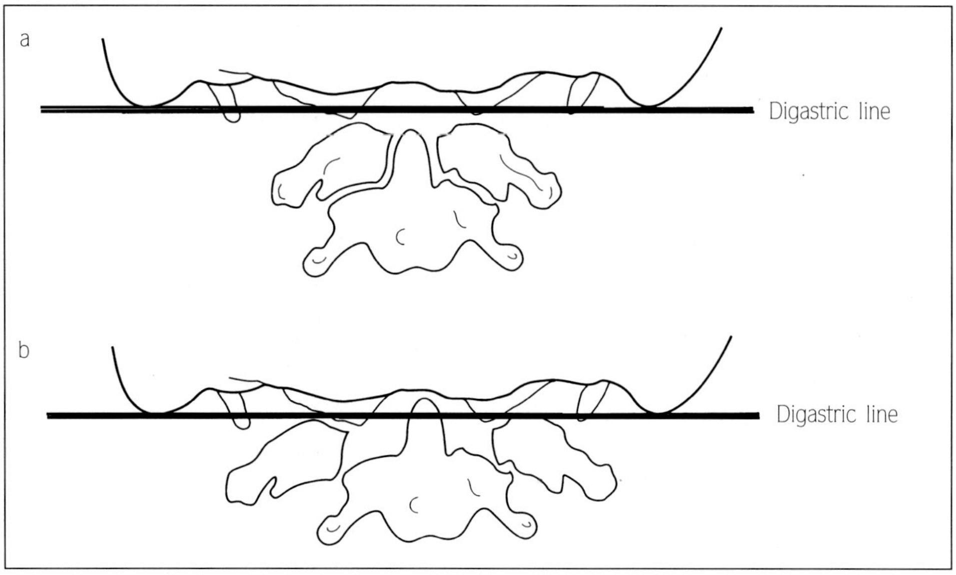

Figure 7.2
Anteroposterior illustration of the upper cervical spine demonstrating the Fischgold–Metzger line. In normal patients (a), the tip of the odontoid lies 10 mm below the digastric line. In patients with basilar impression (b), the odontoid extends above this level

of 4.5 mm is considered the upper limit of normal, although anatomical variations do exist between males and females. Despite these variations, McGregor's line represents a useful screening parameter on routine lateral radiographs.

McRae observed that the lateral radiograph of asymptomatic patients with basilar impression demonstrated that the tip of the odontoid was positioned below a line joining the anterior and posterior lips of the foramen magnum (McRae's line). When the odontoid tip is positioned above this line, patients tend to be symptomatic.

Fischgold and Metzger assessed basilar impression on anteroposterior radiographs. The Fischgold–Metzger line is based between the two digastric grooves and normally lies 10 mm above the odontoid tip and 12 mm above the atlanto-occipital joints. The usefulness of this measurement is reserved for patients in whom lateral radiographs suggest an atlanto-occipital malformation. These varied radiographic methods of assessment are now limited to initial screening. Computed tomography (CT) and magnetic resonance imaging (MRI) have defined the bony anomalies precisely and give direct information with regard to neural compression.

The treatment of symptomatic basilar invagination may require a combined neurosurgical and orthopaedic approach. Asymptomatic patients with basilar impression may be observed with periodic examination. The decision for surgical intervention is based on deteriorating neurologic status and not on the severity of findings observed on imaging studies. Non-operative management has been unsuccessful in symptomatic patients. In those patients with anterior cord impingement, stabilization by posterior fusion of occiput to C2 requires concomitant anterior excision of the odontoid in those patients with an odontoid that is not reduced or with persistent anterior compression. With posterior cord encroachment, suboccipital craniectomy and laminectomy of C1 and C2 may be required. Durotomy with dural grafts is frequently required to relieve compression by posterior dural bands. When concurrent instability exists, fusion of occiput to C2 is also required.

OCCIPITALIZATION OF THE ATLAS

Occipitalization of the atlas, also known as atlanto-occipital fusion or assimilation, is a partial or complete fusion of the atlas to the base of the occiput. The degree of involvement varies from total bony ankylosis to fibrous union. Occipitalization of the atlas occurs in 1.4–2.5 of 1000 children and occurs equally in both sexes. When associated with congenital fusion of C2 to C3, atlantoaxial instability develops in 70% of patients by the fourth decade of life. Associated anomalies occur in 20% of individuals with occipitalization of the atlas and include mandibular anomalies, cleft palate, external ear deformities, cervical ribs, and urinary tract anomalies.

Affected individuals may demonstrate a low hairline, torticollis, short neck, restriction of neck motion, and may resemble the individual with Klippel–Feil syndrome. Although most of these individuals are asymptomatic, they can present with myelopathy and symptoms of chronic atlantoaxial instability in the third or fourth decade of life. In symptomatic patients, weakness and ataxia of the lower extremities are common, and numbness and pain occur in 50% of patients. Physical examination may demonstrate the presence of long tract signs. Posterior column compression may develop when dural bands are present and is frequently accompanied by headache. McRae and Barnum[27] noted that the most important radiographic finding in the symptomatic patient is an odontoid process of abnormal size and position. There may be anterior compression of the medulla oblongata, corresponding signs and symptoms of ataxia, pyramidal tract irritation, and muscle weakness and wasting.[1] Analysis at autopsy has confirmed anterior compression in these patients. Although signs and symptoms of cord compression usually progress slowly from an insidious onset, acute onset of symptoms and sudden death have been reported.[16] Most individuals with occipitalization of the atlas are asymptomatic, being detected incidentally on plain cervical spine radiographs.

Routine radiographs of the occipitocervical junction may be difficult to interpret because of the variable expression of this anomaly, which can range from fibrous union to a complete bony fusion of the occiput to the atlas. Tomography or CT will define the anomaly better; the most commonly observed radiographic pattern is fusion of the anterior arch of the atlas to the occiput. Patients will require flexion–extension lateral radiographs of the cervical spine to rule out C1–C2 instability. McRae and Barnum[27] measured the distance from the anterior arch of the atlas to the posterior lip of the foramen magnum or to the posterior arch of the atlas, whichever was closer (Fig. 7.3); <19 mm of space available for the cord may be associated with neurologic deficit. Measurement should be on the lateral flexion radiograph because maximum encroachment of the spinal canal occurs in this position. The shape, size, and position of the odontoid have been implicated in the pathogenesis of neural deficit in patients with occipitalization of the atlas: the odontoid is frequently larger and angled posteriorly; 60% of patients with atlanto-occipital fusions will exhibit between 3 and 12 mm of space between the anterior arch of the atlas and the odontoid.[27]

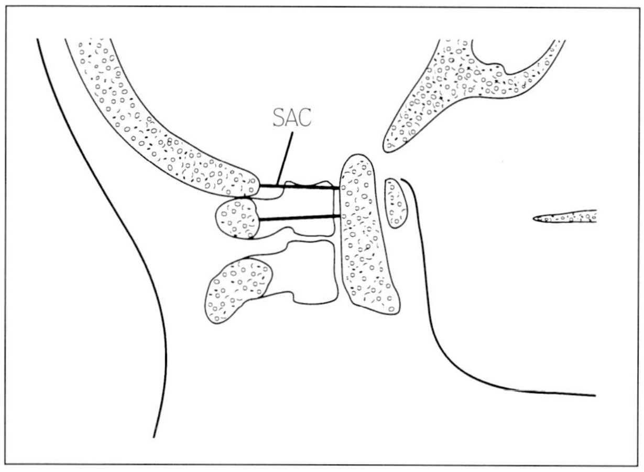

Figure 7.3
McRae's depiction of the space available for the cord in patients with atlanto-occipital fusion. If the space available for the cord (SAC) is <19 mm, neural deficit is usually present

The treatment of patients with symptomatic occipitalization begins with a trial of non-operative management. Either immobilization with a collar or traction may be successful if the symptoms follow minor trauma or infection.

Occasionally, surgical treatment is necessary to relieve compression and correct instability. Anterior symptoms usually originate from a malformed or hypermobile atlantoaxial complex, and instability at this level is corrected by posterior fusion from occiput to C2; its success can be predicted by preoperative traction. If preoperative traction reduces the anatomic odontoid relationship to the arch of the atlas, and enlarges the space available for cord, patients' symptoms will resolve and a successful result is anticipated from fusion alone. If the odontoid remains unreduced despite traction, the prognosis is poor. Surgical reduction is not recommended due to the frequent complication of death.[36] If posterior symptoms predominate, suboccipital craniectomy, excision of the posterior arch of the atlas, and removal of dural band are recommended. Surgical results have been mixed, with some patients gaining complete recovery whereas others have had little to no neurologic improvement or have died in the perioperative period.

ANOMALIES OF THE ODONTOID

Congenital anomalies of the odontoid are rare and are usually detected during routine radiographs taken following trauma. They are clinically important because of associated atlantoaxial instability which may present insidiously or acutely as the result of minor trauma.

Classification of odontoid morphology reveals five types: a normal odontoid, hypoplastic odontoid, ossiculum terminale, os odontoideum, and aplasia of the odontoid.[9] There is considerable controversy over the existence of a true aplasia of the odontoid. McRae noted no proven cases in his review at the Montreal Neurologic Institute up to 1960.[27] In past reports, aplasia was usually confused with hypoplasia; true aplasia, however, requires the absence of the dens below the level of the articular facets. Odontoid malformation occurs in association with other conditions such as Down's syndrome and Klippel–Feil syndrome, and skeletal dysplasias such as Morquio syndrome and spondyloepiphyseal dysplasia.

The etiology of os odontoideum has not yet been determined, and the proposed theories are somewhat controversial. Adherents to a congenital etiology propose failure of fusion of the apex or ossiculum terminale to the body of the odontoid, but this is unlikely because the resultant os terminale is much smaller and does not approximate the size or position of the os odontoideum. The second congenital theory proposes a failure of fusion of the odontoid to the body of C2, but this would leave a large defect in its body, because the odontoid contributes substantially to the anterior body of C2. More commonly, the os odontoideum is a short, flattened ossicle located above the body of C2, and a corresponding defect in the latter is not seen. From this, a congenital origin of os odontoideum has been questioned, leading to the proposal of an acquired mechanism.

Fielding and Griffin[7] suggest that an unrecognized fracture at the base of the odontoid develops into a non-union and results in os odontoideum. Nine cases of os odontoideum have been recorded several years after trauma in patients known to have a normal odontoid. Fielding postulates that, following fracture, only slight separation occurs between the fragments, although with time, contracture of the alar ligaments exerts a force which distracts the fragments. This distraction compromises the arcade-like blood supply to the odontoid and results in poor fracture healing or callus formation. The portion of the odontoid adjacent to the ring of the atlas is maintained by the intact transverse ligament. The blood supply to the displaced fragment is provided by the arterial arcade through the alar ligament. The degree of perfusion involved may be capable only of maintaining part of the odontoid, thus forming the os odontoideum.

Clinical presentation of individuals with anomalies of the odontoid is variable. Symptoms may either develop following minor trauma which aggravates pre-existing atlantoaxial instability or be mechanical with neck pain, torticollis, or headache secondary to irritation at the atlantoaxial articulation. Unlike anomalies of the occipital vertebral junction, cranial nerve involvement associated with odontoid malformations is rare.[29]

The prognosis for patients with anomalies of the odontoid relates to presenting clinical manifestations. If symptoms are limited to neck pain and torticollis with no neurologic involvement, or if transient weakness or sensory changes develop after trauma, complete return of function can be expected. Neurologic deficits are likely to be irreversible in patients with insidious onset of symptoms and slowly progressive neurologic loss.[24] Although weakness and ataxia are common findings, spasticity, hyperreflexia, and sphincter disturbances have been reported. A small percentage of patients will present with signs and symptoms of vertebral artery compression, syncope, seizure, and visual disturbances which can be confused with progressive neurologic disease such as Friedreich's ataxia and multiple sclerosis.[30]

The radiographic evaluation of patients with abnormalities of the odontoid requires anteroposterior open-mouth and lateral radiographs. Voluntary flexion–extension lateral radiographs will demonstrate the presence and degree of instability of the cervical spine (Fig. 7.4). A distance of greater than 4.5 mm between the anterior border of the dens and the posterior border of the anterior arch of C1 (the atlantodental interval – (ADI)) suggests pathologic motion in the immature spine (Fig. 7.5). Lateral tomography or cineradiography is useful to document atlantoaxial instability when neutral lateral radiographs of the cervical spine are difficult to obtain.

Radiographic criteria for the diagnosis of true aplasia of the odontoid requires complete absence of the basilar portion of the odontoid with a resultant defect in the body of the axis well below the superior articular facets. Hypoplasia of the odontoid is depicted radiographically as

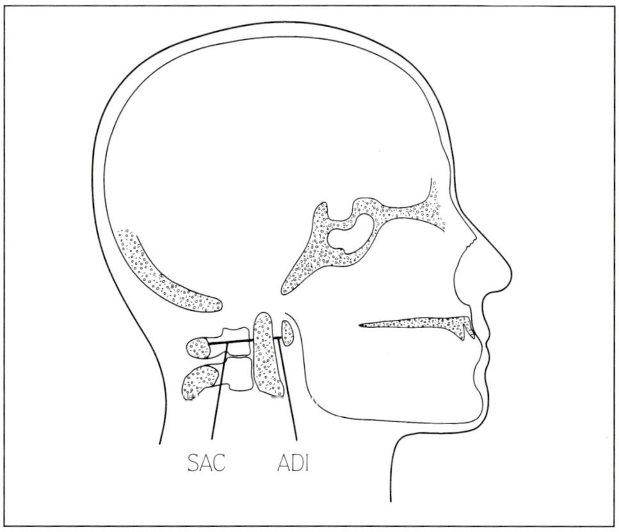

Figure 7.4
Diagrammatic lateral representation of the normal relationship of the C1–C2 articulation demonstrating the atlas–dens interval (ADI) and the space available for cord (SAC)

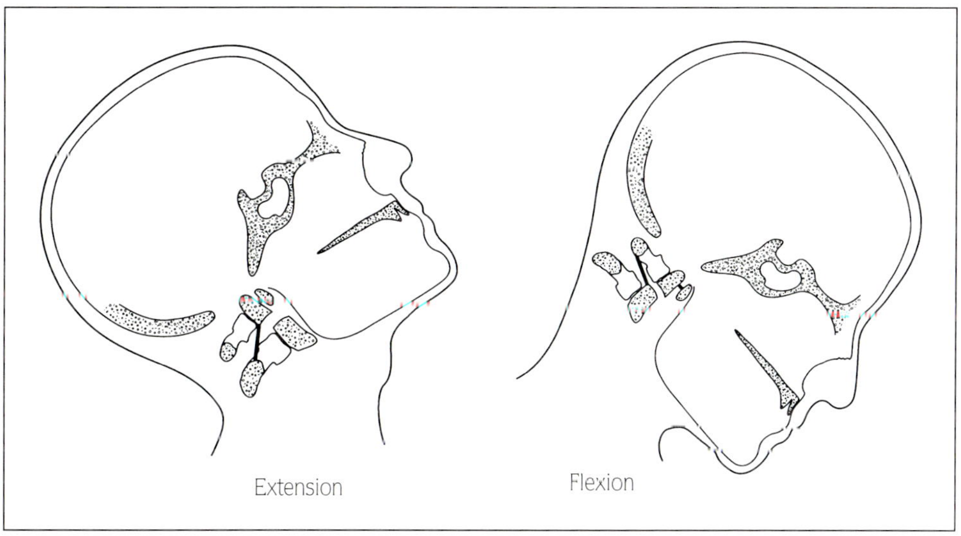

Figure 7.5
Lateral flexion–extension representation of atlantoaxial instability secondary to os odontoideum. Note the maintenance of the atlas–dens interval with a decrease in the space available for cord on extension

a short, flattened odontoid which projects above the lateral facets. CT scans or tomograms will differentiate hypoplastic odontoid from os odontoideum – the latter appears as a round ossicle in association with a hypoplastic odontoid, whereas non union of the base of the dens in the mature spine will exhibit a narrow lucent zone at the odontoid base with a normally shaped dens.

Treatment of patients with odontoid anomalies is directed toward prevention of instability and neurologic compromise. In those patients who present with local irritation or torticollis, and diffuse transient weakness without radicular distribution, cervical traction or orthotic immobilization may resolve the symptoms. The role of prophylactic atlantoaxial fusion in patients with transient symptoms, or in those whose malformation is found incidentally on routine radiographs, is controversial. Deterioration of neurologic status has been reported with surgical fusion, and thus fusion is indicated only in patients who experience episodic symptoms or who demonstrate progressive symptoms.[24,29] Initial management of asymptomatic patients with low-grade cervical instability consists of avoidance of activities that can cause trauma to the head and neck. Shepard[33] believes that adherence to restrictions is unrealistic with potential for catastrophic neurologic injury and recommends elective surgical stabilization.

Surgical indications include neurologic compromise, atlantoaxial instability with ADI >5 mm, progressive instability, or persistent neck complaints.[24] Preoperative evaluation of the posterior ring of C1 is essential because there may be incomplete development in patients with odontoid abnormalities. Preoperative reduction of the atlantoaxial articulation is accomplished by careful positioning or skull traction. Open reduction of C1–C2 subluxation carries the significant risks of respiratory distress, apnea, or death, and is not recommended.[11] Posterior cervical fusion of C1–C2 is the procedure of choice.[9] Wire fixation may be used if C1–C2 reduction had been achieved before operation, although the addition of wire fixation in children has not demonstrated any significant advantages over fusion without wire fixation. Care must be exerted in passing the wire to avoid cord compression. In addition, excessive wire tightening can result in posterior translation of the atlas on the axis with neurologic compromise (Fig. 7.6). In patients with moderate-to-severe neurologic deficit with irreducible translation of C1–C2, fusion of occiput to C2 together with laminectomy of C1 is safer. Postoperative immobilization in extension may be maintained with a Minerva or halo cast.

The management of patients with an irreducible C1–C2 articulation remains a difficult problem. Minderhouse et al[29] reported increased morbidity and mortality with laminectomy alone. Decompression of the posterior arch of the atlas without fusion can aggravate C1–C2 instability and must be accompanied by occiput-to-C2 fusion. In the neurologically intact patient, in situ fusion is the least hazardous option. Several authors have suggested anterior surgical approaches to the cervical spine when reduction is necessary in C1–C2 dislocations, or when posterior stabilization is precluded.[13] Whitesides described the lateral retropharyngeal approach which provides anterior exposure of the C1–C2 articulation for the purpose of decompression or stabilization. Whitesides' approach avoids the increased risk of infection associated with the transoral, mandibular, and tongue-splitting approaches.[39,40]

ATLANTOAXIAL INSTABILITY

Atlantoaxial instability is the consequence of loss of bony or ligamentous integrity about the C1–C2 articulation. Spinal cord impingement may result from an abnormal odontoid, occipitocervical fusion or ligamentous laxity. Atlantoaxial instability is associated with congenital scoliosis, Down's syndrome, neurofibromatosis, and bony dysplasias, and requires radiographic survey of the cervical spine including flexion–extension lateral radiographs before general anesthesia or spinal traction is initiated.

The stability of the C1–C2 articulation, the most mobile in the vertebral column, is based on bony and soft tissue elements. The odontoid prevents hyperextension of the atlas on the axis, whereas the remaining stability is provided by ligamentous and capsular attachments. These stabilizing factors are of great significance because the C1–C2 articulation is positioned between two relatively immobile articulations, the atlanto-occipital and the C2–C3 junctions. In the presence of atlanto-occipital or C2–C3 fusion, additional stress may result in pathologic C1–C2 hypermobility.

The radiographic evaluation of atlantoaxial instability is defined by the ADI which should not exceed 4.5 mm in children or 3 mm in adults (Fig. 7.7).[18,20] This measurement may be difficult to define in the presence of congenital anomalies of the upper cervical spine. In this population, the space available for the cord (SAC), measured from the posterior aspect of the odontoid to either the foramen magnum or the posterior ring of the atlas, is a direct measurement of canal width. In os odontoideum or nonunion of the odontoid, the ADI will remain normal during flexion–extension maneuvers, whereas there is a considerable reduction of the SAC.

The concept of the SAC was first recognized by McRae who reported an association of symptoms in patients with atlanto-occipital fusion who had an SAC of <19 mm.[25] In adults with atlantoaxial instability Greenberg ascertained that an SAC ≤14 mm was uniformly associated with neurologic compromise, 15–17 mm signified potential cord compression, and ≥18 mm was not associated with compression.[13]

The importance of the alar ligaments as a secondary restraint to the odontoid after disruption of the transverse atlantal ligament was reported by Steel.[37] After anatomical studies, Steel proposed the 'Rule of Thirds' to simplify evaluation of this area: in this the spinal canal at the level of the first cervical vertebra can be divided into thirds with one-third occupied by the cord, one-third occupied by the odontoid, and one-third remaining as potential space. Steel observed that displacement of more than one-third the canal width indicates failure of the alar ligaments.

Treatment of atlantoaxial instability involves the reduction and stabilization of the C1–C2 articulation, but open reduction of C1–C2 is not recommended. Preoperative traction or positional reduction is important to decrease spinal cord compression, to prevent further neurologic damage, and possibly to recover neurologic loss.

KLIPPEL–FEIL SYNDROME

Congenital fusion of the cervical spine or the Klippel–Feil syndrome can range from an isolated fusion of two cervical vertebrae to a pattern which involves multiple cervical levels. Neither severity of cervical spine involvement nor

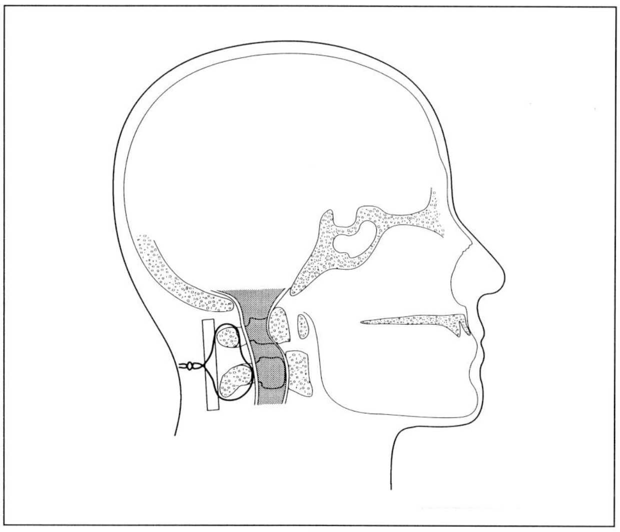

Figure 7.6
Overtightening of the sublaminar wires during C1–C2 posterior fusion for os odontoideum causes retropulsion of the ossicle into the spinal canal, thus compromising the space available for cord

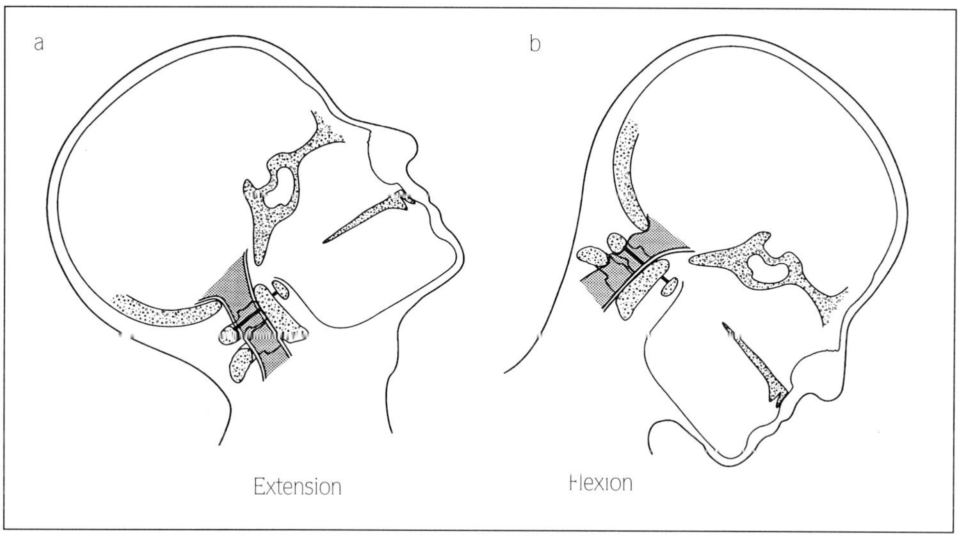

Figure 7.7
Lateral flexion–extension representations of atlantoaxial instability secondary to ligamentous instability. (a) Extension shows the normal relationship of the atlas–dens interval (ADI) and space available for cord (SAC). (b) Flexion causes a decrease in the SAC with an increasing ADI

presence of associated anomalies is considered necessary for inclusion in this syndrome. As yet there is no clear agreement on the anatomic criteria for inclusion in this syndrome, and although occipitalization of the atlas, hemivertebrae, and basilar impression do occur more frequently in patients with the Klippel–Feil syndrome, on the whole their presence in isolation is not generally accepted as part of this anomaly.

The triad of clinical findings in the Klippel–Feil syndrome includes a short neck, a low posterior hairline, and limited range of neck movement. Although this triad occurs in patients with massive cervical spine involvement and is present at birth, it is seen in less than half of all patients with the Klippel–Feil syndrome. Many patients have normal physical appearance[12,15] and are identified as having the syndrome by incidental radiographic studies. A short neck with a low hairline is usually found in patients with severe cervical spine involvement. Other clinical findings such as facial asymmetry, torticollis, or webbing of the neck may facilitate detection, but are present in only 20% of cases.[17] Torticollis secondary to congenital cervical spine anomaly must be differentiated from congenital muscular torticollis. Surgical release of contracted muscles does not benefit those with congenital anomalies of the cervical spine.

The most consistent clinical finding in patients with the Klippel–Feil syndrome is limitation of neck movement. Flexion, extension, and lateral rotation are usually clinically normal. Decrease in lateral bending is found in patients with increasing levels of vertebral involvement. In patients with massive cervical spine involvement, no neck movement may be present, and torticollis and a short neck are frequent. Iniencephaly, a massive enlargement of the foramen magnum with the cervical spine displaying absence of posterior spine elements and congenital fusion of vertebral bodies, must be considered in patients who present with a low posterior hairline and fixed hyperextension of the neck.[35]

The initial radiographic evaluation of patients with the Klippel–Feil syndrome includes anteroposterior, anteroposterior open-mouth, and lateral flexion–extension views of the cervical spine – a series of radiographs that frequently defines the pattern of congenital fusion, and detects coexisting occipitalization of the atlas and atlantoaxial instability, as well as instability at or below the fused vertebrae. Lateral radiographs may appear normal in the young child who has early ossification, but with increasing maturity, ossification and obliteration of the apparent disc space become apparent. An early clue to the presence of congenital fusion in the young is bony union of the posterior elements.[17] The spinal canal is usually normal in width, but the presence of an enlarged canal can indicate syringomyelia, hydromyelia, or the Arnold–Chiari malformation.

Tomography or CT can clarify the details of a more complex fusion pattern, especially when hemivertebrae are involved. Instability can be documented and quantified with cineradiography which allows dynamic evaluation of the spine in axial rotation, lateral bending, and flexion–extension while avoiding the confusion of malrotation. Anterior gaping of the disc space or sudden translation of one vertebral body on another during cineradiographic evaluation may indicate intersegmental instability, and must be differentiated from pseudosubluxation, particularly in patients less than 8 years of age.[4] MRI is helpful in defining concurrent anomalies of the brain stem and spinal cord.

There is no proven theory to explain the development of congenital cervical fusion. It appears that an insult occurs between the fourth and eighth weeks of fetal life. Although teratogenic agents have induced similar spinal changes in animal models, no documentation of teratogenic etiology exists in humans. A report linking the Klippel–Feil syndrome with maternal alcoholism has been suggested, but there is little evidence to support this.[21]

Reports of conditions associated with the Klippel–Feil syndrome are numerous,[17] and include facial malformations such as cleft lip, cleft palate, ptosis, and facial nerve palsy. A high incidence of deafness has been reported suggesting that all Klippel–Feil syndrome patients should undergo audiometric examination.

Anomalies of the thorax, as well as thoracic scoliosis, are associated with the Klippel–Feil syndrome, anomalies in the thoracic spine suggesting the existence of cervical spine malformation. Comprehensive evaluation of patients with congenital scoliosis includes a lateral radiograph of the cervical spine. Cardiovascular anomalies in this syndrome range from the most common ventricular septal defects to mitral insufficiency, coarctation of the aorta, patent ductus arteriosus, dextrocardia, chamber anomalies, and valvular leaflet malformations. Pulmonary complications in the Klippel–Feil syndrome involve restrictive disease caused by rib fusion, scoliosis, or costovertebral deformities. Central respiratory disturbances at the level of the brain stem can render a patient with the Klippel–Feil syndrome susceptible to neurologic injury whenever distraction is applied to the cervical spine. Careful monitoring is required in all such cases.

Sprengel's deformity has been reported in 20% of Klippel–Feil syndrome patients, and may be unilateral or bilateral.[14] Although primarily of cosmetic concern, shoulder movement is affected, especially in those whose omovertebral bone fixes the scapula to the spine. At day 31 of fetal life, the mesodermal scapula is at the level of C4, and by day 42, it descends below the first rib. This period of time coincides with the critical period in the development of the Klippel–Feil anomaly, implying a single insult.

Synkinesia or mirror movement of finger and hand movement is seen in normal children up until the age of 5 years and in 20% of those with Klippel–Feil syndrome. Voluntary movement in one limb is accompanied by involuntary but similar motion of the contralateral limb. This phenomenon is more common in the upper extremity, especially with finger motion, and may hamper bimanual activities. Mirror motions tend to dampen and be less noticeable by the second decade of life.[15] The etiology of synkinesia is unclear; however, incomplete decussation of the pyramidal tracts, noted in autopsy studies, requires alternative and less specific extrapyramidal pathways for the control of limb movement. No physiologic mechanism for this phenomenon has been elucidated to explain the activity recorded by electromyography (EMG) in individuals with the Klippel–Feil syndrome and synkinesia.[31]

Anomalies involving the genitourinary system are frequently found (30%) in the Klippel–Feil syndrome with the most common abnormality being congenital absence of one kidney. The embryological origin of the urogenital system is from the mesoderm in marked proximity to somites destined to form the cervical spine. Girls with the Klippel–Feil syndrome are more frequently affected by anomalies of the kidney, renal collecting system, uterus, and vagina; in boys, the most common finding is small or undescended testicles.[28] Individuals with the Klippel–Feil syndrome require screening of the genitourinary system usually by renal ultrasonography. An intravenous urogram may be needed if structural abnormality is found on initial evaluation.

Scoliosis is the most commonly associated orthopaedic condition, and has been reported in more than 50% of patients with the Klippel–Feil syndrome.[17] There are two forms of scoliosis, the most common being congenital, and the second type being analogous to idiopathic scoliosis. Although the scoliotic spine may be successfully treated with orthosis, in many patients the scoliosis is progressive and will require surgical stabilization.[17]

In the young patient with the Klippel–Feil syndrome, for early detection of instability it is necessary to make serial examinations of the cervical spine, including the occipitocervical junction. The thoracic and lumbar spine must also be examined clinically to monitor the development of scoliosis.

The primary concerns with regard to individuals with the Klippel–Feil syndrome center around the development of intersegmental instability of the cervical spine, degenerative disease, and radiculopathy. Although non-operative therapy for degenerative disease, including non-steroidal medications and physical therapy, is usually successful, surgical fusion may be required. Evaluation of the brain stem and occipitocervical junction is required before surgical intervention is planned. Surgical attempts to make cosmetic improvements have been unsuccessful and do not appear to be warranted.

OCCIPITOCERVICAL FUSION

Surgical decompression or stabilization of cervical spine anomalies requires thorough understanding of the malformation with careful preoperative planning and postoperative care. The patient's age, neurologic status, and the coexistence of associated conditions and malformations must all be considered. Occipitocervical fusion to C1 or C2 may be indicated for congenital occipital–C1 instability, or for C1–C2 instability when the posterior ring of C1 is absent. Three techniques of occipitocervical fusion have been advocated which vary in the technique of grafting. Because of a high failure rate with allograft in the immature cervical spine, posterior fusion should be performed with autograft whenever possible.

Wertheim and Bohlman[38] describe a technique similar to that described by Grantham. Preoperative placement of cranial skeletal traction is followed by turning the patient into the prone position on a Stryker frame. Cross-table lateral radiographs will confirm occipitocervical alignment. Injection of the skin with a 1 : 500 000 solution of epinephrine (adrenaline) along the incision retards bleeding, and a midline incision is made extending from the external occipital protuberance to the base of C4. Sharp subperiosteal dissection is then carried out to expose the occiput and cervical lamina of vertebrae to be included in the fusion mass. The paramedial venous plexus is avoided by midline dissection. The external occipital protuberance is a relatively thick structure in mature individuals and is ideal for the passage of wires so avoiding violation of the inner table of the skull. A high-speed burr prepares a trough on either side of the protuberance at the level of 2 cm above the foramen magnum. Using a towel clip, a hole is made in the outer table, and a 20 gauge wire is passed. A second wire is then passed under the arch of the atlas, and a third at the base of the spinous process of the axis. Three wires are now located on each side of the spine to anchor the bone graft. Iliac crest bone graft is used creating two curved corticocancellous grafts. Careful measurement is taken and three drill holes made in each graft. The occiput and posterior elements are then decorticated, and the graft is anchored using the wires. Additional cancellous graft is used to augment the fusion. After the operation a halo cast is usually worn for 6–13 weeks followed by a soft cervical collar for 6 weeks.

Koop et al[19] described a technique for occipitocervical fusion without the use of wires to anchor the graft. Autologous corticocancellous graft is used together with an occipital periosteal flap which is elevated over the area of the defect of the posterior element. The approach is similar to Bohlman's approach, except a halo cast is applied before the operation. In patients with posterior absence of the atlas ring, care must be taken to avoid exposing the dura. A caudal-based triangular flap is elevated from the occiput and sutured in place over the area of the defect in the posterior element. Decortication of the occiput and posterior elements of the axis is then followed by autogenous cancellous bone grafting. The halo cast is worn until union is evident, usually at 5 months. Lateral flexion–extension radiographs will document union.

ATLANTOAXIAL FUSION

Atlantoaxial fusion is indicated for patients with instability of the C1–C2 articulation resulting from odontoid anomaly, ligamentous instability, post-traumatic instability or rotatory fixation of the atlas on the axis. Two types of fusion have been described with several modifications. The Gallie technique was described by Fielding et al.[8] The patient is placed in the prone position and a midline incision used to expose the bifid spinous process of the axis. The posterior elements of the axis are identified and a longitudinal incision is made over the posterior tubercle of the C1 ring and transversely along each of its laminae. Lateral dissection should be limited to 1.5 cm from the midline in the adult and 1.0 cm in children to avoid the vertebral arteries which pass over the atlas at this level. The anterior part of the posterior arch of the atlas is dissected free of periosteum and a loop of 22 gauge wire is passed under the lamina. A cortical graft is then fashioned to accommodate the posterior ring of C1 and C2, and the wire is passed over the graft and through or around the spinous process of the axis. Cancellous graft is used to augment the fusion. In children, vertebrae that are not to be included in the fusion should not be exposed. Inadvertent extension of fusion to adjacent vertebrae has been reported and further decreases motion of the neck. After the operation, the patient is maintained in traction for 10–14 days, and then fitted with a halo or Minerva cast. This orthosis is kept in place for 6–12 weeks until fusion is demonstrated by radiography.

A second option for atlantoaxial fusion is described by Brooks and Jenkins.[2] The patient position and exposure are similar to those of the Gallie fusion. Two wires are passed on either side of the midline under the ring of the atlas and beneath the lamina of the axis. Two full-thickness bone grafts are then taken from the iliac crest, each approximately 1.25 × 3.5 cm, and then fitted beneath the caudal portion of the atlas and the cephalad portion of the axis. Notches are then created in the superior laminar cortex of the atlas and the inferior laminar cortex of the axis to prevent wire slippage. The wire is tightened over the graft. The advantage of the Gallie fusion is that it requires only one wire under the lamina of C1. Excessive tightening can cause displacement of C1 on C2. The Brooks' fusion requires the passage of two wires under two laminae, and this causes increased resistance to rotation, lateral bending, and extension. In patients under the age of 6 years, fusion can be accomplished without wire fixation. Bone graft should be placed along the decorticated area using a halo or Minerva cast for postoperative immobilization. Down's syndrome patients with posterior cervical fusion have a high complication rate following surgery.[32] Segal et al reported a combined series of Down's syndrome patients with complications including wound infection, graft resorption, and death. As a result of these problems, it is suggested that non-operative management of atlantoaxial instability is used in Down's syndrome patients, although the spinal cord must be protected and newer techniques for fusion are needed.

When adequate reduction through traction cannot be achieved, an anterior cervical approach may be required for atlantoaxial subluxation. In situ posterior fusion is safe and frequently sufficient to protect neural tissue. Posterior decompression by laminectomy without fusion has a high rate of morbidity and mortality due to the increased cervical instability. In these patients, an anterior approach using a transoral,[6] mandibular, and tongue-splitting approach,[34] a lateral retropharyngeal approach,[40] or an anterior retropharyngeal approach[22] can be considered.

REFERENCES

1 Bharucha EP, Dastur HM. Craniovertebral anomalies (a report of 40 cases). *Brain* **87**: 469–480, 1964.

2 Brooks AL, Jenkins EB. Atlantoaxial arthrodesis by the wedge compression method. *J Bone Joint Surg [Am]* **60**: 279–284, 1978.

3 Caetano-DeBarros M, Farias W, Ataide L, Lins S. Basilar impression and Arnold–Chiari malformation: A study of 66 cases. *J Neurol Neurosurg Psychiat* **31**: 596–605, 1968.

4 Cattell HS, Filtzer DL. Pseudosubluxation and other normal variations in the cervical spine in children. *J Bone Joint Surg [Am]* **47**: 1295–1309, 1965.

5 Chamberlain WE. Basilar impression (platybasia): A bizarre developmental anomaly of the occipital bone and upper cervical spine with striking and misleading neurological manifestations. *Yale J Biol Med* **11**: 487, 1939.

6 Fang HSY, Ong GB. Direct anterior approach to the upper cervical spine. *J Bone Joint Surg [Am]* **44**: 1588–1604, 1962.

7 Fielding JW, Griffin PP. Os odontoideum: An acquired lesion. *J Bone Joint Surg [Am]* **56**: 187–190, 1974.

8 Fielding JW, Hawkins RJ, Ratzan SA. Spine fusion for atlantoaxial instability. *J Bone Joint Surg [Am]* **58**: 400–407, 1976.

9 Fielding JW, Hensinger RN, Hawkins RJ. Os odontoideum. *J Bone Joint Surg [Am]* **62**: 376–383, 1980.

10 Fischgold H, Metzger J. Etude radiotomographique de l'impression basilaire. *Rev Rhum Mal Osteoartic* **19**: 261, 1952.

11 Garber JN. Abnormalities of the atlas and axis vertebrae: Congenital and traumatic. *J Bone Joint Surg [Am]* **47**: 1782–1791, 1964.

12 Gray SW, Romaine CB, Skandalakis JE. Congenital fusion of the cervical vertebrae. *Surg Gynecol Obstet* **118**: 373, 1964.

13 Greenberg AD, Scoville WB, Davey LM. Transoral decompression of atlantoaxial dislocation due to odontoid hypoplasia. Report of two cases. *J Neurosurg* **28**: 266–269, 1968.

14 Gunderson CH, Greenspan RH, Glaser GH, Lubs HA. Klippel–Feil syndrome: Genetic and clinical re-evaluation of cervical fusion. *Medicine* **46**: 491–512, 1967.

15 Gunderson CH, Solitare BH. Mirror movements in patients with Klippel–Feil syndrome: Neuropathic observations. *Arch Neurol* **18**: 675–679, 1968.

16 Hadley LA. *The Spine*. Springfield, Ill: Charles C. Thomas, 1956.

17 Hensinger RN, Lang JR, MacEwen GD. Klippel–Feil syndrome: A constellation of associated anomalies. *J Bone Joint Surg [Am]* **56**: 1246–1253, 1974.

18 Hinck VC, Hopkins CE, Savara BS. Diagnostic criteria of basilar impression. *Radiology* **76**: 572, 1961.

19 Koop SE, Winter RB, Lonstein JE. The surgical treatment of instability of the upper part of the cervical spine in children and adolescents. *J Bone Joint Surg [Am]* **66**: 403–411, 1984.

20 Locke GR, Gardner JI, van Epps EF. Atlas–dens interval (ADI) in children. A survey based on 200 normal cervical spines. *Am J Roentgenol* **97**: 135–140, 1966.

21 Lowry RB. The Klippel–Feil anomalad as part of the fetal alcohol syndrome. *Teratology* **16**: 53–56, 1977.

22 McAfee PC, Bohlman HH, Riley LH Jr, et al. The anterior retropharyngeal approach to the upper part of the cervical spine. *J Bone Joint Surg [Am]* **69**: 1371–1383, 1987.

23 McGregor M. The significance of certain measurements of the skull in the diagnosis of basilar impression. *Br J Radiol* **21**: 171, 1948.
24 McKeever FM. Atlantoaxial instability. *Surg Clin North Am* **48**: 1375–1390, 1968.
25 McRae DL. Bony abnormalities in the region of the foramen magnum: Correlation of the anatomic and neurologic findings. *Acta Radiol* **40**: 335–354, 1953.
26 McRae DL. The significance of abnormalities of the cervical spine. *Am J Roentgenol* **84**: 3–25, 1960.
27 McRae DL, Barnum AS. Occipitalization of the atlas. *Am J Roentgenol* **70**: 23–46, 1953.
28 Mecklenburg RS, Krueger PM. Extensive genitourinary anomalies associated with Klippel–Feil syndrome. *Am J Dis Child* **128**: 92–93, 1974.
29 Minderhouse JM, Braakman R, Penning L. Os odontoideum: Clinical, radiological, and therapeutic aspects. *J Neurol Sci* **8**: 521–544, 1969.
30 Nicholson JR, Sherk HH. Anomalies of the occipitocervical articulation. *J Bone Joint Surg [Am]* **50**: 295–304, 1968.
31 Notermans SLH, Go KG, Boonstra S. EMG studies of associated movements in a patient with Klippel–Feil syndrome. *Psychiatria Neurologia Neurochirurgia* **73**: 257–266, 1970.
32 Segal LS, Drummond DS, Zanotti RM, Ecker ML, Mubarak SJ. Complications of posterior arthrodesis of the cervical spine in patients who have Down's syndrome. *J Bone Joint Surg [Am]* **73**: 1547–1554, 1991.
33 Shepard CN. Familial hypoplasia of the odontoid process. *J Bone Joint Surg [Am]* **48**: 1224, 1965.
34 Sherk HH, Pratt L. Transoral approaches. In Bailey RW (ed) *The Cervical Spine*, 1st ed, 527–528. The Cervical Spine Research Society, Philadelphia: JB Lippincott 1983.
35 Sherk HH, Shut L, Chung S. Iniencephalic deformity of the cervical spine with Klippel–Feil anomalies and congenital evaluation of the scapula. *J Bone Joint Surg [Am]* **56**: 1254–1259, 1974.
36 Sinh G, Pandya SK. Treatment of congenital atlantoaxial dislocations. *Proc Aust Assoc Neurol* **5**: 507–514, 1968.
37 Steel HH. Anatomical and mechanical considerations of the atlantoaxial articulations. *J Bone Joint Surg [Am]* **50**: 1481–1482, 1968.
38 Wertheim SB, Bohlman HH. Occipitocervical fusion: Indications, technique, and long-term results in thirteen patients. *J Bone Joint Surg [Am]* **69**: 833–836, 1987.
39 Whitesides TE Jr, Kelly RP. Lateral approach to the upper cervical spine for anterior fusion. *South Med J* **59**: 879–883, 1966.
40 Whitesides TE Jr, McDonald AP. Lateral retropharyngeal approach to the upper cervical spine. *Orthop Clin North Am* **9**: 1115–1127, 1978.

8 Degenerative disc disease of the cervical spine

J. Michael Simpson and Howard S. An

Cervical disc disease is best understood as a spectrum of clinical syndromes reflective of a progressive continuum of degenerative processes. The cervical disc may show anatomic change simply secondary to the aging process or degeneration, with aging generally denoting the progressive accumulation of changes over time. Disc degeneration, however, implies a more significant deterioration or pathologic changes in the tissues, which may lead to impairment of normal disc function. Clinicians should use aging as a term to describe morphologic change alone, whereas degeneration denotes those same changes associated with clinical symptomatology. As physicians, we have the best understanding of the relationship of structural change to clinical pain and dysfunction in the presence of neurocompressive lesions of the cervical nerve roots or spinal cord. Our understanding is least when pain is isolated to the neck as the degree of degenerative change does not correlate well with patient's symptoms.

The term used to describe degenerative change in the cervical spine is 'spondylolysis'. This implies involvement of the entire intervertebral motion segment. Cervical spondylosis includes a spectrum of anatomic change which may be isolated to one component of the motion segment or, more commonly, involve multiple identifiable anatomic structures. Such abnormalities include the alteration of normal disc anatomy, the proliferation of osteophytes about the facet and neurocentral joints with subsequent neuroforaminal impingement or instability.[10,17,19] Additionally, soft disc herniation may occur at any stage of this degenerative process. Each of these anatomic alterations occurs in relationship to disc degeneration. The clinical consequence is dependent upon the specific mechanical alterations and neural structures involved in this process. The pathologic processes involved in disc degeneration form the core of what we know as cervical spondylotic disease.

PATHOGENESIS OF DISC DEGENERATION

In considering the etiology and pathology of disc degeneration, we are confronted with several potential explanations for the disease process, including biochemical abnormalities, biomechanical stress, genetic susceptibility, and autoimmune processes. These degenerative processes presumably start with an alteration in the biochemical integrity of the nucleus pulposus and precede the known structural changes associated with spondylosis. Our basic fund of knowledge of cellular function in biochemical and biophysical terms has progressed to a point at which we may propose specific mechanisms of degenerative change.

Most of what we know of the pathoanatomy of disc degeneration is from the lumbar spine, but the cervical disc structure is the same overall and undergoes the same pathologic change as seen in the lumbar spine. The main structural components of the disc must be identified and the function of each reviewed. These structural components include collagen, proteoglycans, and water, together making up approximately 95% of the volume of the normal disc. The collagen network provides the intervertebral connection with a lamellar structure permitting multidirectional motion. Proteoglycans imbibe water secondary to their osmotic qualities, and maintain hydration of the disc, providing turgor pressure. At the core of the degenerative process is the change and loss of a normal gelatinous nucleus pulposus, and the gradual disappearance of a well-defined border between the nucleus and the annulus fibrosis. The efficient functioning of the nucleus pulposus depends largely on a high concentration of normal proteoglycans which, in turn, account for its hydrophilic qualities. To better understand this, and its relationship to cervical disc disease, the normal biochemical and physiologic properties of the proteoglycans must be reviewed.

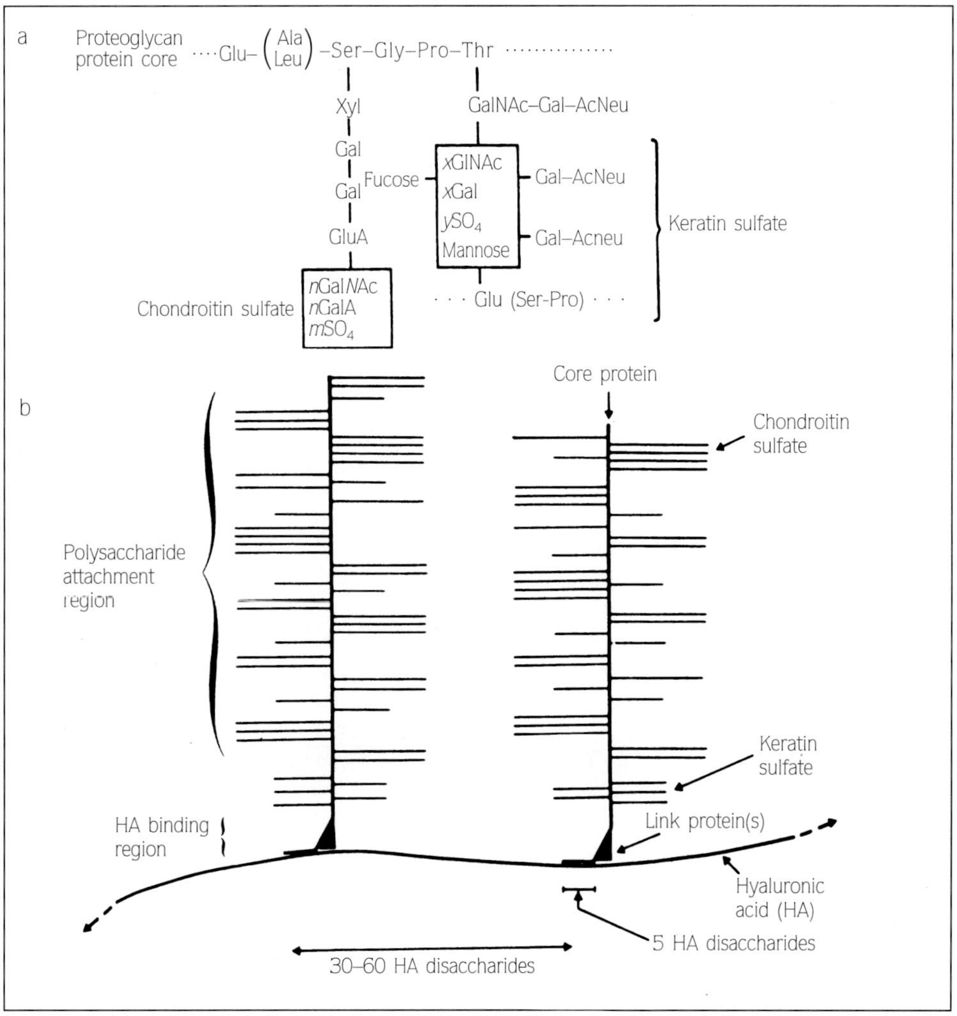

Figure 8.1
(a) Model of keratin sulfate and chondroitin sulfate attached to core protein. (Reproduced from Hopwood JJ, Robinson HC. The structure and composition of cartilage keratin sulfate. *Biochem J* **111**: 517, 1971, with permission.) (b) Model of proteoglycan aggregate: this consists of a core protein to which bulky, sterically active, polysaccharide attachments of keratin sulfate and chondroitin sulfate are attached. These large aggregates are in turn linked to a hyaluronic acid (HA) backbone with the assistance of a link protein. (Reproduced from Hopwood JJ, Robinson HC. Structural studies on keratin sulfate from cartilage. *Biochem J Mol Aspects* 141: 524, 1974, with permission.)

An isolated proteoglycan consists of a core protein which, in turn, allows for binding of bulky, sterically active polysaccharide attachments of glycosaminoglycans, namely chondroitin sulfate and keratin sulfate. These large, negatively charged aggregates are linked to a hyaluronic acid backbone, and are structured much like the attachment of branches to a tree trunk[21,22] (Fig. 8.1).

As a result of the high electronegative qualities of the glycosaminoglycan proteins, water is naturally absorbed and held to them through hydrogen bonding. Within the matrix of these proteoglycan aggregates, a loose fibrillar stroma of type II collagen fibers is interwoven, giving some tensile strength to the nucleus pulposus. Under normal conditions the nucleus pulposus is responsible for the even distribution of all applied forces to the annulus fibrosis and vertebral end-plates (Fig. 8.2).

Urban and McMullin[39] have studied water content of the intervertebral disc in relationship to age, proteoglycan content, and degeneration in the lumbar spine. His study has clearly shown that both proteoglycan content and water content decrease with age, degeneration, and the particular spinal level studied. Such a diminished capacity of the proteoglycans is reflective of a diminished size and number of electronegative glycosaminoglycan proteins. Based on Urban's study, swelling pressure of the disc seems to be more dependent on the proteoglycan/collagen ratio than age or degeneration alone. Furthermore, he found an increase in the ease of extraction of proteoglycans and a decrease in the aggregation of proteoglycans with both age and degeneration. Clearly, both qualitative and quantitative changes in the proteoglycan content of the nucleus pulposus occur with time and degeneration. These changes, by

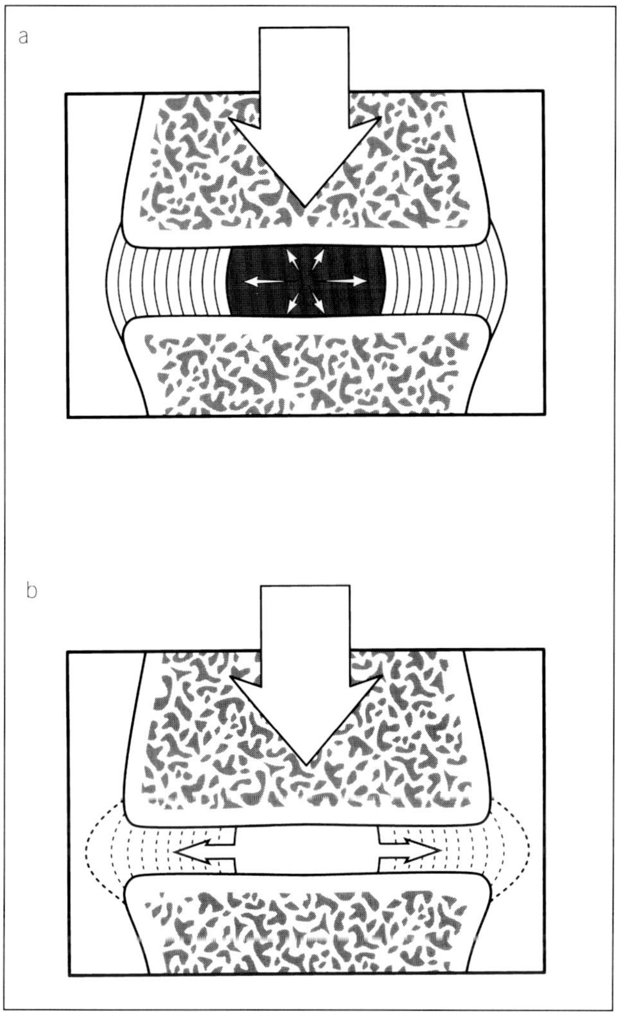

Figure 8.2
(a) Under normal conditions the nucleus pulposus is well hydrated as a result of the high electronegative qualities of the glycosaminoglycan proteins providing even distribution of applied forces across the vertebral end-plates. (b) In degenerative disc disease, qualitative and quantitative changes occur with regard to the proteoglycans leading to a diminished water content and inability to effectively distribute applied force.

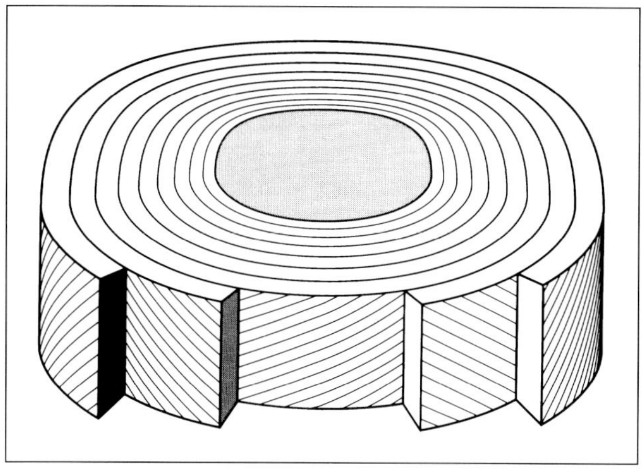

Figure 8.3
The intervertebral disc consists of a nucleus pulposus surrounded by the annulus fibrosis. The annulus is composed of concentric laminated bands of annular fibers. In any two adjacent bands, the fibers are oriented in opposite directions.

definition, lead to a diminished capacity of the disc to hold or bind water, allowing the disc to become more compressible and less elastic.[1,3]

The outer part of the disc, the annulus fibrosis, is made of concentric collagen sheaths loosely bonded together. The fibers are arranged in a helicoid manner, in the same direction for a given band, but in an opposite direction for any two adjacent bands (Fig. 8.3). The annulus is composed of both type I and type II collagen.[15] With degeneration, several changes occur within the collagen of the annulus fibrosis. Type II collagen is slowly replaced with type I collagen; irreducible cross-links among the collagen fibrils increase, and some type III collagen appears. These changes represent a cellular response to a change in the tensile versus compressive loads applied to the disc, which secondarily reflect the quality and quantity of disc hydration.[6,25,26]

As the center of the intervertebral disc dehydrates with age and the nucleus pulposus solidifies, its efficiency in distributing stress from vertical loading decreases. Focal stresses are subsequently created and may lead to tears in the susceptible annulus fibrosis. With time and repetitive microtrauma, the annulus continues to weaken, increasing the potential for herniation of soft disc material.[7] The vertebral end-plates become sclerotic in response to prolonged abnormal stress application.

Such abnormal stresses, which are created in the nucleus pulposus and annulus fibrosis, lead to a loss of the normal mechanical integrity of the cervical disc and may be productive of symptoms initially consistent with mechanical 'instability'. In this early phase of cervical disc degeneration, the involved segment becomes 'unstable', developing excessive, irregular, and asynchronous motion. This 'instability' leaves

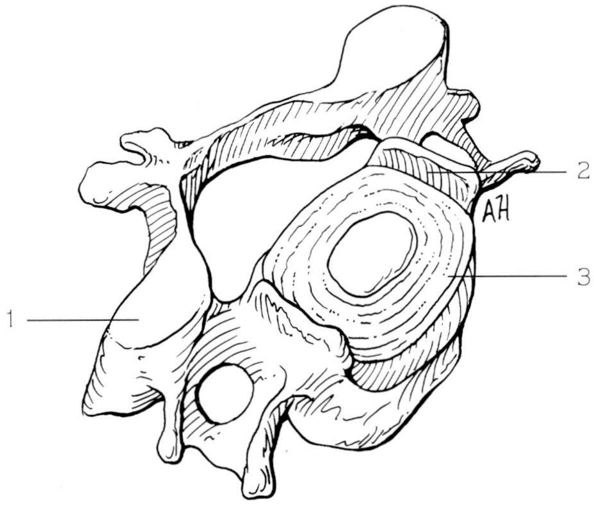

Figure 8.4
There are five joints in the cervical spine to consider: the intervertebral disc, the two facet joints and two neurocentral joints.

1 Facet joint
2 Neurocentral joint
3 Intervertebral disc

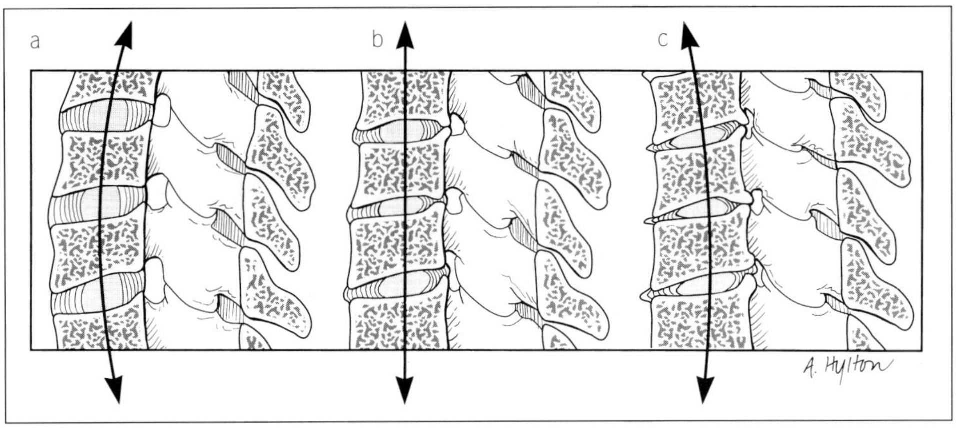

Figure 8.5
(a) Normal cervical lordosis without evidence of degenerative disease. (b) With narrowing of the cervical disc, the neurocentral joints touch and over time lead to the development of osteophytes. (c) Once this occurs, further loss of intervertebral height only occurs anteriorly, leading to a loss of normal cervical lordosis.

the involved intervertebral motion segment and its column of supportive soft tissues vulnerable to injury. Strain of these ligamentous and muscular tissues is often responsible for presenting complaints of neck pain, with referred pain to the shoulder, suboccipital, interscapular, and, occasionally, chest wall regions. Clinical symptoms in this stage are not due to nerve root irritation.

In contrast to the 'three joint complex' of the lumbar spine, the lower five cervical intervertebral articulations must be understood as a 'five joint complex', including the intervertebral disc anteriorly, the two zygoapophyseal joints posteriorly, and the two uncovertebral or neurocentral articulations (Fig. 8.4). With the onset of disc degeneration and subsequent loss of normal hydrophilic qualities of the nucleus pulposus as described, the intervertebral disc loses height, and further stress is applied to both the facet and neurocentral articulations. The bony prominences of the neurocentral joints converge slowly over time as the disc height lessens, and eventually touch, leading to a formation of osteophytes.[28] Thereafter, further loss of intervertebral height can only occur anteriorly, leading to loss of normal cervical lordosis (Fig. 8.5). The resulting combined forces additionally stress the posterior facet joints and their capsuloligamentous support structures. In addition, these joints develop typical hypertrophic changes associated with the degenerative process.

The osteophytic outgrowths that develop about the neurocentral and zygoapophyseal joints may lead to narrowing of the nerve root canal. Symptoms consistent with radiculopathy may evolve with significant impingement and inflammation of the cervical nerve root. Such osteophyte formation producing isolated nerve root impingement is generally referred to as hard disc pathology (Figs 8.6 and 8.7).

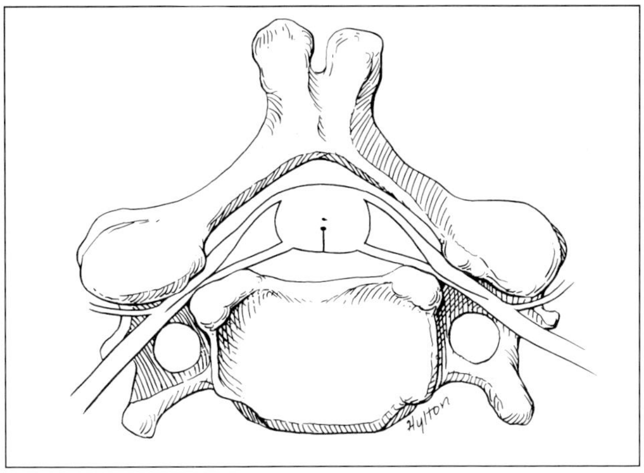

Figure 8.6
Osteophytes formed from the neurocentral and zygoapophyseal articulations produce a narrowing of the neural foramina and subsequent nerve root impingement.

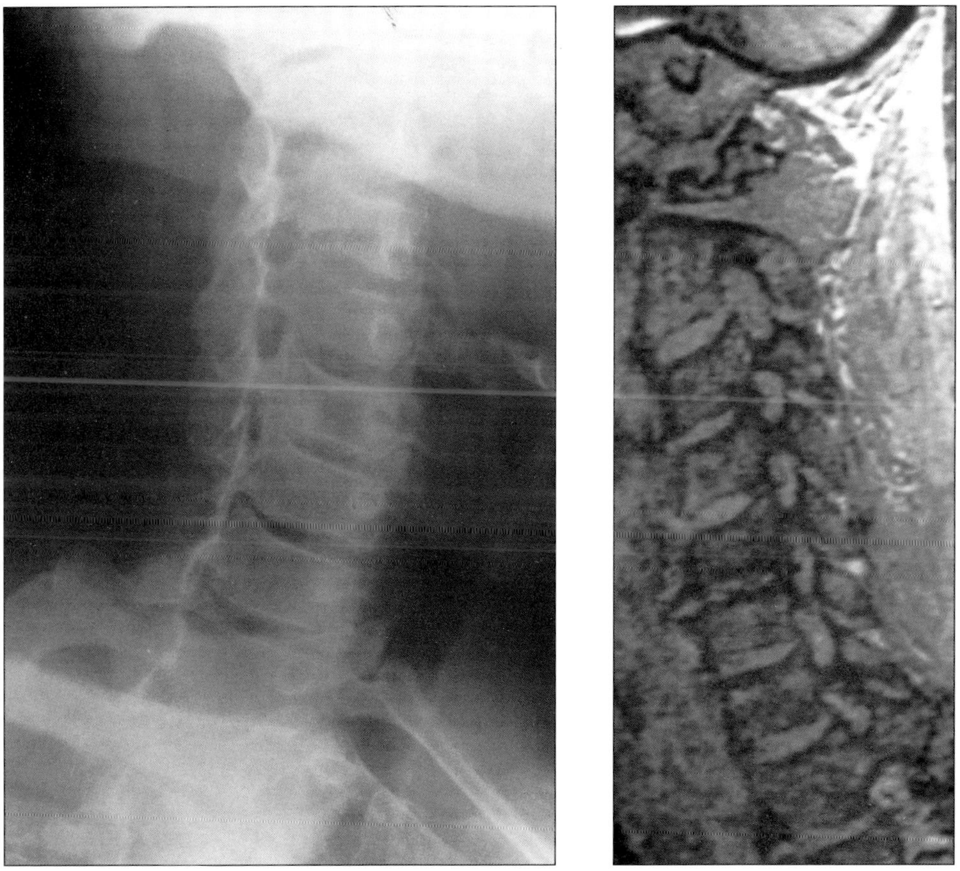

Figure 8.7
(left) An oblique radiograph of the cervical spine showing foraminal narrowing of C5–C6 and C6–C7. (right) A 45° oblique MRI showing C5–C6 neurocentral encroachment of C6 nerve root.

As already alluded to, soft disc herniation may occur at any time in this cascade of degenerative pathologic events. Circumferential and radial tears in the annular ring may allow for the gradual or sudden extrusion of nucleus pulposus. Three types of soft disc herniation have been described by Stookey[37] and Rothman and Marvel[33] (Figs 8.8 and 8.9). An intraforaminal herniation is the most common and frequently gives radicular symptoms in a dermatomal distribution. Posterolateral soft discs produce mostly motor findings of weakness and atrophy, whereas midline herniations may produce a myelopathy. When such soft disc herniation occurs early in the degenerative process, the

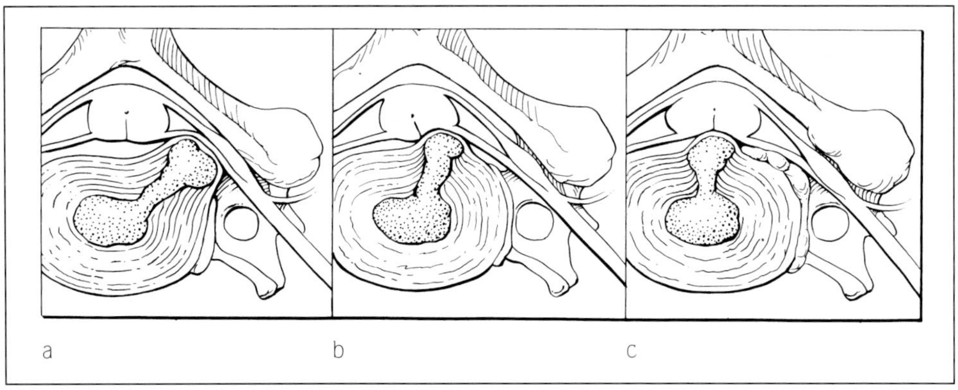

Figure 8.8
Types of soft disc protrusion: (a) intraforaminal is most common; (b) posterolateral produces mostly motor signs; and (c) midline may manifest as myelopathy.

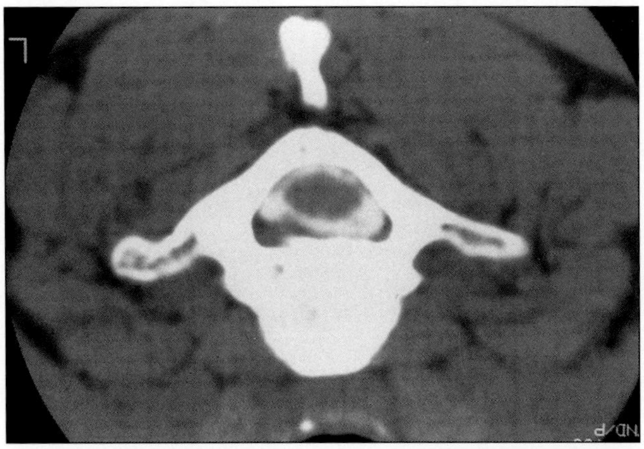

a

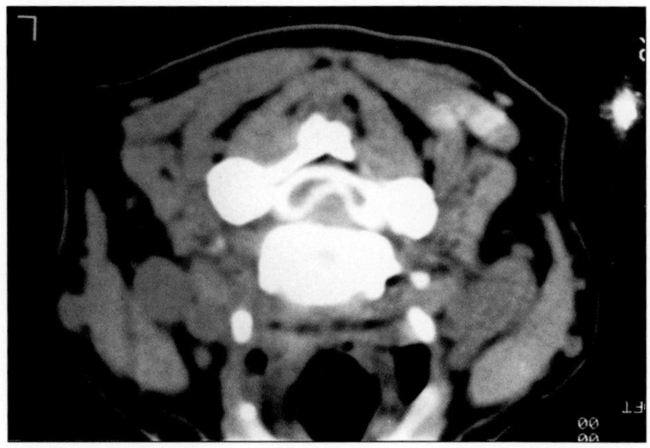

c

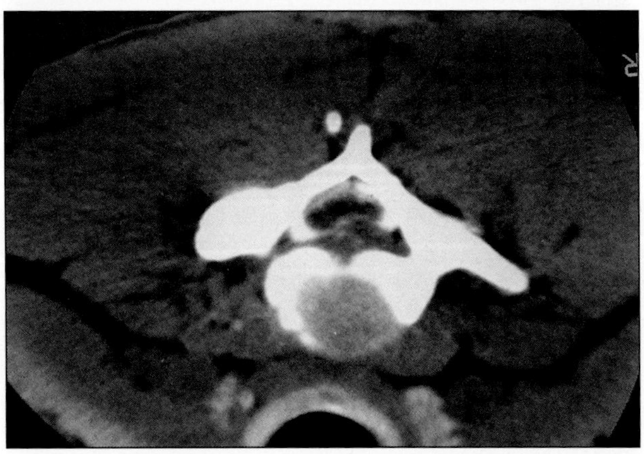

b

Figure 8.9
Post-myelography computed tomogram of soft disc herniation: (a) intraforaminal type; (b) posterolateral type; and (c) midline type.

material will tend to do so in a typical intraforaminal or posterolateral direction producing unilateral radicular symptoms. The posterior longitudinal ligament supplies additional strength and stability to the posterocentral fibers of the annulus, producing a relative weakness in the posterolateral corners of the disc, accounting for such a distribution.

In the later stages of the degenerative process, any concomitant soft disc herniation usually involves a different pathway. Hypertrophic changes in the neurocentral joints act as a protective wall, virtually eliminating any potential for direct posterolateral compression of the nerve root. Rupture of the soft disc at this stage usually occurs centrally and may cause cord compression and long tract findings

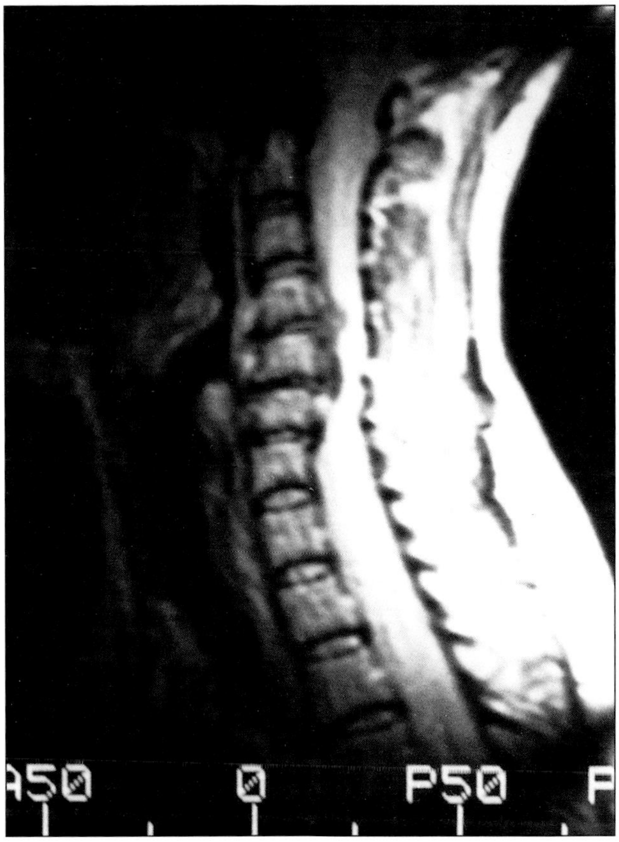

Figure 8.10
T2-weighted sagittal MRI showing spinal cord compression secondary to multi-level cervical spondylosis.

on physical examination. Occasionally, both nerve root and spinal cord may be affected under such conditions and produce a myeloradiculopathy (Fig. 8.10).

More commonly, however, in the advanced degenerative stage, the intervertebral disc tends to have a configuration of a generalized central bulge. This diffusely bulging disc will eventually produce a transverse bar of bone at the discal edge of the vertebral body. With significant posterior protrusion, with or without the combined effects of posterior hypertrophic pathology, the anteroposterior diameter of the spinal canal becomes narrowed. Compression of the spinal cord in this manner may also impair vascular flow to the cord and further the development of a progressive myelopathy.[35]

Under uncommon circumstances, the development of significant lateral hypertrophic changes in the neurocentral joints may impinge upon the vertebral artery foramen. Minor degrees of vertebral artery compression may produce 'vertebral artery syndrome', whereas severe compression or kinking of the artery may result in vertebral artery thrombosis. If such thrombosis does occur, it may then extend in a superior direction and involve the posteroinferior cerebellar artery, occlusion of which can lead to the development of Wallenberg's syndrome with symptoms including palsy of the ipsilateral spinal nerves V, IX, X, and XI, Horner's syndrome, cerebellar ataxia, contralateral loss of pain and temperature sensation, dysphagia, palatal weakness, vocal fold paralysis, and nystagmus.

Attention should also be given to the development of degenerative subluxation of the cervical spine. The 'sloppiness' of the intervertebral disc articulation, and subsequent development of facet joint incompetence through erosion, can lead to subluxation either in the form of spondylolisthesis or retrolisthesis. It is important to realize the potential for dynamic subluxation as well. Evaluation of the cervical spine with flexion–extension radiographs is advised and often helpful to explain the active processes responsible for production of clinical symptoms.

In conclusion, cervical disc disease represents a cascade of events probably initiated through biochemical and physiologic alterations in the intervertebral disc. Quantitative and qualitative changes in the proteoglycans of the nucleus pulposus with subsequent loss of its hydrophilic qualities lead to a sequence of events affecting all five articulations of a given cervical motion segment. Hypertrophic changes in the facet and neurocentral joints, with or without soft disc protrusion, most often occur without symptoms, but may lead to symptoms resulting from these mechanical alterations or compression of the nerve root or spinal cord.

NATURAL HISTORY OF CERVICAL DISC DISEASE

The cervical spine serves two main functions: first, it is responsible for support of the occiput while permitting motion in all three axes; second, it serves as a protective conduit for the spinal cord and cervical nerve roots. The unique and various articulations of the cervical spine provide a high degree of motion at the same time as protecting the neurologic structures from harm. As long as the intervertebral segment maintains its normal structural relationship, the functions are well preserved. However, with the described degenerative processes, both motion and protection of neural structures may be compromised. The clinical symptoms are reflective of the location and type of neurologic compromise or structural injury.

Degenerative change is, by nature, not a reversible process. The morphologic changes as seen and described in this chapter tend to be progressive on a chronic basis. In contrast, however, to this seemingly inevitable course, the various clinical syndromes do exhibit variable natural histories. The very fact that, in most circumstances, significant radiographic evidence of spondylotic disease is not necessarily correlated with clinical symptomatology, is credit to the fact that we understand very little about pain production. The proposed mechanisms of pain production are varied and not completely understood. Potential contributors to the scheme of pain production include the direct compressive effect of osteophytes or herniated disc material, vascular insufficiency, inflammatory mechanisms, mechanical instability, as well as muscular and sympathetic pain. It is probable that all of these stated factors play some role in the production of pain in the various clinical syndromes during the described degenerative process.

When considering cervical disc degeneration, three clinical syndromes can generally be identified and require discussion, including neck pain, radiculopathy, and myelopathy. Although each of these clinical entities share in part a common pathoetiologic pathway, the natural history of each disorder is unique and must be clearly understood by the treating physician.

Successful treatment of degenerative cervical syndromes is usually dependent on identification of the specific problem. By careful elicitation of a complete history of the patient's symptoms and pain, the physician must attempt to correlate these symptoms to physical findings, and appropriate radiographic and other diagnostic testing. With the problem identified, specific treatment can be initiated. Knowledge of the natural history, and medical and surgical therapy options, for each clinical syndrome is necessary to provide both rational and optimal treatment recommendation. Patient education is also quite important, and should not be underestimated. If patients understand their specific medical problem, its potential outcomes, and treatment modalities, many of the anxieties and fears that accompany such disorders may be relieved and treatment expedited.

This section will review the clinical syndromes associated with cervical disc disease and their respective natural histories.

NECK AND REFERRED PAIN

Neck pain or cervical strain is the most common clinical manifestation of underlying cervical spondylotic disease and can be the most frustrating to treat for both physician and patient. It represents the mildest form of cervical disc disease and may be acute or chronic. It is difficult to determine whether alterations in the cervical disc alone are responsible for the production of neck pain. Because of the ubiquitous nature of radiographic findings consistent with disc degeneration and spondylosis, it is an impossible task to correlate these findings directly to isolated symptoms of neck pain. Many patients who complain of axial pain have been subjected to disc excision, fusion, and even laminectomy with variable, and often disturbing, results.

The pattern of pain and complaints among this group of patients is generally consistent. Complaints of neck pain most commonly affect the paramedian musculature of the neck posteriorly, and are usually associated with some stiffness, limited motion, muscular spasm, and headache. Referred pain is common and tends to be distributed into the trapezius, rhomboids, and interscapular regions. These symptoms are generally relieved with rest, immobilization, heat, and massage, and may be made worse by higher levels of activity or stress.

Headaches are a common complaint and affect one-third of all patients with associated symptoms of neck pain. Suboccipital headache or occipital vertex headache may actually be the predominant complaint in a smaller percentage of these patients. How degenerative disc disease of the cervical spine causes headaches is unclear, but these are often attributed to irritation of the greater occipital nerve, which originates from the posterior rami of C2, C3, and C4; headache may develop through irritation of the nerve from reflex spasm in the trapezius muscle with subsequent compression of the greater occipital nerve as it penetrates the cervical spine. Bogduk,[4] however, has shown that the greater occipital nerve does not pierce the trapezius muscle, and therefore it is unclear whether this mechanism can in fact be responsible for these symptoms. Cailliet[8] has suggested that tension myositis was responsible for generating symptoms of headache in both the occipital and suboccipital regions. Again, however, this theory remains unproven.

Neck pain as an isolated complaint is often attributed to abnormalities in the cervical structures innervated by the sinovertebral nerve. Each cervical nerve root gives rise to a sinovertebral nerve near the ramus communicans. This nerve then re-enters the intervertebral foramen and proceeds upwards toward the midline, innervating the posterior longitudinal ligament, the dura, the epidural vasculature, and the spinal periosteum. The facet joints are innervated by a branch of the posterior primary ramus at each spinal segment[5] (Fig. 8.11).

It seems plausible that some of these pain patterns could be mediated by these nerve structures, although this remains unproved. Investigators have performed provocative injections and diagnostic blocks in attempts at better delineation of the source of neck pain with results that generally are less than helpful. Provocative injection of a cervical disc space and facet joints produces only ill-defined patterns of pain and paresthesias. Dwyer et al[14] have recently published a report of provocative zygoapophyseal injections in normal volunteers and derived cutaneous maps of the different segmental pain patterns from these injections. These patterns were then used to treat a group of symptomatic patients with facet blocks. It is not known, however, whether the natural history of neck pain, thought to be secondary to inflammatory changes about the facet

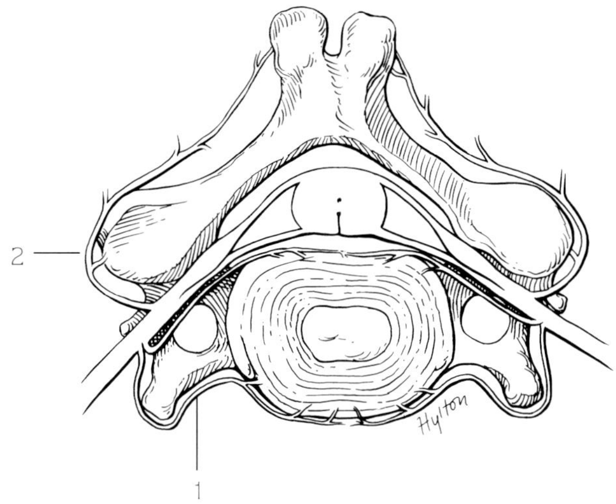

Figure 8.11
Cross-sectional view demonstrating the sinovertebral nerve and posterior ramus.

1 Sinuvertebral nerve
2 Posterior ramus

joint, can be significantly altered using these techniques. Further controlled, randomized, blind studies are needed.

Discography of the cervical disc has also been employed in an attempt to localize neck pain. Whitecloud and Seago[40] have reported 70% good results with anterior cervical fusion in a group of patients with isolated neck pain and positive provocative disc injection. The number of levels operated on ranged from one to three in this study, with better results seen in those patients with symptoms isolated to a single level. Again, however, one must ask whether the reported success rate of 70% is significantly better than the natural history of neck pain secondary to degenerative disc disease alone.

The natural history of untreated neck pain carries with it a guarded prognosis. Gore et al[18] reviewed the long-term follow-up of 205 patients with neck pain, and came to several conclusions. In this 10-year study of neck pain, 79% of those patients were found to be improved, although only 43% of patients were considered pain-free. Thirty-two of those patients, or nearly one-third, had moderately severe residual pain. Patients reporting more severe initial pain were, in fact, found to be more likely to be involved in litigation and frequently found to have an unsatisfactory outcome. Finally, it was also made clear from this study that outcome and treatment are difficult to predict from the clinical and radiographic data on initial presentation. DePalma found that most patients with cervical spondylosis and symptoms of neck pain without radiculopathy can exhibit a reasonable course.[13] After 3 months of non-operative care, in a relatively large group of patients, he found that 21% of all patients had complete relief of their symptoms, 49% had partial relief, and 22% had no relief. Rothman and Rashbaum[34] observed and reported on a similar group of patients for 5 years and found that 23% of them remained partially or totally disabled.

In the absence of controlled studies that indicate whether cervical pain can, in fact, be relieved or improved by removal of degenerated disc, and specific studies indicating to the surgeon which disc should be removed, we are left with the concept that, in most cases, axial pain cannot be treated by surgery on the cervical disc. Surgical intervention has proved successful when degenerative pathology manifests itself through neurologic deficit. However, in the absence of neurologic deficit, surgical intervention for neck pain holds no better prognosis than the natural history of the process itself. Consequently, the remainder of this discussion will consider radiating pain secondary to either nerve root or spinal cord compression.

CERVICAL RADICULOPATHY

Cervical radiculopathy represents the most common symptom complex requiring surgical intervention. Any segment of the lower cervical spine (C2 C3 to C7 T1) may be involved, although most disc herniations occur at either C5–C6 or C6–C7. The clinical complaints and physical findings associated with each of these cervical nerve roots are covered thoroughly in Chapter 4.

Cervical nerve root irritation can be either acute, subacute, or chronic. Nerve roots may be involved unilaterally or bilaterally with varying degrees of symmetry. The onset of such symptoms may be related to some known trauma or occur spontaneously. In the younger patient, the onset of radicular pain is most often isolated to a single nerve root and the result of a posterolateral soft disc herniation near the entrance zone of the foramen. Free or sequestered disc fragments may also be found within the neuroforamen. Epidural migration of the sequestered disc is rare but has been reported. The development of symptoms in the younger patient is often precipitated by some recalled traumatic event.

Older patients with pre-existing cervical spondylosis may present with either monoradicular or polyradicular symptoms. In contrast to the younger patient, these symptoms often develop insidiously with no responsible traumatic event. Spondylosis, manifest by neurocentral joint osteophyte formation, will compress the nerve root anteriorly, causing the radicular syndrome. Less frequently, osteophytes from the tip of the superior articular process may cause symptomatic foraminal narrowing. Loss of disc height additionally leads to reduced neuroforaminal volume, rendering the nerve root more susceptible to compression. More often than not, the process is multifactorial, with each of these anatomic features contributing to the clinical presentation. Failure of such symptoms to improve can lead to the development of a chronic radiculopathy. Conservative care of radicular symptoms under these circumstances often fails.

Classically, manifestations of sensory, reflex, and motor deficits are found within the distribution of the affected nerve root and comprise the symptom complex associated with cervical radiculopathy. Radicular patterns result in some sensory symptoms in nearly all patients. Sensory findings, however, may be in the form of paresthesias, hyperalgesias, or hyperesthesias. Such sensory changes do not always follow discrete dermatomal patterns. Despite the dermatomal charts committed to memory, the degree of functional overlap among the various cervical nerve roots provides for variable findings from patient to patient. In Henderson's large series of 841 patients, he found only 55% of patients to describe a classic distribution of radicular pain, whereas 45% presented with a more diffuse, non-dermatomal pattern.[20] This occurs as each spinal nerve root supplies pain fibers to muscles, joints, and bone over a broad area. The fact that patients' symptoms often do not follow a particular dermatomal pattern does not exclude the existence of a symptomatic nerve root. Such non-dermatomal patterns should be distinguished from pseudoradiculopathy. Patients with pseudoradiculopathy will give a history of radiating upper extremity pain with associated numbness or paresthesias, but without objective physical findings. These patients fail to have any findings of weakness or reflex damage on examination which correlate with their pain. Provocative testing also fails to reproduce or exacerbate pain.

Motor and reflex changes occur frequently, and are more commonly appreciated in those patients with a chronic radiculopathy. Henderson et al[20] and Lunsford et al[27] found specific motor deficits in 68% and 61% of patients respectively. Diminished reflexes are found in approximately 70%. The actual reflex and motor deficits seem somewhat dependent on the degree and position of nerve compression as well as the relative contribution of that root to the musculotendinous unit being tested. In some patients, compression of the C6 nerve will lead to depression or absence of the biceps reflex. In others, an abnormal brachioradialis reflex or wrist extensor reflex can be elicited. Motor weakness is also subject to variability. Given the known and described variations in brachial plexus anatomy, such variability is not surprising. Furthermore, both intradural and extradural anastomoses have been described and may also account for variability in clinical presentation.

Clinically, there are several maneuvers which may in fact elicit or provoke patient symptoms. Spurling's sign is a classic maneuver involving extension of the neck, which leads to further narrowing of the neuroforamen in reproduction of neurogenic arm pain. Extension and lateral rotation to the affected side may further augment neuroforaminal narrowing and worsen patient symptoms.

Other clinical signs just as suggestive of radiculopathy have also been described. Davidson et al[12] described a shoulder abduction relief sign. With this maneuver, patients often get significant relief of their arm pain with the shoulder held in the abducted position. This is considered by many to be a pathognomonic sign shown, for example, when patients enter the physician's office with the shoulder held in the abducted position for relief of symptoms. Beatty et al[2] believe that this sign is highly specific for soft disc herniation, but was not likely to be present in those patients with radiculopathy secondary to spondylosis.

The differential diagnosis of neck, shoulder, and arm pain is extensive and will only be reviewed briefly. Focal upper extremity entrapment syndromes probably represent the most common differential diagnosis to make in patients with such presenting complaints. Entrapments involving the median, ulnar, and radial nerves, as well as the neurovascular structures in the thoracic outlet, may all contribute to a symptom complex similar to but distinguishable from cervical radiculopathy. The concomitant presence of neck pain in patients with these focal upper extremity entrapment syndromes may, however, make this differentiation more difficult, although the absence of positive provocative tests, such as Spurling's maneuver, would be strong evidence against a cervical radiculopathy.

Complaints secondary to shoulder disease usually include some combination of pain, stiffness, instability, or weakness. These symptoms may therefore be found to mimic a proximal cervical radiculopathy. However, findings on physical examination usually give a clear indication of whether one is dealing with a primary shoulder problem rather than a cervical radiculopathy. Common diagnoses in the shoulder which may, in fact, mimic cervical radiculopathy include impingement syndrome, rotator cuff tears, subacromial bursitis, degenerative disease of the acromioclavicular or glenohumeral joints, adhesive capsulitis, calcific tendinitis, or instability. Weakness is a sign that often presents with either a cervical radiculopathy or the painful shoulder. Large tears in the rotator cuff can lead to significant weakness, especially with shoulder abduction. This can easily mimic a C5 radiculopathy. Careful examination may, however, also delineate some weakness in other C5 innervated muscles, namely the biceps and pectoralis major with nerve root compromise.

Both intraspinal and extraspinal tumors may also give rise to symptoms causing confusion with cervical radiculopathy.

These tumors may be either malignant or benign. Intraspinal tumors, such as giant cell tumor, aneurysmal bone cyst, osteoid osteoma, osteoblastoma, fibrous dysplasia, eosinophilic granuloma, and hemangioma may lead to the development of neurologic symptoms with appropriate neurologic compression. Numerous extraspinal tumors may also cause cervical radiculopathy. Tumors of the thyroid, upper esophagus, pharynx, and apical carcinomas of the lung (Pancoast's tumors) may encroach upon the brachial plexus or subclavian vessels, and again mimic symptoms consistent with cervical radiculopathy.

Other potential disorders mimicking cervical radiculopathy include brachial plexus disorders, such as idiopathic brachial neuritis or brachial plexopathy, reflex sympathetic dystrophy, and angina.

The natural history of cervical radiculopathy is well reviewed. Lees and Turner[24] found that cervical radiculopathy only rarely progresses to myelopathy, but generally leads to some persisting symptoms in nearly two-thirds of all patients treated non-surgically. In a 5-year study of non-operative care which included 69% of all patients with both neck and radicular pain and 31% of patients with neck pain alone, the conclusions were that only 45% of these resolved satisfactorily without surgery. Of the 55% who had persistent symptoms, 23% were completely disabled.[34]

In a series of 20 athletes with acute cervical radiculopathy treated conservatively, 17 were able to return to full activity at an average of 17 weeks. Neurologic motor deficits generally improved by 5 months.[35]

Table 8.1 Symptoms and signs at initial presentation of patients with cervical spondylotic myelopathy

Symptoms and signs	*Incidence (%)*
Spasticity	98
Weakness	65
Spinothalamic deficit	58
Posterior column deficit	53
Small muscle atrophy	53
Fasciculations	48
Sphincter disturbances	44
Local cervical pain	42
Radicular pain	39
Paresthetic pain	34
L'hermitte's sign	27
Dermatomal sensory deficit	16
Segmental sensory deficit	11

Adapted from Grandall PH, Batzdorf U. Cervical spondylotic myelopathy. *J Neurosurg* 1966; 24: 57–66, with permission.

CERVICAL MYELOPATHY

Disc degeneration can lead to spinal cord compression in several ways. Most commonly, myelopathy is the result of severe spondylotic changes superimposed on a congenitally narrower spinal canal. In the absence of cervical spondylosis, a large central disc herniation may precipitate myelopathy.

Cervical spondylotic myelopathy has a diverse clinical presentation, with no pathognomonic signs or symptoms. The diagnosis is established by the demonstration of physical signs of upper motor neuron dysfunction resulting from spinal cord compression. Other causes of upper motor neuron disease which may mimic cervical spondylotic myelopathy should be sought.

Cervical myelopathy usually manifests itself as a slowly progressive disability over a period of several months or years. The natural history is nevertheless one of progression. Patients with myelopathy are usually in their sixth or seventh decade of life and present with initial complaints of dysesthesia, weakness, and clumsiness of the hands. Pain is not a dominant complaint. Lower extremity weakness may also be found. More profound weakness of the lower extremity, gait disturbances, and bowel and bladder dysfunction are consistent with a more severe, chronic myelopathy.

In contrast to cervical radiculopathy, pain is not a common presenting symptom. Crandall and Batzdorf[11] noted radicular pain or paresthetic pain in 39% and 34% of their patients respectively, whereas spasticity and weakness were noted in 98% and 65% of their patients respectively (Table 8.1). Patients often find it difficult to express both the discomfort and the dysfunction associated with their disorder. The symptom complex seems to be so widespread in its affect that localizing symptoms are not seen.

The physical signs of myelopathy usually represent a mixture of both upper and lower motor neuron findings. As mentioned earlier, patients' gait is awkward, shuffling, and slow. In severe cases of myelopathy, the patient may be completely ataxic. Deep tendon reflexes can be absent or depressed at the level of compression. Patients may have findings consistent with cervical nerve root impingement in conjunction with their cervical myelopathy. Muscle atrophy may also be evident on examination, especially with advanced hand dysfunction. Muscular fasciculations and motor weakness can be seen and are usually evident in the same involved neurologic distribution.

Long tract findings are seen below the level of the lesions. In a patient with isolated cervical stenosis and cord compression at the C4–C5 segment, examination will usually reveal an absence of the biceps reflex with associated biceps weakness, hyperreflexia of the brachioradialis and triceps reflex, and a positive Hoffman's sign in the same upper extremity. Examination of the lower extremities will usually demonstrate varying degrees of spasticity, hyperreflexia, weakness, clonus, and positive Babinski's sign.

Hand dysfunction has been a subject of interest in patients with cervical myelopathy. Such information has been available only in the last few years. Ono et al[30] have described the myelopathic hand syndrome, including a group of patients distinguished by specific motor and sensory abnormalities. The finger escape sign is characterized by deficient adduction, extension, or both, of the two or three ulnar digits of the affected hand. These same patients may also exhibit an inability to open and close the fist rapidly. A normal patient is capable of opening and closing his or her hand more than 20 times in a period of 10 seconds. The patient with myelopathy finds this maneuver quite difficult and can only perform it slowly and incompletely. These same patients may also exhibit marked hypalgesia in a non-dermatomal pattern extending into the dorsal part of the forearm. In addition, Ono found that 75% of patients with myelopathy of the hand had associated decreased sensation over the lateral aspect of the legs and feet. These symptoms are believed to be indicative of pyramidal tract involvement of the cervical spine above the level of C7.[30]

Myelopathy has been classified in various ways, and the most frequently used classifications include those of Ferguson and Caplan,[16] and Crandall and Batzdorf.[11]

Classification of Ferguson and Caplan

Ferguson and Caplan categorized spondylosis with nerve involvement into four distinct, but somewhat overlapping, syndromes including lateral, medial, combined, and vascular syndromes.

Lateral Syndrome

This syndrome represents a spondylotic radiculopathy rather than a myelopathy. Long tract signs are absent. Patients complain of pain and paresthesias in a typical radicular fashion with possible weakness or reflex change in a muscle group innervated by a specific cervical nerve root. Decrease in pain or temperature sensation, typical of motor neuron nerve involvement, may also be present.

Medial Syndrome

Upper motor neuron symptoms are the predominant feature of this syndrome. Fine motor movements of the upper extremities are clumsy. The patient's gait may be wide-based and spastic, especially in advanced levels of myelopathy. Patients generally complain of weakness in all extremities. Bowel or bladder incontinence is uncommon, but when present, represents a poor prognostic sign.

Combined Medial and Lateral Syndrome

This represents the most common clinical presentation. Patients have combined symptoms and findings as reflected above in both lateral and medial syndromes.

Vascular Syndrome

Patients present with acute onset and rapidly progressive myelopathy. This is known to be in contrast to the insidious onset of symptoms seen in most forms of cervical spondylotic myelopathy. This syndrome is rare, but thought to reflect compression or insufficiency of the anterior spinal artery and its branches to the spinal cord. It appears to be unaffected by surgical intervention.

Classification of Crandall and Batzdorf

The classification of Crandall and Batzdorf subdivides myelopathic patients into groups of spinal cord dysfunction.

Transverse Lesion Syndrome

This syndrome has little effect on the upper extremities. This lesion, which is the most common, reflects involvement of the posterior column, spinothalamic, and corticospinal tracts. Posterior column dysfunction is, however, an uncommon and late feature of cervical spondylotic myelopathy. Anterior horn cells are often involved in this syndrome.

Motor System Syndrome

The motor system syndrome is associated with a predominance of corticospinal tract and anterior horn cell involvement. Sensory complaints are minimal. Upper and lower extremity weakness, gait disturbance, and spasticity predominate. Sensory complaints are minimal. These patients may be wrongly given a diagnosis of amyotrophic lateral sclerosis.

Central Cord Syndrome

The symptoms for this syndrome are analogous to those seen in patients with spinal cord injury. Upper extremities are typically weaker than lower extremities. Hand weakness is often profound. Involvement of the posterior columns may manifest as painful paresthesias and dysesthesias of the hands.

Brown–Séquard Syndrome

This syndrome involves unilateral spinal cord compression or dysfunction, and generally represents an early form of cervical spondylotic myelopathy. Involvement of the corticospinal tract function leads to ipsilateral hemiparesis with pain and temperature analgesia occurring one or two levels below the highest level of motor involvement. This syndrome typically has the best prognosis for recovery.

Brachialgia Cord Syndrome

This syndrome represents combined upper extremity nerve root compression in conjunction with long tract findings secondary to cord compression. This is analogous to Ferguson and Caplan's combined medial and lateral syndrome.

An understanding of the natural history of cervical spondylotic myelopathy is important for assessing the results of treatment modalities. Unfortunately, it is impossible for the physician to predict progression of disease and symptoms. Most clinicians agree, however, that the onset of symptoms is insidious and that the symptoms are generally stable, marked with episodic worsening. Overall, the disease course is one of stepwise degeneration with time.

Clarke and Robinson's[9] report on 120 patients with cervical myelopathy provides the first examination of the natural history of cervical spondylotic myelopathy. In their study, 75% of patients had episodic symptoms, 20% had slow progression, and 5% had a rapid deterioration. Age at presentation and symptom duration were shown in this study to be the most important factors affecting prognosis. Increased age at presentation is associated with overall poorer results. When symptoms of myelopathy have been present for more than one year, the chances for improvement are poor. Spontaneous regression was highly uncommon. However, 50% of the patients improved with immobilization through use of a cervical collar.

Lees and Turner[24] reported on a long-term study of 95 patients with cervical spondylosis. They found that myelopathy rarely develops in patients with radiographic evidence of spondylosis followed for a long period of time. A total of 44 patients in this study were observed for periods of 3–40 years. Most of these patients experienced episodes of worsening symptoms generally followed by a return to baseline symptoms or occasionally mild improvement. Repetitive episodes of progressive symptoms generally left the patients worse with time, establishing a step-like degenerative process. These quiescent periods could be either short or long, depending on the individual. They noted no relationship between prognosis and the age of onset. Lees and Turner concluded from this study that the disease generally had a benign course as only a very few patients experienced steady gradual deterioration. Their recommendation, based on this study, was for conservative therapy.

Nurick[29] reported findings similar to those of Lees and Turner. He noted an initial phase of worsening followed by static periods often lasting several years. The degree of disability seemed to be established early in the disease process and changed little with time. He noted, as did Lees and Turner, an initial phase of worsening symptoms followed by static periods often lasting for many years. The disability associated with the myelopathy generally remained static except in older patients in whom it seemed to progress.

Symon and Lavender[38] have generally disagreed with the findings of Lees and Turner. As opposed to the rather optimistic findings of 55% improvement quoted by Lees and Turner, Symon and Lavender believe that only 18% of those patients actually showed improvement; 67% of Symon and Lavender's patients had steady, progressive deterioration, indicating that cervical spondylotic myelopathy is unlikely to have a benign course.

In short, these studies seem to indicate that the disease of cervical spondylotic myelopathy is benign only in the sense that progression to total disability is generally unusual after a patient's initial presentation. There may be only small changes in disability for a course of several years. However, improvement in the disability status of an individual patient or complete recovery is extremely rare. Episodic worsening is the course to be expected in the untreated individual. Unfortunately, such a natural history makes it difficult for the treating physician to prescribe treatment. The authors have not been able to demonstrate factors identifying the patient at risk for rapid progression. It seems clear that those patients who are experiencing rapid progression are best treated with early surgical intervention. For those patients without rapid progression, treatment should be individualized. For those patients presenting with a moderate-to-severe degree of disability, more aggressive therapy is usually indicated. The unlikely chance of spontaneous improvement in these cases precludes extensive attempts at conservative therapy. It is believed that surgical intervention may, in fact, be able to alter the natural history of the disease process. Studies by Signorini et al,[36] Reale,[32] and Phillips[31] have identified good prognostic indicators for surgical treatment. These include symptom duration of less than one year, unilateral motor deficit, young age at presentation, and the presence of L'hermitte's sign.

SUMMARY

Degenerative disc disease of the cervical spine is a common disorder with an array of clinical syndromes reflective of the anatomic structures involved. Symptoms may range from simple neck pain to a rapidly progressive cervical myelopathy. Each clinical syndrome must be recognized as having its own distinct natural history, clinical symptoms, physical findings, prognosis, and indications for surgical intervention. A thorough understanding of these pathophysiologic processes and clinical syndrome is necessary by the surgeon to optimize recognition of the various disorders and their consequences.

REFERENCES

1 Adams CBT, Logue V. Studies in cervical spondylotic myelopathy. I, II, and III. *Brain* **94**: 557–594, 1971.
2 Beatty RM, Fowler FD, Hanson EJ. The abducted arm as a sign of ruptured cervical disc. *Neurosurgery* **21**: 731–732, 1987.
3 Blumenkrantz N, Sylvest J, Asboe-Hansen G. Local low collagen content may allow herniation of intervertebral disc: Biochemical studies. *Biochem Med* **18**: 283–290, 1977.
4 Bogduk N. The clinical anatomy of the cervical dorsal rami. *Spine* **7**: 319–320, 1982.
5 Borenstein DG, Weisel SW (eds). *Low Back Pain: Medical Diagnosis and Management.* Philadelphia: WB Saunders, 1989.
6 Brickley-Parsons D, Glimcher MJ. Is the chemistry of collagen in the intervertebral disc an expression of Wolff's law? A study of the human lumbar spine. *Spine* **9**: 148–163, 1984.
7 Brown MD. The pathophysiology of disc disease. *Orthop Clin North Am* **2**: 359–370, 1971.
8 Cailliet R. *Neck and Arm Pain*, 37–41. Philadelphia: FA Davis, 1964.
9 Clarke E, Robinson P. Cervical myelopathy: A complication of cervical spondylosis. *Brain* **79**: 483–510, 1956.
10 Coventry MB, Ghormley RK, Kernohan JW. The intervertebral disc: Its microscopic anatomy and pathology. Part III. Pathologic changes in the intervertebral disc. *J Bone Joint Surg [Am]* **27**: 460–474, 1945.
11 Crandall PH, Batzdorf U. Cervical spondylotic myelopathy. J. *Neurosurg* **25**: 57–66, 1966.
12 Davidson RI, Dunn EJ, Metzmaker JN. The shoulder abduction test in the diagnosis of radicular pain in certain extradural compressive monoradiculopathies. *Spine* **6**: 441–446, 1981.
13 DePalma A, Rothman RH, Lewinnek G, et al. Anterior interbody fusion for severe cervical disc degeneration. *Surg Gynecol Obstet* **134**: 755–758, 1972.
14 Dwyer A, Aprill C, Bogduk N. Cervical zygapophyseal joint pain patterns. I. A study in normal volunteers. *Spine* **15**: 453–457, 1990.
15 Eyre DR, Muir H. Type I and II collagens in intervertebral disc. Interchanging radial distributions in annulus fibrosis. *Biochem J* **157**: 267–270, 1976.
16 Ferguson RJL, Caplan LR. Cervical spondylotic myelopathy. *Neurol Clin* **3**: 373–382, 1985.
17 Friberg S, Hirsch C. Anatomical and clinical studies on lumbar disc degeneration. *Acta Orthop Scand* **19**: 222–242, 1949.
18 Gore DR, Sepic SB, Gardner GM. Neck pain: A long-term follow-up of 205 patients. *Spine* **12**: 1–5, 1987.
19 Harris RI, MacNab I. Structural change in the lumbar intervertebral discs. The relationship to low back pain and sciatica. *J Bone Joint Surg [Br]* **36**: 304–322, 1954.
20 Henderson CM, Hennessey R, Shuey H. Posterior lateral foraminotomy for an exclusive operative technique for cervical radiculopathy: A review of 846 consecutively operated cases. *J Neurosurg* **13**: 504–512, 1983.
21 Hopwood JJ, Robinson HC. The structure and composition of cartilage keratin sulfate. *Biochem J* **111**: 517, 1971.
22 Hopwood JJ, Robinson HC. Structural studies on keratin sulfate from cartilage. *Biochem J Molec Aspects* **141**: 524, 1974.
23 Kamano K, Umeyama T. Cervical disc injuries in athletes. *Acta Orthop Trauma Surg* **105**: 223–226, 1986.
24 Lees F, Turner JWA. Natural history and prognosis of cervical spondylosis. *Br Med J* **2**: 1607–1610, 1963.
25 Lipson SJ. Metaplastic proliferative fibrocartilage as an alternative concept to herniated intervertebral disc. *Spine* **13**: 1055–1060, 1988.
26 Lipson SJ, Muir H. Experimental intervertebral disc degeneration. Morphologic and proteoglycan changes over time. *Arthr Rheumat* **24**: 12–21, 1984.
27 Lunsford L, Bissonette DJ, Janetta PJ. Anterior surgery for cervical disc disease. *J Neurosurg* **53**: 1–11, 1980.
28 MacNab I. The whiplash syndrome. *Orthop Clin North Am* **2**: 289–303, 1971.
29 Nurick S. The natural history and the results of surgical treatment of the spinal cord disorder associated with cervical spondylosis. *Brain* **95**: 101–105, 1972.
30 Ono K, Ebara S, Fuji T, et al. Myelopathy hand: New clinical signs of cervical cord damage. *J Bone Joint Surg [Br]* **69**: 215–219, 1987.
31 Phillips DG. Surgical treatment of myelopathy with cervical spondylosis. *J Neurol Neurosurg Psychiatr* **36**: 879–884, 1973.
32 Reale F. Long-term results in 102 cases of cervical myeloradiculopathy operated on for spondylosis and disc herniation. *Ital J Neurol Sci* **3**: 291–296, 1983.
33 Rothman RH, Marvel JP. The acute cervical disc. *Clin Orthop* **109**: 59–68, 1975.
34 Rothman RH, Rashbaum RF. Pathogenesis of signs and symptoms of cervical disc degeneration. In *A.A.O.S. Instructional Course Lectures*, Vol. 27, 1978: 203–215.
35 Rothman RH, Simeone FA (eds). *The Spine*, 2nd ed. Philadelphia: WB Saunders, 1982.
36 Signorini GC, Beltramello A, Pinna G, Dalle Ore G. The significance of preoperative neurologic disorders in predicting outcome of cervical spondylotic myelopathy after surgery. *J Neurosurg Sci* **28**: 89–92, 1984.
37 Stookey B. Compression of spinal cord and nerve roots by herniation of nucleus pulposus in the cervical region. *Arch Surg* **40**: 417–432, 1940.
38 Symon L, Lavender P. The surgical treatment of cervical spondylotic myelopathy. *Neurology* **17**: 117–126, 1967.
39 Urban JPG, McMullin JF. Swelling pressure of the lumbar intervertebral discs: Influence of age, spinal level, composition, and degeneration. *Spine* **13**: 179–187, 1988.
40 Whitecloud TS, Seago RA. Cervical discogenic syndrome: Results of operative intervention in patients with positive discography. *Spine* **12**: 313–316, 1987.

9 Anterior surgical procedures for cervical disc disease

Jeffrey Fischgrund and Harry N. Herkowitz

Degenerative changes within the cervical spine represent ubiquitous radiographic and pathoanatomic findings. Production of clinical symptomatology, however, is less frequent, and generally self-limited. Symptoms may include neck pain with referred pain patterns, radiculopathy, myelopathy, or myeloradiculopathy. Most patients presenting with symptoms that result from degenerative disc disease improve adequately with time or conservative measures, but patients with progressive myelopathy or those with radicular pain refractory to conservative measures become candidates for surgery.

There are always surgical options for any neurocompressive lesion. Anterior, posterior, or combined anteroposterior approaches can be used, depending on the pathoanatomy and evidence of cervical deformity or instability; anterior surgical approaches currently represent the most commonly used approaches. The natural history of cervical disc disease, the indications for surgery, and anterior surgical techniques are reviewed in some detail.

NATURAL HISTORY

Before discussing the surgical treatment of cervical radiculopathy and myelopathy, the natural history of the disease process must be understood. Several authors[12,23,41,43,44,48] have reviewed this subject retrospectively. The results of surgical intervention should be compared to the natural history of the disease before definitive treatment is recommended.

Lees and Turner[41] reported on 95 patients with cervical spondylosis: 51 presented with symptoms of a cervical radiculopathy without evidence of myelopathy. During long-term follow-up (2–19 years), no patient developed myelopathy if it had been absent at initial consultation. Forty-five percent of the study group with radicular pain had only a single episode of pain with no recurrence, 30% continued to have mild symptoms, and 25% had persistent or worsening symptoms. The authors concluded that the symptoms were often relieved by wearing a collar, but that the same final result could be obtained with any or no treatment.

Forty-four of Lees and Turner's patients had radiographic and objective evidence of myelopathy.[41] All patients with a follow-up of more than 10 years had exacerbation of symptoms for at least 1 year followed by either a static period or mild improvement. Patients with myelopathy were graded using Lees and Turner's myelopathy classification as either mild, moderate, or severe.

- Mild: hand and arm symptoms producing some incapacity but not preventing ordinary everyday activities.
- Moderate: considerable difficulty in using hands or legs, sufficient to affect the performance of everyday tasks.
- Severe: ambulatory aids needed for walking, patient often confined to bed, chair, or house.

Those patients with mild disability at initial presentation had the best prognosis with no significant progression during the study period. Of the 15 patients who initially presented with severe disability secondary to myelopathy, 14 remained moderately or severely disabled after 10–20 years of follow-up. Lees and Turner concluded that the course of cervical spondylotic myelopathy may be prolonged and that long periods of non-progressive disability are the rule, with rare instances of progressive deterioration.

Nurick[48] developed his own classification of cervical spondylotic myelopathy based on ambulatory function and reported on 36 patients treated conservatively. Nurick's classification[44] breaks down as:

- No difficulty in walking.
- Slight difficulty in walking, but does not prevent full-time employment.
- Difficulty in walking that prevents full-time employment or ability to do all housework, but not so severe as to require someone else's help to walk.

- Able to walk with someone else's help or with the aid of a frame.
- Chairbound or bedridden.

Twenty-seven patients with mild disability (Nurick grades 1 and 2) at initial presentation were followed for up to 20 years; 18 patients were still graded as mild at final reassessment. Six of nine patients who presented with moderate-to-severe symptoms (Nurick grades 3–5) continued to have moderate-to-severe symptoms at follow-up. The only feature that was often associated with deterioration was the age of the patient at the time of initial presentation, with patients over the age of 60 years having a worse prognosis. Nurick agreed with Lees and Turner, and concluded that the degree of disability is established early in the course of cervical spondylotic myelopathy and, in many instances, the disability is unchanged after long-term follow-up.

Epstein and Epstein[17] combined four large series of patients treated conservatively for cervical myelopathy. Of 114 patients, 36% improved, 38% remained unchanged, and 26% of the patients worsened.

The natural history of neck and cervical radicular pain was reviewed by Gore et al.[23] He retrospectively reviewed 205 patients with neck and arm pain. Approximately 50% of patients who presented with unilateral radicular pain still had radicular symptoms at a mean 15 years of follow-up. The percentage of patients complaining of bilateral radicular pain was relatively unchanged from presentation to long-term follow-up. Gore was also in agreement with Lees and Turner and concluded that conservative treatment of radicular pain may alleviate symptoms without influencing the natural history of the disease.

INDICATIONS FOR SURGERY IN CERVICAL RADICULOPATHY AND MYELOPATHY

The indications for removal of the cervical intervertebral disc and fusion of the cervical spine by the anterior approach were first outlined by Smith and Robinson.[57] They reported that surgery was indicated if either conservative treatment (reduction of activity, collar, traction) failed to relieve upper extremity radicular pain or the pain became excessively burdensome to the patient. The current indications[31] for surgery in cervical radiculopathy are as follows:

- Persistent or recurrent arm pain not responsive to a trial of conservative treatment (3 months).
- Progressive neurologic deficit.
- Static neurologic deficit associated with radicular pain.
- Confirmatory imaging study consistent with clinical findings (computed tomography (CT), myelogram or magnetic resonance imaging (MRI)).

The indications for surgical treatment of cervical myelopathy using Robinson's[52] technique of anterior cervical discectomy and fusion[50] were reported by Bohlman.[5] Surgery was indicated for patients who failed to demonstrate improvement in their myelopathy after cervical immobilization. Surgical decompression is also indicated in patients with progressive impairment of function without sustained remission.[17] Garfin's indications,[1,20] using Robinson's technique, for the anterior surgical approach for the treatment of cervical myelopathy include: (1) one-, two-, or three-level pathology; (2) pathology primarily at the disc level; (3) anterior cord compression; and (4) fairly stable cervical alignment.

Anterior interbody fusions, such as the Smith–Robinson technique, can adequately decompress the spinal cord in many cases. It is recommended that posterior marginal osteophytes be removed at surgery to ensure decompression, but arthrodesis alone has not been shown to ensure resorption of these osteophytes. Anterior interbody fusion techniques, however, cannot be used in cases of congenital cervical stenosis, because the anteroposterior diameter of the canal will remain unchanged.

Anterior vertebrectomy and strut grafting can be used when two or more contiguous interspaces are involved. This technique is useful in cases of ossification of the posterior longitudinal ligament and when cervical spondylotic myelopathy is associated with a short segment of congenital canal stenosis.

SURGICAL TECHNIQUE

Anterior Interbody Arthrodesis in the Cervical Spine

Anterior cervical fusion was first described by Smith and Robinson[57] in 1958. They noted that laminectomy was often not effective when posterior osteophytes compress the nerve root in the intervertebral foramen. Furthermore, if the radicular pain was bilateral, bilateral facet excision was necessary to adequately decompress the roots by a posterior approach, often leading to instability (Fig. 9.1). Therefore, they recommended anterior cervical discectomy and fusion for the relief of radicular symptoms resulting from osteoarthritic spurs (hard discs) impinging on nerve roots. They reported that this operation: (1) has less morbidity than laminectomy combined with foraminal decompression or without posterior fusion of the cervical spine; (2) allows removal of a degenerated disc without

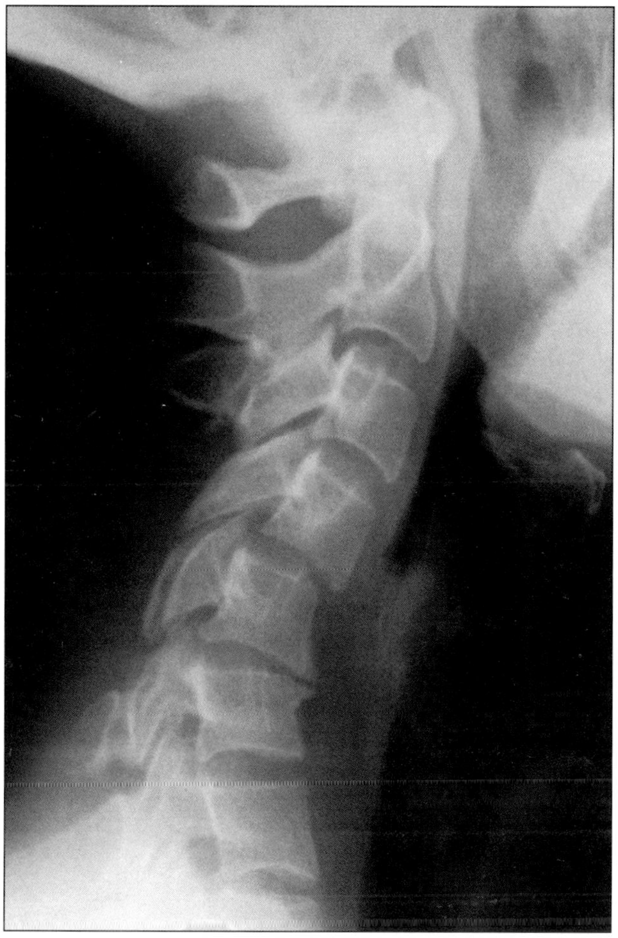

Figure 9.1
Postoperative deformity which developed 5 years after laminectomy for cervical spondylosis. (From Butler JC, Whitecloud TS. Postlaminectomy kyphosis. *Orthop Clin North Am* 23: 505–511, 1992, with permission)

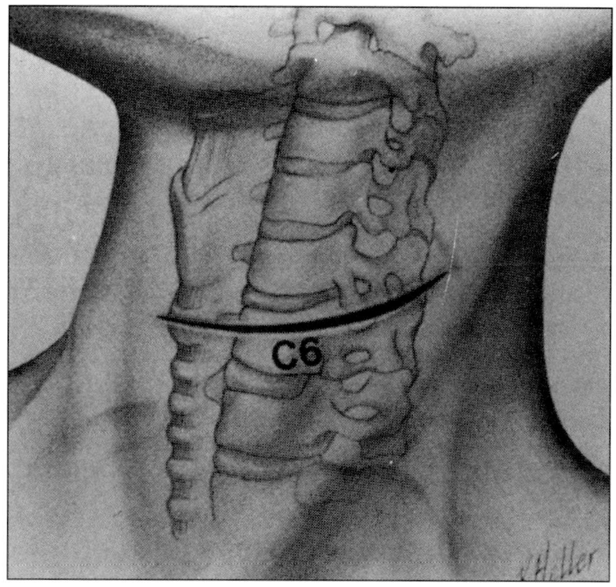

Figure 9.2
Superficial landmarks that are helpful in placing the skin incision: the hyoid bone is at the level of C3, the thyroid cartilage at C4–5, and the cricoid opposite C6. (From Rothman RH, Simeone FA. *The Spine*, 3rd ed. Philadelphia, WB Saunders, 1992, with permission)

disturbing the spinal canal; and (3) permits interbody fusion of the cervical spine at the specific intervertebral level from which symptoms arise.

The surgical approach used by Smith and Robinson was initially described by Lahey and Warren,[40] who used it to expose esophageal diverticula. Before the operation, the surgical level was localized by physical examination and radiographic evidence of degeneration and osteophyte formation. The first 14 patients reported by Smith and Robinson all underwent provocative discograms to precisely localize the involved level.

After induction of general anesthesia, a standard anterior cervical approach is performed. The incision may be transverse or longitudinal and follows the anterior border of the sternocleidomastoid muscle. Knowledge about the anatomical landmarks is helpful in placement of the skin incision: generally, the hyoid bone is at the level of C3, the thyroid cartilage at C4–C5, and the cricoid cartilage lies at the level of C6 (Fig. 9.2). The transverse incision is preferred for a one- or two-level fusion, whereas the longitudinal approach is best for three or more levels. At the cervicothoracic junction, the longitudinal incision may be preferred because inadvertent injury to the inferior thyroid vessels is managed more readily through a longitudinal approach. Once through the skin and platysma muscles, the approach proceeds medial to the sternocleidomastoid muscle. The carotid sheath is retracted laterally, and the esophagus and trachea medially, using hand-held blunt retractors. The superior and inferior thyroid vessels which traverse the carotid artery to the midline structures may limit the extent to which this plane can be opened and may have to be divided. The vertebral bodies and discs can be identified by palpation in the midline. Once the prevertebral fascia and longus colli muscles have been dissected away from the vertebral bodies, a spinal needle should be inserted into the appropriate disc space, and a lateral radiograph of the cervical spine taken to accurately identify the surgical level(s).[30]

A flap of the anterior longitudinal ligament is then raised, starting in the midline, by sharp dissection, and may either be excised or remain attached to the lateral edge of the anterior longitudinal ligament. The longus colli muscles are elevated well above and below the involved disc level by subperiosteal dissection. The sympathetic chain lies directly anterior to these muscles and must be protected. Care should be taken to cauterize encountered vessels using bipolar cautery. With sufficient muscle elevation, retractor blades are then placed under the muscle and secured, protecting the recurrent laryngeal nerve, structures of the carotid sheath, esophagus, and trachea. It may be necessary to remove large osteophytes anteriorly to securely position the retractor blade. Generally the use of dull-tipped blades is preferred. Occasionally, sharp blades are helpful with exposure, but these carry an added risk of injury to any surrounding vital structures dislodged. A second set of retractor blades may be useful in distracting soft tissues superiorly and inferiorly. A no. 15 scalpel blade is then used to enter the disc at both its superior and inferior borders, followed by sequential use of curettes and pituitary rongeurs to actually excise the disc material. After a significant amount of disc material is removed, a small intervertebral body spreader is placed to allow careful distraction of the disc space. Alternatively, the Caspar retractor, using posts secured to the vertebral bodies directly above and below the disc space, provides excellent distraction and visualization. The remainder of the disc as well as the cartilage end-plates are removed with pituitary rongeurs and curettes. Large, overhanging, anterior osteophytes may need to be partially removed to improve the exposure of the disc space and to define the anterior vertebral body border. However, the anterior cortical edges of the adjacent vertebral bodies should be preserved to assist in securing the graft in place. All articular cartilage should be removed but the bony end-plate should not be resected as initially recommended by Smith and Robinson.[57]

The posterior longitudinal ligament (PLL) should be visualized, but not incised routinely. If there is suspicion of a free, sequestered fragment of disc material, then resection of the ligament is performed. Furthermore, in cases of myelopathy, resection of the ligament may facilitate osteophyte removal. This should be performed with an operating microscope to ensure safety of the underlying dura. A no. 15 scalpel blade can be used or, alternatively, special PLL knife blades have now been designed which offer added protection to the dura. It is wise to palpate with a blunt micro-nerve hook behind the PLL to determine whether adhesions exist between the ligament and dura. If free, the ligament can be incised and/or resected, and the region probed for sequestered disc fragments. Removal of posterior osteophytes is not routinely recommended in cases of radiculopathy, because resorption of the osteophytes often occurs with solid fusion,[13,52] and is not absolutely required for nerve root decompression. Foraminal widening through a graft insertion and interspace widening probably accounts for this finding.

Removal of spurs is recommended in cases of myelopathy. A high-speed diamond-tipped burr is recommended to thin the offending osteophytes, with frequent irrigation to minimize the local thermal effects. Once adequately thinned, a small, sharp 5/0 angled curette is used to chip off the remaining bone. This is done only in an anteroposterior direction, thereby minimizing potential injury to the dura and spinal cord.

Once the decompression is complete, the disc space, height, and depth are measured. The space can accept a block of bone up to 10 mm high, 10–15 mm wide, and 12–17 mm deep. The depth is measured by placing a wire into the back of the disc space and measuring the length. To avoid reabsorption, the graft should be a minimum of 5 mm high.[6] The authors prefer use of tricortical autograft from the anterior iliac crest; allograft is an alternative, but healing rates and clinical results are generally worse. Transmission of disease and graft collapse are additional concerns.

In obtaining grafts for an anterior cervical fusion, a small incision is made over the crest of the ilium at least 2 cm behind the anterosuperior iliac spine. Subperiosteal elevation is completed on both the inner and outer tables of the ilium. Cobb elevators are placed along each table of the ilium and used as retractors, while supplying protection to the soft tissues. The size of the initial bone plug should be more than the size of the final trimmed graft. Two vertical parallel cuts, 2 cm deep, are made approximately 10–15 mm apart, with an oscillating saw, along the top of the iliac crest. A half-inch (1.27 cm) curved osteotome is then used to complete a horizontal cut at the base of the graft. After appropriate trimming and removal of any remaining soft tissues, the graft is horseshoe-shaped and consists of cancellous bone surrounded by cortical bone on three sides (tricortical) (Fig. 9.3).

The disc space is then prepared for graft implantation. A burr is used to decorticate, but not penetrate, the subchondral surface. Sometimes it is necessary to 'square off' the surfaces that are to receive the bone graft. A burr or curette is then used to place small holes in the center of the end-plate, into the vertebral body, facilitating vascular ingrowth to the graft. The prepared disc space is then distracted with the addition of weights to a previously placed head halter or cranial tong traction, or by use of the vertebral body spreader or Caspar retractor. Distraction of the disc space can also be done manually by the anesthesiologist who pulls on the cranial tongs. The bone graft is then tapped into position with a bone tamp. The graft should be countersunk 1–2 mm in relation to the anterior cortical edges of the adjacent vertebral bodies (Fig. 9.4).[39] After hemostasis is complete, the flap of anterior longitudinal ligament, if retained, should be repositioned and sutured over the graft.[57]

After the operation, the patient should be placed in a firm cervical collar (e.g. a Philadelphia collar). The orthoses

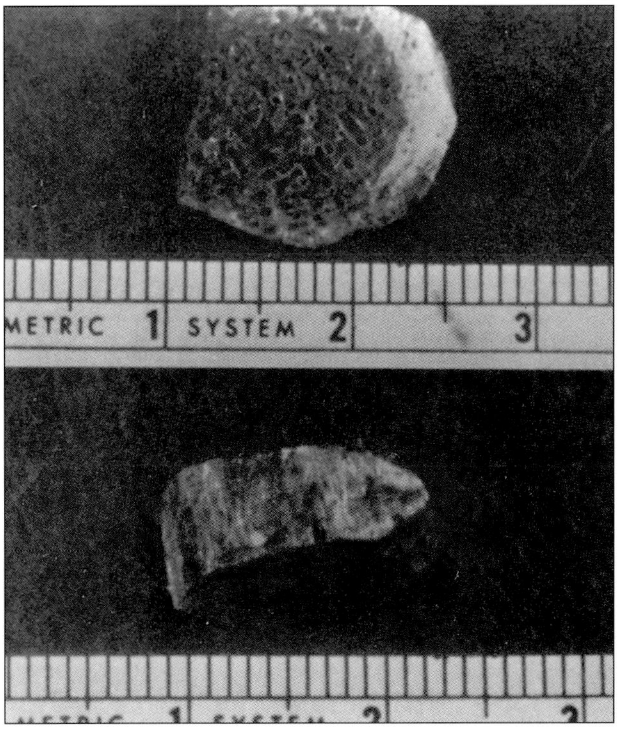

Figure 9.3
Robinson horseshoe graft. (From Rothman RH, Simeone FA. *The Spine*, 3rd ed. Philadelphia, WB Saunders, 1992, with permission)

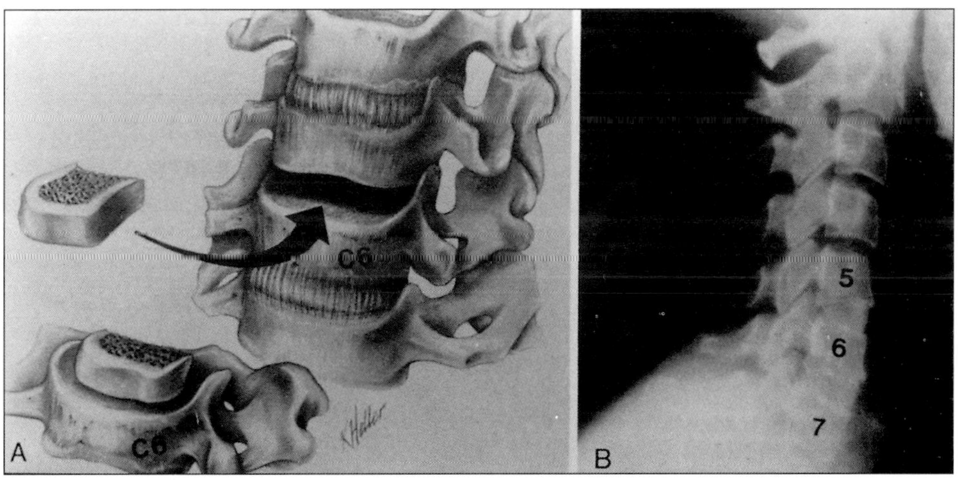

Figure 9.4
(A) The graft harvested from the iliac crest is measured for height and depth. It should be recessed 1–2 mm posterior to the anterior cortex. (B) Lateral radiograph showing correct graft placement. (From Rothman RH, Simeone FA. *The Spine*, 3rd ed. Philadelphia, WB Saunders, 1992, with permission)

can usually be discontinued after 6 weeks, but a longer period may be necessary if fusion has not been demonstrated by radiography at follow-up examination.

Bailey and Badgley[2] described a similar approach to the anterior cervical spine, but used a different configuration of iliac crest bone graft (Fig. 9.5). Their technique recommended cutting a trough in the anterior aspect of the vertebral body ½ inch (12.7 mm) wide and 3/16 inch (4.76 mm) in depth. The trough is cut into the full vertical height of the vertebrae. The intervertebral discs are removed with a rongeur to a depth of 3/16 inch (4.76 mm) and the cartilaginous end-plates on the inferior and superior aspects of the vertebral bodies to be fused are removed.

Iliac crest bone graft is then trimmed to fit in the trough and chips of cancellous bone are packed in the disc space. The neck is then released from its position of extension and sutures placed previously in the prevertebral fascia are tied over the graft. Bailey and Badgley initially recommended 6 weeks of postoperative traction on a Stryker

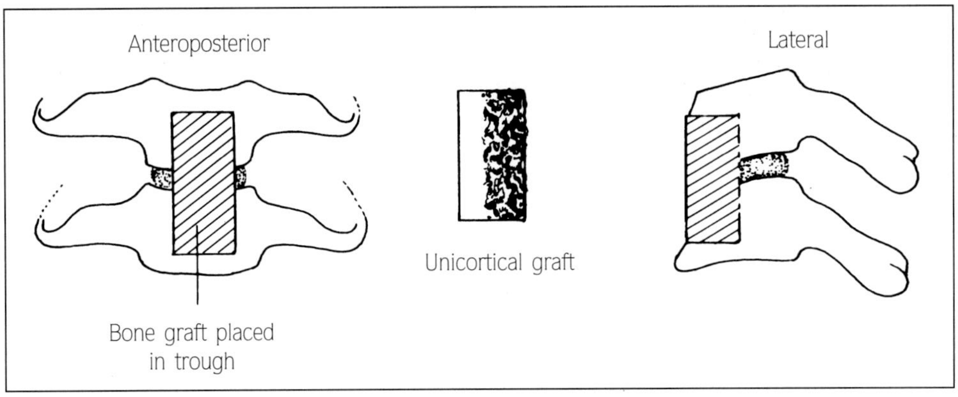

Figure 9.5
Bailey–Badgley graft. (From Wood EG, Hanley EN. Types of anterior cervical grafts. *Orthop Clin North Am* 23: 475–486, 1992, with permission)

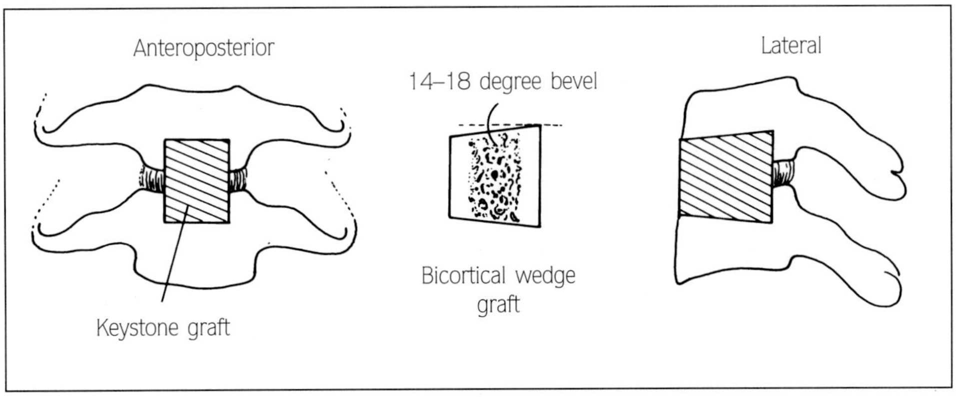

Figure 9.6
Simmons–Bhalla keystone graft. (From Wood EG, Hanley EN. Types of anterior cervical grafts. *Orthop Clin North Am* 23: 475–486, 1992, with permission)

frame followed by immobilization in a brace for 4–6 months.

Simmons and Bhalla[56] developed an additional type of anterior graft to obtain and increase distraction of the disc space. They described a 'keystone' graft which was taken from the iliac crest. After adequate disc removal, the vertebral bodies are chiseled so that the space is beveled upwards into the superior vertebral body and downwards into the inferior vertebral body (Fig. 9.6). Special instruments were designed for precise and safe osteotomies. A rectangular graft was then taken from the iliac crest and beveled up and down to match the cuts made in the vertebral bodies. After insertion of the graft, Simmons and Bhalla performed mechanical studies which indicated that the keystone graft was more stable than a dowel graft under flexion and extension strains. In addition, they emphasized that, as the keystone graft has a large area, the rate of fusion should be higher.

In 1956, Cloward[10] conceived the idea of making a trephine opening in the cervical intervertebral space by an anterior approach. Through this approach all lesions anterior to the spinal cord and nerve roots could be removed. He modified instruments designed for posterior lumbar interbody fusion.[2] A large drill with a guard was used which allowed the intervertebral space and adjacent vertebrae to be drilled to a preset depth. Drilling is continued posteriorly until the posterior cortex of the vertebral bodies is reached. Cloward emphasized the importance of direct visualization of the compressive structures, and removed the protruded disc fragments and posterior osteophytes with curettes and rongeurs.[10] A precut dowel-shaped allograft with cortical bone on both ends is then tapped into place (Fig. 9.7).

The horseshoe-shaped graft of Robinson, the iliac strut graft of Bailey and Badgley, the dowel graft developed by Cloward, and the keystone graft of Simmons and Bhalla[56] all potentially relieve radicular symptoms by distraction and stabilization of the disc space. The benefits of successful fusion include: (1) prevention of further anterior and posterior spur formation; (2) spurs already present will regress secondary to the stability provided by the fusion; and (3) distraction of the disc space will reduce the buckling of the ligamentum flavum, thereby enlarging the neuroforamen and reducing compression of the nerve root.

The compressive strength of the various graft configurations has been studied by White and Hirsch.[59] The horseshoe-shaped graft of Robinson was found to be much more resistant to compressive forces than the other graft shapes, and is therefore preferred by the present authors.

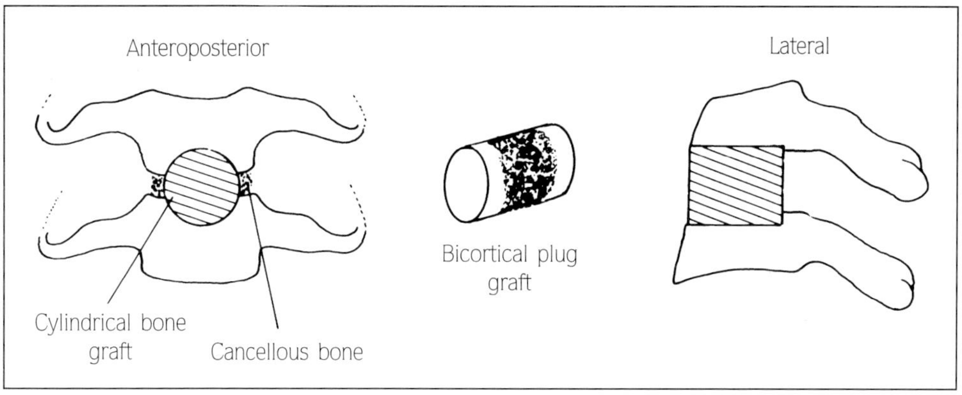

Figure 9.7
Cloward graft. (From Wood EG, Hanley EN. Types of anterior cervical grafts. *Orthop Clin North Am* 23: 475–586, 1992 with permission)

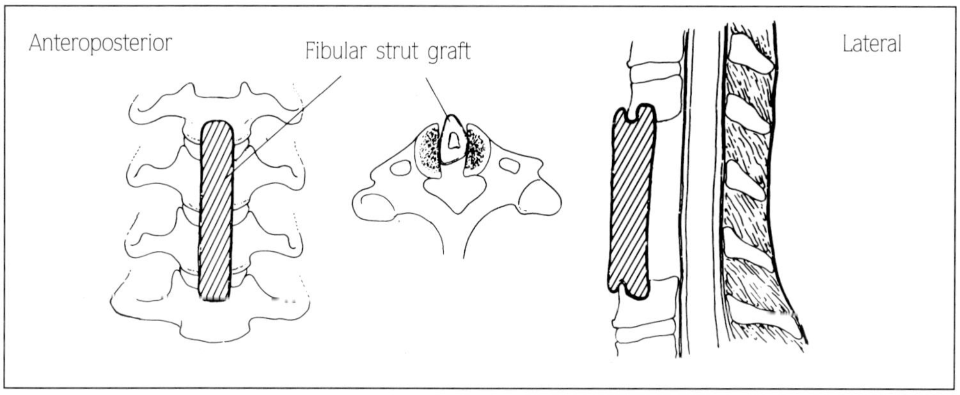

Figure 9.8
Multiple level corpectomy and notched fibular graft. (From Wood EG, Hanley EN. Types of anterior cervical grafts. *Orthop Clin North Am* 23: 475–486, 1992 with permission)

Anterior Cervical Vertebrectomy and Strut Grafting

Both the Smith–Robinson and Cloward techniques become increasingly difficult and time consuming when performed over multiple segments. In addition, the rate of successful fusion decreases as the number of attempted fusion levels increases. For these reasons, many authors[4,7,25] have recommended partial vertebrectomies for multi-level cervical spondylotic myelopathy and myeloradiculopathy. This technique allows for radical anterior decompression over numerous motion segments.

Bernard and Whitecloud[4] reported on 21 patients with either myelopathy or myeloradiculopathy who underwent surgical anterior decompression and stabilization with autogenous fibula strut grafts, using the following technique. After a standard anterior cervical approach, discectomies are completed at the appropriate levels. It is important to identify the uncinate process laterally, to locate the midline of the cervical spine precisely. A trough is created in the vertebral bodies with a small rongeur and a high-speed burr. Only the middle one-third of the vertebral bodies requires resection for spinal cord decompression. The lateral wall is not needed for cord decompression, so maintaining it preserves some intrinsic stability. Bone and disc are removed until the posterior longitudinal ligament is visualized and posterior osteophytes removed after adequate deepening of the trough. In these cases the posterior longitudinal ligament is removed with a small Kerrison rongeur and the lateral margins of the trough undercut to complete the decompression. Bernard and Whitecloud[4] recommended the use of an autologous fibular strut graft. After being harvested, the graft is notched on both ends with a high-speed burr. Traction weight is increased and the graft placed into notches made in the center of the remaining superior and inferior vertebral bodies, with initial insertion of the superior portion of the graft. Once the graft is in place, traction is removed and the graft pulled distally, locking it into place. The preserved anterior portion of the cephalad and caudad vertebral bodies serves as a barrier against dislodgement (Fig. 9.8).

Alternatively, a tricortical anterior iliac crest strut may be used after vertebrectomy. The essentials of the decompression are unchanged. In securing this graft, a 'peg and trough' can be used for additional stability. In the superior vertebrae, the anterior cortex is left intact, and a 'peg hole' drilled well into the substance of the body with a right-angled burr. Care is taken not to disrupt or penetrate the anterior or posterior cortices as this will compromise stability of the construct and may lead to neurologic impingement. In the inferior vertebral body, an 'L-shaped trough' is created using both straight and right-angled burrs. The anterior cortex is obviously violated, although the posterior cortex is left intact. After careful measurement, a tricortical graft is harvested from the anterior iliac crest. The iliac crest fits well with the contours of the cervical spine. The portion of the graft to be inserted superiorly is rounded with a burr into a matching 'peg', whereas the inferior portion is carefully sculpted to fit into the anteroposterior portion of the L-shaped trough. The superior portion of the graft is placed first and cranial tong traction applied. The inferior portion of the graft is then tapped into position and rotated, securely locking the graft into position. Traction is then released. The tricortical iliac crest graft provides more cancellous elements and may facilitate an earlier successful arthrodesis when compared to the fibular strut. However, the fibular strut does provide a more rigid strut when fitted properly.

Boni et al[7] described a technique known as multiple subtotal somatectomy for the anterior decompression of cervical stenosis of three or more levels. He drilled tunnels in the intervertebral spaces using the Cloward[10] technique. The tunnel is deepened (anterior to posterior) until the posterior longitudinal ligament is decompressed by removal of the posterior wall of the vertebral body. The bone bridges linking the tunnels are then removed with bone forceps. The final trench should be 15 mm wide with its height including all the vertebral bodies involved in the arthrodesis. Boni recommended a tricortical iliac crest graft for fusion and found that convexity of the graft adapted well to the normal cervical lordosis. Patients were immobilized after the operation in either a Minerva cast or a SOMI brace.

When using any of these techniques, if the anterior construct is thought to provide insufficient stability, additional stabilization procedures should be considered. Under the circumstances two options exist, including application of a halo device or a concomitant posterior arthrodesis. Many factors need to be considered by the surgeon, including stability of the construct, quality and strength of the patient's bone, the patient's general medical condition, and patient reliability.

RESULTS

The first large series of patients treated with anterior interbody fusion for cervical degenerative disc disease was reported by Robinson et al[52] in 1962. Disc removal and anterior interbody fusion was performed on 107 interspaces in 55 patients. The criteria used by Robinson for rating the results are as follows:

- Excellent: all preoperative symptoms relieved, abnormal findings unchanged or improved.
- Good: minimum residual of the preoperative symptoms, not requiring medication or limiting activity, and abnormal findings unchanged or improved.
- Fair: definite relief of some preoperative symptoms with others remaining unchanged or only slightly improved.
- Poor: symptoms and signs unchanged from preoperative status.

Follow-up ranged from 2 to 73 months. Overall, 46% of the patients were rated as excellent, 27% good, 22% fair, and 6% poor. Patients who had multi-level fusions had worse results than those who had single-level disease. Seventeen of 18 patients who had a significant degenerative disc at a single level had an excellent or good result after fusion, whereas only 8 of 16 patients with three or more involved spaces had an excellent or good result. The poorer results in multiple level fusions may result from the greater severity of disease in those patients with multi-level degenerative disc.

Robinson et al[52] found that there was no clear correlation after operation between the absence of fusion and the clinical results. In all, 13 of the 107 interspaces grafted did not fuse. However, of the nine patients with non-unions, only four continued to have complaints that could possibly have resulted from lack of union. All four patients underwent reoperation. Only one of the 46 patients who had a solid fusion needed additional cervical spine surgery. The value of preserving the subchondral bone plate above and below the graft was also assessed.[52] Of 38 interspaces successfully fused without plate preservation, 26 maintained and 12 lost height. Of the 47 fused with end-plate preserved, 41 maintained and 6 lost space. These findings led Robinson et al to conclude that, by preserving the subchondral bone, a load-bearing surface for the graft remains, preserving the restored height of the intervertebral space during healing.

Connolly et al[13] reported 63 patients who underwent anterior cervical fusion. Follow-up ranged from 7 to 70 months. He used a procedure similar to the standard Smith–Robinson anterior operation, but in most of his cases neuroforamen decompressions were also done. Overall, approximately two-thirds of his patients improved after the operation, with a non-union rate of 21%. Fifteen percent of his one- and two-level decompressions, but 40% of his three-level decompressions, developed a non-union. The results of Connolly et al also showed that the adequacy of the fusion bore no constant relationship to the final clinical result. DePalma and Rothman[16] reported on a large series of anterior interbody fusions for cervical degenerative disc disease. A total of 442 disc levels were fused with the Robinson technique in 229 patients. Follow-up was 13–105 months (mean 57 months). At final follow-up, 63% of the patients were considered to have satisfactory results, rated as excellent or good. There was no tendency for the results to deteriorate or improve as the length of follow-up increased. Follow-up radiographs demonstrated further disc degeneration at adjacent levels (usually below the fusion mass) in 81% of the patients. After the operation, two-thirds of the osteophytes (at 211 levels that fused) had resolved. Pseudoarthrosis occurred in 12% of the patients, although the effect of pseudoarthroses on the quality of the result was of no statistical significance. Lack of correlation between a successful fusion and patient outcome can be explained by the fact that even though bone union does not occur, a stable fibrous union does. In addition, removal of the degenerative disc alleviates mechanical pressure on the nerve root, thus relieving most symptoms. Finally, distraction of the disc space and neuroforamen may still occur, even though much of the initial height of the interspace gained by the bone graft is lost.[31]

Additional factors influencing the late results of anterior interbody fusion were reported by Williams et al.[63] They found that relief of symptoms at long-term follow-up was not as satisfactory as the initial short-term evaluation indicated. Sixty patients with a follow-up of 2–9 years (average 55 months) were reviewed. Preoperative indications for surgery included either radicular or non-radicular (occipital headache, non-radiating, neck, or intracapsular) pain. Seventy-three percent of patients with radicular complaints had a good or excellent result whereas only 26% of those patients with non-radicular pain had good or excellent results. Additionally, the late operative results correlated with the adequacy of decompression. Ten of 13 patients had excellent or good results when the discs removed corresponded to the levels of the preoperative myelographic defect. When several myelographic defects were present before the operation, but discectomy was not done at all levels of compression, only 6 of 11 patients had excellent or good results.

A literature review of series of multiple interbody fusions has shown satisfactory results for the treatment of cervical disc disease, with rates of over 90% in many.[16,22,51,56,61,62,63] As a rule, however, the results tend to deteriorate as the number of levels fused increases. In addition, the success or failure of fusion does not appear to influence the long-term results.

Surgical treatment of myelopathy by an anterior cervical approach was described by Bohlman[5] in 1977. Seventeen patients were treated with a Smith–Robinson anterior cervical discectomy and fusion at one or more levels (Fig. 9.9). Two out of three patients who were bedridden before the operation were ambulatory after surgery. The 14 patients who required walking aids before operation all recovered from their myelopathy and were able to walk independently. Fourteen patients had increased strength in the upper extremities after the operation. In two patients, with severe loss of position and vibratory sense, no recovery occurred. Evidence of posterior column spinal cord dysfunction probably represents a more extensive form of cord compression with a less favorable response to decompression. These excellent results occurred in spite of the fact that Bohlman made no attempt to remove either the lateral or posterior osteophytes. He postulated that the introduction of instruments into a narrow spinal canal could compromise the already compressed spinal cord and produce further deficit. Two patients in his series had repeat myelograms following anterior discectomy and fusion which demonstrated resorption of the posterior osteophytes.

A more radical anterior decompression was described by Boni et al.[7] They performed multiple subtotal somatectomies on 29 patients with spondylotic myelopathy and myeloradiculopathy. The number of levels decompressed ranged from three to six. Good results were reported in 53% of the patients with moderate results reported in 47%. Successful fusion of the iliac crest graft occurred 60–90 days after the operation in all patients. Boni et al advocated this procedure because it allows a full anterior decompression which can be checked visually.

Bernard and Whitecloud[4] performed anterior decompression and stabilization with autogenous fibular graft in 21 patients with either cervical spondylomyelopathy or cervical spondylomyeloradiculopathy (Fig. 9.10). Myelopathy was the dominant feature in all cases. Two to four levels were decompressed in all patients. Before operation, all patients were graded according to Nurick's classification. At follow-up evaluation, 16 of 21 patients had improved one functional grade. Bernard and Whitecloud recommended this approach because it surgically addresses the bony and soft tissue abnormalities responsible for spinal cord and nerve root compression. They suggested that surgical decompression by this method favorably alters the natural history of cervical spondylotic myelopathy and cervical spondylotic myeloradiculopathy. The series of Hanai et al[25] consisted of 30 patients with cervical spondylotic myelopathy who underwent subtotal vertebrectomy and fusion. Three-level vertebrectomies were performed in 18 patients and four-level vertebrectomies were performed in 12 patients. The patients were evaluated by the Japanese Orthopaedic Association (JOA) score before and after the operation. The JOA score consisted of an evaluation of motor, sensory, and bladder functions, with a score of 17 indicating no neurologic deficit. The preoperative score was in the range 5–14 points (mean 8.9). All patients showed postoperative improvement and were satisfied with the surgery. The postoperative score was in the range 9–16 (mean 13.9).

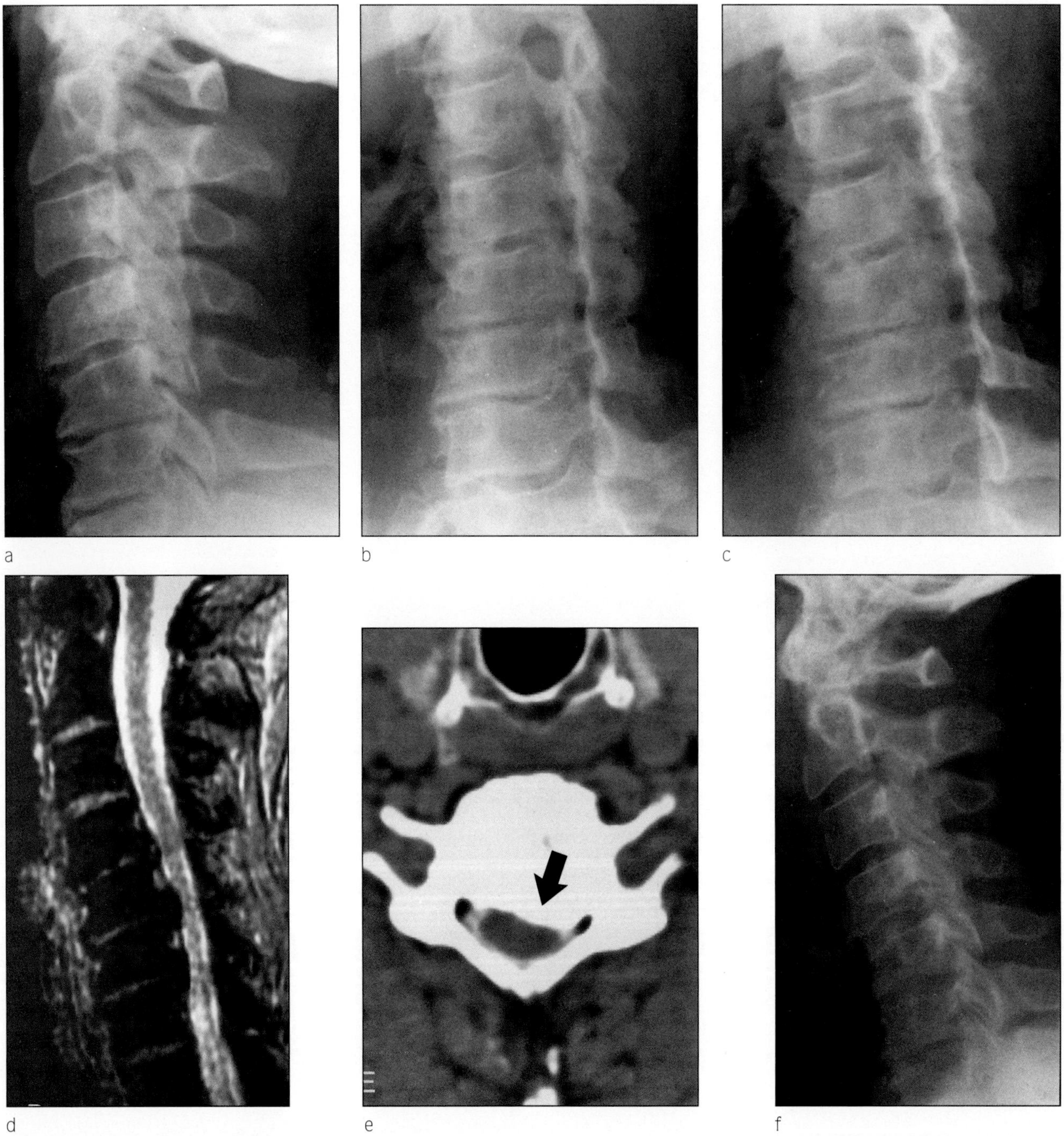

Figure 9.9
A 68-year-old man with cervical myelopathy: (a) preoperative lateral radiograph of the cervical spine demonstrates significant narrowing of the C4–5, C5–6, and C6–7 disc spaces. (b,c) Left and right oblique radiographs show uncinate process osteophytes projecting into the neural foramina. (d) T2-weighted sagittal MRI shows degenerated discs bulging and osteophytes projecting posteriorly from the margins of the end-plates at C4–5, C5–6, and C6–7. (e) Axial contrast-enhanced CT image at the C5–6 level; the arrow denotes a large osteophyte projecting from the margin of the end-plate and causing impingement on the spinal cord. (f) Immediate postoperative lateral radiograph demonstrates distracted disc spaces as well as 1–2 mm recession of the grafts following anterior interbody arthrodesis at C4–5, C5–6, and C6–7. (From Kurz LT, Herkowitz HN. Surgical management of myelopathy. *Orthop Clin North Am* 23: 495–504, 1992, with permission)

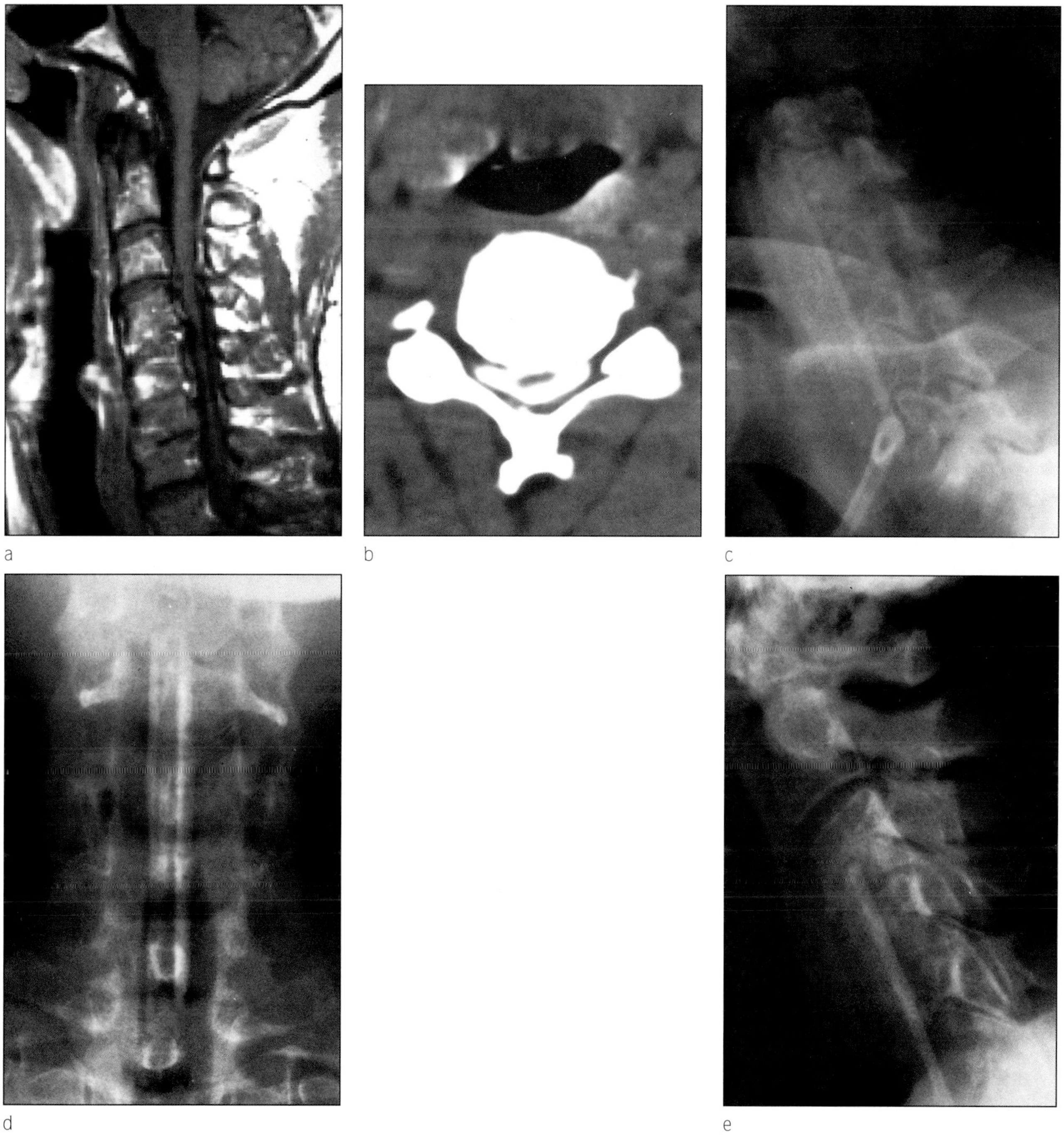

Figure 9.10
A 52-year-old man with quadriparesis from cervical cord compression: (a) T1-weighted sagittal MRI showing cord compression from the lower end of C3 to the upper end of T1. (b) Axial contrast-enhanced CT at the C5–6 level demonstrating marked cord compression. (c,d) Lateral and anteroposterior radiographs of the cervical spine immediately following anterior corpectomy of C4, C5, C6, and C7 followed by fibular strut grafting from C3 to T1. (e) Lateral radiograph demonstrates the interlocking nature of the proximal end of the graft. (From Kurz LT, Herkowitz HN. Surgical management of myelopathy. *Orthop Clin North Am* 23: 495–504, 1992, with permission)

COMPARATIVE STUDIES

Unlike the surgical management of lumbar disc disease, the operative approach to cervical soft disc herniation has remained controversial. Excellent results have been reported using either the posterior[9,55] or the anterior approach.[13,30,52]

Henderson et al[27] reported on 846 patients who had a posterolateral foraminotomy for simple cervical radiculopathy. No distinction of radiculopathy due to soft disc protrusions, hard disc protrusions, or spondylotic spurring or ridging was made. He reported an excellent or good result in 91.5% of all cases. However, recurrent signs of radiculopathy were present in 172 cases (20.3%), and 103 patients (12.2%) ultimately required a second posterior surgical procedure.

Gore and Sepic[22] reviewed 146 patients who underwent an anterior surgical fusion for a degenerative or protruded disc. After the operation, complete pain relief occurred in 78% of patients, with partial relief occurring in 18% of patients. Those patients with an initial diagnosis of soft disc protrusion had less recurrent pain than those with an initial diagnosis of cervical spondylosis.

The decision to perform an anterior discectomy and fusion versus a posterior laminotomy–foraminotomy for a patient with a posterolateral soft disc herniation cannot, for the following reasons, be determined by a review of the previously published series: (1) patient demographics cannot be compared from series to series; (2) prior series include results of surgical treatment for spondylotic radiculopathy (hard disc) as well as that for soft disc herniation; (3) surgical techniques differ among authors and therefore comparisons among series of anterior fusions or posterior laminotomy are not valid; (4) the criteria for a successful result differ from series to series and therefore comparisons cannot be made; and (5) patient follow-up is incomplete and of inadequate length in most series to evaluate the success or failure of the surgical procedure.[31]

Herkowitz et al[32] designed a prospective study to compare the results of anterior fusion versus laminotomy–foraminotomy in patients with a diagnosis of cervical disc herniation. Forty-four consecutive patients with a diagnosis of a one-level cervical radiculopathy or myelopathy were studied. All had a soft disc herniation confirmed by either computed tomography, magnetic resonance imaging, myelogram, or myelogram with computed tomography. Type 1 disc herniations were defined as posterolateral herniations with unilateral nerve root and dural sac compression. Type 2 herniations were defined as central herniations with midline compression of the dual sac with or without nerve root compression. Patients with type 1 herniations were randomly treated with either an anterior discectomy and fusion with a Smith–Robinson horseshoe graft, or a posterior cervical laminotomy and foraminotomy. Patients with type 2 herniations were treated by anterior fusion only. Postoperatively, the follow-up was in the range 1.6–8.3 years (mean 4.3 years). The results were graded as excellent (complete relief of pain and weakness), good (improvement of pain and weakness), fair (improvement of pain and weakness requiring analgesics with lifestyle restrictions), and poor (no improvement of preoperative symptoms and signs).

Overall, patients with a type 1 herniation had a rate for excellent or good results of 85%. For the 17 patients who had undergone an anterior fusion in this group, the results were excellent or good in 94%. The 16 patients who had undergone laminotomy–foraminotomy had excellent or good results in 75% of the cases. Although the results were not statistically significant ($p<0.175$), a definite trend was observed for better results when an anterior discectomy and fusion were performed rather than a laminotomy and foraminotomy. For patients with a type 2 herniation, excellent results were noted in six patients, good results in four patients, and fair results in one patient.

Herkowitz concluded that the recommended procedure for the surgical management of cervical anterolateral or central soft disc herniation is anterior discectomy and fusion. Posterior laminotomy–foraminotomy may be considered in the following situations: (1) technical limitations of the anterior approach; and (2) prior anterior surgery restricting access to the surgical level.

Herkowitz[28] also reviewed the results of anterior surgical fusion, cervical laminectomy, and cervical laminoplasty for the surgical management of multi-level cervical spondylotic radiculopathy. A retrospective study of 45 patients who had nerve root compression resulting from spondylosis at three or more levels was carried out. Eighteen patients had an anterior fusion through a left anterior longitudinal incision as previously described by Robinson et al.[52] Twelve patients had a complete laminectomy with bilateral partial facetectomy. The amount of facet joint removed per level and side was variable, with sufficient bone to decompress the nerve root being removed. Fifteen patients had a surgical laminoplasty following the principles of Hirabayashi et al[33] with some modifications.[28]

With a minimum 2-year follow-up, the anterior fusion group reported 92% excellent to good results, whereas the laminectomy group recorded 66% excellent to good results. Excellent to good results were seen in 86% of the laminoplasty patients, although those patients undergoing laminectomy for bilateral radiculopathy had statistically poorer results. Postoperative pseudoarthrosis developed in 22 of 58 levels in the anterior fusion group. However, the presence of a pseudoarthrosis had no relationship to the clinical result. Cervical kyphosis developed in three patients (25%) who underwent cervical laminectomy. Two patients undergoing laminoplasty developed closing of the hinge with subsequent necessity for anterior fusion.

Herkowitz made the following conclusions concerning the surgical treatment of multiple level cervical radiculopathy: the procedure of choice for multi-level spondylotic radiculopathy is anterior cervical discectomy and fusion. The laminoplasty procedure is preferred for patients with developmental canal stenosis, for those with continued nerve root symptoms after anterior fusion, or for those with prior anterior neck surgery for other reasons. Cervical laminectomy may be considered for patients with failed laminoplasty or for those with anterior bony ankylosis due to degenerative or inflammatory disorders.

There are currently no prospective, randomized studies available which compare surgical approaches and results for cervical myelopathy. Many of the available studies[14,15,24,34,35,38] represent restrospective reviews of various procedures performed at the same institution. Guidetti and Fortura[24] compared the results of anterior cervical fusion versus laminectomy in the treatment of cervical spondylomyelopathy: 51% of patients who had an anterior approach improved, compared to 42% of patients who underwent laminectomy and foraminotomy. Additionally, patients who were older and had had myelopathic symptoms for longer had worse results compared to younger patients and those who had disease for less than 6 months. They concluded that 'age and the severity of the clinical syndrome are less important factors than the duration of the disease and the type of operation performed; it means that an appropriate operation performed at an early stage can yield an excellent result even in an elderly patient with severe cord damage'.[24]

Hukuda and associates[34] compared the results of 269 patients who underwent six different operative procedures for cervical spondylotic myelopathy. Patients were grouped before the operation into five clinical categories according to the Crandall and Batzdorf classification:[14] 34% of the patients had transverse spinal cord lesions characterized by involvement of the corticospinal and spinothalamic tracts, and the dorsal column; 20% of the patients had a motor syndrome which primarily involved the corticospinal tract and the anterior horn cells; central cord syndrome was seen in another 20% of the patients with motor deficits affecting the arms more than the legs; 17% of the patients had radicular pain in the arm associated with long tract signs, and the smallest group (9%) had a Brown–Sequard syndrome.

Of the 214 anterior operative procedures, the Cloward operation was performed on 156 patients, the Smith–Robinson approach on 46, and subtotal spondylectomy followed by strut bone grafting on 12. Thirty-eight patients had a posterior approach to the cervical spine; 14 had a conventional laminectomy, and 7 underwent a French window laminectomy as described by Kirita.[38] In addition, 17 patients underwent a French window laminoplasty. The selection of the surgical technique was based on radiographic findings. When a myelographic defect was confined to the level of one or two discs without accompanying stenosis of the canal, either the Cloward or the Smith–Robinson operation was performed. Subtotal spondylectomy was performed when there was involvement at the level of two or three discs complicated by a narrow spinal canal. When three or more levels required decompression, the posterior approach was used, unless there was extreme instability of any involved spinal segment.

In the analysis of results, Hukuda et al excluded those patients who had either a central cord or a radicular syndrome with long tract signs. The patients with these two syndromes generally demonstrated a less severe myelopathy and were treated, in most cases, by an anterior approach. Comparison of the surgical results in patients in the three remaining categories (transverse lesion, Brown–Sequard syndrome, motor syndrome) was then performed. Using the JOA scoring system, the patients on whom anterior operations had been performed had significantly better preoperative function than those who had posterior operations. After the operation, this difference in function became statistically insignificant, indicating that posterior decompressive procedures improved function in cases with more advanced myelopathy to the level achieved by anterior surgery in less advanced cases. Overall, however, their results showed no definite superiority of any individual anterior or posterior operative procedure. Hukuda[34] currently recommends the Smith–Robinson approach to either the Cloward or subtotal spondylectomy because of the excellent mechanical strength of the horseshoe-shaped graft. Of the posterior operations, he currently only uses the laminoplasty technique.

Yonenobu et al,[88] through a retrospective study of 95 cases, analyzed the surgical results of three procedures: extensive laminectomy, anterior interbody fusion using the Cloward or Smith–Robinson technique, and subtotal spondylectomy and fusion. All patients had myelopathy secondary to multi-segmental spondylosis. Patients with a lesser degree of compression (two-level disease) had either an anterior interbody fusion or spondylectomy. Laminectomy was performed when four or more levels of compression existed. Three-level involvement had any one of the three procedures performed according to the preference of the surgeon. As severity of the disease dictated the surgical procedure, it is difficult to compare the postoperative results. For two- and three-level decompressions, the results of spondylectomy were significantly ($p < 0.01$) better than those of anterior interbody fusion. Examination of only the three-level decompressions showed that the results of spondylectomy appeared better than those of laminectomy. Additionally, 25% of patients who had a laminectomy had late neurologic deterioration due to instability of the cervical spine.

COMPLICATIONS

Complications of anterior surgery for cervical disc disease can be divided into those occurring at the graft site and those occurring in the neck. The initial report of Robinson et al[52] described no complication in 48 of 56 patients. Four patients had a temporary unilateral paralysis of the vocal folds, two patients had marked dysphagia, and two patients had a transient Horner's syndrome. In the large series of De Palma et al,[16] the most common complication occurred at the graft donor site. Hematomas developed in 9% of the patients, and 36% had persistent donor site pain 1 year after surgery.

Flynn[19] compiled the replies of 704 neurosurgeons describing 36 657 anterior cervical interbody fusions. The single largest neurologic complication was recurrent laryngeal nerve palsy, which occurred in 52 cases, and this compromised almost 17% of all neurologic complications. The risk to the recurrent laryngeal nerve can be decreased by using a left-sided approach because, on the left, the nerve enters the thorax within the carotid sheath which then loops under the aortic arch and ascends into the neck beside the trachea and esophagus. On the right side it may leave the carotid sheath at a higher level, and of course anteriorly behind the thyroid, thus leaving itself more susceptible to injury (Fig. 9.11).

The most dangerous neurologic complication is that of spinal cord injury. Flynn[19] reported that there were 100 cases of significant permanent myelopathy or myeloradiculopathy in his large series; 75% of these patients had an immediate postoperative deficit, whereas 25% of the patients developed a neurologic deficit during the postoperative recovery period. Analysis of the data led Flynn to conclude that, regardless of the etiology of the myelopathy, reoperation had little effect on the ultimate status of the neurologic deficit. In addition, most surgeons were unable to determine the etiology of the neurologic deterioration.

The most common problems seen after the operation include a transient sore throat and difficulty in swallowing.[29,60] Certainly, the vast majority of these complaints are minor and resolve within a few days or weeks. More severe, penetrating injuries to the esophagus and trachea may occur, although the risk of such injury may be decreased by using dull retractors. Perforating injuries to the esophagus are rarely reported, but can be life threatening. Newhouse et al[47] reported an incidence of perforation of 0.25% in over 10 000 cases of anterior cervical surgery. One-third of the perforations occurred at the time of surgery, and were related to sharp or motorized instruments. Late perforation was usually related to the use of anterior plates and screws, often used for fracture stability.

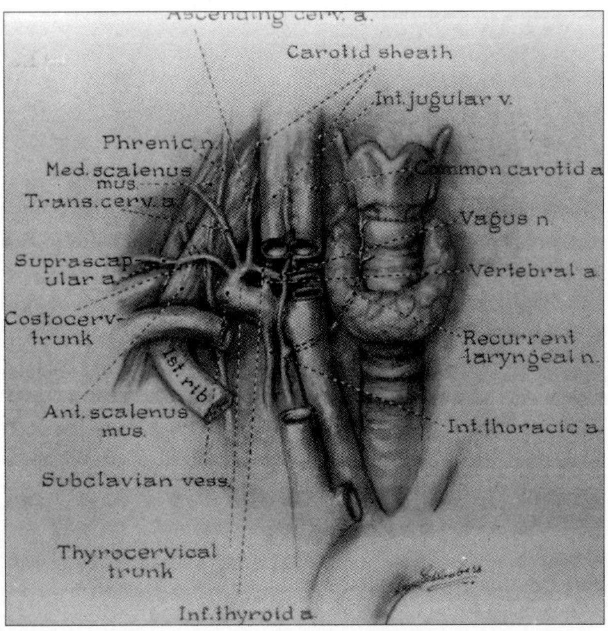

Figure 9.11
Arteries and nerves at the base of the neck on the right side. The right recurrent laryngeal nerve arises from the vagus nerve at the level of the subclavian artery, loops beneath it, and ascends between the trachea and esophagus. The nerve can recur above the level of the subclavian artery and be injured in an approach to the middle cervical spine from the right side. (From Rothman RH, Simeone FA. *The Spine*, 3rd ed. Philadelphia, WB Saunders, 1992, with permission)

ANTERIOR DISCECTOMY WITHOUT FUSION

Anterior discectomy without fusion developed as an alternative to cervical fusion based on the premise that, if successful results of anterior fusions occur with pseudoarthroses, then discectomy can be performed without fusion. Several papers have advocated anterior cervical discectomy without fusion, reporting success rates similar to those with fusion.[46,49,53]

Murphy and Gado[46] reported on 26 patients who underwent one- or two-level anterior cervical discectomy for 'radiculitis' secondary to a herniated cervical disc without concomitant fusion. Good results (improvement of neurologic deficit, alleviation of pain, and patient able to return to normal activities) were reported in 24 of 26 patients. The two patients with poor results required reoperation within 2 weeks of the initial procedure. Seventy-two percent of patients developed a spontaneous fusion at the discectomy level. Twenty patients developed some degree of postoperative kyphosis.

O'Laoire and Thomas[49] also performed anterior discectomy without fusion in 26 patients. All patients had a myelopathy secondary to cervical disc protrusion. He reported that all patients improved after the operation with 100% excellent to good results. Results were graded only according to neurologic recovery. The minimum follow-up in this study was only 1 year.

The studies of both Murphy and Gado[16] and O'Laoire and Thomas[49] neglected specific mention of the postoperative incidence of neck pain. Transient, but severe, neck pain after anterior cervical discectomy has been reported by several authors.[3,37,64] Although 82% of patients in one series[36] noted symptomatic relief after anterior cervical discectomy, 12% reported the development of cervical pain after an average follow-up of 3.5 years.

Yamamoto et al[65] reported on 55 patients who underwent anterior cervical discectomy without fusion for either an acute soft disc herniation or spondylosis. At 3 months follow-up, all but one patient with spondylosis had improved. However, a final follow-up, 2–3 years after surgery, showed that only 47% had actually improved. An overall satisfactory result was present in 82% of the patients who had surgery for an initial diagnosis of soft disc herniation. In the experience of Yamamoto et al, the incidence of cervical and/or intracapsular pain, not present preoperatively, was 49% within 1 month of anterior cervical discectomy. One year after surgery, 9% of the patients with soft disc herniations and 34% of the spondylotic patients continued to have neck or scapular pain.

Anterior cervical discectomy without fusion defeats many of the principles of anterior cervical fusion, which includes distraction of the neuroforamen and stretching of the buckled ligamentum flavum. In addition, by its very nature, this surgery is designed to create a pseudoarthrosis, which may lead to a less satisfactory result. Although results of surgery for soft disc herniation are better than those with spondylosis, there is a relatively high rate of persistent postoperative neck pain. Most series, to date, have limited clinical and radiographic follow-up needed to determine the development of instability or kyphotic angulation. This procedure cannot be recommended until better long-term follow-up studies are available.[31]

AUTOGRAFT VERSUS ALLOGRAFT

In an attempt to eliminate donor site problems while maintaining acceptable fusion rates, many surgeons have substituted allograft for autogenous bone in anterior cervical fusions.[8,11,18,26] Allograft eliminates the necessity for additional surgery to obtain the bone graft, thereby decreasing operative time, morbidity, and pain at the donor site.

One of the first studies comparing allograft versus autograft bone for anterior cervical fusion was reported by Brown et al[8] in 1976. He reported no difference in fusion rates between the two types of graft. However, a difference in graft collapse was noted. Twenty-eight percent of patients receiving allografts had collapse of the graft compared to 16% of the patients receiving autograft. This trend was only true for multi-level fusions. Brown found no difference in collapse rate for one-level cervical fusions.

Fernyhough et al[18] retrospectively reviewed 126 patients who underwent autogenous or allograft fibular strut grafting (Fig. 9.12) after decompression for multi-level cervical spondylosis. The combined non-union rate for both groups ranged from 21% for a two-level fusion up to 50% for a four-level fusion. Overall, the allograft group had a statistically significant higher rate of non-union (41%) than the autograft group (27%). However, no correlation between the clinical results and the rate of union was presented in this study.

Zdeblick and Ducker[67] reviewed 88 consecutive patients who underwent a Smith–Robinson anterior cervical fusion: 60 patients had autologous iliac crest graft placed, whereas freeze-dried iliac crest grafts were inserted in 27 patients. The delayed union and non-union rate was significantly higher in the allograft group compared to the autograft group. However, when one-level fusions were considered, the non-union rates at 1 year were similar. In two-level fusions the union rate was dramatically lower with allograft (38% versus 83%). In addition, the freeze-dried allograft bone collapsed more frequently during the healing process. The clinical results for the two patient groups were similar. The authors concluded that the use of freeze-dried iliac crest allograft bone in Smith–Robinson cervical fusions is

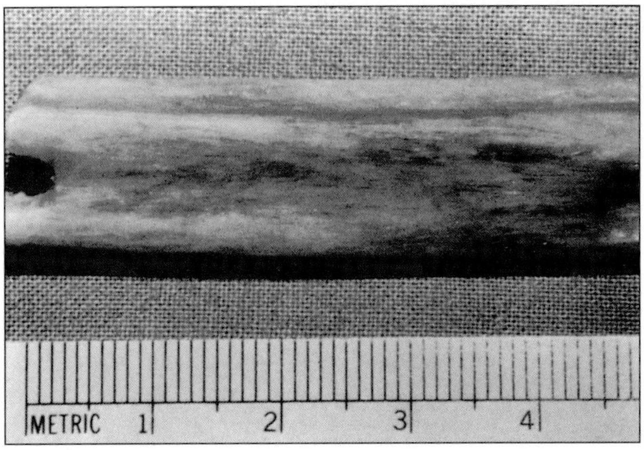

Figure 9.12
Contoured fibular strut graft reconstituted after freeze-drying. (From Rothman RH, Simeone FA. *The Spine*, 3rd ed. Philadelphia, WB Saunders, 1992, with permission)

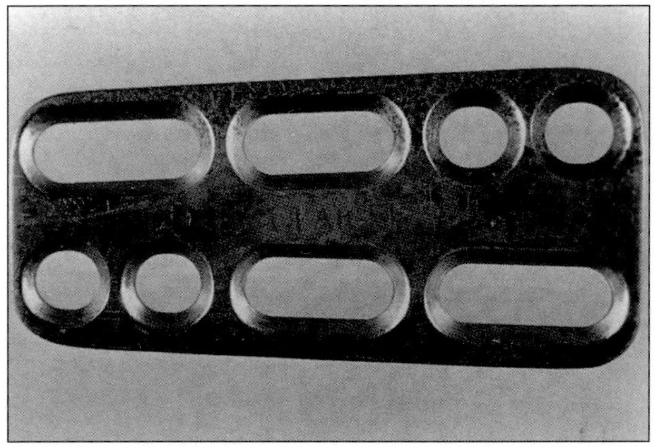

Figure 9.13
The Caspar anterior cervical plate

not recommended in multi-level fusions; when used for one-level fusions, radiographic collapse or lucency may persist despite clinical success.[7]

ANTERIOR CERVICAL INSTRUMENTATION

In an attempt to increase the success rate in anterior cervical fusions, several authors[21,45,54,58] have advocated the use of anterior cervical instrumentation. The anterior cervical plate theoretically provides increased postoperative stability after anterior decompression. In addition, the plate can act as a buttress to prevent graft extrusion in the immediate postoperative period, before bone fusion occurs.

Gassman and Seligson[21] used an anterior cervical plate for 13 anterior cervical fusions in adults undergoing surgery for traumatic and degenerative lesions. All patients showed radiographic evidence of progressive or complete fusion at 1 year follow-up. One patient required plate and screw removal approximately 2 months after the initial surgery because of screw loosening that caused dysphagia. Both this report and that of Tippets and Apfelbaum[58] used a plating system which requires penetration of the posterior cortex of the vertebral body for adequate screw fixation. Although no new neurologic deficits were reported in either study, penetration of the screws into the spinal cord carries the potential for neurologic injury.

Seifert and Stolke[54] combined spondylectomy, microsurgical decompression, and osteosynthesis using the Caspar plate (Fig. 9.13) in 22 patients with multi-segmental cervical spondylosis. In all patients, satisfactory bony fusion was achieved. Because of the immediate stability provided by the osteosynthesis, Seifert and Stolke felt that the application of a halo vest was not necessary, and immobilized their patients in either a hard or soft cervical collar. Recently, Morscher et al[45] developed a titanium plate system that is MRI compatible and does not rely on posterior vertebral body cortical penetration for stability. Currently, there are no long-term studies available to evaluate this system or the plate of Lesoin et al[42] which affords some medial–lateral and cephalocaudal variability in screw placement. Until prospective studies are available which use anterior plating systems, it is difficult to state the indications for their use in degenerative cervical spine disease.

In summary, as clinical information on cervical degenerative disorders becomes increasingly available, it is clear that the anterior approach represents the procedure of choice in many cases. Familiarity of the surgical anatomy, adequate decompression through discectomy or vertebrectomy, followed by solid arthrodesis, are essential for success. Adherence to basic spinal surgery principles of anterior cervical techniques, as outlined in this chapter, will lead to success in most patients while minimizing the potential of complication.

REFERENCES

1 Abitol JJ, Garfin SR. Surgical management of cervical disc disease: Anterior cervical fusion. *Seminars in Spine Surgery* **1**(4): 233–238, 1989.

2 Bailey RW, Badgley CE. Stabilization of the cervical spine by anterior fusion. *J Bone Joint Surg [Am]* **42**: 565–594, 1960.

3 Benini A, Krayenbuhl H, Bruder R. Anterior cervical discectomy without fusion: microsurgical technique. *Acta Neurochir* **61**: 105–110, 1982.

4 Bernard TN, Whitecloud TS. Cervical spondylotic myelopathy and myeloradiculopathy: Anterior decompression and stabilization with autogenous fibula strut graft. *Clin Orthop* **221**: 149–160, 1987.

5 Bohlman H. Cervical spondylosis with moderate to severe myelopathy. *Spine* **2**: 151–162, 1977.

6 Bohlman H. Degenerative arthrosis of the lower cervical spine. In Evarts CM (ed) *Surgery of the Musculoskeletal System*, vol. 2, 4:25–4:55. New York: Churchill Livingstone 1983.

7 Boni M, Cherubino P, Benazzo F. Multiple subtotal somatectomy: Technique and evaluation of a series of thirty-nine cases. *Spine* **9**: 358–362, 1984.

8 Brown MD, Malinin TI, Davis PB. A roentgenographic evaluation of frozen allografts versus autografts in anterior cervical spine fusions. *Clin Orthop* **119**: 231–236, 1976.

9 Chestnut R, Abithol JJ, Garfin SR. Surgical management of cervical radiculopathy. Indication, technique, and results. *Orthop Clin North Am* **23**: 461–474, 1992.

10 Cloward RB. The anterior approach for removal of ruptured cervical discs. *J Neurosurg* **15**: 602–614, 1958.

11 Cloward RB. Gas sterilized cadaver bone grafts for spinal fusion operations. *Spine* **5**: 4–10, 1980.

12 Connell M, Wiesel S. Natural history and pathogenesis of cervical disc disease. *Orthop Clin North Am* **23**: 369–380, 1992.

13 Connolly ES, Seymour RJ, Adams JE. Clinical evaluation of anterior cervical fusions for degenerative cervical disc disease. *J Neurosurg* **23**: 431–437, 1965.

14 Crandall PH, Batzdorf U. Cervical spondylotic myelopathy. *J Neurosurg* **25**: 57–66, 1966.

15 Crandall PH, Gregorius FK. Long-term follow-up of surgical treatment of cervical spondylotic myelopathy. *Spine* **2**: 139–146, 1977.

16 DePalma A, Rothman RH, Lewinnek G, Carole S. Anterior interbody fusion for severe cervical disc degeneration. *Surg Gynecol Obstet* **134**: 755–758, 1972.

17 Epstein JA, Epstein NE. The surgical management of cervical spinal stenosis, spondylosis, and myeloradiculopathy by means of the posterior approach. In Sherk HH, Dunn EJ, Eismont FJ, et al (eds) *The Cervical Spine*, 2nd ed, 625–643. Cervical Spine Research Society, Philadelphia: JB Lippincott 1989.

18 Fernyhough JC, White JI, LaRocca H. Fusion rates in multilevel cervical spondylosis comparing allograft fibula with autograft fibula in 126 patients. *Spine* **16** (suppl): S561–S564, 1991.

19 Flynn TB. Neurologic complications of anterior cervical interbody fusion. *Spine* **7**: 536–539, 1982.

20 Garfin S. Cervical spine stenosis and myelopathy. Presented at the American Academy of Orthopaedic Surgeons Summer Institute, Monterey, California, September 1990.

21 Gassman J, Seligson D. The anterior cervical plate. *Spine* **8**: 700–707, 1983.

22 Gore DR, Sepic SB. Anterior cervical fusion for degenerated or protruded discs: A review of one hundred forty-six patients. *Spine* **9**: 667–671, 1984.

23 Gore DR, Sepic SB, Gardner GM, Murray MP. Neck pain: A long-term follow-up of 205 patients. *Spine* **12**: 1–5, 1987.

24 Guidetti B, Fortuna A. Long-term results of surgical treatment of myelopathy due to cervical spondylosis. *J Neurosurg* **30**: 714–721, 1969.

25 Hanai K, Fujiyoshi F, Kamei K. Subtotal vertebrectomy and spinal fusion for cervical spondylotic myelopathy. *Spine* **11**: 310–315, 1986.

26 Hanley EN, Harvell JC, Shapiro DE, Kraus DR. Use of allograft bone in cervical spine surgery. *Seminars in Spine Surgery* **1**(4): 262–270, 1989.

27 Henderson CM, Hennessey H, Shuey H, Shackelford E. Posterior–lateral foraminotomy as an exclusive operative technique for cervical radiculopathy: A review of 846 consecutively operated cases. *J Neurosurg* **13**: 504–512, 1983.

28 Herkowitz HN. A comparison of anterior cervical fusion, cervical laminectomy, and cervical laminoplasty for the surgical management of multiple level spondylotic radiculopathy. *Spine* **13**: 774–780, 1988.

29 Herkowitz HN. The surgical management of cervical spondylotic radiculopathy and myelopathy. *Clin Orthop* **239**: 94–108, 1989.

30 Herkowitz HN. Anterior cervical surgery in cervical spondylosis. Presented at the American Academy of Orthopaedic Surgeons Annual Meeting in Washington, DC, February 1992.

31 Herkowitz HN. Surgical management of cervical radiculopathy: Anterior fusion. In Rothman RH, Simeone FA (eds) *The Spine*, 3rd ed, 597–606. Philadelphia: WB Saunders 1992.

32 Herkowitz HN, Kurz LT, Overholt DP. Surgical management of cervical soft disc herniation: A comparison between the anterior and posterior approach. *Spine* **15**: 1026–1030, 1990.

33 Hirabayashi K, Watanabe K, Wakano K, et al. Expansive open-door laminoplasty for cervical spinal stenotic myelopathy. *Spine* **8**: 693–699, 1983.

34 Hukuda S, Mochizuki T, Ogata M, Shichikawa K, Shimomura Y. Operations for cervical spondylotic myelopathy. *J Bone Joint Surg [Br]* **67**: 609–615, 1985.

35 Hukuda S, Shichikawa K, Mochizuki T, Ogata M. Cervical hyperostotic myelopathy and its surgical treatment. *Rheumatologie* **33**: 81–88, 1981.

36 Husang L, Probst C. Microsurgical anterior approach to cervical discs: Review of 60 consecutive cases of discectomy without fusion. *Acta Neurochir* **73**: 229–242, 1984.

37 Kadoya S, Nakamura T, Kwak R. A microsurgical anterior osteophytectomy for cervical spondylotic myelopathy. *Spine* **9**: 437–441, 1984.

38 Kirita Y, Miyazaki K, Hayashi T, et al. Clinical findings and surgical results of the ossification of the posterior longitudinal ligament in the cervical spine. *Rinsho Seikeigeka* **10**: 1077–1185, 1975.

39 Kurtz LT, Herkowitz HN. Surgical management of myelopathy. *Orthop Clin North Am* **23**: 495–504, 1992.

40 Lahey F, Warren K. Esophageal diverticula. *Surg Gynecol Obstet* **98**: 1–28, 1954.

41 Lees F, Turner JWA. Natural history and prognosis of cervical spondylosis. *Br Med J* **2**: 1607–1610, 1963.

42 Lesoin F, Viavel C, Jumin M. Universal plate for anterior cervical spine osteosynthesis. *Acta Neurochir* **70**: 60–61, 1985.

43 Lipson SJ. Cervical disc disease: Pathogenesis and natural history. *Seminars in Spine Surgery* **1**(4): 190–193, 1989.

44 Montgomery DM, Brower RS. Cervical spondylotic myelopathy. Clinical syndrome and natural history. *Orthop Clin North Am* **23**: 487–493, 1992.

45 Morscher E, Sutter F, Jenny H, Olerud S. Die vordere verplatung der halswirbelsaule mit dem hohlschraubmplattensystem aus titanium. *Chirurgie* **57**: 702–707, 1986.

46 Murphy M, Gado M. Anterior cervical discectomy without interbody bone graft. *J Neurosurg* **37**: 71–74, 1972.

47 Newhouse KE, Lindsey RW, Clark CR, et al. Esophageal perforation following anterior cervical spine surgery. *Spine* **14**: 1051–1053, 1989.

48 Nurick S. The natural history and the results of surgical treatment of the spinal cord disorder associated with cervical spondylosis. *Brain* **95**: 101–105, 1972.

49 O'Laoire SA, Thomas DGH. Spinal cord compression due to prolapse of cervical intervertebral (herniation of nucleus pulposus). *J Neurosurg* **59**: 847–853, 1983.

50 Phillips DG. Surgical treatment of myelopathy with cervical spondylosis. *J Neurol Neurosurg Psychiat* **36**: 879–884, 1973.

51 Riley LH, Robinson RA, Johnson KA, Walker AE. The results of anterior interbody fusion of the cervical spine. *J Neurosurg* **30**: 127–133, 1969.

52 Robinson RA, Walker AE, Ferlic DC, Wieking DK. The results of anterior interbody fusion of the cervical spine. *J Bone Joint Surg [Am]* **44**: 1569–1587, 1962.

53 Rosenorn J, Hansen E, Rosenorn M. Anterior cervical discectomy with and without fusion. *J Neurosurg* **59**: 252–255, 1983.

54 Seifert V, Stolke D. Multisegmental cervical spondylosis treatment by spondylectomy, microsurgical decompression, and osteosynthesis. *Neurosurgery* **29**: 498–503, 1991.

55 Simeone F. Surgical management of cervical disc disease: Posterior approach. *Seminars in Spine Surgery* **1**(4): 239–244, 1989.

56 Simmons EH, Bhalla SK. Anterior cervical discectomy and fusion (Keystone technique). *J Bone Joint Surg [Br]* **51**: 225–237, 1969.

57 Smith GW, Robinson RA. The treatment of certain cervical spine disorders by anterior removal of the intervertebral disc and interbody fusion. *J Bone Joint Surg [Am]* **40**: 607–624, 1958.

58 Tippets R, Apfelbaum R. Anterior cervical fusion with the caspar instrumentation system. *Neurosurgery* **22**: 1008–1013, 1988.

59 White A, Hirsch C. An experimental study of the immediate load-bearing capacity of some commonly used iliac bone grafts. *Acta Orthop Scand* **42**: 482–490, 1971.

60 Whitecloud TS. Complications of anterior cervical fusion. In American Academy of Orthopaedic Surgeons, *Instructional Course Lectures*, Vol. XXVII, 223–227. St Louis: CV Mosby 1978.

61 Whitecloud TS. Anterior surgery for cervical spondylotic myelopathy: Smith–Robinson, Cloward, and vertebrectomy. *Spine* **13**: 861–863, 1988.

62 Whitecloud TS. Management of radiculopathy and myelopathy by the anterior approach in the cervical spine. In Sherk HH, Dunn EJ, Eismont FJ, et al (eds) *The Cervical Spine*, 2nd ed, 644–658. Cervical Spine Research Society, Philadelphia: JB Lippincott 1989.

63 Williams JL, Allen MB, Harkes JW. Late results of cervical discectomy and interbody fusion: Some factors influencing the results. *J Bone Joint Surg [Am]* **50**: 277–286, 1968.

64 Wilson DH, Campbell DD. Anterior cervical discectomy without bone graft. *J Neurosurg* **47**: 551–555, 1977.

65 Yamamoto I, Ikeda A, Shibuya N, Tsugane R, Sato O. Clinical long term results of anterior discectomy without interbody fusion for cervical disc disease. *Spine* **16**: 272–279, 1991.

66 Yonenobu K, Fuji T, Ono K, et al. Choice of surgical treatment for multisegmental cervical spondylotic myelopathy. *Spine* **10**: 711–716, 1985.

67 Zdeblick TA, Ducker TB. The use of freeze-dried allograft bone for anterior cervical fusions. *Spine* **16**: 726–729, 1991.

10 Surgical management of cervical disc disease: posterior approach

J. Michael Simpson
and
Frederick A. Simeone

INTRODUCTION

The term 'cervical disc disease' is an all-encompassing term suggesting anatomic alteration in the cervical disc with subsequent structural and clinical manifestations. Cervical spondylosis is a form of cervical disc disease. At the gross anatomic level, spondylosis includes an alteration of the normal disc anatomy and biomechanics, proliferation of osteophytes about the uncovertebral and facet joints, with subsequent narrowing of the neural foramina, ligamentous thickening, and the potential for instability. In addition, soft disc herniation may occur perhaps as a stage of the overall degenerative process. Each of these alterations of normal anatomy occurs in relation to disc degeneration with the clinical consequence being dependent upon the specific mechanical alterations and neurologic structures involved. To a large extent the degenerative changes seen radiographically remain asymptomatic. However, the clinical spectrum of symptomatology associated with cervical disc disease may include radiculopathy, myelopathy, or simply neck pain. It is obviously important to delineate the primary complaint and neurologic involvement for every patient as each condition warrants specific intervention.

By far the most common presentation to the physician is neck pain. A course of conservative care, including immobilization, anti-inflammatory medications, cervical traction, exercise and/or physical therapy modalities, can be helpful. However, the prognosis is guarded for patients with symptoms of isolated neck pain. In a 10-year follow-up study on patients with neck pain only, 43% considered themselves pain free.[8] Surgery is rarely indicated for these patients. With no randomized, prospective studies to prove that cervical disc surgery can be of benefit in relief of axial pain, the surgeon should be quite reluctant in offering this as a treatment modality.

Patients who present with radicular symptoms will generally respond to a course of conservative measures over a period of several days to a few weeks. If, however, a patient presents with weakness, more acute intervention may be recommended. This is particularly true with either C5 or C8 nerve root involvement. Loss of deltoid function or hand intrinsic weakness can represent a functionally disabling problem for the patient and surgery should generally be recommended. Biceps or triceps weakness is well tolerated in most patients, unless the weakness is profound. Patients with persistent, disabling arm pain over a course of 6–8 weeks should generally be further evaluated either with a myelogram followed by computed tomography (CT) or with magnetic resonance imaging (MRI). Patients with radiographic evidence of pathology which corresponds to their level and distribution of pain would represent surgical candidates. These patients are conservatively treated, however, for 3 months before contemplating surgery as a treatment alternative.

Cervical myelopathy is a graded process with highly variable clinical manifestations. The anatomic location of cord compression, ischemic changes in the cord, and dynamic factors contribute to the wide spectrum of symptomatology. It is important to realize that myelopathy is treatable in its earliest stages, so clinical suspicion, careful history taking, and thorough neurologic evaluation are essential in the treatment of patients with these disorders.

In review of the literature, the natural history of cervical spondylotic myelopathy remains somewhat unclear. Clarke and Robinson's report of 120 patients with cervical myelopathy provides the first careful examination of the natural history of the disease.[3] Age at presentation and duration of symptoms before treatment were shown to be the most important factors affecting prognosis, with increased age at presentation being associated with poorer results overall. If the symptoms of myelopathy have been present for more than 1 year, the chances of improvement are significantly reduced. Very few patients with cervical myelopathy reverse their symptoms with conservative care.[20,25,29,32] In most patients, myelopathy seems to have progression in a step-wise course with poorly defined periods of non-progression. A small percentage of patients present with rapid progression of neurologic compromise leading to severe disability. The factors initiating such progression are unknown, but may involve a vascular insult to the spinal cord. It is clear that cervical spondylotic myelopathy is a completely different entity from radiculopathy: given the natural history of slow progression, early surgical intervention is generally recommended.

The surgical approach for cervical radiculopathy or myelopathy is still a controversial one in the literature. A purely posterior approach to these problems is not recommended, but there are specific indications for the posterior approach with either condition which are outlined below in some detail.

POSTERIOR SURGICAL APPROACH FOR CERVICAL RADICULOPATHY

The diagnosis of cervical disc disease with radiculopathy is very specific. Pain, loss of reflex, weakness, and sensory deficits are included in the clinical spectrum. Pain can be quite severe and usually has a sharp lancinating or burning character. The failure of non-operative treatment, as indicated above, or the rapid development of neurologic deficit encourages operative decisions.

Cervical radiculopathy, secondary to either soft or hard disc pathology, may be addressed either anteriorly or posteriorly. Many factors contribute to the individual surgeon's choice of operation in a given patient, with influential factors reflecting not only the specific nature of the disease but the idiosyncrasies and training of the individual surgeon. A competent spine surgeon must be able to perform all approaches safely.

Anterior surgery plays a role in the treatment of all forms of cervical spine pathology. The present authors reserve the anterior approach for the following disorders:

- Midline soft disc herniation with symptomatic myelopathy at one or more levels.
- Midline hard disc protrusion at one or two levels.
- Disc herniation with bilateral radiculopathy at the same level.
- Resection of a disease process in the vertebral body.
- Spinal cord decompression in a kyphotic cervical spine.

A posterior approach is used for the following:

- Unilateral radiculopathy at one or more levels (posterior keyhole foraminotomy).
- Cervical myelopathy with spinal cord compression at three or more levels (posterior laminectomy or laminoplasty).
- Spinal cord compression secondary to degenerative subluxation (posterior laminectomy with facet joint fusion).
- Spinal cord compression secondary to congenital spinal stenosis or acquired stenosis from posterior compression due to cervical hyperlordosis.

In addition, if the patient has significant axial pain plus radicular pain, anterior discectomy and fusion are the preferred technique.

Technique: Posterior Keyhole Foraminotomy for Cervical Radiculopathy

In general, posterior approaches to the cervical spine are performed with the patient either prone or in a sitting position. The advantage of the sitting position is the reduction in blood loss secondary to collapse of the epidural vessels. The major disadvantage of the sitting position is the risk of air embolus. However, for posterior decompressive procedures to the cervical spine such a risk is quite small, and it can be reduced by proper positioning of the patient. Placement of the knees higher than the heart and prophylactic use of compression stockings are helpful. Routine placement of a Swan–Ganz catheter in monitoring for air has generally been recommended in the use of this position. However, the present authors prefer an intermediate position: the patient is placed in a kneeling position with the head slightly flexed and held in a Mayfield pin-holder headrest or allowed simply to rest on a well-padded horseshoe-shaped headrest (Fig. 10.1).

Meticulous attention should be paid to protection of the eyes which should be taped shut after instillation of a protective ointment, and it should be ensured that no part of the pin-holder headrest is in contact with the patient's face. When using the horseshoe headrest, the padding should be carefully checked to ensure that no undue pressure is placed about the orbit and that no localized pressure is placed upon the face. The authors recommend the use of the Mayfield pin-holder headrest because it seems to offer more rigid control of the head during the operative procedure with complete alleviation of any potential pressure points on the face of the patient. With the patient secured, the operating room table is then tilted so that the cervical spine is roughly parallel to the floor (Fig. 10.1). This allows for partial collapse of the epidural veins, although the surgeon can be free of concern of air embolism. In the series of the present authors, no signs or symptoms of air embolism have ever occurred in this position.

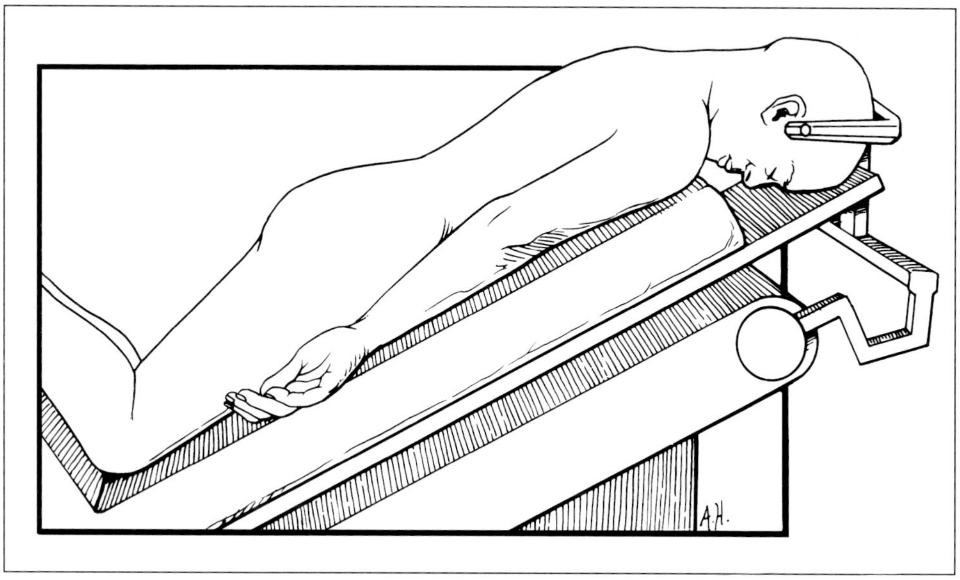

Figure 10.1
Position of the patient for any posterior cervical surgical procedure. The patient's face rests on a well-padded horseshoe-shaped headrest, and the operating table is tilted in a reverse Trendelenburg fashion so that the cervical spine is parallel to the floor. This technique decreases blood flow and reduces risk of air embolism associated with the sitting position. A pin-holder headrest is preferred by the present authors, allowing complete relief of all potential pressure points

The appropriate spinal level is identified by inserting a needle through the skin into a spinous process. A radiograph is then taken while the neck is prepped. An incision (approximately 3–4 cm) is then made in the midline covering the two spinous processes between which the offending disc lies. The dissection is then carried down to the spinous processes using electrocautery. Continuous, meticulous hemostasis is completed as the dissection proceeds. With a spinous process clearly visualized, a second radiograph is obtained for identification of the operative level. The dissection is then carried laterally over the laminae and a Taylor retractor placed lateral to the articular mass for soft tissue retraction. Great care is taken not to disrupt the facet capsule. A weight may be hung from the Taylor retractor or gauze wrapped from the retractor to the surgeon's foot. Gentle traction may then be applied with excellent exposure. With a thin 1-mm Schlessinger rongeur, a circular laminotomy defect is then made approximately 8 mm in diameter (Fig. 10.2). Half of this defect is placed on the superior lamina and the other half on the inferior lamina. This laterally placed laminotomy forms the circular portion of the 'keyhole'.

With clear visualization using magnification in the form of either loupes or an operating microscope, a high-speed air drill and a 3-mm diamond-tip burr are used to thin the bone directly over the nerve root. For the best delineation of the particular pathway required for decompression, the nerve root should be palpated with a fine dental probe in the foramen (Fig. 10.3). Because the nerve root leaves between the two laminae, the drilling involves partial excision of the facet joint. During the

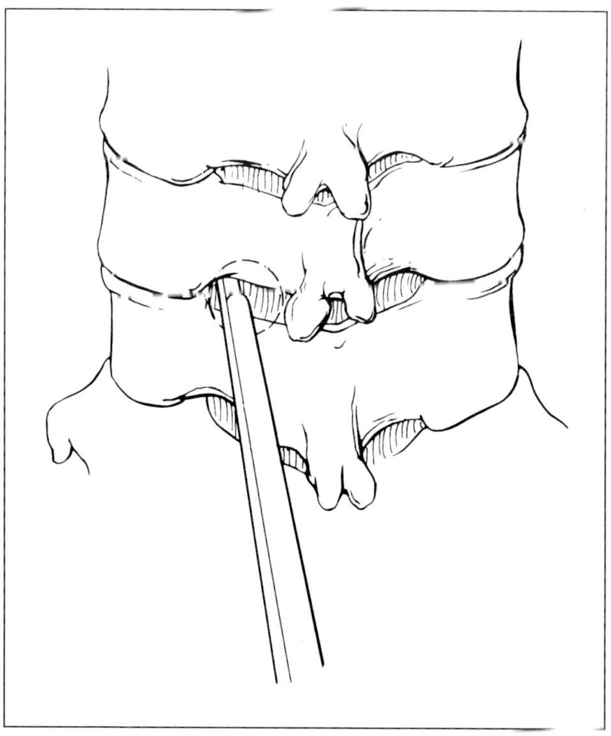

Figure 10.2
After the appropriate interspace is identified, a 1-mm Schlessinger rongeur is used to create a circular defect approximately 8 mm in diameter. One-half of this laminotomy is made on the superior lamina and the other half on the inferior lamina, forming the circular portion of the keyhole. Care is taken to preserve as much of the facet capsule as possible

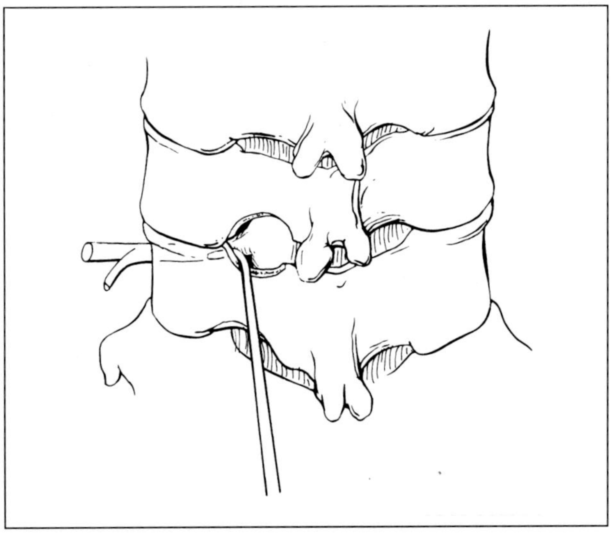

Figure 10.3
Under the operating microscope or 3.5 × magnifying loupe, the exiting nerve root is palpated with a fine dental probe. This allows the surgeon to identify the pathway for the foraminotomy

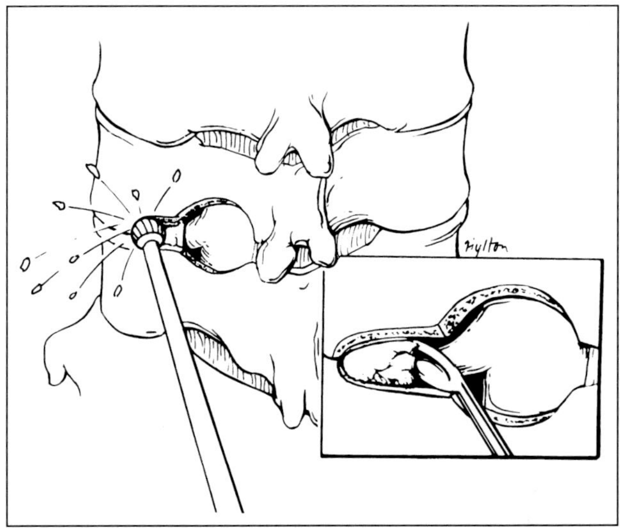

Figure 10.4
A high-speed air drill with a 3-mm diamond tip is used to thin the bone over the nerve root. Because the nerve root leaves between the laminae, the drilling straddles the facet joint. Superior and inferior extension of the drilling process goes from pedicle to pedicle. Inset: once the bone is adequately thinned, a fine angled curette is used to remove the layer of remaining bone over the nerve root

drilling process, the surgeon will first encounter the outer cortical table, which is quite dense and hard, followed by cancellous bone which is easily thinned; the second cortical table will then be encountered. Drilling at this point must proceed slowly and with caution as the nerve is approximated. Drilling must be completed in a medial-to-lateral direction. Continuous irrigation is used to prevent thermal injury.

Once this anterior cortical rim is thinned appropriately, a fine angled curette is then used to chip off the thin layer of remaining bone in an anterior-to-posterior direction, thus minimizing potential for mechanical injury to the underlying nerve root (Fig. 10.4). Surgeons find themselves alternating constantly between burr and curette during the decompression. As the bone is chipped away, it can be appreciated how tight the nerve root is against the inferior surface of the facet joint. The lateral extent of the foraminotomy is determined by passing a thin, angled instrument such as a fine, blunt, nerve hook or dental probe out through the neural foramen. Proper lateral decompression of the nerve root generally requires 5 mm of root exposure. Cranial-to-caudal exposure should extend from pedicle to pedicle. With hard disc pathology, if the instrument can pass comfortably around the shoulder, axilla, and foramen of the root, the foraminotomy is complete. If, however, any resistance is felt, the foraminotomy is extended as needed to effect decompression of the involved neural structure.

For most soft disc herniations, bony decompression through laminotomy and foraminotomy is adequate. However, with diminished mobility or feeling of incomplete freeing of the nerve, the vascular cuff enveloping the nerve root should be removed, and both the root and the soft discs explored (Fig. 10.5). Once this vascular cuff is removed with electrocautery, the root can be gently retracted cephalad and the disc space entered with a Rosen knife or microsurgical Penfield dissector (Fig. 10.6). If the herniated disc appears substantial and soft, the annulus can then be cut with a no. 11 scalpel blade, being careful not to involve the dura of the nerve root sheath which can be severely thinned under pressure. Incision of the annulus is then usually associated with extrusion of disc material. If this does not occur, the Rosen knife can be placed under the ventral portion of the nerve root and the disc material pressed through the opening in the annular fibrosis. Incision of the annulus is generally created over the apex of the disc protrusion. This can be seen either over the shoulder of the root or in the axillary region. In some

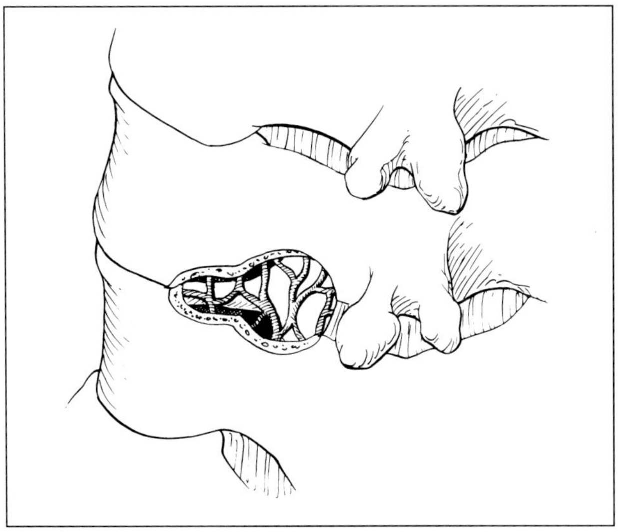

Figure 10.5
With large soft disc herniations, removal of the disc fragment may be necessary for adequate decompression of the nerve root. The vascular cuff enveloping the nerve root must first be removed using electrocautery with continuous irrigation, and the nerve root mobilized

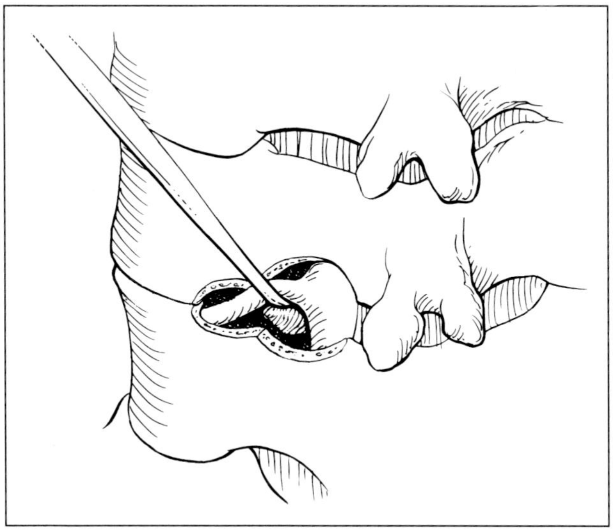

Figure 10.6
The nerve root is gently retracted, and the disc fragment identified and removed. If the disc is contained by fibers of the annulus, the space may be entered at its apex with a Rosen knife or microsurgical Penfield dissector. This usually results in the automatic extrusion of disc material which can then be easily removed.

instances, this maneuver can yield substantial portions of soft disc material, although the yield is disappointing, particularly in instances of chronically degenerated disc. Once this is completed the surgeon generally finds increased mobility of the root when palpated in all directions. If no soft disc material is produced, no further attempt at bony decompression is made. The nerve root is then covered with a small portion of fat. The paraspinous muscles are approximated with no. 1 Vicryl (polyglactin 910). A two layer skin closure is completed with a running subcuticular suture of 3/0 Vicryl. After the operation, the patient does not require immobilization, although immobilization in a soft collar is often of benefit for the first few days.

The development of acute instability after foraminotomy has been investigated in several previous studies. A recent study by Zdeblick et al[38] studied the effect of a progressive, staged foraminotomy on cervical stability. Physiological loads were applied to human cadaveric cervical spines following resection of 25, 50, 75, and 100% of the facet joint and capsule unilaterally. It is clear from this study that segmental hypermobility can be created if the foraminotomy involves resection of more than 50% of the facet joint, and also that the remaining portion of the facet joint capsule must be left intact. It therefore seems reasonable that, with decompressions involving more than 50% of the joint, concomitant fusion should be completed.

The present authors have achieved excellent results with this operative procedure in a non-compensation, non-litigation group of patients. In a recent review by the authors of 65 patients with a 6-year follow-up, 95% of patients reported a good to excellent result.[31] A small subgroup of these patients allowed follow-up radiographic evaluation to determine development of instability. Flexion–extension views were obtained in 25 patients with over 6 years of follow-up. No evidence of instability was seen in any patient. Similar good results have been reported by Henderson et al.[12] In this study, it is evident that excision of the offending soft disc material is not necessary for good outcome. He reported excellent results in 96% of a series of 846 patients with posterior decompression and no disc removal.

Complications

Reported complications with the keyhole foraminotomy have been few. Potential problems include failure to operate at the correct level, dural tear, nerve root injury, inadequate foraminotomy, and iatrogenic instability. These problems become less common as surgeons develop their skill with the technique. Use of careful intraoperative radiographs, magnification, and repeated palpation of the nerve root for 'looseness' is necessary. Nerve root injury is commonly a result of direct mechanical injury to the root. Forcing a Kerrison rongeur into the foraminal zone should not be done. Thinning of the bone with the burr, followed by chipping of the remaining bone with a small angled curette, is safe and efficient with little risk to the underlying root. Direct injury to the root with the burr is also possible. Two hands should always be used to control this instrument, and the surgeon's hands should rest on the patient's neck for stability purposes. A diamond-tipped burr, although slower, is preferred. Continuous irrigation is necessary to prevent thermal injury.

Dural tears, although uncommon, also represent a potential complication of this procedure. Repair of dural tears is generally recommended. This should be performed under microscopic visualization using a 4/0 or 5/0 suture. If closure is not possible, then use of Surgicel or Gelfoam soaked in some of the patient's blood often suffices. A watertight closure of the fascia is required and no drains would be used under these circumstances.

The question of iatrogenic instability has already been addressed. Careful adherence to the surgical principles as outlined is required. If a decompression requires more than 50% excision of the facet joint at any level, a concomitant fusion should be completed.

In general, patients recover from surgery without arm pain and can be discharged on the second postoperative day. Most of these patients are discharged without any form of immobilization, although, occasionally, a soft collar is preferred by the patient for a few days. This freedom from complication and the rapid return to normal activity compare favorably with anterior disc surgery where reported results for arm pain relief are approximately the same. However, the present authors feel that the complications associated with the anterior approach are potentially more severe and common than those seen posteriorly.

POSTERIOR CERVICAL LAMINECTOMY FOR CERVICAL STENOSIS AND MYELOPATHY

There are a variety of surgical techniques available to the surgeon for patients with symptomatic cervical stenosis with or without myelopathy. It is obviously clear that consideration of surgery for a given pathologic process is predicated on the natural history of that disease. Likewise, the risk-to-benefit ratio determines which particular surgical or non-operative treatment is chosen. The history, physical examination, and radiographic work-up must correlate to confirm the diagnosis of cervical spondylotic myelopathy.

In review of the literature, there has been no adequate study of the conservative treatment of cervical spondylotic myelopathy. There are, however, numerous reports describing the course of cervical spondylotic myelopathy and the effects of various treatment forms on this disease process.[4,5,11,14,16,17,20,25,29,32] Clarke and Robinson's report of 120 patients with cervical spondylotic myelopathy provides the most clear examination of the disease's natural history.[3] From their study, it was clear that 75% of patients underwent a course defined by episodes of worsening symptoms and signs. Two-thirds of this 75% showed ongoing deterioration between acute clinical episodes and the remaining one-third showed stabilization between the episodes of acute clinical deterioration. These periods of stability lasted from just a few weeks to several years. One-fifth of all patients showed a slow, steady progression without periods of remission. Five percent of patients were characterized as having a rapid onset of myelopathy, and progression of signs and symptoms to a point of stabilization. Deaths related directly to cervical spondylotic myelopathy occurred in 5% of patients, usually secondary to pulmonary or urinary complication. In conclusion, Clarke and Robinson determined that the clinical course of a patient with cervical spondylotic myelopathy is quite variable, although generally of slow progression. True improvement in the patient's clinical symptomatology is rare.

Additional studies looking at cervical spondylotic myelopathy are available, but limited in their ability to truly assess the natural history of the disease. These studies include those by Lees and Turner in 1963,[20] Nurick in 1972,[25] Phillips in 1973,[27] and Symon and Lavender in 1967.[32] Although no two studies used the same criteria in evaluating outcomes and different studies have used a wide variety of conservative and surgical techniques, there appears to be a common thread of available information. Age and duration of symptoms appear to be the most important factors affecting prognosis. Increased age of presentation and myelopathic symptoms present for more than a year are associated with poorer results.

Surgical treatment for cervical spondylotic myelopathy can be accomplished either anteriorly or posteriorly dependent upon the extent and type of pathology. Four basic procedures are available for the surgical treatment of cervical spondylotic myelopathy: a posterior cervical laminectomy, posterior cervical laminoplasty, anterior cervical discectomy with interbody arthrodesis, and anterior cervical vertebrectomy and strut graft fusion.

In patients presenting with a pure myelopathy, spinal cord impingement is usually due to bulging of degenerated disc or osteophytes projecting posteriorly from the margins of the end-plates. This results in anterior compression of the spinal cord. Hypertrophy and buckling of the ligamentum flavum are also generally appreciated under these conditions and may contribute to posterior compression of the spinal cord.

Anterior cervical discectomy, with removal of posterior marginal osteophytes, and interbody fusion can be used in a large number of cases of cervical spondylotic myelopathy. The pathology, however, should be limited to two or three surgical levels and there should be no evidence of a congenital canal stenosis. Both union rate and results diminish as the number of operative levels increases.[30] The bone graft, through distraction, may also provide an indirect decompression by stretching out the buckled ligamentum flavum.

Anterior cervical corpectomy and arthrodesis is used when only two or more consecutive levels are involved in which spinal cord compression is at the level of the vertebral body, as well as the intervertebral disc margins. As this decompression is more radical, it may be used in cases with a congenital canal stenosis and in ossification of the posterior longitudinal ligament (OPLL). Distraction of the created space with the strut graft potentially provides an indirect posterior decompression through stretching of the buckled ligamentum flavum. The incidence of surgical complications with this procedure is high. Yonenobu et al[36] reported a 29.3% complication rate with anterior cervical corpectomy and strut grafting in a series of 41 patients. They reported 10 graft complications (dislodgement, fracture, and non-union), one esophageal fistula, and one retrolisthesis. Four of these complications were associated with neurologic deterioration. These results were compared to those in a group of 42 patients undergoing laminoplasty.[36] The complication rate was 7.1% with three patients experiencing neurologic deterioration.

Either of these anterior techniques affords cervical nerve root decompression, which may be required in cases of myeloradiculopathy. Direct decompression is accomplished by removal of offending osteophytes and disc material. An indirect decompression is obtained through distraction, so widening the neuroforamina.

Laminectomy and laminoplasty can be used for multilevel cervical spondylotic disease, with or without concomitant radicular symptoms or congenital cervical stenosis, particularly in those cervical spines with hyperlordosis. Either posterior procedure permits an increase in the anteroposterior canal diameter and effectively removes spinal cord decompression due to pathologic ligamentum flavum. An indirect spinal cord decompression is presumed through posterior translation of the spinal cord. Foraminotomies may be completed with either posterior procedure in cases of myeloradiculopathy.

In this section, cervical laminectomy and laminoplasty are considered in the treatment of cervical stenosis and cervical spondylotic myelopathy.

Technique: Posterior Cervical Laminectomy

The space available for the spinal cord can be greatly increased by cervical laminectomy, which represents the definitive treatment for disorders that compromise the spinal cord posteriorly such as congenital or degenerative cervical stenosis. The posterior approach can also be used for anterior pathology. This is particularly true for cervical spondylotic myelopathy involving three or more levels. Ideally, these problems could be approached anteriorly. However, a multi-level anterior operation can be quite complicated and time consuming. In such cases, a posterior decompression is generally recommended. In OPLL producing cervical spondylotic myelopathy, an anterior approach may also be contemplated. However, this may involve resection of several vertebral bodies and require subsequent reconstruction. Such reconstruction needs prolonged halo immobilization with its inherent disability and lower rate of success with fusion. There has been a gradual return in the literature to the use of laminectomy or laminoplasty in the treatment of OPLL.

For patients with cervical spondylotic myelopathy, fiberoptic intubation while awake is required. Attempts to hyperextend the neck for placement of an endotracheal tube certainly put the patient at grave risk for spinal cord injury. It is well known that, under the effects of neuromuscular blocking agents and general anesthesia, the neck can be extended to a greater degree than that achieved voluntarily.

The options for patient positioning are the same as those indicated for cervical foraminotomy, although the patient's head should be kept in a neutral position. Hyperextension or -flexion for long periods of time will probably not be tolerated by the patient, and neurologic compromise may result. Physicians should not depend on preoperative bending films of the cervical spine for determination of the extent of flexion or extension tolerated by the patient. Placement of the patient's head in an extreme position for a period of several hours under general anesthesia is obviously quite different from holding it in one of these positions for a few minutes in an office setting.

Once the patient is positioned and the neck region properly prepped, the involved spinous processes are exposed through a midline incision and hemostasis obtained. The appropriate levels can usually be identified by palpation of the prominent C2 spinous process. If there is any question, an intraoperative radiograph is taken. Dissection is then completed by exposing the appropriate laminae bilaterally. Care is taken not to disrupt the facet joint capsules. (If a patient with cervical spondylotic myelopathy has concomitant root involvement, foraminotomies may be first completed as previously described. Once the foraminotomies are completed, the laminec-

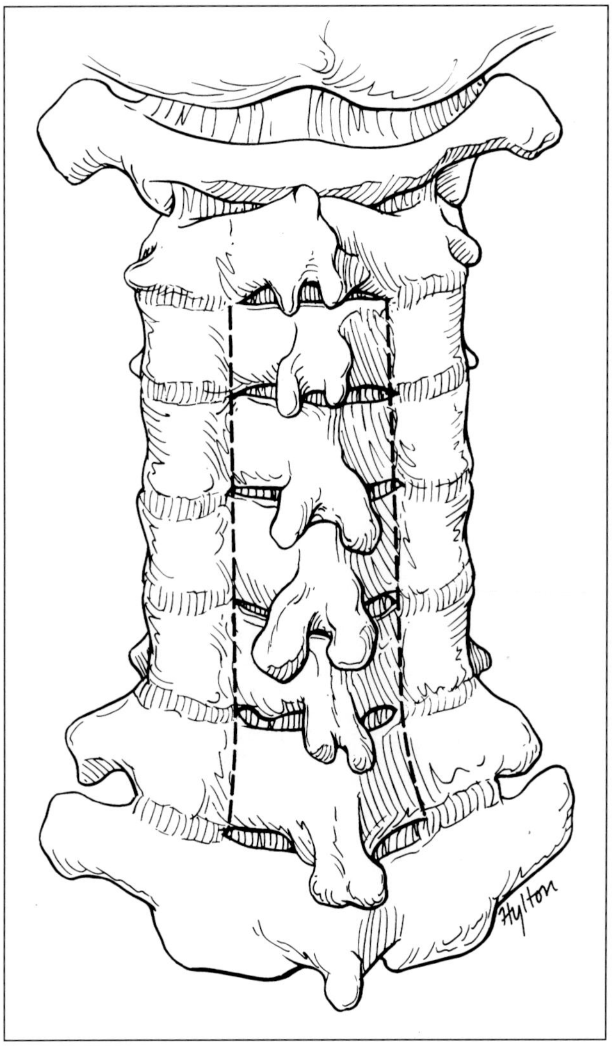

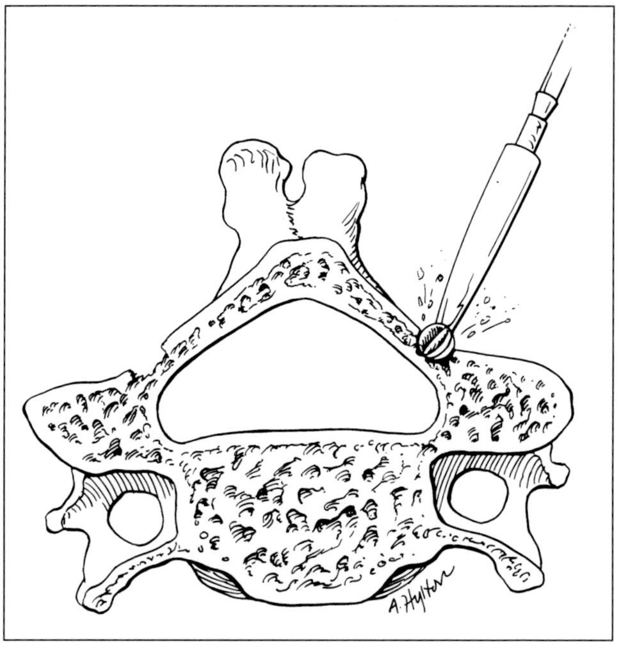

Figure 10.8
The vertical line described in Fig. 10.7 shows the location of the trough. This trough is created using a round 4-mm cutting burr just medial to the lateral border of the facet joint. Drilling is completed in a caudal-to-cranial direction. Three layers of bone will be encountered during the drilling process. The inner cortical layer is thinned but not penetrated with the burr. Continuous irrigation is used to prevent thermal injury

Figure 10.7
Operative view of the posterior cervical spine for a patient undergoing a multi-level laminectomy or laminoplasty procedure. The vertical lines on each side of the laminae indicate the pathway for drilling and creation of the troughs

tomy may proceed.) The spinous processes can be removed with a rongeur if preferred by the surgeon, and the laminectomy then completed in a piecemeal fashion similar to that generally carried out in the lumbar spine. This does, however, tend to be time consuming and requires passage of instruments central to the spinal cord which can further compromise the canal and potentiate neurologic injury.

The present authors prefer an *en bloc* resection of the involved laminae: two lateral troughs are created with the use of a round cutting burr just medial to the lateral border of the facet joint (Figs 10.7 and 10.8). A diamond cutting burr may be used, but tends to be slow and creates more heat. The drilling process is completed under loupe magnification, beginning at the lower lamina to be excised and extending in a cranial fashion. Once again the surgeon will encounter three layers of bone (Fig. 10.8). The outer cortical layer of the lamina is removed with the burr; the cancellous elements are encountered and easily removed with the burr; then the inner cortical table is seen and thinned with the burr, although the rim is not penetrated. Overaggressive drilling may cause injury to the dura or underlying nerve root. Continuous irrigation is used to prevent thermal injury and to maintain proper operative visualization.

Once these troughs have been thinned appropriately, a small 1-mm Kerrison rongeur can be used to complete the trough (Fig. 10.9). This requires resection of the bony elements as well as the ligamentum flavum. Once the troughs are completed bilaterally, the ligamentum flavum must be resected at the proximal and distal poles of the laminectomy, which can be done simply by placing a towel clip into the spinous process of the most superior and inferior involved segments. The spinous processes are then lifted, and the ligamentum flavum resected using a no. 12 scalpel blade or fine scissors (Fig. 10.10). Be careful not to allow any portion of the resected laminae to dip or translate anteriorly potentially compressing the spinal cord. Once completed, it is possible to remove the entire block of excised laminae. When this portion of the procedure is properly carried out, the lateral margins of the dura are visible with the facet joints intact (Fig. 10.11). Often, bleeding lateral epidural veins are encountered, and these are generally managed with bipolar cautery. Individual nerve roots are palpated for adequate decompression. The paraspinous muscles are then approximated tightly, usually using running no. 1 Vicryl sutures. The skin and subcutaneous tissue are then approximated in two layers, and the skin closed with a running subcuticular suture.

Attention must be given before operation to pre-existing deformity or evidence of instability. For those patients with evidence of degenerative subluxation at any level, a concomitant fusion across that segment is strongly encouraged. Preoperative flexion–extension views are necessary to delineate instability. Internal fixation methods with facet wiring or posterior plating may be used to obtain fusion, or else only grafting can be done with appropriate postoperative immobilization in a Minerva brace or cervical halo. The development of a postlaminectomy kyphosis is an added concern, and it should be noted that this deformity may occur in any age group, although it is most frequently found in children and young adults. In older adults, kyphosis is most often seen in traumatic disorders and patients requiring foraminotomy in addition to laminectomy. After the operation, patients undergoing laminectomy may prefer short-term immobilization with a soft cervical collar, which can be discontinued several days later based on patient symptoms.

Reports reviewing cervical laminectomy for spondylotic myelopathy are variable, and on review of several studies, it appears that 68–85% of patients undergoing laminectomy, with or without foraminotomy for myelopathy or myeloradiculopathy, can be expected to have a good or excellent outcome.[1,6,7,22,25] In comparing anterior cervical discectomy and fusion to laminectomy and laminoplasty for multi-level cervical spondylotic radiculopathy, Herkowitz found 92% good to excellent results with anterior fusion, 86% in the laminoplasty group and only 66% in the laminectomy group.[13] Complications reported in the cervical laminectomy group were the development of cervical kyphosis in 25% of patients and anterior subluxation (less than 2 mm) in nearly 40% of the operative levels.[13] These complications appear secondary to the multiple foraminotomies required for adequate decompression.

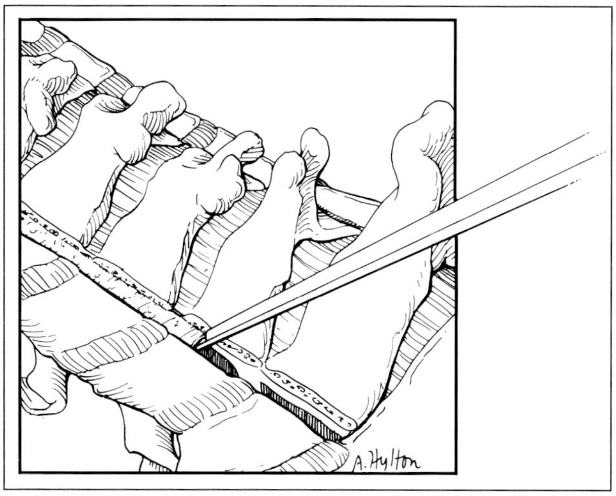

Figure 10.9
Once troughs are appropriately thinned a 1-mm Schlessinger rongeur is used to complete the trough. This requires resection of the bony elements and ligamentum flavum. The surgeon will feel a 'freeing' of the laminar block to be resected

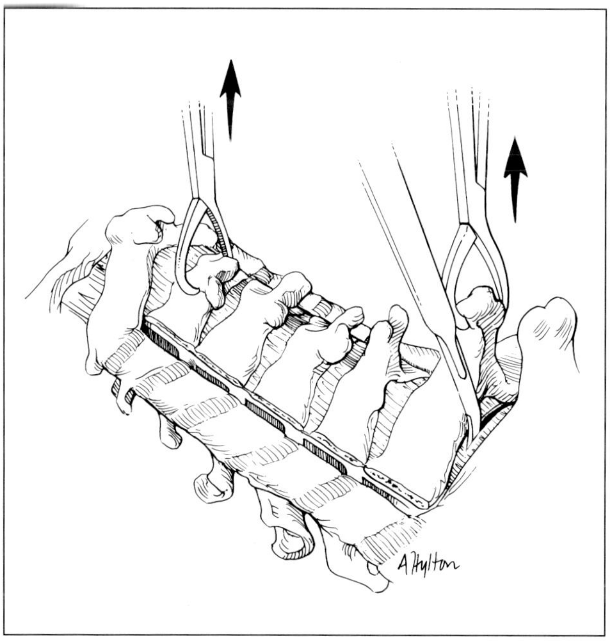

Figure 10.10
Towel clips are placed in the spinous processes at the proximal and distal poles of the laminectomy. Gentle upward traction is applied as the ligamentum flavum at each pole is resected using either a no. 12 scalpel blade or fine scissors

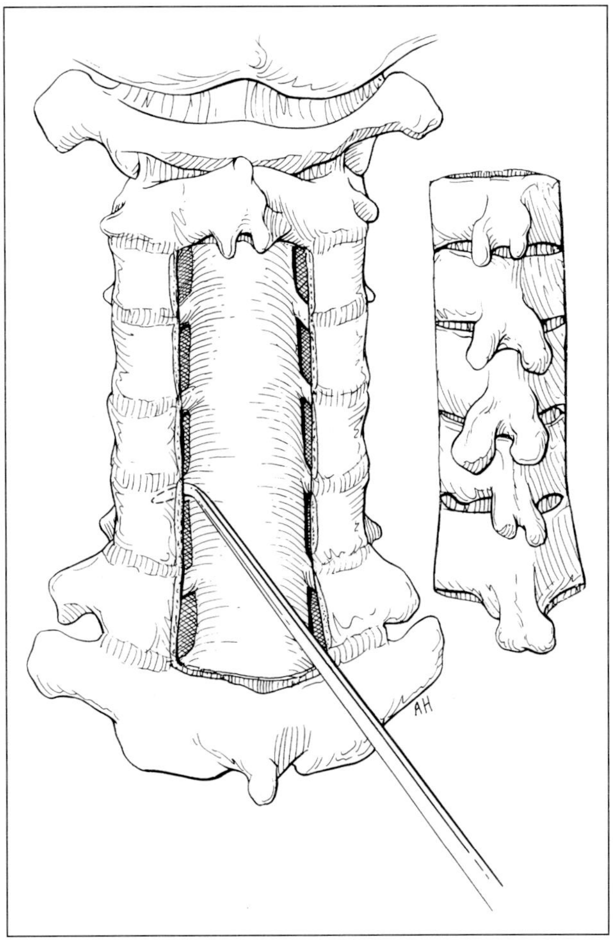

Figure 10.11
Left: The dura is decompressed after removal of the cervical laminae. The lateral margins of the dura are visible with the facet joints intact. Individual nerve roots are palpated for adequate decompression. Right: The block of five resected cervical laminae connected by ligamentum flavum

POSTERIOR CERVICAL LAMINOPLASTY FOR MULTI-LEVEL RADICULOPATHY, MYELOPATHY, AND MYELORADICULOPATHY

The laminoplasty technique was first described by Hirabayashi et al in 1968,[16] and was originally described for the surgical management of multi-level cervical radiculopathy. Certain refinements in the technique have occurred since the original description. Current surgical indications for use of laminoplasty include multi-level radiculopathy, multi-level cervical spondylotic myelopathy, and myeloradiculopathy.[8]

Although laminoplasty appears to be a viable alternative for multi-level bilateral radiculopathy, the present authors prefer the anterior approach in most of these cases. However, for patients with multi-level cervical spondylotic myeloradiculopathy or myelopathy *with* preoperative evidence of instability, laminoplasty represents the procedure of choice. Laminectomy alone, especially in the younger patient or in patients requiring multiple foraminotomies, may lead to a deformity and instability. Postoperative progressive instability does not appear to be a problem with laminoplasty. In fact, contrary to logic, excellent results have been achieved regardless of whether associated radicular symptoms were unilateral or bilateral, and despite foraminotomies not being performed on the hinged side. Opening of the spinal canal seems to be sufficient to relieve symptoms without formal nerve root decompression on this side.[19]

Technique: 'Open Door' Laminoplasty

The patient is positioned in the fashion described for cervical foraminotomy. Again, use of the Mayfield pin-holder headrest is preferred. For patients with myelopathy, an awake intubation is performed. The 'open door' portion of the laminoplasty is made on the most symptomatic side for the patient. For example, the open door will be made on the right side of a patient with predominant right-sided arm pain. In patients with an equal distribution of pain into both upper extremities, the opening is made on the side exhibiting the greatest compression on radiographic studies. In cases of myeloradiculopathy, foraminotomies are first completed as necessary on the patient's most symptomatic side before the laminoplasty is created, because greater protection of the spinal cord is then maintained during the drilling process for the foraminotomy. The foraminotomies are carried out in the fashion described earlier, and once the foraminotomies are completed, the laminoplasty can then be performed.

Two bony gutters are first made with a high-speed burr, as described for a cervical laminectomy; the burring proceeds in a caudal-to-cranial direction, and is performed just medial to the facet joint and pedicle. On the side that is to be opened, the burr is taken through the outer cortical table and through the cancellous elements to the inner cortical table of the laminae, which is thinned but not penetrated (Fig. 10.12). On the opposite, hinged side, the burr is used to go through the outer cortex only, although occasionally, it may be necessary to burr through the cancellous elements to the inner cortex. Next, a 1-mm Kerrison rongeur is used to remove the inner cortex of the 'open door' side in a caudal-to-cranial direction. Once

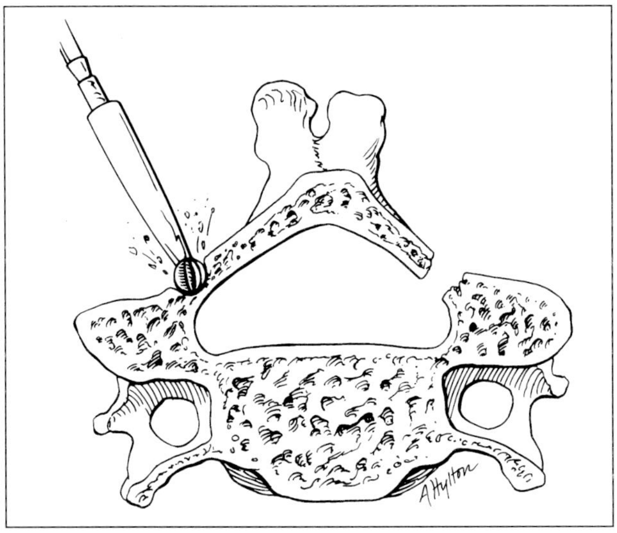

Figure 10.12
On the laminar side to be opened, the burr is taken through the outer cortical table and cancellous elements. The inner cortical table is then thinned with the burr as completed in the laminectomy technique. On the opposite 'hinged' side, the burr is taken through the outer cortical table only

this gutter is completed, gentle pressure is then applied to the spinous processes in an attempt to 'open the door'. Usually 'greensticking' of the hinge occurs, allowing the door to be opened, and it is commonly necessary to release a portion of the ligamentum flavum at the proximal and distal poles of the laminoplasty with a scalpel or Kerrison rongeur (Figs 10.13 and 10.14). When the hinge is finally opened, it is essential to make sure that adhesions are not present between the dural sac and the undersurface of the lamina; a Penfield elevator or a Woodson-type instrument may be used to release these adhesions. The laminar opening should be approximately 10–12 mm. A laminar opening of 10 mm has been shown to expand the sagittal diameter of the canal by 4–5 mm.[18]

Once this expansion has been completed, it must be maintained in this position by use of a non-absorbable suture. The tips of the spinous processes are removed using a rongeur, and the suture is then placed through the base of the spinous process. It is usually easier to place these burr holes across the spinous process before elevation of the laminae in which case the suture is passed through the base of each of the involved spinous processes and secured to the facet capsules at each segment. These sutures, once again, should maintain the laminar opening at 10–15 mm. Occasionally this 'fixation' of the hinge may be insecure and inadequate. In this case, instead of a non-absorbable suture at the proximal and distal poles of the laminoplasty, 20 or 22 gauge wire is passed through the spinous process and secured to the facet via a drill hole as for routine facet wiring (Fig. 10.15).

Following this, the bone from the spinous process tips is cleaned of remaining soft tissues, fashioned into small strips and placed in the hinged gutter. The exposed dura is usually covered with a thin layer of fat removed from the subcutaneous tissues. If this is not available, a strip of Gelfoam may be used. After the operation, the patient is kept in a Minerva brace for 6 weeks, at which time, the patient is instructed about the range of movement possible and isometric exercises.

The present authors are in agreement with Herkowitz that bilateral foraminotomies are not required for patients with bilateral radicular symptoms. For reasons that have not been clarified, these patients appear to have good relief of radicular symptoms on the hinged side, which may be related to improvement in the vascular supply of the nerve root.

Various modifications of the laminoplasty operation have been developed. Hirabayashi et al[15] have described a spinous process splitting form of laminoplasty for bilateral symptomatology. Hase et al[11] describe a similar technique in which a bilateral open laminoplasty is secured in the open position with ceramic laminae to prevent late closure and recurrent stenosis. The present authors, however, feel that these procedures are technically more difficult to perform and generally not required.

COMPLICATIONS ASSOCIATED WITH LAMINECTOMY AND LAMINOPLASTY

The commonly reported complications after posterior cervical laminectomy include development or progression of deformity (kyphosis), instability (spondylolisthesis), and inadequate decompression.[13] Postlaminectomy kyphosis is most frequently seen in children and young adults. Haft et al [10] found a 59% incidence of kyphoscoliosis in children undergoing cervical laminectomy for tumor. Cattel and Clark[2] described three children with cervical kyphosis and instability following laminectomy. Lonstein et al[21] found a 100% incidence of spinal deformity at the level of cervical laminectomy in a series of immature patients. Yasouka et al[34] reported development of postoperative kyphosis with no pre-existing deformity or surgical disruption of facet joints. It is believed that the greater tendency for ligamentous stretching and secondary vertebral body wedging in children leads to a higher percentage of such deformity in this group compared to adults.[33]

In adults with normal preoperative alignment and stability, laminectomy is usually not associated with a significant

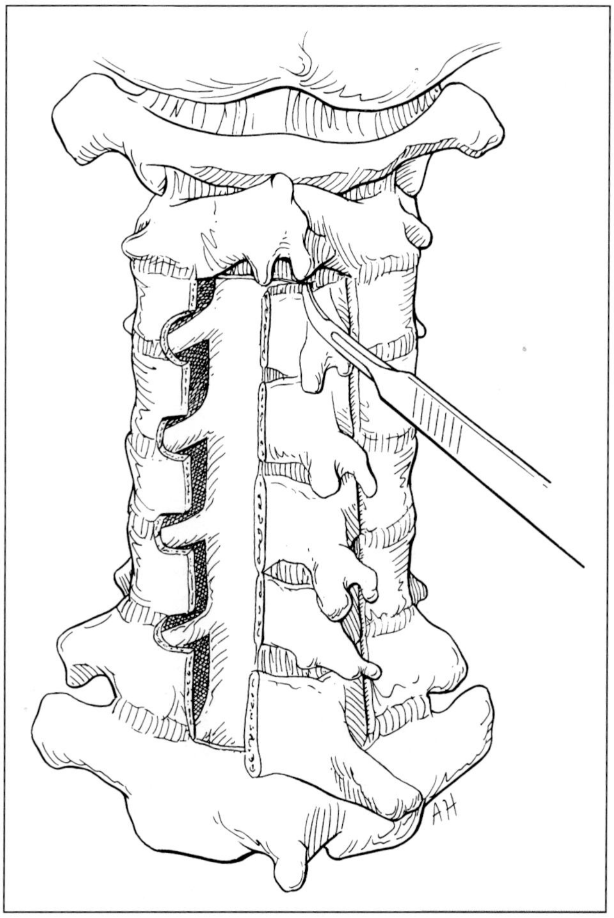

Figure 10.13
Diagram illustrating the opening of the laminoplasty: a Schlessinger rongeur or no. 12 scalpel blade is used to release the ligamentum flavum at proximal and distal poles of the laminoplasty

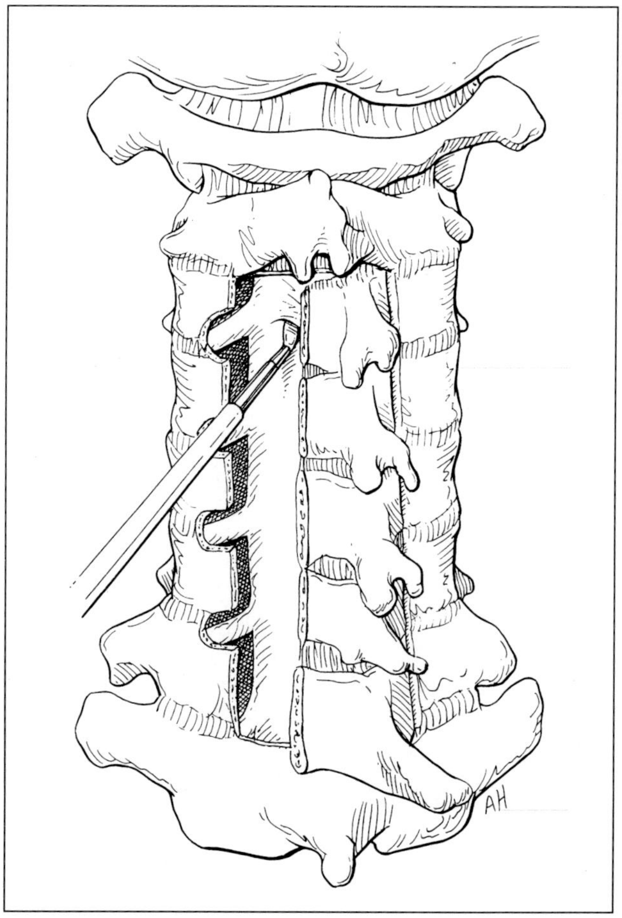

Figure 10.14
Schematic demonstration of laminoplasty with multiple foraminotomies, performed on the 'open' side, before creation of the trough to afford protection of the spinal cord. A Woodson or Penfield elevator is used to release adhesions connecting the dura from the undersurface of the lamina

rate of progressive kyphosis, but preoperative deformity or instability will be potentiated. In a report reviewing laminectomy and fusion in a group of patients with cervical spondylotic myelopathy plus preoperative deformity, Miyazaki et al[23] found that 50% of their patients developed either a new deformity or a worsening of the pre-existing malalignment.

The effect of partial or complete facetectomy or development of instability must be emphasized. Several clinical and biomechanical studies have demonstrated the importance of facet integrity to cervical spine stability.[5,24,26,28,37,38] Clearly, the surgeon must recognize both preoperative deformity and the potential for development of postoperative deformity or instability. The addition of stabilization procedures at the time of these posterior decompressive procedures should be based on an understanding of these principles.

Inadequate decompression of the spinal cord is usually the result of persistent anterior compression. This is most often true in cases with significant preoperative loss of the normal cervical lordosis and subsequent draping of the spinal cord over the posterior marginal osteophytes of the vertebral bodies and bulging disc. In such cases consideration should be given to anterior decompression.

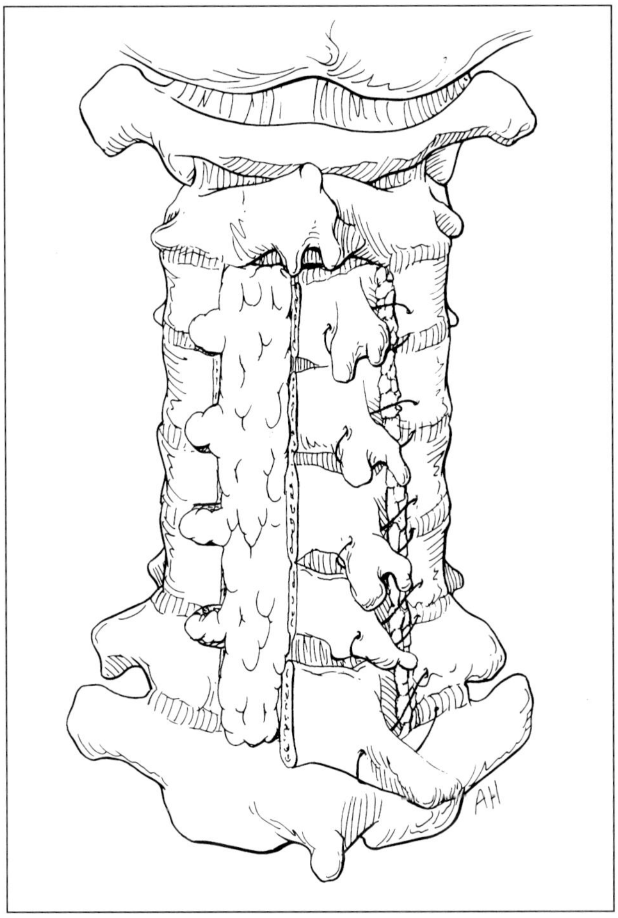

Figure 10.15
Non-absorbable suture, or preferably 22 gauge wire, is placed through each spinous process and secured to either the facet capsule or through a drill hole in the facet itself. Fat may be gently placed over the exposed dura. A few pieces of morselized bone from the very tips of the spinous processes are placed in the hinged gutter as shown

Other potential complications, inherent with any spinal procedure, include neurologic complications due to iatrogenic cord or nerve root compression, dural tears, and infection. Care must be taken in handling power instruments with exposed dura. Forced placement of hand-held instruments, such as Kerrison rongeurs, into a tight spinal canal is ill-advised and may potentiate neurologic injury. Repair of dural tears should be attempted preferably with an operating microscope. Yonenobu et al[35] reported four neurologic complications in a series of 85 patients undergoing laminectomy. One of these involved a transient C5 paresis, whereas three resulted in permanent quadriparesis – in two of these, an epidural hematoma was found at exploration. Routine use of drains is strongly urged.

Complications resulting from laminoplasty are similar, although the potential for development of postoperative instability is not so profound. One complication specific to laminoplasty is closure of the hinge. This can be alleviated by wire suturing of the proximal and distal poles of the 'door'. Neurologic complication rate is similar to laminectomy as reported by Yonenobu et al.[35] Four of 95 patients undergoing laminoplasty experienced C5 nerve root paresis; there were no patients with spinal cord dysfunction.

REFERENCES

1 Allen KL. Cervical spondylosis with accompanying myelopathy: Its alleviation by removal of the bony spur. *S Afri J Surg* **6**: 5, 1966.
2 Cattell HS, Clark GL Jr. Cervical kyphosis and instability following multiple laminectomies in children. *J Bone Joint Surg [Am]* **59**: 991–1002, 1977.
3 Clarke E, Robinson P. Cervical myelopathy: A complication of cervical spondylosis. *Brain* **79**. 483–510, 1956.
4 Crandall PH, Gregorius FK. Long term follow-up of surgical treatment of cervical spondylotic myelopathy. *Spine* **2**: 139–146, 1977.
5 Epstein JA. The surgical management of cervical canal stenosis, spondylosis, and myeloradiculopathy by means of the posterior approach. *Spine* **13**: 864–869, 1988.
6 Epstein JA, Carras R, Lavine LS Epstein BS. The importance of removing osteophytes as part of the surgical treatment of myeloradiculopathy in cervical spondylosis. *J Neurosurg* **30**: 219–226, 1969.
7 Epstein JA, Janin Y, Carras R, Lavine LS. A comparative study of the treatment of cervical spondylotic myeloradiculopathy: Experience with 50 cases treated by means of extensive laminectomy, foraminotomy, and excision of osteophytes during the past ten years. *Acta Neurochir (Wien)* **61**: 89–104, 1982.
8 Gore DR, Sepic SB, Gardner GM. Neck pain: A long term follow-up of 205 patients. *Spine* **12**: 1–5, 1987.
9 Gorter K. Influence of laminectomy on the course of cervical myelopathy. *Acta Neurochir* **33**: 265–281, 1976.
10 Haft H, Ransohoff J, Carter S. Spinal cord tumors in children. *Pediatrics* **23**: 1152–1159, 1959.
11 Hase H, Watanabe T, Hirasawa Y et al. Bilateral open laminoplasty using ceramic laminas for cervical myelopathy. *Spine* **16**: 1269–1276, 1991.
12 Henderson CM, Hennessey R, Shuey H. Posterior lateral foraminotomy for an exclusive operative technique for cervical radiculopathy: A review of 846 consecutively operated cases. *J Neurosurg* **13**: 504–512, 1983.
13 Herkowitz HN. A comparison of anterior cervical fusion, cervical laminectomy, and cervical laminoplasty for the surgical management of multiple level spondylotic radiculopathy. *Spine* **13**: 774–780, 1988.

14 Herkowitz HN. The surgical management of cervical spondylotic myelopathy radiculopathy, and myeloradiculopathy. *Clin Orthop* **239:** 94–108, 1989.
15 Hirabayashi K, Miyakawa J, Satomi K, et al. Operative results and post-operative progression of ossification among patients with ossification of cervical posterior longitudinal ligament. *Spine* **6**: 354–364, 1983.
16 Hirabayashi K, Watanabe K, Wakano K, et al. Expansive open-door laminoplasty for cervical spinal stenotic myelopathy. *Spine* **8**: 693–699, 1983.
17 Kadoya S, Nadamura T, Kwak R. A microsurgical anterior osteophytectomy for cervical spondylotic myelopathy. *Spine* **9**: 437–441, 1984.
18 Kimura I, Oh-Hama M, Shingu H. Cervical myelopathy treated by canal-expansive laminoplasty. *J Bone Joint Surg [Am]* **66**: 914–920, 1984.
19 Kurz LT, Herkowitz HN. Surgical management of myelopathy. *Orthop Clin North Am* **23**(3): 495–504, 1992.
20 Lees F, Turner J. Natural history and prognosis of cervical spondylosis. *Br Med J* **2**: 1607–1610, 1963.
21 Lonstein JE, Winter RB, Bradford DB, et al. Postlaminectomy spine deformity. *J Bone Joint Surg [Am]* **58**: 727, 1976.
22 Mayfield FH. Cervical spondylosis: A comparison of the anterior and posterior approaches. *Clin Neurosurg* **13**: 181–188, 1965.
23 Miyazaki Y, Tada, K, Matsuda Y, et al. Posterior extensive simultaneous multisegment decompression with posterolateral fusion for cervical instability and kyphotic and/or S-shaped deformities. *Spine* **14**: 110–117, 1989.
24 Munechica Y. Influence of laminectomy on the stability of the spine: An experimental study with special reference to the extent of laminectomy and the resection of the intervertebral joint. *Nippon Sei Keigeka Gakkai Zasshi* **47**: 111–126, 1973.
25 Nurick S. The natural history and the results of surgical treatment of the spinal cord disorder associated with cervical spondylosis. *Brain* **95**: 101–105, 1972.
26 Panjabi MM, White AA, Johnson RM. Cervical spine biomechanics as a function of transection of components. *J Biomech* **8**: 327–336, 1976.
27 Phillips DG. Surgical treatment of myelopathy with cervical spondylosis. *J Neurol Neurosurg Psychiatry* **36**: 879–884, 1973.
28 Raynor RB, Pugh J, Shapiro I. Cervical facetectomy and its effect on spine strength. *J Neurosurg* **63**: 278–282, 1985.
29 Roberts AH. Myelopathy due to cervical spondylosis treated by collar immobilization. *Neurology* **16**: 951–954, 1966.
30 Robinson RA, Walker AE Ferlic DC, Wieking DK. The results of anterior interbody fusion of the cervical spine. *J Bone Joint Surg [Am]* **44**: 1569–1587, 1962.
31 Simpson JM, Silveri CP, Simeone FA, Balderston RA. Cervical disc disease and the keyhole foraminotomy: Proven efficacy at extended long term follow-up. *Spine* in press, 1994.
32 Symon L, Lavender P. The surgical treatment of cervical spondylotic myelopathy. *Neurology* **17**: 117–126, 1967.
33 Yasouka S, Peterson HA, Laws ER, et al. Pathogenesis and prophylaxis of postlaminectomy deformity of the spine after multiple level laminectomy: Difference between children and adults. *Neurosurgery* **9**: 145–152, 1981.
34 Yasouka S, Peterson HA, MacCarty CS. Incidence of spinal column deformity after multilevel laminectomy in children and adults. *J Neurosurg* **57**: 441–445, 1982.
35 Yonenobu K, Hosono N, Iwasaki M, Asano M, Ono K. Neurologic complications of surgery for cervical compression myelopathy. *Spine* **16**: 1277–1282, 1991.
36 Yonenobu K, Hosono N, Iwasaki M, Asano M, Ono K. Laminoplasty versus subtotal corpectomy. A comparative study of results in multisegmental cervical spondylotic myelopathy. *Spine* **17**: 1281–1284, 1992.
37 Zdeblick TA, Bohlmann HH. Myelopathy, cervical kyphosis, and treatment by anterior corpectomy and strut grafting. *J Bone Joint Surg [Am]* **71**: 170–182, 1989.
38 Zdeblick TA, Zou D, Warden KE, McCabe R, Kunz D, Vanderby R. Cervical stability after foraminotomy. *J Bone Joint Surg [Am]* **74**: 22–27, 1992.

11 Traumatic injuries of the adult upper cervical spine

Alexander R. Vaccaro and Jerome M. Cotler

Traumatic injuries of the adult upper cervical spine and cervicocranium represent a special subgroup of cervical spine disorders resulting from the unique anatomy, the multitude of potential injury patterns, and various treatment options.[57,101,106,134,153,154,198] Injuries to the upper cervical spine, the occiput–C1–C2 complex, are most frequently responsible for traumatic, fatal, spinal injuries. Injuries to the axis are responsible for most of these fatalities, followed by the atlas and atlanto-occipital articulations.[5] These injuries are usually the result of motor vehicle accidents, falls, or other miscellaneous trauma.[4,179] However, as a result of the capacious volume of the spinal canal at this level and the relatively small ratio of cord size to canal volume, many surviving patients who sustain injury in this region have minimal or no neurologic deficit despite severe soft tissue and bony disruption. It is important for the treating physician to have a high index of suspicion for injuries at this level in all patients with a history of significant trauma. Outward evidence of head or facial contusion, loss of consciousness, chest injury, or complaints of neck and suboccipital pain should always be managed as cervical spine injury until proved otherwise. The standard in-field management of these patients must be strictly adhered to including the ABCs (airway, breathing, circulation) of trauma care, strict spinal immobilization and careful, complete, spinal radiographic assessment once the patient arrives in the emergency room.

This chapter reviews the various fracture patterns and injury complexes that occur in the adult upper cervical spine. Discussion includes the initial management, diagnosis, radiographic assessment, injury classifications, and various treatment options available to the managing spinal injury team.

OCCIPITAL CONDYLES

Fracture of the occipital condyles may occur as an isolated entity or in combination with injuries to the odontoid, atlanto-occipital complex, or other multiple non-contiguous injuries to the cervical spine.[118,132,192] Fracture of the occipital condyle was first described by Bell in 1817[20] with the rarity of this entity reflected by the fact that, as of 1988, only 27 cases[124,200] have been reported in the world's literature.[87] Over one-third of occipital condyle fractures have been reported in patients with traumatic atlanto-occipital dislocations.[87] The severity of neurological compromise associated with this injury varies from no deficit to complete quadriparesis with respiratory compromise. In Goldstein's review of occipital injuries prior to 1981, he noted frequent severe neurologic deficits. Of injuries to the occipital condyles 44% resulted in fatality, and an additional 22% of patients demonstrated lower cranial nerve deficits.[87]

Diagnosis

The most common mechanism of injury involves a high-speed deceleration force resulting in axial compression and anterior or lateral shear forces, with or without a rotatory component. Many surviving patients experience a period of unconsciousness and, as noted above, may have isolated neurologic injury to the lower cranial nerves.[52,87,95] Injuries to cranial nerves IX (glossopharyngeal) and XII (hypoglossal) occur most frequently as a result of the proximity of their foramen to the occipital condyles. Injury to cranial nerve VI may also occur as a result of compression at some point along its extensive intracranial course or direct injury to the anterior brain stem (Fig. 11.1).[27,52]

Radiographic Evaluation

Identification and evaluation of injuries to the occipital condyles through plain radiographs is difficult due to

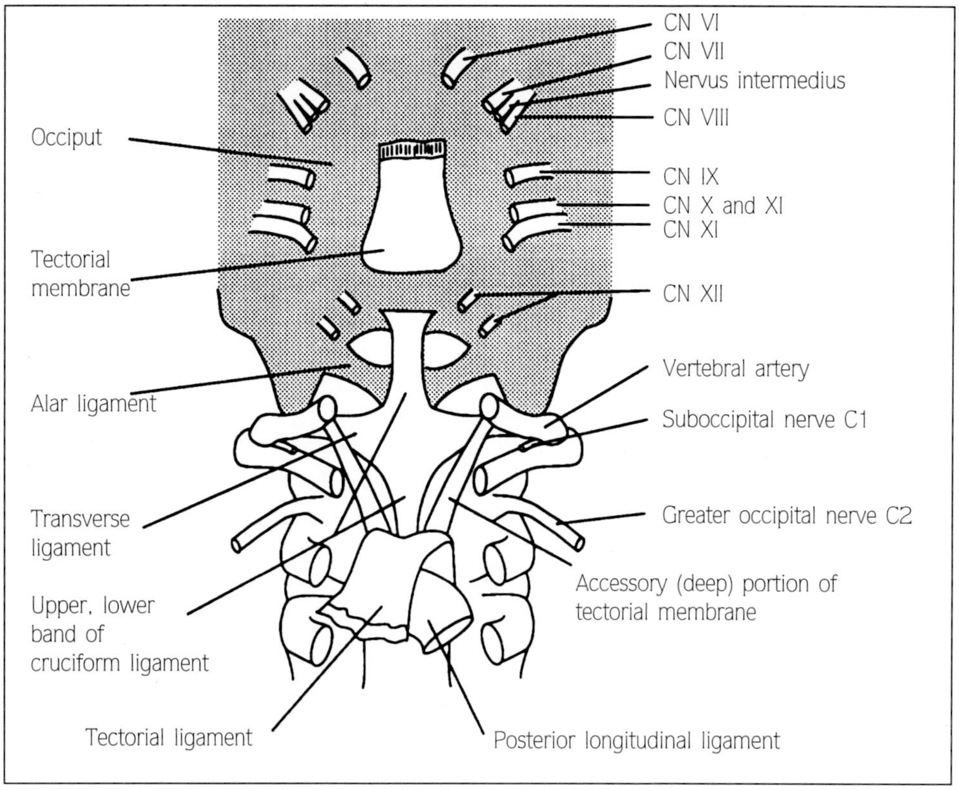

Figure 11.1
A schematic diagram with the posterior cervical bony elements and spinal cord removed revealing the bony, neural, and ligamentous structures of the ventral surface of the spinal canal. Note the close approximation of the cranial nerves to the occipital condyles. CN = cranial nerve

superimposition of the overlying facial bones.[87] The most sensitive plain radiographic study enabling visualization of this area is a frontal projection of the atlanto-occipital joint through the maxillary sinus.[87] More complex imaging modalities, such as complex motion[87] or hypocycloidal tomography,[52] and computed tomography (CT) with reformatted images in the sagittal and coronal planes, are invaluable. Mariani[124] recommends routine CT scan evaluation of the cervicocranium in all patients with unexplained prevertebral swelling. This general recommendation is in agreement with that of the authors.

Classification and Treatment

To date, only one paper[13] has attempted to classify these injuries in terms of mechanism of injury, fracture configuration, and stability based on injury to soft tissue and osseous structures (Fig. 11.2). In 1988, Anderson and Montesano[13] developed a three-part classification with type I injuries representing impacted, comminuted fracture of the occipital condyle with minimal or no displacement, resulting from a pure axial load to the skull. Ligamentous stability is maintained through an intact tectorial membrane and contralateral alar ligament, although the ipsilateral alar ligament may be functionally compromised. This is a stable injury which should be treated with rigid halo immobilization for approximately 3 months. Once the halo is removed, dynamic flexion and extension radiographic studies should be performed to evaluate soft tissue ligamentous stability. Type II injuries result from a direct blow to the occiput and upper cervical spine. Such trauma generally results in a basal skull fracture with subsequent propagation of the fracture line through the occipital condyles into the foramen magnum. This pattern of injury is also stable without significant disruption of the alar ligaments or tectorial membrane, and is treated similarly to type I injuries. Type III injuries are more ominous and are the result of shear, lateral bending or rotatory forces alone, or in combination. These forces invariably cause bony avulsion injury of the occipital condyles through the alar ligament, which is the primary ligamentous constraint to atlanto-occipital rotation and lateral bending. This injury may result in the displacement of a bony fragment toward the tip of the odontoid. These are potentially unstable injuries[52] and should be rigidly immobilized in a halo vest followed closely for evidence of displacement. The integrity

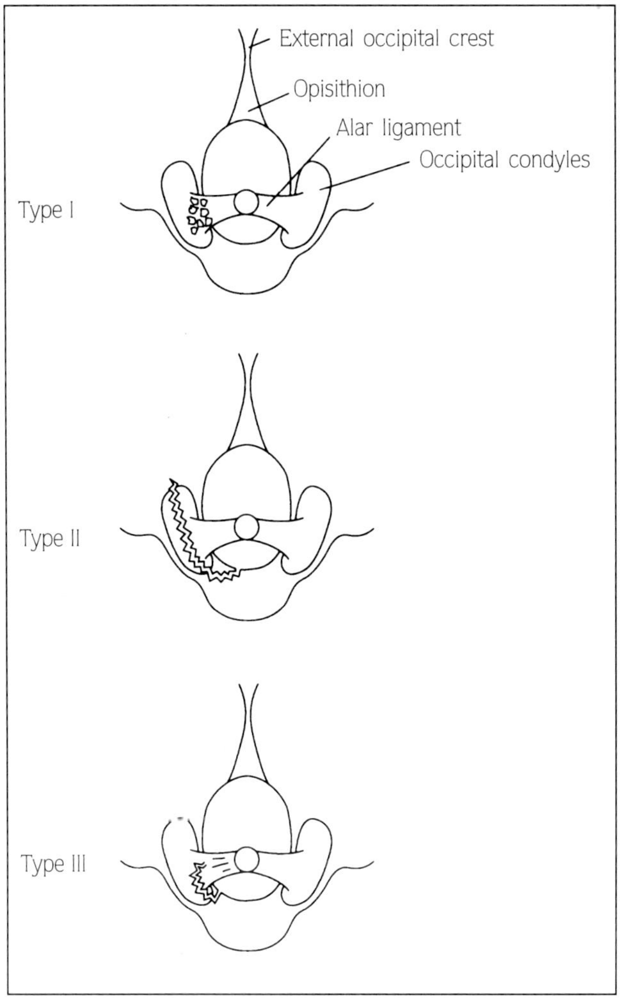

Figure 11.2
Anderson classification of occipital condyle fractures. Type I – impacted comminuted fracture of the occipital condyle with minimal or no displacement. Type II – basilar skull fracture with fracture propagation through the occipital condyle into the foramen magnum. Type III – an avulsion fracture of the occipital condyle through the attachment of the alar ligament

of the soft tissue supporting structures should be evaluated after 3 months of halo immobilization with dynamic radiographic evaluation.

The indications for surgical intervention are unclear in the literature. With no evidence of brain-stem compression[124] or instability noted during immobilization, most of these patients have done well with conservative treatment.[27,95,118,124]

ATLANTO-OCCIPITAL INJURIES

Injuries of the atlanto-occipital joint are extremely rare in the literature with only 21 cases reported as of 1989.[26,118,136,201] Of these, four patients eventually died secondary to either injury to their central nervous system or associated injuries during their initial hospital stay. Thirteen patients had significant initial neurologic deficits with variable improvement in recovery and four patients were neurologically intact. The true incidence of this injury is probably underestimated, as most are fatal.

Alker et al[5] performed post-mortem examinations on 312 victims of multiple trauma and found 19 patients to have succumbed through fatal atlanto-occipital dislocations. Most of these patients were pedestrians struck by a motor vehicle. Alker postulated the mechanism of injury to be primarily a hyperflexion force, although careful scrutiny of the literature shows little support for this mechanism. Bucholz and Burkhead[33] performed similar post-mortem studies on 112 victims of traumatic deaths and found 9 cases of atlanto-occipital dislocation. They determined the mechanism of injury to be one of distraction and hyperextension, often associated with injuries to the scalp, mandible, submental region, and posterior pharyngeal wall. On post mortem analysis of one patient, the posterior atlanto-occipital membrane was intact, supporting their hypothesis. Other authors have suggested a complex combination of forces ranging from hyperextension, distraction, lateral flexion with an associated rotatory component, to hyperflexion.[136,137]

As relatively little rotation occurs at the atlanto-occipital articulation, forced rotation at this level may cause significant disruption of the supporting capsular and ligamentous structures resulting in subluxation or pure dislocation.[25,136] However, as a result of the intrinsic strength of these ligaments, fractures at the base of their attachments usually occur before ligamentous disruption.[179] Rotatory dislocation at this level may also be associated with compensatory rotation in the opposite direction at the C1–C2 articulation.

Fatal atlanto-occipital injuries in Bucholz and Burkhead's series[33] were more commonly seen in children (15%) than in adults (6%), which may reflect the relatively shallow inclination of the atlanto-occipital articulation in the child or the fact that more children were involved in motor vehicle versus pedestrian incidents. Overall, 67% of these injuries were the result of motor vehicle accidents, whereas in the remaining 103 patients, the cause of death was similar in nature in only 18%.

In summary, injuries to this level may not be rare, although they are frequently fatal.[176] With more advanced and aggressive in-field care of victims of multiple trauma, particularly regarding airway management and respiratory support, an increase in survival may be seen with future injuries to this level.[208]

Diagnosis

Patients surviving injury to the atlanto-occipital junction generally present with significant neurologic deficits, although patients with radiographically documented atlanto-occipital dislocations may be neurologically intact.[118,211] Injuries to the caudal 7–10 pairs of cranial nerves – brain-stem, spinomedullary junction, upper cervical spinal cord, and the upper three cervical nerves – have been reported in survivors.[59,60,118,136] If compression occurs to the proximal medullary cord above the decussation of the foraminal tracts, total spastic quadriplegia may result. If compression occurs proximal to the substance of the foraminal tracts involving only the upper extremity fibers, only the upper extremities will be involved. Confusion may occur with midline compression of the foraminal tracts when upper extremity motor fibers are primarily involved and lower extremity fibers are compressed to a lesser degree. This may resemble a central cord injury, suggesting injury to the lower cervical spinal cord.[60]

Unilateral injury to the vertebral basilar artery system represents a rare, but morbid, complication of atlanto-occipital dislocation known as Wallenberg's syndrome. This injury is caused by cervical hyperextension and rotation, resulting in stretching and intimal damage to the ipsilateral vertebral artery. With diminished arterial flow through the vertebral artery, Clinical symptoms may include may result with deficits of the ipsilateral cranial nerves of V, IX, X, XI, contralateral loss of pain and temperature, ipsilateral Horner's syndrome, and cerebellar ataxia. Once diagnosis is confirmed by subtraction angiography, patients may be anticoagulated to prevent further clot formation and propagation. Supplemental oxygenation of the patient is also recommended to increase cerebral oxygenation.[125]

In patients who present without evidence of neurologic compromise, the diagnosis of atlanto-occipital injury may be difficult. A history of significant upper cervical spine trauma in an awake and alert patient, with evidence of a suboccipital hematoma and complaints of posterior occipital neck pain, should be thoroughly investigated by appropriate imaging studies. Three of the four patients reported in Motane and Eismont's series[136] were overlooked by the initial examiner at presentation. Those patients who present with a similar mechanism of injury and with evidence of cardiopulmonary arrest or signs of a high or mixed quadriplegia should also be suspected of this diagnosis.[118]

Radiographic Evaluation

The radiographic stigmata of bony and soft tissue injury to this level of the spine are often subtle and may be overlooked by those unfamiliar with the normal soft tissue and bony relationships which exist in the adult cervical spine.[37,88,99,129,162] A primary indicator of injury to this level is an increase in prevertebral soft tissue swelling seen on a plain lateral radiograph. The normal documented retropharyngeal space in adults at the C2 level may range from 1 to 7 mm, whereas at the level of C4–C5 it may range from 9 to 22 mm.[34,63,84,118] Any enlargement of the retropharyngeal space beyond these norms should raise concern of underlying injury to the cervical spine.

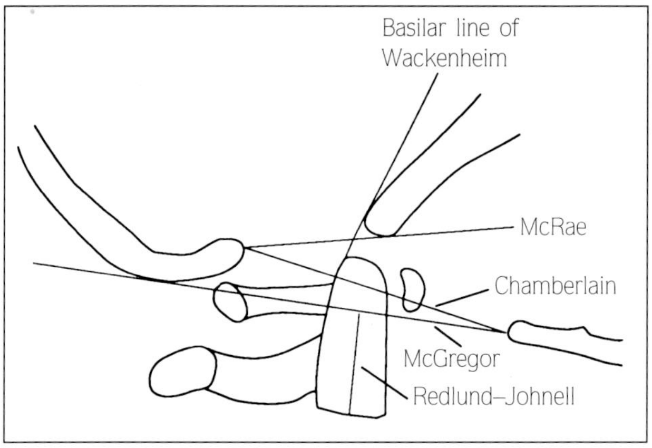

Figure 11.3
An illustration of various linear measurements used to establish normal cervicocranial relationships, i.e. the basilar line of Wackenheim, McRae's line, Chamberlain's line, McGregor's line, and the Redlund–Johnell line

There are several bony relationships and measurements that can be used to evaluate the atlanto-occipital articulation. The tip of the odontoid is used as a guide in evaluation of anteroposterior or vertical subluxation of the atlanto-occipital joint. The anterior aspect of the dens should be in line with the tip of the basion[159] and the distance between these two structures should be no more than 4–5 mm in the child and 1 cm in the adult.[89] This relationship should change 1 mm or less with voluntary flexion and extension.[118,135] Another useful indicator of alignment is the basilar line of Wackenheim[200] which is drawn along the posterior surface of the clivus and is normally at a tangent to the posterior cortex of the dens (Fig. 11.3).

The most commonly used measurement for injuries of the atlanto-occipital joint is Power's ratio.[158] This ratio is determined by measuring the distance from the basion to the anterior border of the posterior arch of the atlas, divided by the distance from the opisthion to the posterior border of the anterior atlas arch (Fig. 11.4). The

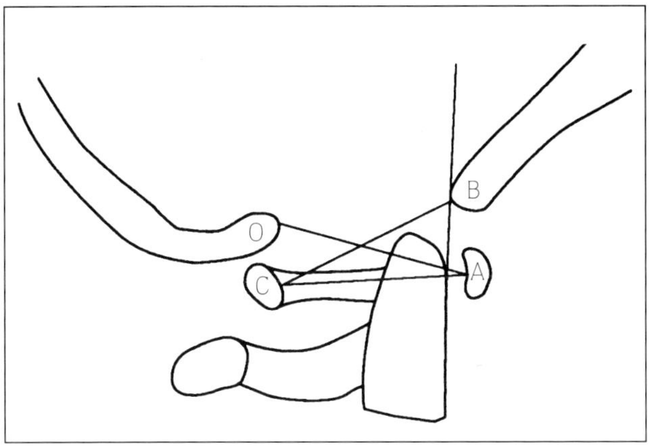

Figure 11.4
An illustration of Power's ratio at the atlanto-occipital joint for discerning the presence of anterior or posterior atlantoaxial subluxation. The ratio BC/OA should be approximately 0.77 with a ratio of 1 being the upper level of normal

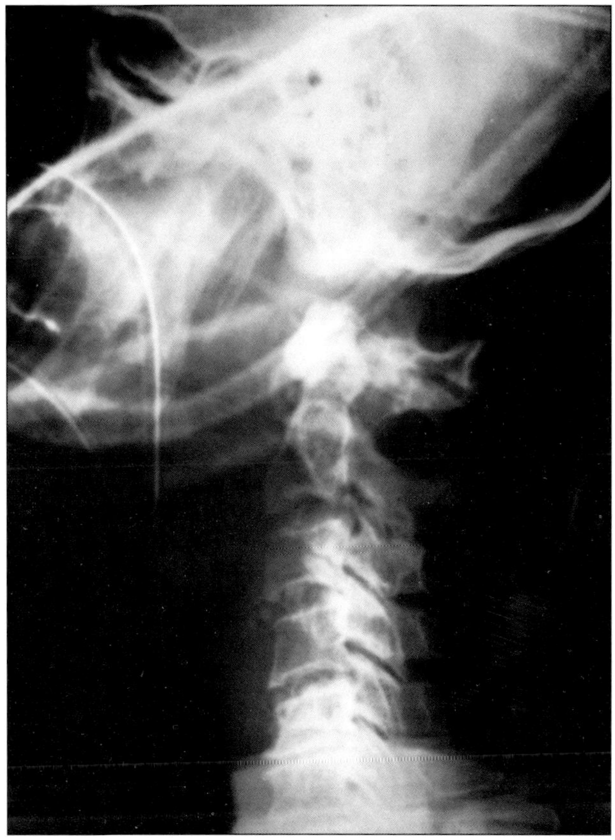

Figure 11.5
A plain lateral radiograph revealing pathological vertical diastasis of the atlanto-occipital articulation. (Courtesy of G Scuderi, MD)

normal ratio at this level should be 0.77, with 1 being the upper level of normal. If this measurement is greater than 1, significant anterior atlanto-occipital subluxation or dislocation has occurred. Anteroposterior and lateral tomography greatly assists in identifying these specific bony landmarks.[157]

These injuries are sometimes associated with disruption of the posterior pharyngeal wall allowing air to be seen on plain radiographs or on CT evaluation of this area. At postmortem examination, Bucholz and Burkhead found that three of nine cadavers had complete lacerations of the posterior pharyngeal wall with air noted in the cranium and vertebral veins on plain radiography.[33] Arteriography may demonstrate stenosis or disruption of the vertebral vessels secondary to severe distraction. Meningeal disruption will be evident on spinal myelography.[34]

Fracture Classification and Treatment

Traynelis[197] has classified these injuries into three groups: type I injuries present with radiographic evidence of pure longitudinal distraction of the atlanto-occipital articulation without dislocation (Fig. 11.5); type II injuries consist of anterior subluxation or dislocation and represent the most common form of atlanto-occipital disruption;[131] type III injuries are represented by either posterior subluxation or dislocation.

Management of these injuries is directed toward immediate stabilization of the atlanto-occipital articulation through reduction and restoration of normal alignment, thus protecting and/or decompressing the surrounding neural structures.[118] For type I injuries, reduction maneuvers are not required. Immediate halo-vest immobilization is needed, however, to prevent inadvertent injury during patient handling and transport. For type II and type III injuries, closed reduction should be attempted, initially accomplished with light traction of 0.9–1.35 kg applied through cranial tongs. The weight may then be increased to 1.35–2.25 kg with the appropriately applied force vectors to accomplish reduction.[176] Once reduction is obtained, traction weight is reduced to maintain stability. This process should be accomplished through meticulous radiographic surveillance and serial neurologic examinations.[136] Some authors have written about the risk of traction in these injuries and have only advocated immediate halo immobilization. The present authors feel, however, that stability and neurologic protection are achieved better through reduction.

Due to the tenuous stability of these injuries, most subluxations/dislocations of the atlanto-occipital complex require immediate occipitocervical fusion.[118,157] In those patients treated exclusively with halo immobilization, persistent instability has been documented after as long as 5 months.[34] It is imperative to maintain stability of this injury in the perioperative period. Halo immobilization is strongly recommended with a C ring during all phases of patient positioning for any cervical operative procedure on this injury,[176,208] and the technique described by Wertheim and Bohlman[204] for occipitocervical arthrodesis is the one recommended; it is described later in this chapter.

ATLAS FRACTURES

Fractures of the atlas are relatively uncommon[34] and comprise approximately 3–13% of all injuries to the cervical spine,[77,92,111,114,122,147] 25% of all injuries to the atlantoaxial complex,[119] and roughly 2% of injuries to the entire spine.[118,132] Associated cervical spine injuries occur in up to 53% of cases. Most of these associated injuries involve the odontoid process or other portions of the axis.[60,92,105,118,119,147] Fracture of the posterior arch represents the most frequent fracture of the atlas, and has the highest incidence of associated cervical vertebral injuries. Most of these associated injuries are incurred through a similar mechanism of hyperextension.[118]

Diagnosis

In patients who survive transport to the hospital, the incidence of neurologic compromise is low because of the capacious spinal canal and the tendency for fractures of the atlas to displace in a decompressive or centrifugal manner.[92,111,118,119,177] Cranial nerve palsies, however, have been reported with these injuries, especially the abducens (VI), glossopharyngeal (IX), vagus (X), spinal accessory (XI), and hypoglossal nerves (XII). This is most probably a reflection of the anatomic location of cranial nerves IX, X, and XII, which lie just medial to the styloid process at the level of the occiput and cross the transverse process of C1. With burst-type injuries of C1, the lateral masses can disperse laterally and impinge on these nerve structures.[132] Patients with combined cervical spine injuries at this level, especially those with an associated displaced odontoid fracture, report the highest incidence of neurologic deficit.[92,119] Some patients may incur significant intracranial damage at the time of the accident,[119] thereby confusing the presenting neurologic picture and its relationship to the atlas injury.[118] Myers found 4 of 15 patients in his series to present with significant neurologic compromise. Two of these patients were found to have an incomplete spinal cord injury and two patients had a complete cord deficit.[14] Symptoms of basilar impression have also been reported as a result of C1 lateral mass displacement, and subsequent cranial settling and brain-stem compression.[50]

Mechanism of Injury

As with other injuries to the cervicocranial region, most atlas fractures reesult from motor vehicle accidents, falls, and other miscellaneous trauma.[92,111,114,177] The fracture mechanism is primarily one of axial compression to the vertex of the skull sometimes associated with secondary forces of hyperextension, lateral bending, or rotation.[92,131,132] If an associated odontoid fracture is present with these injuries, this is suggestive of an additional flexion or extension force being applied at the time of injury.[111] An axially applied load causes compressive approximation of the occiput–C1 and C1–C2 articular processes. This force is channeled through the obliquely oriented C1–C2 facet joints, and the relatively rigid anterior C1–C2 odontoid process–transverse ligament complex, resulting in failure of the atlas in tension with lateral spreading of the articular processes. This results in a vertical fracture at the narrowest cross-sectional area of the anterior arch at one or two locations, usually where the anterior arch joins the lateral masses.[114] A similar unilateral or bilateral fracture occurs in the posterior arch. If extension occurs, the atlas posterior arch finds itself compressed between the occiput and C2 spinous process[119] with a fracture line appearing at its weakest point in the sagittal plane, which is usually in the groove of the vertebral vessels bilaterally.[135] The fractured posterior arch may be displaced superiorly as the result of an upward pull by the posterior inferior oblique musculature of the cervical spine.[179] Kahanovitz has reported a case where a fragment of the posterior arch actually became entrapped within the foramen magnum.[109] Fowler et al[77] have noted an increased incidence of posterior arch fractures in the elderly with pre-existing cervical degenerative disease in the mid to lower cervical spine.

Associated Transverse Ligament Injuries

Fractures in the anterior and posterior arch of the atlas may allow lateral spreading of the articular processes; the degree of spread is dependent on the integrity of the transverse ligament. Spence et al[191] performed biomechanical studies

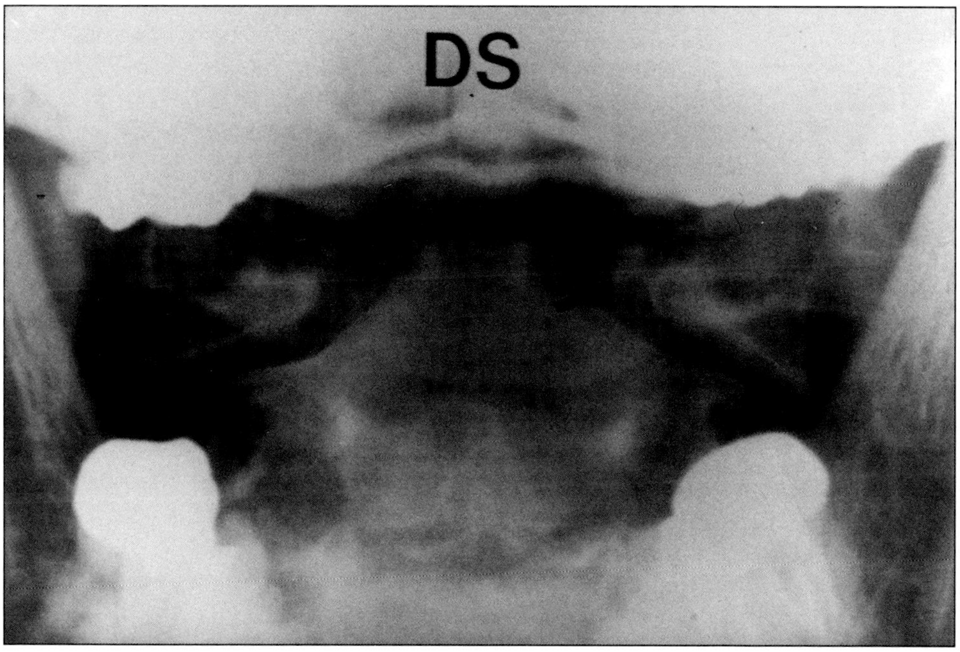

Figure 11.6
An open-mouth plain radiograph revealing an atlas burst fracture with obvious diastasis of the atlas lateral masses and evidence of a transverse ligamentous bony avulsion of the medial tubercle of the C1 lateral mass (arrow). (Courtesy of JJ Abitbol, MD)

on ten cadaveric cervical spines and correlated the degree of lateral mass displacement to the integrity of this ligament. They found a high probability of transverse ligament integrity with a lateral mass spread of <5.7 mm. A spread of >6.9 mm is usually indicative of complete transverse ligament disruption.[132,157] Disruption of the transverse ligament may be diagnosed through either excessive spreading of the lateral masses on an anteroposterior open-mouth radiograph or an increase in the atlantodental interval of more than 3.5–4 mm on a lateral radiograph in the adult, or through direct observation on an axial CT scan (Fig. 11.6).[147]

Although most clinical and biomechanical studies[58,177] suggest that injury to this ligament occurs through a periosteal avulsion of the medial tubercle of the C1 lateral mass or comminution of the ipsilateral C1 ring with a floating C1 articular facet,[208] Fielding found 75% of these disruptions to represent a midsubstance ligament injury in a cadaveric model.[69] However, even with complete disruption of this ligament, Fielding found the alar ligaments and facet capsules to be intact. As a result, only minimal atlantoaxial instability was demonstrated on lateral flexion and extension radiographs with an atlantodental interval of about 5 mm.[118] Panjabi and associates[149] experimentally produced atlas fractures in ten fresh cadaveric human spines. Of the eight specimens with an associated transverse ligament disruption secondary to axial loading with or without an extension moment, all had intact alar ligaments, tectorial membranes, and C1–C2 capsular ligaments. Dvorak et al[58] performed biomechanical testings on seven human cadaveric spines and showed that the transverse ligament was the strongest ligament of the C1–C2 joint complex, with disruption always occurring at its insertion into the medial tubercle of the atlas. The incidence of rupture of this ligament is far less frequent in fractures of the dens, suggesting a superiority in strength over the dens, although this was not borne out in cadaveric studies by Fielding and colleagues.[63,69]

The transverse ligament is actually part of the more extensive cruciform ligamentous complex, which consists of upper and lower extensions into the basion of the occiput and midportion of the inferior dens respectively. The transverse ligament resides in a shallow groove on the posterior surface of the odontoid. Other supporting soft tissue structures in this area include the bilateral alar ligaments, which span from the lateral superior portion of the dens to each occipital condyle, and the articulating facet joint capsules of the occiput–C1 complex. The integrity of the alar ligaments contributes some inherent stability in the presence of an atlas burst injury with an associated transverse ligament rupture. Patients with pure transverse ligament disruptions as a result of excessive flexion tend to be older than those with other upper cervical injuries (i.e. fifth decade versus third decade). Those patients with a greater degree of lateral mass spread (i.e. 7.5–11 mm) have a higher incidence of neurologic dysfunction than patients with a lesser degree of lateral mass separation (i.e. 5–6.5 mm).[69,118]

Radiographic Evaluation

Plain radiographs represent the mainstay in the initial evaluation of suspected C1 fractures. However, plain radiographs may often miss subtle arch fractures, especially if they occur at the junction of the lateral masses without evidence of significant soft tissue swelling. As a result of the often innocuous presentation of these injuries, they may be missed by the initial examiner and lead to a significant delay in diagnosis.[111] Keterson[111] reported a delay in diagnosis in three of seventeen patients due to an initial low index of suspicion and inadequate radiographic evaluation. Isolated posterior arch fractures may easily be overlooked as a result of the lack of anterior soft tissue swelling on lateral radiographs,[118,119] whereas anterior arch fractures should always be suspected in the presence of any anterior retropharyngeal swelling without obvious bony injury (Fig. 11.7).[119] Sherk suggested a useful way of offsetting the arches of the atlas on plain lateral radiography by focusing the beam of the X-ray tube over the body of C3, allowing thorough visualization of C1.[181]

The open-mouth view is useful in illustrating spread of the lateral masses, although difficult to obtain in the uncooperative or intubated patient.[111] This view also does not allow precise localization of anterior or posterior arch fractures. The imaging modality of choice for C1 burst injuries is CT, but only if proper gantry alignment in the plane of the C1 ring is performed. Levine found that CT scan missed the diagnosis of a C1 injury in four of seventeen patients with atlas fractures due to inaccurate gantry alignment.[119] CT scanning may also miss an associated transverse odontoid fracture in the plane of imaging, although it is better than lateral tomography in detecting central anterior arch fractures which may be missed as a result of imaging outside the plane of the fracture. Anteroposterior tomograms are useful in detecting anterior arch fractures as well as lateral mass and odontoid injuries, whereas lateral tomograms are efficacious in posterior arch injuries as well as odontoid fractures.[119] If transverse ligament instability is not implied by these imaging modalities, physician-supervised voluntary flexion and extension radiographs may be performed to assess stability.[147]

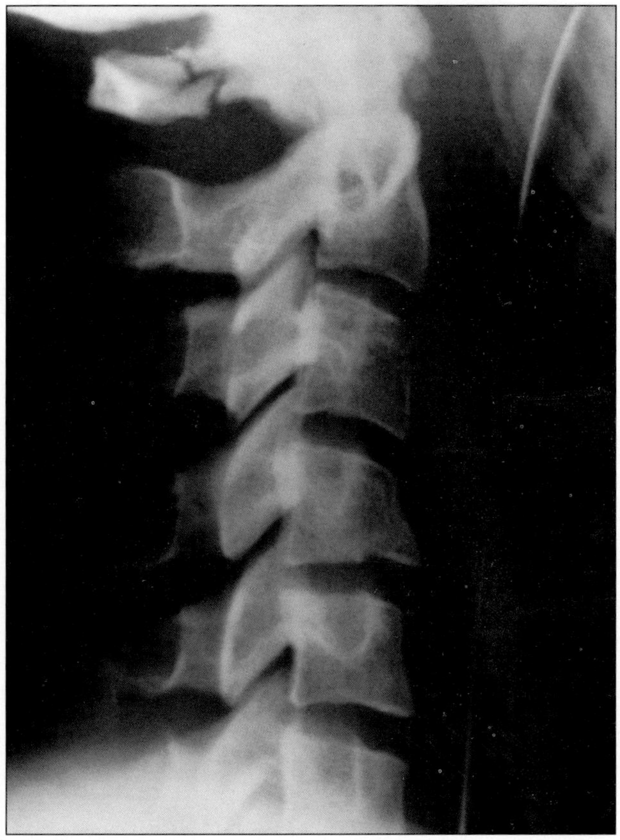

Figure 11.7
A plain lateral radiograph revealing a bilateral posterior arch fracture of the atlas. (Courtesy of JJ Abitbol, MD)

Diagnosis

Most responsive patients with C1 injuries present with significant suboccipital discomfort, a sense of subjective instability, associated posterior paracervical muscle spasm, and marked restriction of cervical motion.[34,111,179] The greater occipital sensory nerve (C2) appears most vulnerable to injury as it courses through the atlantoaxial membrane, although the suboccipital nerve (C1) is also at risk of injury as it passes over the ring of C1.[111] Less frequently reported symptoms include isolated cranial nerve injuries with associated visual alterations, changes in phonation, or disturbances in taste. Injury to the vertebral basilar system, resulting from vertebral artery stretch or transection as it crosses the posterior arch of the atlas, may present with findings of posterior fossa ischemia such as loss of consciousness or, again, visual disturbances.[111]

Classification

Many classification systems have been proposed to describe injuries to the atlas (Fig. 11.8).[92,105,131,135,142] However, as a result of the almost universal acceptance of primary, nonoperative treatment in isolated atlas injuries, the relative importance in subgrouping these injuries, outside the implication of a proposed mechanism of injury, is less important

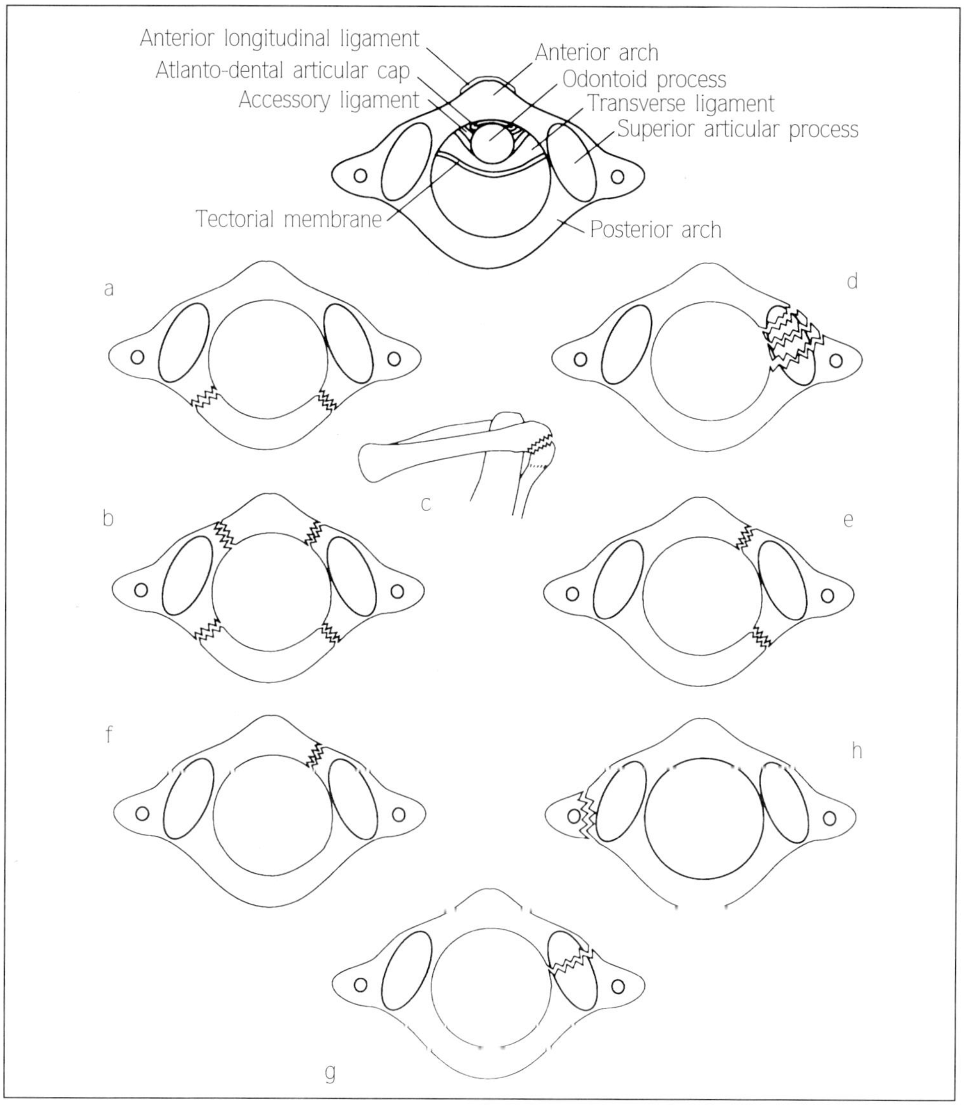

Figure 11.8
A schematic illustration demonstrating the bony and ligamentous anatomy of the atlas as well as various fracture patterns encountered in clinical settings. (a) Bilateral posterior arch fracture; (b) classic burst fracture; (c) hyperextension avulsion fracture of the anterior arch; (d) comminuted lateral mass fracture; (e) ipsilateral anterior and posterior arch fracture; (f) unilateral anterior arch fracture; (g) lateral mass fracture; (h) transverse process fracture

than for other fractures in the cervical spine. Most classification systems have not stressed any importance of prognosis in their fracture subgroups with most authors finding that these fractures have similar outcomes regardless of treatment or residual displacement at follow-up.

Levine and Edwards[117,119] have subgrouped these injuries into three types depending on the mechanism of injury as well as the position of the head at the time of injury: type I fractures include bilateral fractures of the posterior arch; type II includes a unilateral lateral mass fracture with fracture lines passing both anterior *and* posterior to one lateral mass, with or without an associated fracture of the contralateral posterior arch; and type III fractures include the typical Jefferson three- or four-part burst fracture with either two anterior and posterior arch fractures or one anterior arch fracture with two associated posterior arch fractures. Type I injuries tend to have the highest incidence of neurologic deficit at presentation.

Landells and Peteghem[114] attempted to correlate fracture type with long-term symptoms in their three-part classification system which is similar to that of Levine. In this classification scheme, type I injuries consist of fractures confined to a single arch without crossing the equator, type II injuries consist of fractures involving both anterior and posterior arches, such as the Jefferson burst fracture, and type III fractures consist primarily of lateral mass fractures with extension into only one arch. Landells and Peteghem found late symptoms of pain developing in 50% of patients with type I fractures, 70% with type II fractures, and 33% with type III fractures.

Segal et al[177] expanded on Gehweiler's original classification system, describing five injury patterns. According to Gehweiler's scheme, type I fractures consist only of fractures of the anterior arch; type II fractures consist only of fractures to the posterior arch; type III fractures consist of fractures to the lateral masses; type IV fractures represent the classic four-part burst fracture; and type V fractures consist of fractures of the transverse process.[84] To this, Segal et al. added the 'comminuted type' of fracture pattern which they stated has significant prognostic value. This fracture pattern includes double breaks in the ring, or one anterior and one posterior to a unilateral mass, similar to Levine's lateral mass injury. Patients with this fracture configuration had a 50% non-union rate in their series of four patients, with one patient having a poor and one a fair functional result at follow-up.

Stewart,[196] in 1977, described a horizontal anterior arch fracture resulting from a hyperextension avulsion injury at the insertion of the longus colli muscle and anterior longitudinal ligament. As of 1989, only 15 cases of this injury have been reported in the literature[118,196] with most patients having no neurologic deficit and symptoms limited only to localized neck pain. However, 70% of these patients also had additional cervical spine fractures resulting from hyperextension; 50% of these injuries involved fracture of the odontoid.[34]

Treatment

Isolated Transverse Ligament Injuries

Many authors have stressed the importance of primary surgical stabilization for injuries of the transverse ligament regardless of whether injury occurs in its midsubstance or at its periosteal insertion.[34,69,131,191] Spence et al[191] noted midsubstance disruption in six of ten cadavers with cervical spine injuries, and thought that aggressive surgical treatment was imperative. This has been echoed by Fielding[69] through his clinical and biomechanical observations of transverse ligament disruptions. He performed primary surgical stabilization in nine of eleven patients with this injury and believed that associated injuries at this level, such as attenuation of the alar ligaments or joint capsules, put the patient at risk for subsequent neurologic damage if immediate stabilization was not undertaken.

Levine[117] has stressed the importance of evaluating clinical stability once protective spasm disappeared, and feels that instability results not only from injury to the transverse ligament, but must also include injury to the alar ligament and joint capsules. Other authors have contested the views of Spence and Fielding and found no significant sequelae at follow-up from treating this injury non-operatively. Fowler et al[77] reported four patients with transverse ligament avulsion injuries. Three of these patients showed no evidence of instability at follow-up. Hadley et al[92] reported on five patients with displacement of the lateral masses of >6.9 mm, none of which demonstrated instability at follow-up. Landells also found that five of six patients with lateral mass spreading of >6.9 mm did well with conservative treatment.[114] Therefore, it appears prudent to treat patients with injuries to the transverse ligament in a conservative fashion and consider surgical stabilization only if objective instability is demonstrated during the course of treatment or at follow-up.

Atlas Injuries

Isolated injuries to the atlas with minimal soft tissue disruption and less than 6.9 mm of lateral mass diastasis can usually be treated with a range of braces including a cervical orthosis, sternal occipital mandibular immobilization (SOMI) brace, or the more rigid halo apparatus for approximately 2–4 months until healing is appreciated.[92,111,131,147,157] The halo vest cannot, however, apply any traction force which is sometimes necessary for stabilizing moderately displaced atlas fractures. Koch and Nickel[113] have actually demonstrated that, in certain positions, an axial compression force is applied to the head with the use of the halo device, and may be counterproductive. If reduction is deemed appropriate, axial skeletal traction up to 9.0–13.5 kg may be used.[118]

Some authors have advocated use of skeletal traction for 6–8 weeks, even with minimally displaced injuries, followed by halo immobilization.[119,146] Controversy, however, exists as to the necessity of fracture reduction, as there are no long-term studies with adequate patient numbers that prove the benefits of anatomic reduction. Segal et al[177] suggested that the degree of initial fracture displacement had an effect on healing outcome. Three of eighteen patients in their series with significant spread of the lateral masses and rupture of the transverse ligament went on to non-union, with two of these having a poor clinical result at follow-up. Fowler et al[77] reported on 48 consecutive patients with atlas injuries and found patients whose fractures were reduced anatomically, or were initially non-displaced, had a better outcome than those with residual displacement. Unfortunately, Fowler reported that only three of thirteen patients were reduced successfully with traction. Landells[114] reported on 35 patients with atlas injuries and found that varying treatment modalities had no real effect on long-term symptoms or stability. Five of six patients in their series treated non-surgically with significant diastasis of the lateral masses had no evidence of instability at follow-up, although four of these patients complained of significant symptoms, i.e. pain referable to this region. Levine and Edwards[119] noted that even with skeletal traction in three patients, they were only able to achieve partial reduction with residual displacement averaging 3.9 mm from an original displacement of 12.3 mm. Of six patients with a mean lateral mass displacement of 7.6 mm treated with only 7 days of skeletal traction, Levine and Edwards noted no evidence of atlantoaxial instability or degenerative change at 4.5 years follow-up. Hadley et al[92] followed 5 of 57 patients with atlas injuries with lateral mass displacement of >6.9 mm for an average of 2.5 years. They also found no evidence of instability at follow-up. Some authors have noted an increased incidence of cervical discomfort with restrictive range of motion at follow-up thought to result from an incongruity of opposing articular surfaces. This contrasts with the findings of Sherk and Nicholson[181] and Hinchey and Bikel,[100] who state that most patients with a fibrous non-union report an excellent outcome.[26] In fact, many investigators believe that the primary cause for symptomatic degeneration at this level is the initial trauma to the occiput–C1–C2 complex at the time of injury and not the joint incongruity or instability at follow-up.[118,119]

For those who choose to attempt anatomic reduction, axial traction is used for an average of 4–6 weeks or until bony healing is seen radiographically, followed by halo-vest immobilization for an additional 1–2 months. At the conclusion of treatment, dynamic flexion and extension radiographs are performed to evaluate stability.[92] If moderate-to-severe instability persists despite evidence of bony union of the atlas, surgical stabilization of the C1–C2 or occiput–C2 level can be undertaken.[135,208] Occiput–C2 fusion is required only when significant damage has occurred to the occiput–C1 articulation, with marked displacement of joint surfaces or when extensive degenerative changes are present.[129] Non-union of the atlas ring can result from displaced burst-type fractures. An isolated posterior fusion of C1–C2 can be performed if there is bony integrity of the posterior arch of C1 at the site of wire placement; occiput–C2 fusion must be performed with posterior arch non-union. Minimal instability with an atlantodental interval of <5 mm can be accepted with no long-term reports indicating any adverse consequences or symptoms with these findings.[118]

Unfortunately, if the functional outcome of patients with all types of injuries to the atlas is examined, a good proportion of these patients, regardless of fracture type, report symptoms of suboccipital discomfort and decreased motion, even if they are able to participate fully in activities of daily living.[26] Segal et al[177] found that most patients who had sustained burst-type fractures were able to participate fully in their daily lives; however, two-thirds reported either fair or poor range of motion. Patients with 'comminuted fractures' reported fair or poor range of motion with limited return to activities of daily living. In the series of Levine and Edwards,[119] 88% of patients complained of neck pain, not requiring fusion, at 4.5 years follow-up. Hadley et al.,[92] however, reported that only 6 of 57 patients had significant symptoms of neck pain or restricted motion at 2.5 years follow-up.

In summary, isolated fractures of the atlas are relatively innocuous and can be managed effectively with conservative treatment. It remains to be seen through well-designed, controlled prospective studies whether reduction is necessary in terms of long-term symptomatology and stability, given the morbidity associated with prolonged bedrest and applied axial skeletal traction.

ATLANTOAXIAL ROTATORY SUBLUXATION AND DISLOCATION

Atlantoaxial rotatory abnormalities have been referred to by many names in the literature, including atlantoaxial rotatory subluxation or dislocation, rotatory deformity, spontaneous hyperemic dislocation, and atlantoaxial rotatory fixation.[70,73,118,179] Most of these lesions have been reported in children, although such abnormalities can be seen in the adult resulting from trauma,[102] tumor, infection, or other miscellaneous conditions.

The primary stabilizer of the atlantoaxial articulation is the transverse ligament, which prevents anterior subluxation of the ring of C1 on C2, although allowing the atlas to pivot concentrically around the dens process. The alar ligaments function as secondary ligamentous restraints preventing excessive C1–C2 rotation. Studies on cadavers by Werne[203] have shown that dislocation of the C1–C2 facets occurs at 63° of rotation, with the spinal canal significantly narrowed by any further rotation.

The etiology of deformities affecting the soft tissues and bony elements of the C1–C2 junction is multifactorial and can be classified as congenital or acquired. In the child, acquired subluxation or dislocation generally follows some minor trauma after a recent upper respiratory tract infection or retropharyngeal inflammatory process such as an adenoiditis, mastoiditis, or tonsillitis.[159] Other reported causes include the following: inflammatory processes such as rheumatoid arthritis, tuberculosis, or ankylosing spondylitis;[34,159] tumors of the surrounding musculature, especially the sternocleidomastoid; ocular or vestibular dysfunction;[70] and metabolic bone disease with pathologic remodeling of abnormal bone, including osteogenesis imperfecta, rickets, renal osteodystrophy, and Paget's disease. Additionally, genetic disorders of collagen formation and bone growth, and development such as Klippel–Feil syndrome, neurofibromatosis, Down's syndrome, achondroplasia, metaphyseal–epiphyseal dysplasia, spondyloepiphyseal dysplasia, Morquio's disease, and metatrophic dwarfism, can all be associated with upper cervical spine ligamentous laxity and/or odontoid hypoplasia. Trauma is an important causative factor of C1–C2 disruption. In children, even minor trauma may lead to ligamentous injury and instability, whereas adults generally require more significant energy forces, i.e. motor vehicle accidents. Any traumatized patient should undergo careful clinical and radiographic investigations, and be stabilized to prevent inadvertent iatrogenic injury to neurologic structures.[70,118,159]

Diagnosis

Patients with a C1–C2 rotatory deformity secondary to trauma usually present with significant suboccipital pain and marked restriction of cervical rotation. The patient's head usually presents in the characteristic 'cock robin' position. The skull is rotated approximately 20° in one direction and tilted 20° in the opposite direction with minimal cervical flexion. This posturing differs from congenital muscular torticollis which presents with shortening instead of lengthening of the sternocleidomastoid on the side to which the head rotates. With significant subluxation or dislocation and transverse ligament disruption, rapid neurologic deterioration may ensue as a result of proximal cord compression or transection. Vertebral artery compromise within the normal range of cervical rotation is rare. With excessive rotation, however, these vessels may be compressed with resultant brain-stem and cerebellar ischemia.[73] Fielding has reported that, with an intact transverse ligament, complete-dislocation of the C1–C2 lateral articulations occurs at about 65° of cervical rotation, with resultant narrowing of the anteroposterior spinal canal to approximately 7 mm. With transverse ligament insufficiency and 5 mm of anterior displacement of C1 on C2, unilateral C1–C2 facet dislocation will occur at 45° of rotation and with resultant anteroposterior canal narrowing of 12 mm.[73] With significant rotatory displacement, asymmetry of the anterior articulation between C1 and C2 may be palpated in the retropharyngeal space anteriorly.[179]

An interesting compensatory rotatory phenomenon may occur with this disorder, consisting of atlanto-occipital rotation in the opposite direction from the original atlantoaxial subluxation. This may result from either upper paracervical spasm on attempting to correct the perceived rotational deformity or the original traumatic injury itself.[8] This can be appreciated on a lateral radiograph of the cervical spine demonstrating rotation of the skull in relationship to C1 but possibly in profile with the C2 vertebral body. On an anteroposterior view, the chin and C2 spinous process are aligned in the midline, but with obvious rotation of the C1 vertebra.[8] Such compensatory rotation can also occur in the lower cervical spinal segments, decreasing any apparent clinical deformity.[34] Patients with long-standing rotatory deformities may develop flattening of the skull or plagiocephaly on the involved side, a condition that tends to correct itself on long-term follow-up with appropriate treatment.[70,73] In these patients it is important to elicit a careful history of trauma, of transient loss of neurologic function, or of any preceding constitutional symptoms or predisposing factors to upper cervical spine rotatory deformities. The potential seriousness of fixed deformities at the C1–C2 level has been highlighted in a report by Fielding and Hawkins[73] where a patient with significant anterior displacement of C1 on C2 expired while in traction for 10 days although voluntarily rotating her head in the direction of the deformity.

Radiographic Evaluation

The radiographic analysis of patients with C1–C2 rotatory deformities is difficult and often delayed due to problems with patient positioning and discomfort, and the presence of bony and soft tissue overlap obscuring often subtle, but important, anatomic landmarks.[70,73,76,161] The typical findings on an anteroposterior open-mouth radiograph include displacement of the C1 lateral masses in relationship to the odontoid. The anteriorly displaced lateral mass appears closer to the midline, and is broader and more superior than the posteriorly displaced lateral mass, which appears narrower and further displaced from the midline. The inferior border of the posteriorly displaced lateral mass becomes obscured by overlap of the ipsilateral C2 superior articular process, creating the so-called 'wink' sign (Fig. 11.9)[10,34,118] With lateral tilt of the head, this posteriorly displaced C1 lateral mass appears even further from the midline in the direction of the head tilt. Normally, the occiput and C1 rotate as a single entity because C1 rotates on C2 with 50% of the rotation of the cervical spine occurring at the C1–C2 articulation. The midline deviation of the C2 spinous process becomes visible when >50% of the normal physiologic rotation of C1 and C2 occurs. The deviation is further accentuated by any lateral tilting of the head with the chin and C2 spinous process both lying on the same side of the midline.[10,157]

The lateral plain radiograph is useful for evaluating prevertebral soft tissue swelling as well as the atlantodental interval. This allows inference of the integrity of the transverse ligament as well as the presence of any rotatory displacement of the C1 arches.[69,132] With overlap of the cranium on C1 when the head is tilted laterally, assimilation of C1 to the skull may be suggested.[10] With significant rotation, loss of the normal superimposition of the posterior or anterior arches may be observed with one lateral wedge-shaped mass appearing anterior to the odontoid in place of the normal appearing round anterior arch ring.[10] Other more illustrative imaging modalities include tomography, CT, MRI, and cineradiography (Fig. 11.10).[10] Reformatted axial CT scanning is an optimum imaging tool which allows visualization of the rotatory deformity of C1–C2 as well as any subluxation or dislocation present. Cineradiography, 3-mm axial CT scanning parallel to the C1 ring,[159] or plain radiographs with the head rotated 15–20° to the right and then to the left allow

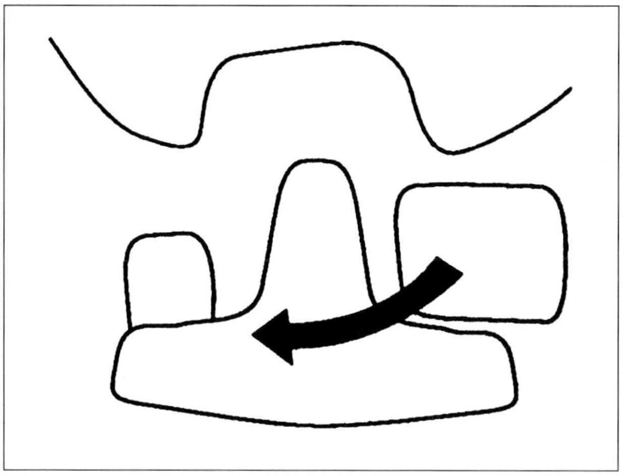

Figure 11.9
A schematic anteroposterior illustration revealing the relationship of the lateral masses of C1 to the odontoid with atlantoaxial rotation. The lateral mass rotating forward in the anteroposterior plane appears broader, more cephalad, and closer to the midline odontoid process than the lateral mass rotating posteriorly which appears narrower and further from the odontoid, with its inferior border obscured by the C2 superior articular process

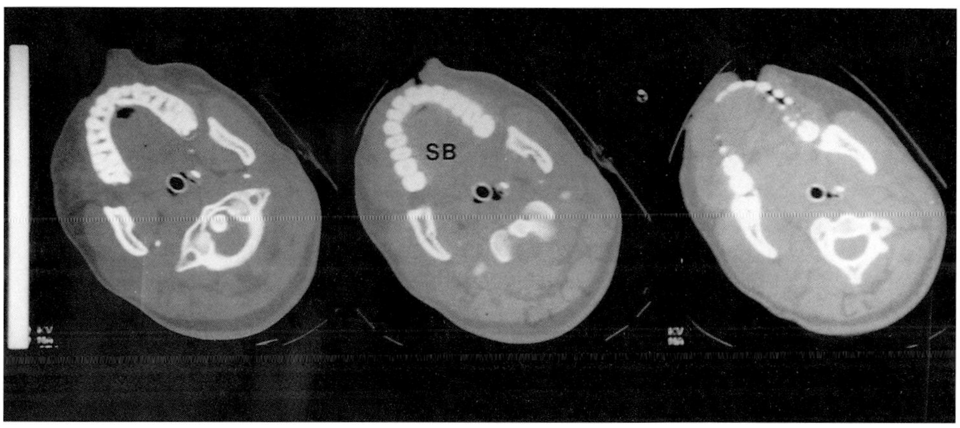

Figure 11.10
Successive caudal transaxial CT scan slices of the atlantoaxial articulation revealing significant atlantoaxial rotation. The relationship of C1 to C2 did not change with maximum cervical rotation in opposite directions. (Courtesy of JJ Abitbol, MD)

the visualization of the presence of C1–C2 rotatory fixation, which may occur in long-standing deformities.[34,132] Rotatory displacement without subluxation is not pathognomonic for injury at this level unless fixation is demonstrated on dynamic imaging studies.[34]

A small number of patients with rotatory displacement will develop fixed deformities at this level. The etiology of this condition is not clear as a result of the lack of clinical pathologic post-mortem correlation, but many authors believe that, once the deformity persists for a certain period of time, then the stretched and attenuated C1–C2 capsular complex begins to contract and scar, preventing future realignment of this articulation. Weakening and stretching of the supporting soft tissue structures may be a reactive response to an inflammatory process which results in development of a significant synovial capsular effusion. Grisel's syndrome,[152] primarily known to occur in the pediatric population but also found in adults, is a result of drainage of inflammatory agents from the posterior nasopharynx through pharyngeal lymphovenous channels to the venous plexus surrounding the atlantoaxial joint capsule. A possible accompaniment to such an effusion may be the interposition of synovial folds in the atlantoaxial joint as well as rupture and possible entrapment of one or both alar ligaments, preventing reduction. Soft tissue contracture may ensue resulting in a fixed deformity. Post-mortem findings in infants and small children have confirmed the discovery of meniscus like synovial folds in the atlanto-occipital and atlantoaxial joints which may prevent reduction of these articulations.[159] Other factors predisposing to fixed deformity include accompanying hyperemic decalcification of the surrounding ligaments, significant sternocleidomastoid muscle contracture in response to an upper respiratory tract infection, traumatic injury to the atlantoaxial articulation or some combination of these factors.[34,70,179]

Classification

Fielding and Hawkins,[73] in their classic article describing 17 patients with C1–C2 rotatory fixation, classified atlantoaxial rotatory fixation into four groups according to severity (Fig. 11.11). Type I is the most common and is usually seen in children. This type was seen in eight patients in Fielding's study. Here, rotation is fixed within the normal physiologic range of C1–C2 motion, without evidence of significant soft tissue disruption. Only mild anterior displacement (<3 mm) is noted on the lateral radiograph. Type II injuries were the second most common deformity seen in five patients. Here, rotatory fixation occurs with anterior displacement of one C1 lateral mass by 3–5 mm, pivoting on the non-displaced contralateral C1–C2 articular process. The transverse ligament is deficient in these patients although marked instability (>5 mm) is not present. Type III fixation is more severe and was described in three patients. Here anterior displacement of >5 mm of both C1 articular masses occurs with a marked increase in the atlantodental interval demonstrated on the lateral radiograph. This signifies complete disruption or severe attenuation of both the primary and secondary soft tissue restraints, i.e., the transverse ligament and capsular structures, with one articular mass subluxating or dislocating more than the other. Type IV rotatory fixation is rare and is usually seen in patients with deficiencies of their odontoid and posterior displacement of the ring of C1 on C2, with one articular mass displaced more than the other, allowing rotation to occur. This occurred following trauma in one patient, in the study of Fielding et al. with rheumatoid arthritis. Although displacement or subluxation can occur anteriorly, posteriorly, or in combination with rotation, Fielding et al were more commonly able to produce anterior displacement with transection of the transverse ligament in cadaveric studies.[69,135]

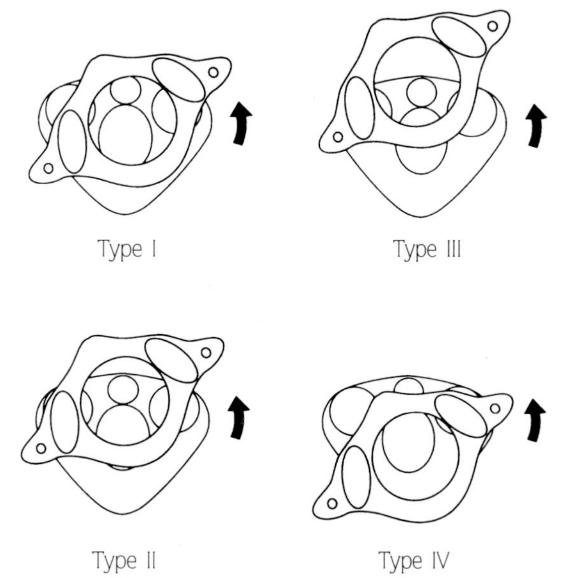

Figure 11.11
A schematic illustration of the four-part classification of Fielding and Hawkins of atlantoaxial rotatory fixation. Type I – atlantoaxial rotatory fixation within a normal physiologic range of motion without evidence of subluxation. Type II – atlantoaxial rotatory fixation with anterior displacement of a unilateral C1 lateral mass of 3–5 mm. Type III – atlantoaxial rotatory fixation with bilateral lateral C1 mass anterior subluxation of more than 5 mm. Type IV – atlantoaxial rotatory fixation with posterior C1 subluxation on C2

Treatment

The treatment and prognosis of rotatory injuries of the C1–C2 level depend on the severity of displacement, presence of neurologic deficit, patient age, and the duration of deformity.[159] Most of these injuries are fairly benign and resolve with either observation or bedrest. A soft cervical collar may be used for comfort, provided trauma is minimal or non-existent.[70,73,118] More significant trauma or prolonged deformity requires a more detailed work-up with appropriate imaging studies. These injuries, if persistent, tend to be diagnosed late because of the difficulty in obtaining accurate imaging studies and confusion on the part of the treating physician in understanding the precise nature of the disorder. All such factors may lead to development of a fixed deformity. Fielding and Hawkins[73] reported that the average delay in diagnosis in his series was 11.6 months.

If a patient presents and is properly diagnosed within 1 week of the appearance of the deformity, treatment with head-halter traction of 1.35–2.25 kg, depending on age, as well as analgesics and sedation for discomfort may be instituted.[159] For those who do not respond to treatment or present 1 week to 1 month after injury, admission to a hospital with skeletal traction is useful.[159] Fielding and Hawkins[73] found that deformities with no evidence of subluxation were stable and could be treated conservatively, whereas those with anterior or posterior subluxation usually required surgery. Often, those patients with symptoms of short duration can usually undergo reduction within 24 hours of injury. The patient will usually feel a 'pop' on reduction and immediate relief of symptoms.[132] Skeletal traction with weights of 3.15 kg for children and

6.75 kg for adults may be used initially. Weights can then be increased gradually every 3–5 days to a maximum of 6.75 kg in children and 9.00–15.75 kg for adults, as needed.[70,73,159] Traction is usually continued at the completion of reduction for 1 or 2 weeks until cervical rotation is symmetrical. The patient may be placed either in a cervical orthosis or halo brace, depending on the severity of injury, until capsular healing occurs.[70] The success and duration of treatment are generally predicated on the duration of symptoms. For those reporting the presence of deformity for more than 1 month, a poor response to conservative treatment can be expected.[73,159]

It is often difficult with axial traction to correct the rotatory deformity efficiently. It is necessary to be additionally cognisant of any pre-existing compensatory atlanto-occipital rotatory deformity which may also be exacerbated in attempting to realign a fixed atlantoaxial subluxation.[40,118] In these circumstances, Clark et al[40] have recommended lightweight skeletal traction (i.e. 4.5 kg) followed by an in situ posterior cervical fusion from the occiput to C2. Altongy and Fielding[8] have tried to preserve the available motion at the occiput–C1 level by limiting any necessary fusion to the atlantoaxial joint, believing such occipital rotation to be compensatory and probably self-correcting. Little correction is usually achieved with deformities present for more than 1 month which makes fusion the only available treatment option. Although not uniformly accepted as absolute indications for surgery, most authors reserve posterior cervical fusion for those who present with symptomatic instability, the presence of deformity over more than 3 months, the recurrence of deformity after previous correction, or deformity resistive to conservative treatment.[118] Children with an atlantodental interval >5 mm and adults of >3–4 mm on lateral plain radiographs usually have significant soft tissue instability; more aggressive measures, such as surgical fusion, are therefore usually warranted.

The average adult patient may manifest symptoms of spinal cord compression with an atlantodental interval of ≥7.5 mm. Signs of neurologic compromise usually appear before symptoms of pain and discomfort if rotation is not associated with deformity.[69,132,159] Anterior displacement of the anterior ring of C1 by more than 1 cm leaves very little area available for the spinal cord unless a coexistent fracture of the odontoid with anterior displacement is present at the time of injury.[135]

Posterior displacement of C1 on C2 with an intact odontoid may exist as a consequence of a severe hyperextension force, especially if the applied force occurs when the cervical paraspinal muscles are relaxed.[209] As of 1991, only four cases with survival have been presented,[135,170] all four cases presenting without major neurologic deficit; they were treated successfully with traction, followed by posterior cervical fusion in three. The method of closed reduction for these special injuries includes a three-stage maneuver. Stage I consists of axial distraction with weights not exceeding 6.75 kg in an adult. Slight flexion is needed to allow the anterior border of the anterior ring of C1 to remain opposed to the posterior border of the dens preventing cord impingement, while also allowing the ring to slip over the odontoid once adequate distraction has occurred. In stage II, once reduction has occurred, traction is then realigned to a more extended position allowing the posterior cortex of the anterior ring of C1 to be closely approximated to the anterior border of the dens. At the completion of this phase, traction is gradually released to a maintenance weight of about 2.25 kg until a decision for possible surgical fusion is made (stage III).[138]

Closed reduction of atlantoaxial rotatory deformities under general anesthesia and traction with direct palpation through the oral cavity under local anesthesia have been cited as alternatives in reducing these injuries. Such maneuvers, however, may increase the chance of neurologic injury.[118] Fielding and Hawkins[73] strongly deter the use of manipulation of fixed deformities for fear of catastrophic neurologic compromise. If conservative treatment with skeletal traction is effective, the patient should be immobilized in a halo brace for 6–12 weeks to allow for soft tissue capsular healing.[73] When performing surgery, some authors recommend preoperative skeletal traction for 1–2 weeks to regain as much alignment as possible, followed by postoperative skeletal traction of 4.50–6.75 kg to prevent possible recurrence of deformity as the fusion mass matures.[73] This is then followed by halo immobilization. It is important to remember that the halo brace is less effective in immobilizing rotatory deformities and, therefore, these injuries should be carefully followed during the postoperative period.[118,159] At the conclusion of halo treatment, the patient may be placed in a Philadelphia collar until dynamic studies confirm a stable arthrodesis.

ODONTOID FRACTURES

Fractures of the odontoid process are the subject of much renewed interest in the literature. A significant rise in the number of motor vehicle accidents over the last two decades has led to an increase in the number of these fractures. Additionally, anterior fixation techniques, common in Europe, are the subject of new enthusiasm in the USA. The incidence of odontoid fractures, although not precisely known because of a lack of post-mortem confirmation of fatal accidents, is reported to range in the literature from 5% to 15% of all cervical spine injuries.[1,9,11,12,24,33,41,82,103,122,132,133,148,155,169,180,185,189] The incidence in the last two decades has increased as a result of an increased number of motor vehicle accidents as well as improved resuscitation and triage measures to regional trauma centers. The average patient age in most series is in the middle forties,[12,150,171] with men involved three times as often as women.[12,15,150,171]

Mechanism

The mechanism of injury responsible for producing odontoid fractures has been studied in both cadaveric[33] and clinical studies. Althoff,[6] in cadaveric studies, postulated that fractures of the dens were the result of axial compression and vertical shear, with the type of fracture varying with the direction of force in the sagittal plane. Mouradian et al[139] tested 34 cadavers biomechanically and noted that laterally applied forces were necessary to produce consistent odontoid fractures and concluded that head rotation or oblique impact loading was necessary. These findings do not agree, however, with those of other authors who were unable to reproduce such consistent fracture patterns using a cadaveric model.[11,135] In a review of the literature, anterior displaced odontoid fractures are approximately seven times more frequent than posteriorly displaced fractures.[11,15,80,103,150] This, however, differs from the authors' experience at Thomas Jefferson University Hospital where Craft and associates found that most displaced odontoid fractures treated between 1980 and 1990 (38 of 62, or 61%) were displaced posteriorly.[46]

The mechanism of injury reported in retrospective studies suggests that an axial load coupled with a flexion–anterior translation vector is needed to produce anteriorly displaced fractures. Axial loading, extension, and a posterior translation vector are required for posteriorly displaced fractures.[5,11,46,135,189] Rotation appears to play a role especially in certain avulsion type injuries. The position of the ring of C1 may also play a role in fracture location and displacement in extension, posterior translation injuries.[135] In flexion, the strong and taut transverse ligament assists in displacing the odontoid anteriorly, whereas in extension the strong bony anterior arch of C1 assists in displacing the odontoid posteriorly.[125]

Fractures of the odontoid tip appear to be related to ligamentous avulsion by the alar ligaments,[12] although the isolated existence of these injuries is now under investigation.[176] Many authors are suggesting that such avulsion injuries represent only a component of a more global and serious injury to the atlanto-occipital articulation with potential for atlanto-occipital subluxation or dislocation.[176] Traynelis has suggested that injury to the alar and tectorial ligaments may be more common than usually suspected.[197] He feels that it is necessary to be suspicious of injury to the atlanto-occipital joint especially in cases of avulsion and waist fractures of the odontoid. Scott et al.,[176] in reporting a case of an odontoid tip avulsion fracture in association with both an atlanto-occipital and atlantoaxial dislocation resulting in death, found only six cases of such avulsion injuries reported in the literature up to 1990. He postulated, from the radiographic appearance of these injuries, that there must be disruption of at least the occipital portion of one alar ligament and partial disruption of the tectorial membrane. Similar observations were reported by Eismont and Bohlmann[60] when describing a patient who survived a traumatic posterior atlanto-occipital dislocation associated with an odontoid tip avulsion injury and C1 ring fracture.

Blood Supply

Several authors have performed both cadaveric and in vivo injection animal studies to characterize the arterial network supplying the upper cervical spine, especially the odontoid process.[6,7,11,151,172,173] It appears from these studies that the odontoid is the recipient of a rich anastomosing network of dense intraosseous and extraosseous vessels, contesting the notion that extrinsic vascular paucity is responsible for the high rate of non-union in certain odontoid fractures. Schiff and Parke,[173] using barium injection studies, demonstrated the existence of bilateral anterior and posterior ascending arteries which exit from the vertebral arteries at about the level of the C3 vertebra. These vessels send penetrating branches to the base of the dens and travel superiorly to anastomose in a rich apical arcade at the tip of the dens. Additional vessels supply the body of the dens as well as the apical arcade, including cleft perforators, inferior and superior horizontal arteries from each internal carotid artery, ascending pharyngeal vessels and meningeal vessels of the occipital artery (Fig. 11.12). Althoff and Golde[7] and Schatzker and associates[171] noted similar findings in their cadaveric investigation. It appears that the odontoid process does not suffer from the physiologic consequences of an end-vessel supply, thereby preventing the occurrence of ischemia from either low or high odontoid fractures. Schatzker et al[172] performed in vivo dog studies confirming human cadaveric findings of central ascending vessels within the body of the dens, as well as a rostral apical arcade with vessel contributions to both the apical and accessory ligaments. He found that, in dogs, if the odontoid was fractured above the insertion of the accessory ligaments, the odontoid usually failed to unite properly as a result of distraction by the apical and alar ligaments, whereas fractures below the accessory ligaments usually healed. He could not find any association between fracture level and quality of healing in 37 patients with odontoid fractures who were followed, and postulated that displacement may be the primary cause of non-union.[171]

Ligamentous and Bony Anatomy

The odontoid process is surrounded by bony and soft tissue elements affording stability to the C1–C2 articulation (Fig. 11.13). Posteriorly, the dens is held firmly to the anterior arch of C1 by the transverse ligament which arises

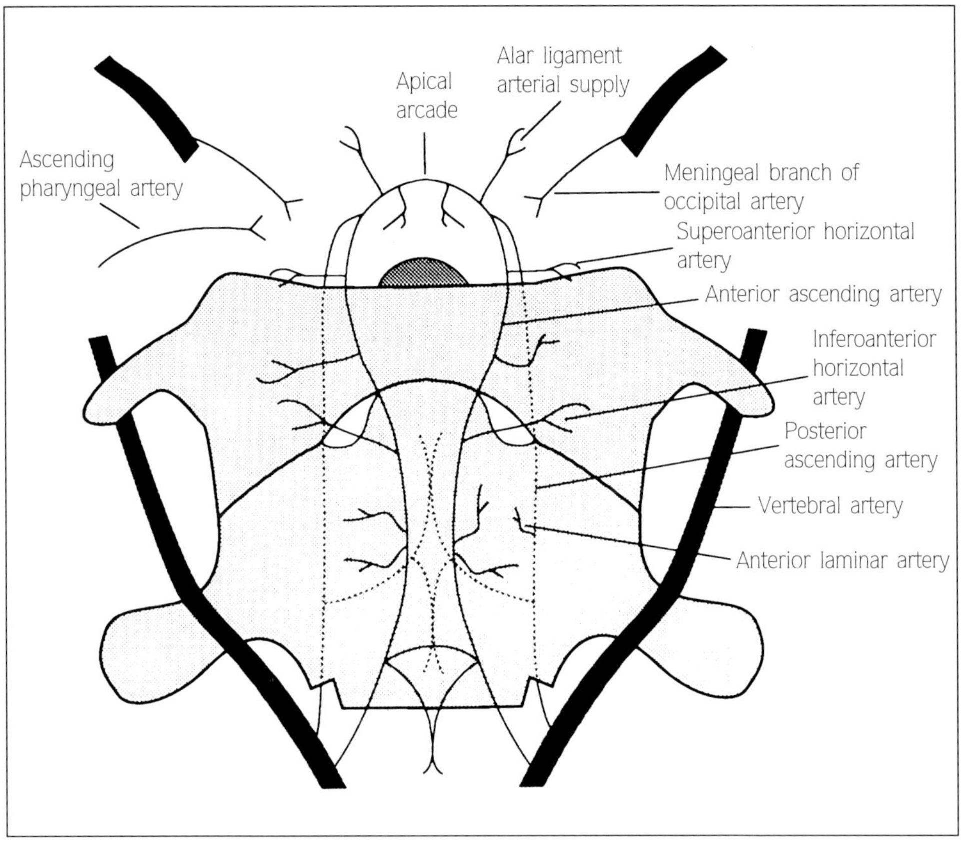

Figure 11.12
An anteroposterior and lateral schematic illustration of the extensive blood supply of the odontoid process

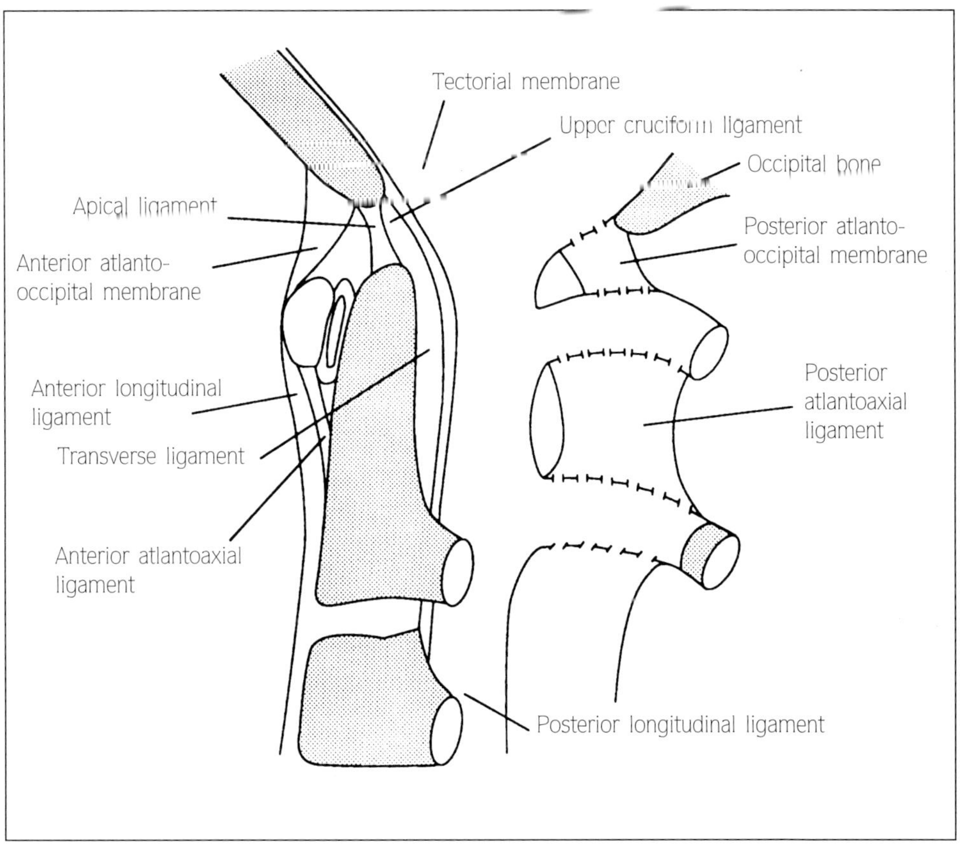

Figure 11.13
A schematic lateral diagram revealing the bony and ligamentous structures of the upper cervical spine

bilaterally from the medial tubercles of the lateral masses of the atlas. The transverse ligament also sends a superior attachment to the occiput and an inferior attachment to the posterior inferior dens, referred to respectively as the upper and lower cruciform bands. The transverse ligament is the primary stabilizer of the odontoid to the anterior ring of C1 in flexion, as well as allowing the odontoid to act as a stable pivotal point for C1 rotation. The odontoid functions to limit posterior translation of the atlas in extension. Anterior to the transverse ligament's attachment to the atlas lie the accessory ligaments which arise in conjunction with or anterior to the transverse ligament from both lateral masses of C1 and attach to the anterior lateral surface of the dens. This ligament also assists the transverse ligament in stabilizing the odontoid in flexion, extension, and lateral bending. Superiorly, the dens is attached to the occipital condyles by paired alar ligaments arising bilaterally from its superolateral apex, with a central apical ligament attaching its tip to the basion of the occiput. These ligaments are important in lateral bending and axial rotation.[11,39] The observed increase in non-union rates of odontoid waist fractures compared to other locations on the odontoid may result from superior or partial lateral displacement of the dens by the apical, accessory, and transverse ligaments as illustrated by Schatzker.[132,172] The inherent elasticity of the apical and alar ligaments allows superior displacement of the cephalad portion of the odontoid in fractures above the accessory ligaments.[169,171] The superior and inferior articular facets of C2 are located in different vertical planes with the superior facets lying anterior and with less vertical inclination than the inferior facets, allowing rotation to occur between C1 and C2.[35]

Classification

At present, five different classification systems have been popularized for odontoid fractures.[6,12,19,91,156,171] The most commonly used fracture classification is the three-part system of Anderson and D'Alonzo, which was developed after their study of 60 patients with odontoid fractures between 1964 and 1972 at the Campbell Clinic (Fig. 11.14).[12] In their classification system, the type I fracture is an oblique fracture at the tip of the dens caused by an avulsion of the alar and, possibly, the apical ligaments.[189] This fracture must not be confused with an unfused apical secondary center of ossification which may be present in a minority of cases. To date, there have only been six reported cases of this injury in the literature, and four of these are clearly related to injuries to the atlanto-occipital and atlantoaxial articulations.[12,35,54,60,96,169,176] Therefore, these injuries may simply be a radiographic marker for an occult injury to the atlanto-occipital joint. Burke and Harris,[35] after a thorough review of reported cases of isolated type I injuries, noted the obvious ambiguity in their description and concluded that they do not exist and that all odontoid fractures should therefore be classified as either high or low. A worrisome complication of a displaced type I odontoid fracture, although extremely rare, is superior migration of the dens tip into the foramen

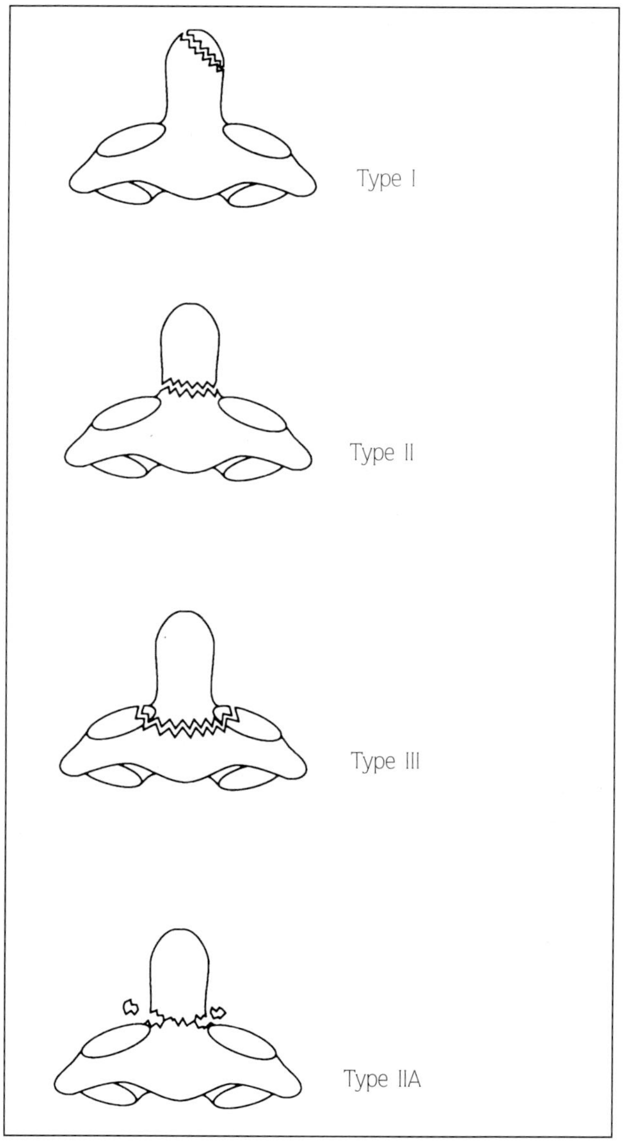

Figure 11.14
The Anderson and D'Alonzo three-part odontoid fracture classification with the addition of Hadley's type IIA fracture. Type I – an oblique ligamentous avulsion fracture of the tip of the odontoid. Type II – a fracture at the base of the dens with its juncture with the C2 body. Type III – a fracture of the dens with extension into the body of C2. Type IIA – type II fracture with comminution of the anterior and posterior cortical fracture margins

magnum causing significant compression of the ponto-medullary junction of the brain stem.

A type II fracture is the most commonly reported odontoid fracture in the literature and is located at the base of the dens at its junction with the C2 body. This fracture should not be confused with an injury to the neurocentral synchondrosis in a skeletally immature child, which occurs much lower in the centrum of the C2 vertebral body.[39,125] Fielding and associates[72,75] have suggested that an occult type II fracture from minor trauma may be the etiologic cause for the os odontoideum found incidentally in patients with cervical discomfort. An os odontoideum can be differentiated from an acute fracture by its smooth cortical outline and significant distance between itself and the remaining portion of the dens. A type III fracture occurs within the body of C2 and courses through one or both of the superior articular surfaces.

Hadley et al,[91], in 1988, noted that 3 of 62 patients who have type II fractures have noticeable fragmentation at the anterior and posterior aspects of the odontoid base, preventing appropriate alignment by closed manipulation and traction. He postulated that such fragments were indicative of additional injury to the alar and transverse ligamentous complexes and demanded more aggressive treatment (i.e. fusion). He classified these as type IIA fractures.

Diagnosis

Injuries to the upper cervical spine are frequently missed on presentation as a result of lack of suspicion in those patients without neurologic deficit or whose other injuries may overshadow cervical insult.[11,15,39] Therefore, in all unconscious or intoxicated patients, particularly with trauma above the clavicles or with complaint of cervical pain, thorough radiographic evaluation to rule out possible injury to the upper cervical spine should be undertaken. Symptoms and findings relating to fractures of the odontoid tend to be non-specific. In the absence of any neurocompromise, most patients complain of poorly localized posterior occipital pain which may be a result of irritation of the greater occipital nerve, localized muscular trauma, or cervical paravertebral muscle spasm. A decreased range of motion and subjective sense of instability may be seen.[46,189] The incidence of neural injury is reported to occur in 15–25% of all cases, and ranges from irritation of the greater occipital nerve or isolated nerve root deficits to tetraplegia with respiratory center involvement.[11] In contrast to neural injury, associated severe injuries are reported in up to 50% of cases,[103,150] including cerebral concussions, scalp lacerations, and facial and extremity fractures. Fractures of the arch of C1 are also frequently reported and should be closely looked for when a fracture of the odontoid exists. The reported incidence of mortality from injuries to the odontoid is difficult to determine due to a multitude of unknown variables, but is thought to occur in 3.3–8% of all cases.[9,11,12,15]

RADIOGRAPHIC EVALUATION

Apart from standard anteroposterior, lateral, and open-mouth plain radiographs, anteroposterior and lateral polytomography, as well as CT with sagittal reconstruction, appear to be beneficial in the evaluation of odontoid fractures. CT scanning in the transaxial plane must be interpreted with caution because of the chance of missing a fracture completely within the plane of imaging.[11,63]

Treatment

The primary goal of treatment for patients with odontoid fractures should be immediate restoration of spinal stability through appropriate realignment of bony displacement and immobilization.[16] Many authors have tried to elucidate important prognostic factors affecting fracture healing in an attempt to develop appropriate treatment algorithms. Variables such as age, neurologic status, degree of fracture displacement,[93,133] comminution or angulation, and delay in diagnosis may be important in deciding between initial non-operative versus operative intervention.[91] At Thomas Jefferson University Hospital the approach is to apply gentle, low-weight (2.25 kg) skeletal traction to all patients with odontoid injuries while further studies are completed for better elucidatation of the fracture type. If a type I fracture is associated with injury to the atlanto-occipital joint, such low-weight traction, under close supervision, will safeguard against iatrogenic injury before appropriate treatment.

Type I Injuries

Isolated type I injuries without evidence of atlanto-occipital instability are, by definition, stable injuries, and can be treated with a cervical orthosis for approximately 3 months, followed by dynamic flexion–extension radiographs for evaluation of residual instability.[11,46,131] There have been no reported non-unions or complications of this fracture in the literature.

Type II Injuries

Type II fractures of the odontoid have a more ominous outcome than the more stable and predictable type I and type III injuries. Controversy exists over the suggested initial treatment of these fractures, with some advocating primary cervical stabilization and others recommending strict initial conservative treatment.[9,12,26,38,41,43,54,55,69,79,180,182,189] Unfortunately, the answer is not clear because the literature supports both arguments. Several authors have noted poor results in certain patients or fracture subgroups and, as such, have suggested more aggressive treatment modalities in some situations.

Clark and White[41] performed a multicenter retrospective view of 144 odontoid fractures of which 96 were of the type II variety. Their overall non-union rate with type II fractures was 32%. They found a statistically significant ($p \leq 0.05$) increase in non-union or malunion in fractures that were displaced >5 mm or angulated >10°. Halo treatment was successful in eventually obtaining stability in only 70% of patients with type II fractures, whereas those treated with posterior cervical fusion were stabilized successfully in 96% of cases. Stability in the study of Clark and White was defined as lack of movement at the fracture site on follow-up flexion–extension films. The authors recommended that all type II and type III fractures should be treated initially with skeletal traction followed by halo immobilization. Primary posterior cervical fusion should be considered only in those fractures that are significantly displaced and/or angulated.

Anderson and D'Alonzo[12] recommended primary cervical fusion in all patients with type II fractures, although they found no difference in union rates between displaced and undisplaced fractures. Their overall non-union rate for type II fractures was 36.4%, although only 80% of patients treated with posterior cervical fusions obtained a stable union.

Bell and Meyer[21] had remarkable success (3% non-union) in their series of type II fractures treated with initial skeletal traction for 4–6 weeks followed by SOMI bracing for 3 months. Husby and Sorensen[103] treated 32 patients with odontoid fractures and grouped them according to high (type II) versus low (type III) fractures. Injuries of a high type were treated by primary posterior cervical fusion with a 100% fusion rate. They, therefore, recommended primary fusion for all high fractures as well as for low unstable fractures. Donovan[54] treated 28 of 54 patients with type II and type III fractures by halo immobilization and noted a 75% union rate. He found no correlation between the patient's age or degree of fracture displacement, and thus recommended primary fusion for all type II injuries. Hadley et al[91,93] reported on 68 acute type II fractures and noted a 78% incidence of non-union with fractures displaced >6 mm compared to a 10% non-union rate with fractures displaced <6 mm. These patients were all treated with extended immobilization regardless of their alignment status in post-injury traction radiographs. There was no significant influence on healing rate of patient's age, neurologic status, or direction of displacement. Hadley also termed type II fractures with comminution at the base anteriorly and posteriorly 'type IIA fractures' and noted the inability to align these fractures adequately with traction. Early surgical stabilization was recommended for this fracture group.

Fujii et al[79] reported on a series of 58 odontoid fractures, 31 being type II fractures. They recommended surgical stabilization for all acute type II fractures, significantly displaced type III injuries, and any non-unions of type II or type III fractures. Fujii and colleagues further recommended the use of anterior compression screw fixation in all acute type II fractures, as well as for significantly displaced type III injuries; posterior cervical fusion was reserved for missed cases, fractures with residual displacement, or cases of non-union. Dunn and colleagues[52] evaluated 128 odontoid fractures and recommended primary posterior cervical fusion in patients over 65 years of age with type II fractures (78% non-union), fractures with more than 3 mm of posterior displacement (100% non-union), fractures with a delay in diagnosis of 7 days or more, or fractures which redisplaced while undergoing closed treatment (100% non-union). In 1981, Ekong et al[62] noted a 41% non-union rate in type II fractures with an especially poor prognosis in patients over the age of 55, and evidence of posterior displacement or anterior displacement >4–6 mm. Ryan and Taylor[169] pointed to the need for adequate fracture overlap and contact, and suggested the need for at least 60% fracture contact for adequate healing to occur.

Several authors have commented on treatment success with odontoid injuries without mention of or correlation to an acceptable fracture classification. Roberts and Wickstrom[164] noted an overall non-union rate of 20% in their series with displaced fractures experiencing a higher rate of non-union than undisplaced fractures (30% versus 17%). They recommended initial traction for all fractures followed by Minerva casting for approximately 20 weeks. Schatzker et al[171] noted a 64% incidence of non-union in 22 patients treated with 4–6 weeks of traction followed by 4–6 weeks of casting or bracing. They believed non-union was more common in displaced fractures, especially if displaced posteriorly, and in those patients over 60 years of age. Schatzker cited an 86% fusion success rate in 15 patients and therefore recommended primary atlantoaxial fusion after a 1- to 2-week period of skeletal traction for edema control. Apuzzo et al[15] followed 45 patients treated at Los Angeles County Hospital between 1969 and 1974, and he noted an increased incidence of non-union in displaced fractures in patients over 40 years old. He recommended conservative treatment in undisplaced fractures and primary atlantoaxial fusion for those fractures displaced >4 mm. Blockley and Purser[22] followed 35 adult patients with odontoid fractures and noted a 63% non-union rate; they found no relationship between the direction and degree of displacement, but did note a high degree of non-union in elderly patients. Amyes and Anderson[9] published one of the most successful series describing 63 patients all treated with traction for approximately 1 month followed by casting or collar immobilization. They reported only three cases of non-union (5%) with conservative treatment.

It is obviously difficult to assimilate all the presented data into a concise treatment plan because of variations in classification and treatment protocols. The present authors have, therefore, reviewed their data[46] at the Regional Spinal Cord Injury Center of Delaware Valley (RSCICDV) of Thomas Jefferson University Hospital. Of 70 consecutive patients treated between 1980 and 1990, 30 patients went on to non-union (43%). Of those with type II fractures treated by halo immobilization, 75% went on to eventual non-union compared to 100% union for patients primarily fused. Of the original 38 fractures with posterior displacement treated with halo immobilization, 70% went on to non-union. Of 24 patients with anterior displacement treated solely with halo immobilization, 33% went on to non-union. Of those fractures displaced >5 mm, 81% of the posteriorly displaced fractures and 100% of the anteriorly displaced fractures failed to unite. This compared with 43% and 0% respectively for fractures displaced <5 mm. Post-reduction alignment had no influence on overall fusion rate. It was also noted that there was an increased incidence of non-union in significantly displaced fractures in patients over the age of 60 (68%) compared to those under 60 years of age (33%). All ten patients treated with primary cervical fusion went on to non-union regardless of age or fracture displacement, whereas 58% of all patients treated by halo immobilization went on to non-union. Four fractures displaced while undergoing halo treatment with three of these eventually going on to non-union. Four of seven patients with a delay in diagnosis of 10 or more days also failed to unite. A 45% incidence of non-union (5 of 11 patients) was also seen in patients with an initial neurologic deficit on presentation. It was therefore concluded that patients with non-displaced type II fractures, or fractures displaced <5 mm, should be reduced with skeletal traction, if necessary, followed by halo-vest immobilization. For displaced type II fractures of >5 mm, patients over the age of 60 years, and loss of previous reduction are both considered to be major risk factors for non-union and deserve consideration for primary surgical fixation. Gapping at the fracture site, delay in diagnosis of more than 10 days, unstable C1–C2 fracture combinations, and significant fracture angulation all appear to be minor risk factors for non-union.

Traction for short periods of time (i.e. 1–2 weeks) allows acute symptoms of neck pain and paracervical spasm to subside, and further safeguards the spinal cord from unnecessary movement which may potentiate cord swelling. Cervical or head to thorax braces are inadequate for immobilization of the upper cervical spine because of the indirect forces of jaw motion.[189] It is therefore preferable to use the more rigid fixation provided by the halo device. Studies have shown that the halo effectively restricts 75% of atlantoaxial joint motion, whereas a cervical orthosis only limits 45% of motion.[107,189] However, use of the halo device has not been universally accepted because of the infrequent, but sometimes ominous, complications reported with its use. Such complications include facial scars, draining sinuses, skull penetration, abscess formation, difficulties with activities of daily living, poor radiographic imaging, potential for sensory neuropathy from pin impingement, degenerative changes secondary to prolonged rigid immobilization, and difficult access to the thoracic cavity in cases of cardiopulmonary emergencies. Koch and Nickel[113] have studied dynamic forces of the cervical spine immobilized in a halo vest or cast. They have noted distraction forces up to 9 kg in a halo vest and 13.6 kg in a halo cast in patients changing from the supine to the sitting position. This is in direct contrast to desired compression forces in the treatment of odontoid fractures. In general, the average quoted rate of non-union for all variations of type II fractures is approximately 33%.[11,194] Great care must be applied to the placement of a halo device to avoid complications, and to minimize the potential for distractive forces at an already unstable interface.

Type III Fractures

Although type III fractures of the odontoid are not as benign as once thought, most authors continue to favor conservative management because of the large cancellous overlap of fracture surfaces and generally high rate of union.[11,25,39,46] Clark and White[41] suggested a need for more aggressive methods of external immobilization after experiencing four cases of malunion and one case of non-union in 10 patients treated with cervical orthoses. They have recommended halo immobilization as the method of choice in these patients.[41,86] Their overall rate of non-union in the treatment of 48 type III fractures was 13% with a 15% malunion rate. Forty percent of fractures displaced >5 mm and 22% of fractures angulated >10° went on to non-union in their series. Paridis and Jones,[150] at the Mayo Clinic, treated 13 of 17 acute low fractures with 4–5 weeks of traction followed by bracing with only two non-unions. They recommended a total period of immobilization of 4–5 months. Husby and Sorensen,[103] in 1950, used non-operative treatment for 21 of 23 low fractures and achieved a non-union rate of only 14%. Apuzzo and associates,[15] however, reported a 54% rate of non-union in a series of 13 patients with type III fractures treated with halo immobilization. They did not agree with the prognostic significance of the Anderson and D'Alonzo classification system and suggested primary posterior cervical fusion for elderly patients with fractures displaced >4 mm.

At Thomas Jefferson University Hospital, 16 of 18 patients with type III injuries were treated with halo immobilization after an initial period of skeletal tong traction. Four of the conservatively treated patients (25%) went on to non-union, and three of these had significant posterior displacement on initial radiographic evaluation. Nevertheless, the authors believe that all type III fractures, regardless of displacement, should be treated with initial skeletal traction (2–6 weeks) in an attempt to restore and maintain reduction, followed by halo immobilization for approximately 3 months. At the end of this treatment period, dynamic flexion–extension radiographs should be obtained to evaluate for residual instability. White has, in adults, described a subgroup of type III fractures in which there is evidence of stable impaction of cancellous elements across the fracture site; he has suggested that these may be treated adequately with cervical orthosis immobilization. In general, it appears that posteriorly displaced fractures have a more ominous prognosis than anteriorly displaced injuries. This may be due to the fact that posteriorly displaced fractures are more difficult to reduce and maintain in traction with the head in a flexed position compared to traction in extension for anteriorly displaced fractures.

Combined C1–C2 Fractures

Many series reviewing fractures of the cervicocranium cite a high incidence of associated contiguous and non-contiguous fractures of the cervical spine. The odontoid represents the most common secondary fracture seen with fracture of the atlas. Many authors recommend careful scrutiny of both C1 and C2 when any fracture is noted in this region. Jefferson,[105] in his original treatise on burst fractures of the atlas, noted that, of 19 combined C1–C2 fractures, 15 involved fracture of the odontoid. However, Levine and Edwards[119] noted only four cases of combined atlas and odontoid fractures in 34 patients with atlas fracture. Hadley et al[92] found that 10 of 25 patients with atlas fractures had type II odontoid fractures. Dickman[53] found 43% of his 58 reported acute atlas fractures to have combined C1–C2 injuries, whereas Anderson and D'Alonzo[12] only reported one case in 32 to have an associated atlas and type II odontoid injury. In the present authors' series at Thomas Jefferson University Hospital, 16 of 70 patients (23%) with odontoid fractures had an associated atlas injury.[111,157] It has been suggested that patients with combined C1 and odontoid injuries have a higher incidence of neurologic deficit at presentation compared to other upper cervical spine injuries. Others argue this claim, however, citing that a burst fracture of C1 actually decompresses an already capacious upper cervical spine and gives the cord more room, especially in the presence of a displaced odontoid fracture. The mechanism of injury for combined C1 and odontoid injuries appears similar to that described for isolated odontoid fractures combined with either an axial load to produce an atlas burst fracture or hyperextension to produce a posterior arch fracture.

Treatment of combined C1–C2 injuries is usually determined by the type of C2 fracture present. Traditionally, an unstable odontoid fracture with an associated C1 ring injury has been treated with rigid halo immobilization allowing the atlas to unite before attempting any necessary treatment for an ununited odontoid fracture.[122,157] If significant displacement of the lateral masses of the atlas exists with evidence of transverse ligament insufficiency and an associated type II odontoid fracture, Ketterson[11] has recommended primary occiput–C2 fusion to avoid prolonged immobilization in light of the potential for fracture non-union and/or instability. Recently, surgeons have approached combined C1 and C2 fractures more aggressively to avoid the potential morbidity of prolonged immobilization. In the present authors' series, five of ten patients with combination C1–odontoid fractures went on to non-union requiring further surgical stabilization. Many surgeons, especially in Europe and Japan, have recommended anterior screw fixation for these injuries to preserve motion.[2,23,24,64,65] If posterior cervical fusion is attempted, Meyer and Cotler,[131] as well as Hadley et al.[92] emphasize the fact that only C1–C2 levels should be fused as long as the integrity of the C1 posterior arch is maintained or the fracture line is not in the location of C1 sublaminar wire placement.

COMPLICATIONS OF ODONTOID FRACTURES

Non-union

As stated previously, the non-union rate of odontoid fractures in various series ranges from 5% to 88%.[55] Although a precise etiology is not known, many factors, including lack of stability at the fracture site,[131] age of the patient, mechanism of injury, direction or degree of displacement, angulation, delay in treatment and associated injuries, all contribute to the potential for non-union and must be considered carefully when formulating treatment recommendations.[2,23,64,65]

Neurologic Deficit

Patients who survive transfer to a regional trauma center after sustaining odontoid injuries have a low incidence of neurologic deficit due to the capacious nature of the upper cervical spinal canal. Steel's ratio of thirds in the upper cervical canal divides this region into three equal regions with 1 cm allocated for the odontoid, 1 cm for the spinal cord, and 1 cm of available space for the spinal cord.[194] Anderson and D'Alonzo[12] have reported a 25% incidence of neurologic deficit in patients with type II and type III dens fractures. However, as a result of the unavailability of post-mortem reports for patients who die from upper cervical spine fractures, the mortality rate of odontoid injuries is not precisely known, but is estimated between 5% and 18%.[9,12,15,55,90,148,188,189]

Late-onset myelopathy has been reported in cases of unstable odontoid non-unions.[121] Schwartz and Wigton reported two patients with late developing myelopathy 5–18 years after the original injury. Osgood and Lund[148] noted that 10 patients in their series of 55 developed such symptoms. Anderson and D'Alonzo, in a review of the literature, found 50 reported cases of late-onset myelopathy with symptoms ranging from urinary and fecal incontinence, Brown–Séquard syndrome and spastic hemiparesis, to complete quadriplegia.[12] In fact, they presented one patient in their series who developed symptoms 19 years after the original injury date. Paradis and Jones[150] reported on 29 patients with documented non-union of the odontoid 4 months to 15 years post-injury, with 76% of them demonstrating some degree of neurologic compromise. Such neurologic compromise is thought to result from either displacement or hypertrophy of the odontoid non-union site with subsequent neural impingement.[11,91] In the present authors' series, only one patient with a posteriorly displaced odontoid non-union developed a progressive myelopathy requiring decompression. It is imperative from these observations that early stability be established to avoid late neurologic compromise.[11]

AXIS FRACTURES

The term 'traumatic spondylolisthesis' was first introduced in 1964 by Garber[82] in describing a bilateral fracture through the pars interarticularis of the axis. Frequently, this entity is inaccurately described as a fracture through the pedicle of the axis. This is technically incorrect because of the unusual anatomy of the C2 vertebra which actually has no well-defined pedicle.[35] The bony anatomy of this injury was first described by Wood–Jones in 1912.[34,210] He correctly correlated the effect of knot placement during hanging and the resultant fatal fracture–dislocations which occurred through violent hyperextension and distraction. Today, fractures of the axis occur primarily as a result of motor vehicle accidents, falls,[174] or diving accidents,[71] with a significant portion (25–40%) of these injuries resulting in immediate death of the patient. In an evaluation of fatal multiple trauma victims at the Dallas County Medical Center, Bucholz and Burkhead[33] found 8 of 170 patients to have a traumatic spondylolisthesis of the axis, second in incidence only to atlanto-occipital dislocations. Six of these eight injuries were thought to be incompatible with life.[32]

Axis fractures comprise 12–18%[93,132] of all acute cervical spine fractures. Of patients who survive these injuries, only 3–10% sustain neurologic injury,[32,59,78,93] which is partly a reflection of the mechanism of injury, where primary forces of hyperextension and axial loading are involved. This is unlike judicial hangings, where significant axial stretching and cord transection occurs.[97,135] Meyer and Cotler[131] reported on 59 patients with axis fractures: 10 patients (17%) were found to have an incomplete cord lesion, and one sustained a complete cord injury. In the series of Levine and Edwards[116] of 52 patients, only four (7.7%) presented with any signs of neurologic deficit. Hadley et al[93] reported on 229 patients with acute axis fractures and found only 13 patients (5.7%) to have evidence of neurologic deficit. This low rate of neurologic deficit in surviving patients is also a manifestation of a spacious canal at the C2 level which has a diameter of approximately 1.95 cm,[131] while housing a spinal cord of diameter only 1 cm. With bilateral vertebral element separation at the pars interarticularis and anterolisthesis of C2 on C3, there is actually an increase in the total cross sectional area of the spinal canal and neuroforamina.[32,83] This fact, coupled with the lack of distraction normally associated with a fatal judicial hanging,[71] leads to the paucity of neurologic deficits seen in these patients. Most surviving patients with permanent spinal cord injury incur a fracture of the pars interarticularis with dislocation of the C2–C3 facet joints, resulting in spinal cord impingement. As with all injuries to the cervicocranium, associated spinal fractures are common.[131] The most commonly seen associated fractures include C1 or C3 arch fractures, C2–C3 avulsion fractures, type II odontoid injuries, and occasionally burst fractures of the midcervical spine.[80,131] The reported frequency of these associated injuries is 14–33%.[59,71,78] Associated non-spinal injuries are extremely common[34,59,71] and include facial and scalp lacerations, tracheal disruptions, thoracic cage trauma, and closed head injuries.[78] Francis et al[78] reported a 79% incidence of associated head and cervical spine injuries in his group of patients, and also noted a low incidence (6.5%) of neurologic deficit.

Diagnosis

The signs and symptoms reported in surviving patients are usually non-specific and consist of localized discomfort at the cervicocranial junction, possibly in the distribution of the greater occipital nerve (C2), an unusual subjective sense of instability, and associated physical signs of head and neck trauma.[83]

Radiographic Evaluation

As with other areas of the cervical spine, fractures of the axis may be extremely subtle on plain radiographic survey. Additional imaging modalities, such as CT scan or anteroposterior and lateral tomography, may be necessary in their evaluation.[118,160]

Classification

Francis and associates,[78] in 1981, developed a five-part classification system based on the stability criteria of White and Panjabi:[205] >3.5 mm sagittal plane translation or >11° angulation compared to adjacent levels suggests instability. Unfortunately, this system fails to reflect the implied mechanism of injury and therefore does not offer coherent treatment alternatives. The three-part classification system of Effendi et al.[59] as modified by Levine and Edwards,[116] is generally more useful (Fig. 11.15). In this system, a type I fracture represents a fracture through the pars interarticularis bilaterally, or adjacent portions of the superior or inferior articular facets, with <3 mm fracture displacement and without angulation or gross stability on voluntary flexion and extension lateral radiographs.[131] The C3 vertebral body below is always intact without evidence of compression. This particular fracture has a high association with other cervical spine fractures, especially C1 posterior arch fractures, atlas burst fractures, odontoid injuries, and C1 lateral mass fractures.[116]

Type II fractures have >3 mm displacement or significant angulation and are associated with a wedge compression fracture of the anterosuperior portion of the C3 vertebral body, and possible avulsion fracture of the posteroinferior body of C2.[120] Associated cervical spine injuries occur less frequently with type II fractures. Levine and Edwards[116] have described a type IIA fracture which has slight or no fracture displacement, but is significantly angulated (Fig. 11.16). With this injury, the anterior longitudinal ligament remains intact; however, the posterior longitudinal ligament and posterior disc space between the C2 and C3 vertebral bodies is completely disrupted.[59] This is further differentiated from a type II injury by the presence of significant fracture fragment distraction on application of axial traction.

Type III fractures are extremely unstable injuries; they are similar to type I injuries, with fracture of the pars interarticularis or the lamina posterior to the facet joints, with severe displacement and angulation and an associated unilateral or bilateral facet dislocation of C2 on C3. This usually results in disruption of both the anterior and posterior longitudinal ligaments, making closed reduction virtually impossible unless the fracture is posterior to the facet dislocation. If reduced, this fracture is extremely difficult to maintain and therefore generally requires open reduction and internal fixation. Unlike type I fractures, these fractures have a low incidence of associated cervical spine injuries.[120]

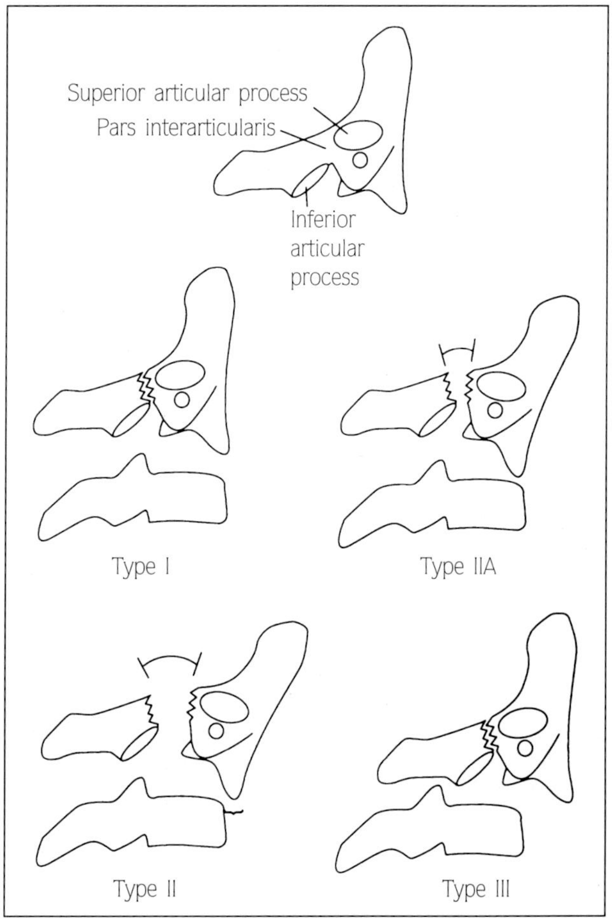

Figure 11.15
A schematic illustration of Effendi's three-part classification system of traumatic spondylolisthesis of the axis with a modification by Levine and Edwards. Type I – fracture of the pars interarticularis with <3 mm fracture displacement without angulation. Type II – fracture of the pars interarticularis with >3 mm displacement with significant angulation. Type IIA – fracture of the pars interarticularis with no or slight translation but with significant angulation. Type III – usually a type I fracture of the pars interarticularis with a unilateral or bilateral facet dislocation of C2 on C3

Burke and Harris,[35] in 1989, described an atypical variant of the hangman's fracture where the fracture line courses through the posterior cortex of the C2 vertebral body allowing the body of the axis to separate from the posterior neural arch. This, according to Burke, allows for an extremely unstable situation which is difficult to reduce by

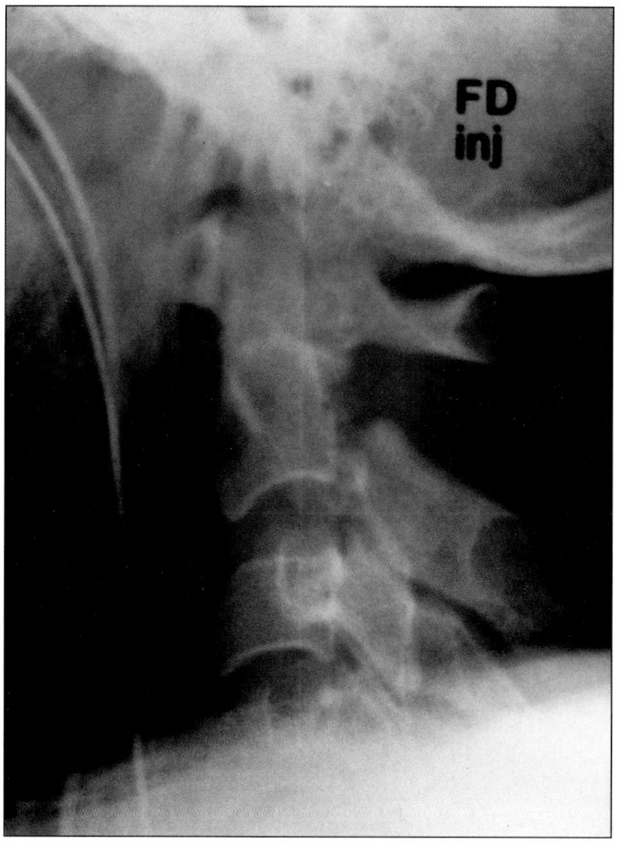

Figure 11.16
A type IIA hangman's fracture revealing marked angulation at the fracture site with minimal evidence of anterior subluxation of C2 on C3. (Courtesy of JJ Abitbol, MD)

closed means as a result of significant soft tissue interposition and instability. Other fracture configurations can occur and are important to recognize as treatment prognosis is variable. Isolated lateral mass fractures are usually stable and result from axial compression with associated lateral bending. These patients usually have no neurologic deficit and complain only of isolated pain in the cervical region.[35]

There are two forms of axis body fractures. The first is a hyperextension teardrop-type fracture, and the second represents an avulsion body fracture resulting from a hyperextension–dislocation injury. In hyperextension teardrop injuries, the vertical height of the body fracture is more than or equal in length to the horizontal component. This injury is caused by an avulsion fracture of the anteroinferior body of C2 by the anterior longitudinal ligament. This is usually seen in elderly, osteoporotic patients and is usually associated with minimal localized prevertebral swelling on lateral radiographs. The hyperextension fracture–dislocation results from avulsion of Sharpey's fibers of the anterior annulus at its insertion into the anteroinferior body of C2, resulting in a fracture whose transverse width is always more than the vertical height. This fracture, unlike hyperextension teardrop fractures, is associated with extensive prevertebral swelling on lateral radiographs.[35] Isolated laminar or spinous process fractures may also be found at the level of C2 after cervical spine trauma.

Mechanism of Injury

Although flexion and axial loading have previously been suggested as the primary force vectors involved in the production of these injuries,[120] cadaveric and clinical studies have revealed hyperextension to be the primary vector force in type I, type II, and type IIA injuries. These injuries, common during motor vehicle accidents, occur as a result of deceleration–acceleration forces, with a resultant hyperextension and axial load applied to the cervicocranium and compression of the posterior facet joints.[31] This allows shear forces to be specifically concentrated on the pars interarticularis, the adjacent articular masses, and foramen transversarium.[83,120,131,132] This asymmetric force distribution is the result of the unique elongated shape of the pars interarticularis, its transverse orientation, and anatomic location midway between the C2 superior and inferior facets, which occupy different vertical planes.[35,71,120] The resultant fracture is usually bilateral but asymmetric, implying a degree of cervical rotation at the time of injury. If minimal or no displacement exists without injury to the disc or compromise of the anterior or posterior longitudinal ligaments, this represents a type I injury.[116] With continued extension, the C2–C3 disc begins to disrupt with the anterior longitudinal ligament failing in tension with or without an avulsion fracture of the anterosuperior margin of C3 or, less frequently, the anteroinferior margin of C2.

Continued extension results in separation of the C2–C3 disc from the superior end-plate of C3 or, less commonly, the inferior end-plate of C2, with eventual rupture of the posterior longitudinal ligament allowing marked separation of the bony elements. At this stage, significant neural compression may occur resulting in neurologic deficit.[78] If a rebound flexion force occurs before anterior longitudinal ligament failure, anterior translation of the C2 body on C3 may occur, as commonly seen in type II fractures. With this injury, the anterior longitudinal ligament will not rupture in tension but may be stripped off the superior body of C3 in an anterior direction. This occurs in association with partial or full disruption of the posterior longitudinal ligament and posterior C2–C3 disc space, allowing a variable degree of angulation. An intact anterior and posterior longitudinal ligament will allow successful closed manipulation of these injuries through skeletal traction and cervical extension. However, if the posterior longitudinal ligament and posterior annulus are disrupted, hinging will occur at the stretched and elongated anterior longitudinal ligament causing extensive distraction and angulation as seen in type IIA fractures. If a pure flexion force is initially involved, a unilateral or bilateral C2–C3 facet fracture–dislocation may occur before fracture of the pars interarticularis or other posterior elements.[83,116]

The fracture line in type I and type II fractures is usually oriented in a vertical direction at the junction of the anterior pars interarticularis and C2 body. Type IIA fractures are more oblique, and type III fractures may occur in one of two locations: the midportion of the pars interarticularis or through the lamina in an oblique orientation running from anterosuperior to posteroinferior just behind the inferior facet joint.

Treatment

The treatment of traumatic spondylolisthesis of the axis is guided by a basic understanding of the injury mechanism, effectively represented by the fracture classification of Effendi et al[59] as modified by Levine.[47,116] Before coherent fracture type grouping, authors presented conflicting views on effective treatments of these injuries. Schneider et al,[174] in 1965, recommended prolonged traction for all patients followed by cast or brace immobilization with successful outcomes in seven of eight patients. Cornish,[44] in 1968, disagreed with traction immobilization and recommended immediate C2–C3 stabilization of these injuries, although he reported a significant rate of complication with this approach. Fortunately, it is now known that most of these fractures can be treated closed with excellent results.[41,48]

Type I fractures are stable injuries which can be treated effectively with rigid cervicothoracic immobilization or a cervical orthosis[116] for 3 months or until osseous union is present. Some authors have advocated cranial tong traction for 4–6 weeks[132] before application of a halo or other cervical orthosis, although this appears to be unusually aggressive for such non-displaced injuries. If there is a question of fracture stability, physician-supervised, voluntary, flexion–extension, lateral radiographs should be performed.

Type II injuries present with more extensive soft tissue damage and, in general, can be treated with short-term (1–2 weeks) skeletal traction of 4.5–9.0 kg.[116,132] Use of a posterior cervical roll at C4–C5 allows for distraction with slight extension, simulating lordosis and therefore aiding reduction. Others have successfully managed these injuries with closed manipulation, through cervical hyperextension, followed by halo immobilization for approximately 3 months.[83] It is clear from published reports of displaced type II injuries that short-term skeletal traction does not necessarily result in long-term fracture reduction. Unfortunately, however, no long-term follow-up studies have correlated residual fracture displacement or angulation with non-union or instability.[19,71,78,116,120] Some authors have recommended closed manipulative reduction under general anesthesia with fluoroscopic guidance, although the inherent risk of this procedure may not be justified because of the reported benign consequences of fracture displacement at follow-up.[83] Levine and Edwards[116] recommended axial traction for 4–6 weeks if reduction was lost, but reported 3 mm residual fracture translation and 4.5° angulation, or 60% of the original fracture translation and 40% of the original angulation, in 16 of 22 patients treated in this manner. He also recommended immediate halo application with translation <4.5 mm or <15° of angulation.[120] Effendi et al[59] cautioned against the use of traction of more than 4.05 kg for fear of C2–C3 disc space widening, and suggested anterior C2–C3 fusion if instability was present 6 weeks after the injury. Brashear et al[30] originally recommended 6 weeks of skeletal traction followed by 2–3 months of immobilization, but at follow-up discovered a high incidence of union regardless of immediate immobilization or prolonged traction. Unfortunately, Brashear did not correlate residual displacement with eventual outcome. Francis et al,[78] and later Fielding et al,[71] in reporting on a similar group of patients, found satisfactory results with either immediate halo application, short-term traction (around 8 days), or traction for 6 weeks, with a healing success rate of 94.5% (116 of 123 patients). They did, however, observe that six of the seven non-unions in their series had >11° angulation at follow-up. It is interesting that a good number of these injuries (70% of type II fractures) resulted in spontaneous anterior C2–C3 interbody fusion with inherent stability. This is the result of extensive disc injury with elevation of the anterior longitudinal ligament and associated hematoma formation, as well as damage to the anterosuperior body of C3.[32,116] Brashear et al[30] reported on long-term follow-up of 29 patients with traumatic spondylolisthesis of the axis. He found significant C2–C3 disc space narrowing in 24 patients, large bridging anterior osteophytes in 15 patients, and complete C2–C3 interbody fusion in 7 patients. Type I fractures, resulting from less significant soft tissue injury, tend not to autofuse, and have a higher degree of symptomatic degeneration at the C2–C3 disc level (up to 30% of patients) at follow-up. For symptomatic degeneration at the C2–C3 level, many authors[68,78] have chosen to perform an anterior C2–C3 fusion in order to avoid posterior procedures, thereby preserving atlantoaxial rotatory motion.[34]

Type IIA injuries can be recognized by their fracture orientation, presence of significant angulation without translation, excessive widening of the posterior C2–C3 disc space, and hinging on an intact, anterior, longitudinal ligament with axial traction. These injuries should not be treated with traction, but with gentle cervical extension and compression followed by halo immobilization.[116,120]

Type III injuries may be approached from one of two vantage points. If a unilateral or bilateral dislocated facet is present with a fracture to the pars, closed reduction is usually impossible. An open reduction with spinous process wiring of C1 or C2 to C3[116] must be performed under these circumstances, followed by rigid halo immobilization of the pars fracture. If the fracture site is posterior to the pars, closed reduction may be attempted with success. However, bilateral laminar fracture is usually impossible to hold in a closed fashion, and requires internal fixation through oblique facet wiring of the inferior facet of C2 to the spinous process of C3.[116] An anterior cervical fusion for this injury would compromise the anterior longitudinal ligament, the only viable intact soft tissue structure. With bilateral inferior facet fractures of C2 and a neural arch fracture, a posterior arthrodesis of C1 to C3 must be performed.[120] A unilateral facet fracture with an associated pars fracture may be successfully treated with closed reduction and halo immobilization.[120]

In general, indications for surgical intervention in these injuries include unreduced facet dislocations in type III injuries, symptomatic degeneration of the C2–C3 disc, and objective instability at follow-up after conservative treatment.[78] Fortunately, regardless of treatment, these injuries have a remarkably low non-union rate of approximately 5.5% and are uncommonly associated with development of long-term neurologic deficits in only 6.5% of patients.[78]

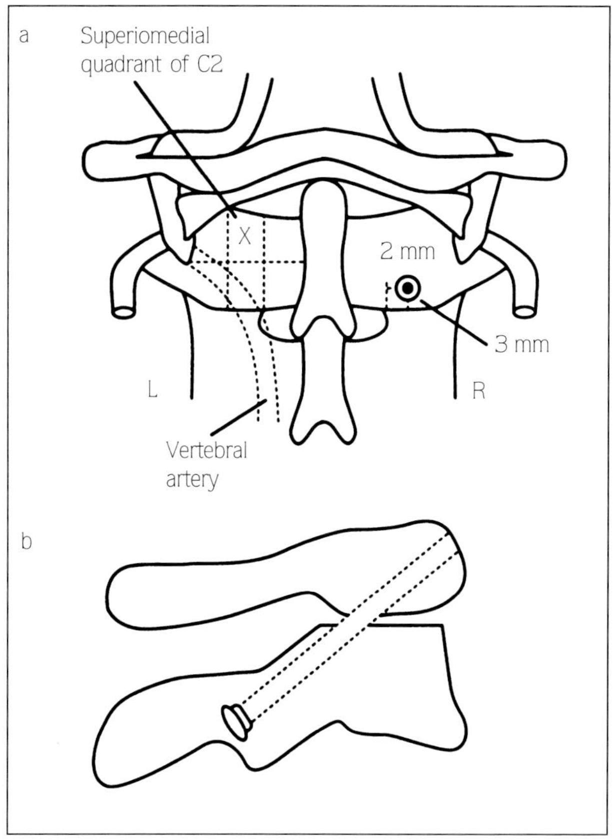

Figure 11.17
A schematic illustration revealing (a) the starting screw fixation point for a C2 isthmic (pedicle) screw on the left avoiding the vertebral artery and the starting point for a C1–C2 transarticular facet screw by the technique of Magerl on the right. (b) A lateral schematic drawing illustrating the Magerl posterior cervical transarticular facet screw fixation of the atlantoaxial joint

SURGICAL APPROACHES TO THE UPPER CERVICAL SPINE

General Considerations: the Posterior Approach

In attempting posterior surgical stabilization of the upper cervical spine, certain principles must be followed and surgical techniques mastered to ensure a safe and successful result.[132,133,168] The skin incision should be long enough to allow ample room for entry of instruments from the inion of the occiput to the level of C3. It is important when stripping laterally at the level of C1 to go no more than 1.5–2 cm in adults and 1 cm in children from the midline to avoid damage to the vertebral artery and accompanying venous plexus.[10,141] Also, it is necessary to be careful to avoid injury to the C2–C3 interspinous ligaments to ensure as much soft tissue stability as possible.[141]

The passage of sublaminar wires in the upper cervical spine can be dangerous, particularly with ligamentous instability or canal compromise from subluxation or stenosis. A useful technique of sublaminar wire passage in the upper cervical spine after ligamentum flavum removal is through the use of an aneurysmal needle (with its pointed removed with a wire cutter) threaded with a no. 1 silk suture. This method involves passing the eye of the needle, in a sublaminar fashion, from an inferior to superior direction, following the superior insertion of the ligamentum flavum along the undersurface of the superior lamina. Once passage of the no. 1 silk suture is complete, it is then tied securely to the looped end of a gauge 16–24 stainless steel wire. The wire is then advanced slowly under the lamina in an inferior-to-superior direction. It is most important that the surgeon apply a continuous posterior force vector with the suture-wire to prevent inadvertent pressure on the underlying spinal cord.[125,132,157] Sublaminar wires should not be used below the level of C3 in intact patients for fear of possible cord contusion.[132]

If C2 pedicle screw, or more appropriately isthmus, fixation is chosen, the starting landmark for screw insertion is the superomedial quadrant of the C2 lateral mass avoiding injury to the greater occipital nerve and vertebral artery (Fig. 11.17). Direction of screw passage is approximately 15° superior and 15° medial, which allows passage of the screw away from the vertebral artery and into the subchondral bone of the C2 superior articular facet. It is useful to palpate the medial border of the C2 isthmus (pedicle) during screw insertion with a small Penfield or microsurgical dissector, after opening the posterior capsule of C1–C2, to avoid spinal cord damage.[167] The screw length used is approximately 22–26 mm in most cases.[140,167]

Posterior Cervical Fusion: Atlantoaxial Joint

Injuries to the odontoid and symptomatic instability of the atlantoaxial joint can be treated effectively with an isolated posterior fusion of the C1–C2 level.[127,167] Theoretically, this preserves motion of the occiput–C1 level, where 50% of total cervical flexion is known to occur. Over the years, many techniques have been developed to fuse the posterior atlantoaxial joint such as the Gallie technique[81] and its modifications,[132] the technique of Brooks and Jenkins[31] with its modifications,[90] and posterior C1–C2 facet screw fixation.[10,61,74,128,132]

Gallie Technique

The time-honored approach for fusion of the posterior atlantoaxial joint is the Gallie technique with its various modifications.[10–14] This consists of placing the looped end of a gauge 16–20 wire under the arch of C1, with both free ends of the wire passed through the wire loop grasping the arch of C1. After placing a block-shaped corticocancellous graft contoured to the upper surface of the C2 spinous process and over the posterior lamina, one free end of the wire is placed through the spinous process of C2 and twisted to itself, securing the graft in place. Many authors have reported a high success rate with this technique,[208] advocating its use over C2 sublaminar wire techniques, especially in flexion injuries.[10,28] Biomechanically, this configuration protects against flexion forces,[10] but provides little stability against rotational or lateral force vectors.[35]

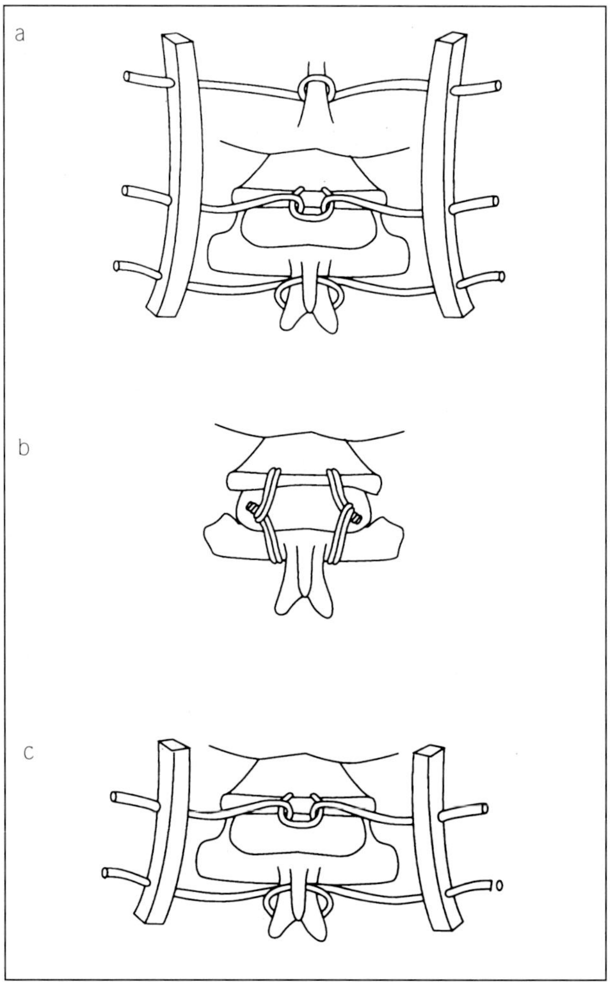

Figure 11.18
Schematic illustrations revealing (a) the triple-wire technique of Wertheim and Bohlman for posterior occipital C2 fusions; (b) a modification of the Brooks C1–C2 posterior cervical fusion with bilateral looped C1–C2 sublaminar wires; and (c) a modified Gallie posterior C1–C2 cervical fusion with a C1 sublaminar wire and a C2 spinous process wire threaded through bilateral corticocancellous bone struts

There are multiple variations of Gallie's original technique. Fielding's modification uses an H-shaped graft that is locked around the spinous process of C2, establishing some degree of rotational control. Extension is prevented by graft contact with the spinous process of C2.[135] Other authors have modified the grafting procedure by using two separate parallel corticocancellous strips, one on each side of the neural arches (Fig. 11.18c). Wilbur has documented a modification of this procedure for the treatment of hangman's fracture, placing separate wires through the spinous process of C2 and C3 and a sublaminar wire at C1.[208] The problems noted with this technique have included rare graft resorption and the potential for pivoting or translation at the C1–C2 level as a result of the posterior location of the fusion mass in relationship to the C1–C2 articular facets.[208] Additionally, the technique tends to oppose the posterior arches of C1 and C2 making it ideal for reducing an anterior displaced odontoid fracture, but possibly further displacing or redisplacing a posterior displaced type II odontoid fracture.[131,135] In this situation, the posterior fusion technique of Brooks and Jones is more prudent.

Brooks Technique

In 1978, Brooks and Jenkins[31] described a technique of sublaminar wire fusion at the C1–C2 level in 12 patients and reported successful results in 11 of them. The original description by Brooks included a horseshoe-shaped tricortical wedge graft placed between the inferior lamina of C1 and superior spinous process of C2 secured by bilateral C1–C2 sublaminar wires (Fig. 11.18b).[31,132] This allows for increased rotational and lateral stability over the Gallie technique and is useful in preventing posterior translation of the C1 ring and overcompression of the posterior laminae of C1 and C2.[132,135,168] Callahan modified the Brooks technique to avoid the potential neurologic risk of C1 sublaminar wire placement by drilling holes perpendicular through the lamina of C1 for wire passage.[36,132] Others have used double or twisted wires as far from the midline as possible with corresponding notches in the posterior cortex of the wedge bone graft for better rotational stability, but with increased risk of neurologic damage. Also, two equal-sized wedge-shaped grafts can be used on either side of the midline instead of one large horseshoe-shaped graft. Some authors have placed drill holes through the bone graft for better graft fixation.[10,132]

The authors believe that the biomechanical advantages of the Brooks technique make this the procedure of choice in most cases where a posterior C1–C2 arthrodesis is deemed appropriate. A looped gauge 16 or 18 wire is passed on either side of the midline in a sublaminar fashion as described earlier in a caudal-to-cranial direction. The loop is then removed with a wire cutter, resulting in four sublaminar wires. These wires are then secured around two wedge-shaped grafts placed on either side of the midline and sequentially tightened. This technique affords excellent stability in flexion, extension, lateral bending, and rotation, but with the inherent risk of sublaminar wire placement.[132,141] In cases where the spinal canal is compromised, spinal cord monitoring is beneficial to detect inadvertent injury to the spinal cord.

Posterior Facet Screw Fixation

Posterior facet screw fixation of C1–C2 is gaining popularity and is a particularly useful technique in cases of laminar deficiency. C1–C2 facet screw fixation has been found to be biomechanically superior to the Gallie procedure in preventing rotation, and can be used successfully.[28,123,202] Image intensification is used to assist in placement of bilateral 3.5 mm screws from an inferior-to-superior direction through the posterior portion of the isthmus and superior articular facet of C2 into the lateral mass of C1, while avoiding anterior cortical penetration. The screw insertion starting point is 2 mm lateral to the laminar lateral mass junction at the posteroinferior border of the C2 inferior facet. The screw is guided upward and forward 50–60° in the sagittal plane and somewhat medial to avoid damage to the vertebral arteries (see Fig. 11.17).[28,45,167] The atlantoaxial membrane may be opened to allow probing of the medial isthmic border of C2 in evaluation of cortical integrity. Care to avoid damage to the greater occipital nerve and vertebral vessels must be taken at all times. Magerl et al have strongly recommended the addition of a Gallie fusion if the C1 lamina is intact (Fig. 11.19).[123]

Halifax Interlaminar Clamp

By using the Halifax interlaminar clamp, the surgeon avoids the potentials of neurologic injury associated with sublaminar wire passage.[45,49] This construct relies on clamp fixation of the superior laminar border of C1 and inferior laminar border of C2, with compression applied through a screw mechanism joining both clamps at the C1–C2 interspace. Clamps are applied unilaterally or bilaterally depending on the instability pattern. Unfortunately, only short-term follow-up is available on its use in patients with cervical trauma, and many question its ability to control axial rotation and lateral bending, while citing its tendency to overcompress the C1 and C2 posterior elements.[45] Cybulski reported on eight patients, but with an average follow-up of only 6 months, showing adequate stability with no instrument failure.[49] Holness et al[102] reported on its use in 51 patients treated after the operation with just a Philadelphia collar. All patients obtained successful fusion and only two patients demonstrated clamp dislodgement. The weakness of the system lies in its bulky nature, decreasing the area available for graft placement, and therefore increasing the possibility of pseudoarthrosis. Also, potential for instrument slippage has been noted with usage.[10]

The present authors feel that the Halifax clamp, although inherently safer than sublaminar wire placement, provides inferior fixation of the C1–C2 complex. Difficulties in obtaining good laminar purchase with the clamp, overcompression of the posterior elements, limited

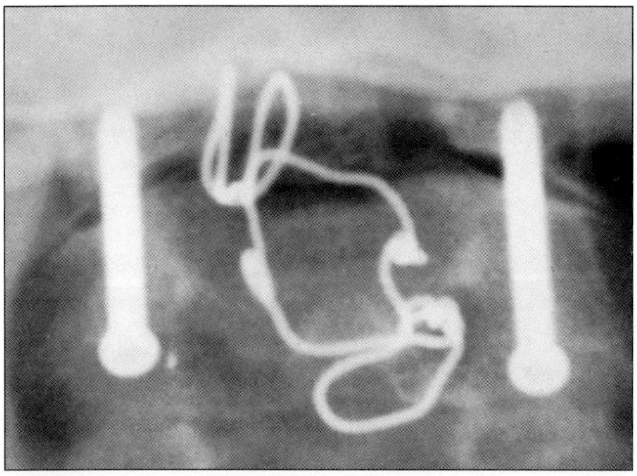

a

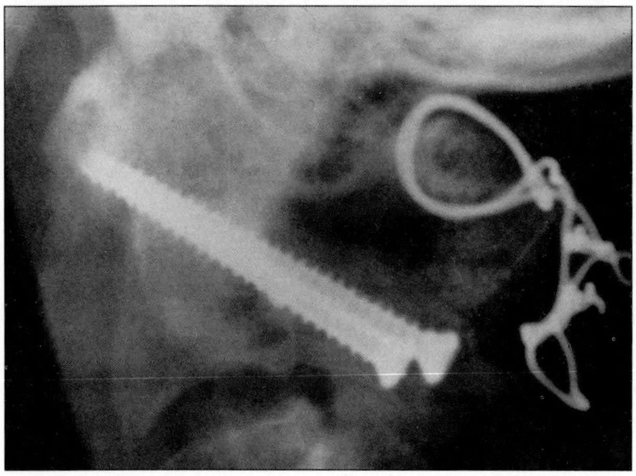

b

Figure 11.19
(a) A plain anteroposterior radiograph and (b) lateral radiograph revealing posterior C1–C2 transarticular facet screw fixation with the addition of a Gallie posterior fusion supplementation. (Courtesy of S Garfin, MD)

space for graft, and potential for clamp dislodgement appear to outweigh the benefit.

Posterior Occipitocervical Fusion

If fusion is deemed necessary to the occiput,[28] there are several potential techniques including in situ onlay bone grafting,[135,144] wire or plate fixation,[167] and Luque rod constructs.[161] In rare circumstances, methylmethacrylate[127,208] may be used adjunctively to create an acceptable stable construct of the occipitocervical region.[88] In situ onlay bone grafting suffers from the potential of prolonged immobilization as well as a high documented rate of pseudoarthrosis. Therefore some form of internal fixation is advised in most cases.[10]

The passage of wires through the occipital bone can be performed by one of two methods: the first involves drilling holes completely through both cortices of the calvarium, 5 mm lateral to the apex of the occipital protuberance, but with risk of injury to both the epidural veins and dura; the second involves burring a trough through only the outer cortex along each side of the inion and using a right-angled burr or towel clip to form a hole for passage of gauge 16–24 stainless steel wire through the outer cortex of the skull.[108,204] The level of wire passage should be approximately 2.5 cm above the inferior rim of the foramen magnum.[131,141] This wire may be looped on itself and passed again through the inion for greater holding strength.

Roy-Camille has popularized plate fixation to the occiput with prebent plates of 105° conforming to the natural contour of the posterior occipital cervical juncture. He recommends bicortical screw fixation to the occiput with 3.5 mm screws. A protected drill depth of 13 mm is used in the drilling process. Cervical lateral mass screws are inserted at the midportion of the lateral masses in both the superoinferior and medial–lateral directions with the drill guided 10° laterally to avoid possible damage to the vertebral vessels. The Roy-Camille plates come in two sizes with the holes approximately 13 mm apart. The lateral mass screws come in two sizes of 16 mm or 19 mm.

Cotrel-Dubousset has a modified system that also uses screw fixation into the occiput, but uses hook fixation below into the cervical spine.[115,195] Others have used the Luque rectangular rod and wire construct in performing arthrodesis of this region.[104] Itoh and associates[104] reported a 92% fusion rate in 32 patients with rheumatoid arthritis treated with the Luque rod and wire technique. However, the risk of sublaminar wire passage in these patients must be carefully considered before its use.[10] All of these plate and rod systems offer excellent stability, but at the expense of decreased surface area for bone graft applications (Fig. 11.20).[45]

A commonly used method by surgeons for occipitocervical fusion is the three-wire technique originally described by Grantham in 1969 and later modified by Wertheim and Bohlman (see Fig. 11.18a).[131,150,204] This technique is especially useful with congenital flattening of the occipital bone or in the presence of significant basilar impression.[131] With this technique, one wire is placed either through one or both cortices of the occipital bone on either side of the occipital protuberance. Another wire is placed under the lamina of C1, and a third wire looped through the spinous process of C2 with the respective ends placed through two laterally placed corticocancellous bone struts measuring approximately 1–1.5 × 4 cm.[132] The grafts are placed laterally over the posterior elements and along the posterior

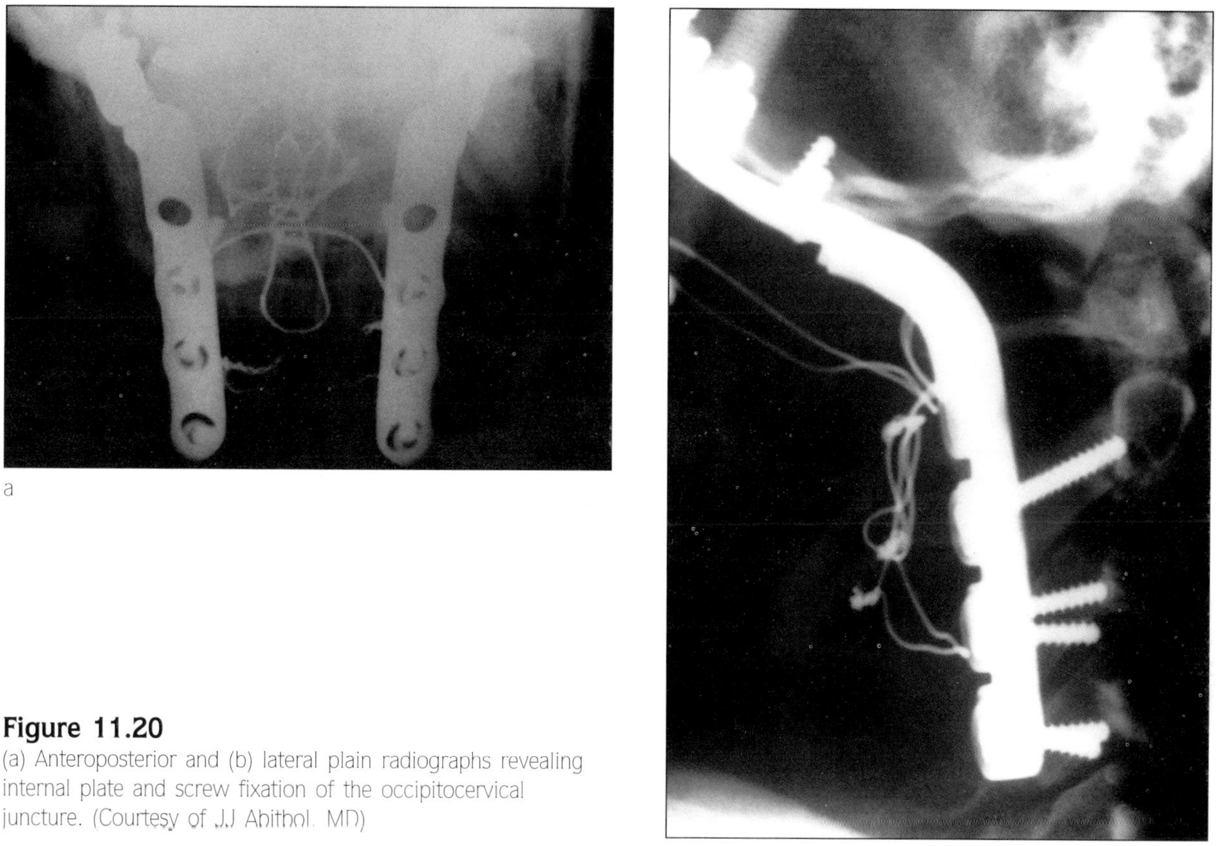

Figure 11.20
(a) Anteroposterior and (b) lateral plain radiographs revealing internal plate and screw fixation of the occipitocervical juncture. (Courtesy of JJ Abitbol, MD)

surface of the occiput. This technique proved successful in all 13 patients treated by Wertheim and Bohlman.[204] The bicortical strut grafts may be shaped into diagonal wedge grafts to better conform to the posterior cervical spine.[36]

Other variations of wire passage and bone graft shaping for stabilization of the occiput to the C1 or C2 level have been published with similar success rates.[36,127,204,208] Meyer and Cotler[131] use an H-shaped graft with its superior limbs placed within a 4 cm transverse trough in the occipital bone and a central hole in its transverse limb for wire loop passage to assist in graft stabilization. The inferior H-shaped portion of the graft allows easy straddling of the C2 spinous process to ensure greater stability.

In most traumatic cases requiring occipitocervical fusion, the technique of Wertheim and Bohlman proves to be simple, although providing excellent fixation. Wires of gauge 16 or 18 are placed through the unicortical trough of the occiput, spinous process of C2 and sublaminarly at C1. Drill holes are placed through the corticocancellous strips and tightened as seen in Fig. 11.18a. A tricortical graft obtained from the posterior iliac crest is divided and generally conforms nicely to the contours of the occipitocervical region. Use of more rigid constructs, although of potential benefit in the rheumatoid patient population, is generally not required in the typically younger traumatic victim.

Loss of motion is a significant consequence of this operation. Rogers,[166] in 1957, stated that patients whose fusions extended to the occiput lost approximately 80–90% of cervical rotation, while fusion isolated to the atlantoaxial joint compromised rotation by 50%. Similar results have not been obtained by others.

Non-union is another potential problem associated with attempted occipitocervical arthrodesis. However, recent literature does not support the once-held theory that occipitocervical fusion has a significantly higher failure rate than isolated C1–C2 fusions.[111] Other complications of occiput to C2 or C1–C2 posterior fusions have included neurologic injuries from sublaminar wire or screw placement, especially in irreducible subluxations, vertebral artery injuries, and spinal wound infections.[45,145,187] Nordt and Stauffer[145] reported two patients with anterior C1 on C2 subluxations who incurred significant cord damage with quadriplegia from C1 sublaminar wire passage. Smith and associates[125] found perioperative neurologic complications to be common in patients with significant atlanto-occipital instability, unreduced dislocations, or the presence of a preoperative neurologic deficit. In 47 patients undergoing a posterior cervical fusion consisting of either an occipitocervical, atlantoaxial, or C1–C3 fusion, only 11 patients had an uncomplicated course. In this series 45 patients had C1 sublaminar wires placed. This high complication rate has not been universally experienced by other authors who report few to no complications from upper posterior cervical spine fusions.[12,73,74,90]

Anterior Approaches

Surgical stabilization of the upper cervical spine after trauma can usually be approached safely and efficiently through a posterior route.[160,183] In special circumstances, however, such as variations in anatomy, iatrogenic deficiency of the posterior elements or fixed flexion deformities, or in an attempt to limit the number of cervical spine segments fused,[126,127,163] other more technically difficult approaches[135] may be used. These include the anterior, anterolateral or lateral retropharyngeal, transoral, mandibular osteotomy and tongue-splitting approaches to the upper cervical spine with their many variations.

Anterior Retropharyngeal Approach

The most popular approaches to the upper anterior cervical spine represent cephalad extensions of the anterolateral approach originally described by Southwick and Robinson in 1957,[190] Smith and Robinson in 1958,[186] and Bailey and Badgley in 1960.[17] These approaches may traverse one of two paths, either anterior or posterior to the carotid vessels.[42,165,193,199] The approach described by DeAndrade and MacNab,[51] and later popularized by McAfee et al[126] is an extrapharyngeal approach which develops the plane between the sternocleidomastoid muscle and pre-tracheal strap muscles superficially, and the carotid vessels and hypopharynx posteriorly, through an incision starting above the angle of the mandible and ending below the cricoid cartilage. This approach is especially useful for anterior cervical corpectomies of C2 and C3 with easy access for resection of the odontoid and C1 anterior arch with or without bone grafting and internal fixation.[51] Incision is usually made on the right side well above the recurrent laryngeal nerve which is at risk usually at or below the level of C5. After traversing the platysma, the marginal mandibular branch of the facial nerve is protected at the superior portion of the wound, during mobilization and ligation of the various superficial veins at this level. Then the spinal accessory nerve may be encountered as it enters the anterior portion of the sternocleidomastoid at the level of the transverse process of the atlas. The deep cervical fascia investing the sternocleidomastoid is divided along its medial border, mobilizing the pre-tracheal strap muscles medially and the sternocleidomastoid laterally exposing the carotid sheath. This approach is sometimes limited by the angle of the mandible and subglottal structures, especially in patients with short muscular necks.[108,138] Nothing should be placed in the oral cavity to keep the mandible away from the operative field. The submandibular and salivary glands along with associated lymph nodes are resected, exposing the posterior belly of the digastric muscle as well as the stylohyoid muscle, which are then both divided. This allows the hyoid bone with its attached muscles to be retracted medially, assisting in protection of the underlying alimentary structures. The hypoglossal nerve is visualized at the superior portion of the approach and is mobilized anterosuperiorly for better visualization, allowing ligation of the superior thyroid, lingual, ascending pharyngeal, and facial arteriovenous branches of the external carotid vessels. Care must be rendered in mobilizing the hypoglossal nerve which exits approximately 2 cm from the midline through the anterior condyloid foramen.[51] The retropharyngeal space is then bluntly dissected from the level of C3 to the clivus. The superior laryngeal nerve courses from its origin near the nodose ganglion to the larynx and is at risk for injury during this approach, especially its external branch that tends to be closely approximated to the superior thyroid artery.[126] Cranial nerves IX, X, XI, and XII, as well as the internal carotid and jugular veins, are anchored laterally by their passage into the occiput. The pharyngeal and laryngeal branches of the vagus which arise somewhat inferior to this level may also be injured by overzealous medial or lateral retraction during surgery.[108]

DeAndrade[51] recommended this approach for patients with cervical myelopathy and instability when posterior bony arch sufficiency secondary to previous laminectomy makes posterior fusion difficult. They did not report the use of this approach in any patients with instability secondary to trauma and all patients experienced temporary hoarseness thought to be secondary to retraction of the superior laryngeal nerve. McAfee et al[126] reported on 17 patients who underwent this approach; 15 patients obtained a solid arthrodesis whereas one developed a malunion of an odontoid fracture with C1–C2 subluxation, and one developed a non-union of a hangman's fracture with C2–C3 subluxation. They reported three cranial nerve neurapraxias, one permanent unilateral hypoglossal nerve injury, and one perforation of the hypopharynx repaired without incidence at surgery. This approach allows optimum exposure for placement of a bone graft as compared to the transoral route if surgical arthrodesis is chosen.[127]

Anterolateral Retropharyngeal Approach

In individuals with slender necks, it may be possible through the standard Smith–Robinson approach to retract the superior soft tissues with a long blade retractor placed over the anterior tubercle of C1, avoiding any unnecessary resection of soft tissues or surgical ligation of the branches of the external carotid artery.[138,186] Another useful, but technically difficult, approach is the (anterior) lateral retropharyngeal approach of Whitesides[206] with dissection posterior to the carotid sheath. This approach had originally been described by Henry[98] for exposure of the vertebral artery. This approach is useful for lesions below C1, avoiding the risk of infection associated with transoral routes, but limited by its inability to allow adequate room for bone graft application.[18,56,184] Although the surgeon may gain access as high as C1 with this approach, if a more cephalad extension is desired, the anterolateral approach with dissection medial to the carotid vessel should be chosen. For this approach, the incision is made along the anterior margin of the sternocleidomastoid muscle with extension superolaterally over the mastoid prominence. Dissection is then taken medial to the sternocleidomastoid muscle with the option of detaching this muscle from its mastoid process insertion as well as taking down the styloid process in order to get better exposure of the carotid sheath. The splenius capitus muscle may also be resected below the sternocleidomastoid for better exposure. The spinal accessory nerve should be identified as it enters the sternocleidomastoid muscle, and the sternocleidomastoid branch of the occipital artery located and ligated. The carotid sheath can then be retracted medially allowing the dissection to proceed posterior and lateral, avoiding ligation or damage to branches of the external carotid vessels or associated neural structures, especially the superior laryngeal nerve. The cephalad extent of this exposure is somewhat limited by the ring of C1 due to the location of the surrounding neurovascular structures and their passage into the occiput, thus preventing an extension of the fusion mass to the occiput.[108] It is then possible to palpate the transverse process of C1 and C2 allowing dissection medially between the alar and prevertebral fasciae.[108]

Lateral Retropharyngeal Approach

A variation of the anterolateral retropharyngeal approach is a bilateral exposure of the lateral masses of C1 and C2 through a lateral approach described by Barbour,[18,56,133,167,184] in patients without short stocky necks or platybasia, making internal fixation technically difficult.[133] This approach is similar to that of Whitesides and McDonald[207] except that the route of dissection is either through or posterior to the sternocleidomastoid muscle with retraction of this muscle anteriorly, along with the carotid sheath to access the lateral masses of C1 and C2. Bilateral incisions are made, starting at the tip of the mastoid apophysis and coursing along the anterior border of the sternocleidomastoid muscle. Once at the level of the C1 transverse apophysis 1 cm below the mastoid, all soft tissues are cleared anteriorly off the C1–C2 transverse processes and lateral masses allowing the C1–C2 facet joint to be opened in preparation for bone grafting. The intertransverse muscle is preserved in order to protect the underlying vertebral vessels. It is now possible to place transarticular screws across the C1–C2 articular facets with the starting point of screw insertion being the anterior base of the C1 transverse process. Screw orientation is directed lateral to medial 25° obliquely inferior from the horizontal in the coronal plane and 10° posteriorly, with the drill directed in line with the mastoid process and the C1 transverse process starting point.[28] The average screw length is approximately 25–35 mm. Other means of fixation through this exposure include use of a staple or anterior plate across the anterior C1–C2 articular process.

Transoral Approach

The transoral route is a straightforward and relatively avascular approach, but it has been condemned in the past for its high incidence of postoperative infectious complications, reported in some series as high as 50%.[126,193] The incidence of perioperative morbidity, particularly infection, has reportedly decreased in contemporary series as a result of more meticulous handling of soft tissues, use of an operative microscope, broad-spectrum prophylactic antibiotics,[16] more effective retraction, and intraoperative neurophysiologic monitoring.[188] This approach allows immediate and adequate access to the anterior bony elements of the upper cervical spine, especially for odontoid resection, but as a result of its confining borders, such as the temporomandibular joint and depth of the wound, bony fusion with adequate stability is difficult.[135,193] The transoral approach was first described by Kanavel in 1919[110] with a series of patients subsequently reported by Fang and Ong in 1962.[67] This approach, with various modifications, allows access to all upper cervical midline structures including the tip of the clivus, anterior arch of C1, atlantoaxial joint, odontoid process, and upper cervical vertebral bodies down to the superior end-plate of C4.[16,67,138] After routine tracheotomy and packing of the hypopharynx, the soft palate is retracted and sewn to its junction with the hard palate or tied with 0/0 silk to two red rubber catheters placed through the nostrils to allow its retraction into the upper nasopharynx. The need for tracheotomy may be deferred with a special

McGarver three-ring retractor, or variant thereof,[16,138] which parts the lips and gums widely and depresses the tongue and endotracheal tube caudally for adequate visualization.[188] It is now possible to palpate the anterior tubercle of the atlas through the pharynx. The incision may be longitudinal over the C1 anterior arch measuring approximately 5 cm long. Dissection is taken sequentially through the pharyngeal mucosa, pharyngeal constrictor muscles, buccopharyngeal fascia, retropharyngeal space, prevertebral fascia, and prevertebral space down to the anterior longitudinal ligament, allowing access to the anterior bony elements of the upper cervical spine.[124] Stripping may be performed laterally as far as 14 mm from the midline before risk of injury to the vertebral vessels is encountered.[16,67]

Early reports of the use of the transoral route for surgical treatment of the upper cervical spine revealed marked morbidity primarily as a result of infection that is usually related to the addition of bone grafting through this approach. Fang and Ong[67] reported on five patients with atlantoaxial dislocation who were reduced successfully with this approach; three subsequently developed a postoperative infection with one dying secondary to damage to the vertebral vessels. Sonntag et al[188] used the transoral approach on 27 extradural procedures with only one postoperative complication. Ashraf, Moskovich, and Crockard[16,138] reported the use of the transoral approach in over 133 patients with only four pharyngeal wound breakdowns,[138] none requiring resuturing. Menezes[130] reported the use of this approach in 72 patients with rheumatoid arthritis and found it to be safe and effective, even in the debilitated elderly patient population, but noted difficulties attempting bone grafting with this method because of the potential of graft resorption and infection.

Other variations of the transoral approach for more extensive anterior bony decompression, i.e. clivus to C6, include the transmandibular tongue-splitting approach[178,193] or the transmandibular swing approach, allowing more inferior extension of the operative field. These approaches have reported low incidence of infection, probably due to decrease in tissue tension through greater exposure, although others have not found this to be the case.[94,133]

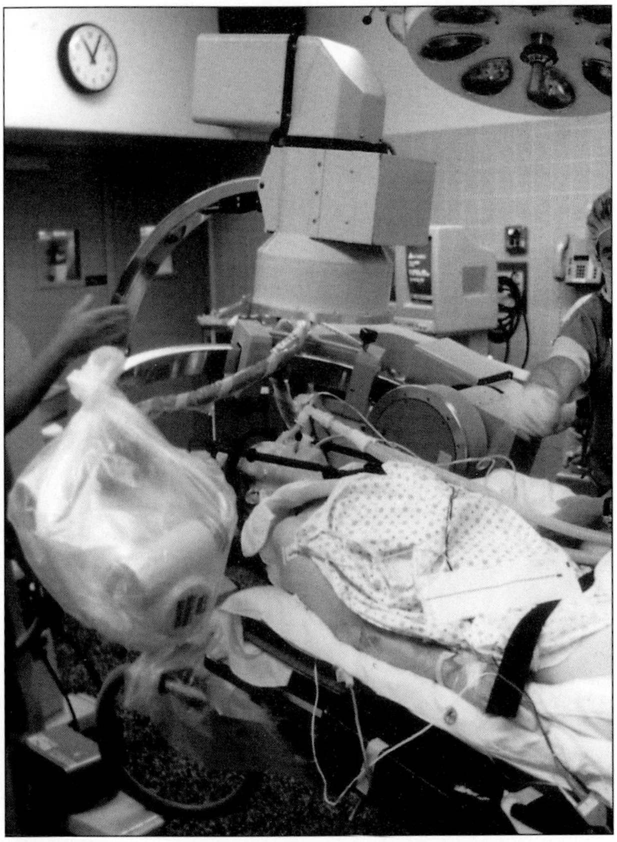

Figure 11.21
An example of biplanar fluoroscopic imaging necessary for safe and accurate anterior screw fixation of the odontoid.

Anterior Screw Fixation of the Dens

Screw fixation of the dens from the anterior approach has evolved into a favored procedure in both the European and Japanese orthopaedic and neurosurgical circles with slow, but increasing, acceptance in the USA. This method offers rigid internal fixation, preserves axial rotation at the C1–C2 facet articulation,[45] restores anatomy, and avoids potential complications or failures of autograft or allograft bone grafting procedures.[3,20,24,29,45,123,133,143] The procedure, first described by Bohler in 1975,[24] uses the standard Smith and Robinson[186] anterior approach to the midcervical spine with the patient supine and nasally intubated, allowing access to the anterior inferior endplate of C2. The approach may be performed on the right side with the head rotated slightly to the left. The optimum fracture for this procedure is a reduced acute type II or high type III odontoid fracture in a neurally intact patient,[25,133,137,167] with a non-prominent thoracic rib cage and an associated C1 fracture or other defect limiting posterior fusion. Some authors have advocated the procedure in displaced fractures that cannot be reduced by closed means, with reduction being performed at the time of surgery, before guide wire placement.[85,133] To ensure adequate visualization, biplanar imaging is necessary during guide wire placement in preparation for two 3.5 mm lag or cortical screws (Fig. 11.21). Knoringer[112] has reported the use of a screw with a variably threaded pitch allowing compression on insertion similar to the Herbert

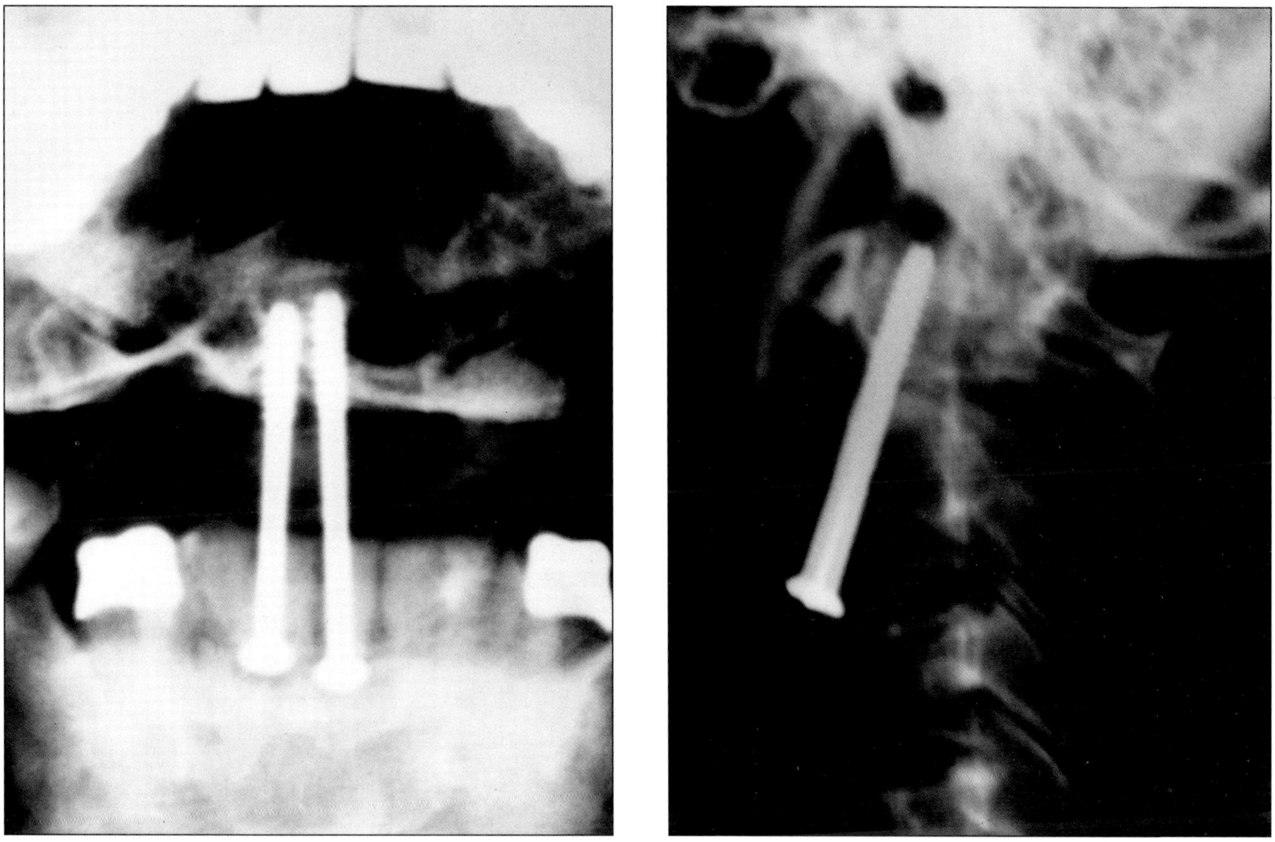

a b

Figure 11.22
(a) Anteroposterior and (b) lateral plain radiographs of an anterior screw fixation of a type II dens fracture. (Courtesy of S Garfin, MD)

screw used in the upper extremity. It is important to have accurate preoperative transaxial computed tomography measurements to determine the diameter of the odontoid waist which is usually found to be about 8 mm.[25] The starting point for guide wire placement is the anteroinferior border of the C2 end-plate just lateral to the midline to allow placement of two 3.5 mm screws. For ease of guide wire insertion, the point of wire insertion may be prepared by removing a portion of the C2–C3 anterior disc space or trimming the anterosuperior border of the C3 vertebra.[112,133] Under biplanar visualization, both guide wires are inserted through the anterior portion of the C2 body and dens toward the posterosuperior tip of the odontoid with cortical tip penetration.[25,167,208] The screw lengths are usually around 32–40 mm and one may prefer to use washers for better screw head stability (Fig. 11.22).[133]

CONCLUSION

In managing acute spinal trauma, a high degree of suspicion for upper cervical spine disorders must be afforded to all patients who present after injury with significant suboccipital pain, limited range of cervical motion, and no evidence of neurologic deficit. As a result of the often high incidence of associated spinal injuries with upper cervical spine fractures, the entire spinal column should be radiologically investigated using all available imaging modalities necessary to make an accurate diagnosis. Knowledge of the anatomy, biomechanics, and clinical significance of the various classification systems for each injury pattern will assist the treating physician in determining an appropriate level of aggressiveness in the management of these often difficult complex injuries.

REFERENCES

1 Ackerson TT, Patzakis MJ, Moore TM, Korze T, Harvey JR Jr. Fractures of the odontoid: A ten-year retrospective study. *Contemp Orthop* **4**: 54–67, 1982.
2 Aebi M, Etter C, Coscia M. Fractures of the odontoid process: Treatment with anterior screw fixation. *Spine* **14**: 1065–1070, 1989.
3 Aebi M, Mohler J, Zaech GA, Morscher E. Indications, surgical techniques, and results of 100 surgically treated fractures and fracture dislocations of the cervical spine. *Clin Orthop* **203**: 244–257, 1986.
4 Alker GJ Jr, Oh YS, Leslie EV. Post mortem radiology of head and neck injuries in fatal traffic accidents. *J Neuroradiol* **114**: 611–616, 1975.
5 Alker GJ Jr, Oh YS, Leslie EV. High cervical spine and craniocervical junction injuries in fatal traffic accidents. *Orthop Clin North Am* **9**: 1003–1010, 1978;
6 Althoff B. Fracture of the odontoid process. An experimental and clinical study. *Acta Orthop Scand Suppl* **177**: 1–95, 1979.
7 Althoff B, Goldie IF. The arterial supply of the odontoid process of the axis. *Acta Orthop Scand* **48**: 622–629, 1977.
8 Altongy JF, Fielding JW. Combined atlanto-axial and occipito-atlantal rotatory subluxation. A case report. *J Bone Joint Surg [Am]* **72**: 923–926, 1990.
9 Amyes EW, Anderson FM. Fracture of the odontoid process. *Arch Surg* **72**: 377–393, 1956.
10 An HS. Posterior instrumentation of the cervical spine. In An HS, Cotler JM (eds) *Spinal Instrumentation*, 37–47. Baltimore: Williams & Wilkins, 1992.
11 Anderson LD, Clark CR. Fractures of the odontoid process of the axis. In Sherk HH, Dunn EJ, Eismont FJ, et al. (eds), *The Cervical Spine*, 2nd ed., 325–343. Cervical Spine Research Society. Philadelphia: J.B. Lippincott, 1989.
12 Anderson LD, D'Alonzo RT. Fractures of the odontoid process of the axis. *J Bone Joint Surg [Am]* **56**: 1663–1674, 1974.
13 Anderson PA, Montesano PX. Morphology and treatment of occipital condyle fractures. *Spine* **13**: 731–736, 1988.
14 Aprin H, Hart R. Stabilization of atlantoaxial instability. *Orthopaedics* **11**: 1687–1693, 1988.
15 Apuzzo, MLK, Heiden JS, Weis MH, Ackerson TT, Harvey JP, Kurze T. Acute fractures of the odontoid process. *J Neurosurg* **48**: 85–91, 1978.
16 Ashraf J, Crockard HA. Transoral fusion in high cervical fractures. *J Bone Joint Surg [Br]* **72**: 76–79, 1990.
17 Bailey RW, Badgley CE. Stabilization of the cervical spine by anterior fusion. *J Bone Joint Surg [Am]* **42**: 565–594, 1960.
18 Barbour JR. Screw fixation in fracture of the odontoid process. *Southern Australian Clinic* **5**: 20–24, 1971.
19 Barros TEP, Fielding JW. Traumatic spondylolisthesis of the axis with unusual distraction. *J Bone Joint Surg [Am]* **72**: 124–125, 1990.
20 Bell C. Surgical observations. *Middlesex Hosp J* **4:** 469, 1817.
21 Bell W, Meyer P. Non-halo/non-surgical management of C1–C2 fractures. *Orthop Trans* **7**: 481, 1983.
22 Blockley NJ, Purser DW. Fractures of the odontoid process of the axis. *J Bone Joint Surg [Br]* **38**: 794–816, 1956.
23 Bohler J. An approach to nonunion of fractures. *Surg Ann* **14**: 299–315, 1982.
24 Bohler J. Anterior stabilization for acute fractures and nonunions of the dens. *J Bone Joint Surg [Am]* **64**: 18–28, 1982.
25 Bohler J. Lecture. Fifty-second American Orthopaedics Course (Spine), Davos, Switzerland, 1990.
26 Bohlman HH. Acute fractures and dislocations of the cervical spine. An analysis of three hundred hospitalized patients and review of the literature. *J Bone Joint Surg [Am]* **61**: 1119–1142, 1979.
27 Bolender N, Cromwell LD, Wendling L. Fracture of the occipital condyle. *Orthop Clin North Am* **131**: 729–731, 1978.
28 Bolester MJ, Bohlman HH. Late complications of cervical fractures and dislocations and their management. In Frymoyer JW (ed) *The Adult Spine*, 1107–1126. New York: Raven Press, 1991.
29 Borne EM, Bedow GL, Pinaudeau M, Cristino G, Hussein A. Odontoid process fracture osteosynthesis with a direct screw fixation technique in nine consecutive cases. *J Neurosurg* **68**: 223–226, 1988.
30 Brashear HR, Venters GC, Preston ET. Fractures of the neural arch of the axis. *J Bone Joint Surg [Am]* **57**: 879–887, 1975.
31 Brooks AL, Jenkins EB. Atlanto-axial arthrodesis by the wedge compression method. *J Bone Joint Surg [Am]* **60**: 279–284, 1978.
32 Bucholz RW. Unstable hangman's fractures. *Clin Orthop* **154**: 119–124, 1981.
33 Bucholz RW, Burkhead WZ. The pathologic anatomy of fatal atlanto-occipital dislocations. *J Bone Joint Surg [Am]* **61**: 248–250, 1979.
34 Bunders DA, Rechtine GR, Bohlman HH. Upper cervical spine injuries. *Orthop Rev* **13**: 23–32, 1984.
35 Burke JT, Harris JH. Acute injuries of the axis vertebrae. *Skelet Radiol* **18**: 335–346, 1989.
36 Callahan RA, Lockwood R, Green B. Modified Brooks fusion for an os odontoideum associated with an incomplete posterior arch of the atlas. A case report. *Spine* **8**: 107–108, 1983.
37 Chamberlain WE. Basilar impression (platybasia). A bizarre developmental anomaly of the occipital bone and upper cervical spine with striking and misleading neurologic manifestations. *Yale J Biol Med* **11**: 487–496, 1939.
38 Chan BPK, Morwessel RM, Leung KYK. Treatment of odontoid fractures with halo cast immobilization. *Orthop Trans* **5**: 118–119, 1981.
39 Clark CR. Dens fractures. *Semin Spine Surg* **3**: 39–46, 1991.
40 Clark CR, Kathol MH, Walsh T, El-Khoury GY. Atlantoaxial rotatory fixation with compensatory counter occipito-atlantal subluxation. A case report. *Spine* **11**: 1048–1050, 1986.
41 Clark CR, White AA. Fractures of the dens: A multicenter study. *J Bone Joint Surg [Am]* **67**: 1340–1348, 1985.
42 Cloward RB. The anterior approach for rupture cervical disc. *J Neurosurg* **15**: 602–614, 1958.
43 Cooper PR, Maravilla KR, Sklar FH, Moody SF, Clark WK. Halo immobilization of cervical spine fractures. Indications and results. *J Neurosurg* **50**: 603–610, 1979.
44 Cornish BL. Traumatic spondylolisthesis of the axis. *J Bone Joint Surg [Br]* **50**: 31–44, 1968.
45 Cotler JM, Simpson JM, An HS. Principles, indications, and complications of spinal instrumentation: A summary chapter. In An HS, Cotler JM (eds) *Spinal Instrumentation*, 435–456. Baltimore: Williams & Wilkins, 1991.

46 Craft DV, Cotler JM, Bauerle WB. A rational approach to the management of Type II and Type III odontoid fractures. Presented at the American Academy of Orthopedic Surgeons Annual Meeting, Washington, DC, February 1991.

47 Craig JB, Hodgson BF. Superior facet fractures of the axis vertebra. *Spine* **16**: 875–857, 1991.

48 Crockard HA. Anterior approaches to lesions of the upper cervical spine. *Clin Neurosurg* **34**: 389–416, 1988.

49 Cybulski GR, Stone JL, Crowell RM, Rifai MH, Gandhi Y, Glick R. Use of Halifax interlaminar clamps for posterior C1–C2 arthrodesis. *Neurosurgery* **22**: 429–431, 1988.

50 Day GL, Jacoby CG, Dolan KD. Basilar invagination resulting from untreated Jefferson's fracture. *AJR Am J Roentgenol* **133**: 529–531, 1979.

51 DeAndrade JR, MacNab I. Anterior occipital cervical fusion using an extrapharyngeal exposure. *J Bone Joint Surg [Am]* **51**: 1621–1626, 1969.

52 Desai SS, Coumas JM, Danylevich A, Hayes E, Dunn EJ. Fracture of the occipital condyle: Case report and review of the literature. *J Trauma* **30**: 240–241, 1990.

53 Dickman CA, Hadley MN, Browner C, Sonntag VKH. Neurosurgical management of acute atlas-axis combination fractures. *J Neurosurg* **70**: 45–49, 1989.

54 Donovan MM. Efficacy of rigid fixation of fractures of the odontoid process and retrospective analysis of fifty-four cases. *Orthop Trans* **3**: 309, 1979.

55 Dunn ME, Seljeskog EL. Experience in the management of odontoid process injuries. An analysis of 128 cases. *Neurosurgery* **18**: 306–310, 1986.

56 DuToit G. Lateral atlanto-axial arthrodesis: A screw fixation technique. *S Afr J Surg* **14**: 9–12, 1976.

57 Dvorak J, Panjabi MM. Functional anatomy of the allyl ligaments. *Spine* **12**: 183–189, 1987.

58 Dvorak J, Schneider E, Sladinger P, Rahn B. Biomechanics of the craniocervical region. The alar and transverse ligaments. *J Orthop Res* **6**: 452–461, 1988.

59 Effendi B, Roy D, Cornish B, Dussault RG, Laurin CA. Fracture of the ring of the axis. A classification based on the analysis of 131 cases. *J Bone Joint Surg [Br]* **63**: 319–327, 1981.

60 Eismont FJ, Bohlman HH. Posterior atlanto-occipital dislocation with fractures of the atlas and odontoid process. Report of a case with survival. *J Bone Joint Surg [Am]* **60**: 1397–1399, 1978.

61 Eismont FJ, Bohlman HH. Posterior methylmethacrylate fixation for cervical trauma. *Spine* **6**: 347–353, 1981.

62 Ekong CEU, Schwartz ML, Tator CH, Rowed DW. Odontoid fracture: Management with early mobilization using the halo device. *Neurosurgery* **9**: 631–637, 1981.

63 El-Khoury GY, Kathol MH. Radiographic evaluation of cervical spine trauma. *Semin Spine Surg* **3**: 3–23, 1991.

64 Esses SI, Bednar DA. Screw fixation of odontoid fractures and nonunions. *Spine* **16S**: 483–485, 1991.

65 Etter C, Coscia M, Jaberg H, Aebi M. Direct anterior fixation of dens fractures with a cannulated screw system. *Spine* **16S**: 25–32, 1991.

66 Evarts CM. Traumatic occipito-atlantal dislocation. Report of a case with survival. *J Bone Joint Surg [Am]* **52**: 1653–1660, 1970.

67 Fang HSY, Ong GB. Direct anterior approach to the upper cervical spine. *J Bone Joint Surg [Am]* **44**: 1588–1604, 1962.

68 Fardon DF, Fielding JW. Defects of the pedicle and spondylolisthesis of the second cervical spine. *J Bone Joint Surg [Br]* **63**: 526–528, 1981.

69 Fielding JW, Cochran G, Lawsing JF III, Hohl M. Tears of the transverse ligament of the atlas. A clinical and biomechanical study. *J Bone Joint Surg [Am]* **56**: 1683–1691, 1974.

70 Fielding JW, Francis WR, Hawkins RJ, Hensinger RN. Atlantoaxial rotatory deformity. *Semin Spine Surg* **3**: 33–38, 1991.

71 Fielding JW, Francis WR, Hawkins RJ, Pepin J, Hensinger RN. Traumatic spondylolisthesis of the axis. *Clin Orthop* **239**: 47–52, 1989.

72 Fielding JW, Hawkins RJ. Roentgenographic diagnosis of the injured neck. In American Academy of Orthopaedic Surgeons *Instructional Course Lectures*, Vol. 25, 149–169. Chicago: CV. Mosby, 1976.

73 Fielding JW, Hawkins RJ. Atlanto-axial rotatory fixation. *J Bone Joint Surg [Am]* **59**: 37–44, 1977.

74 Fielding JW, Hawkins RJ, Ratzan SA. Spine fusion for atlanto-axial instability. *J Bone Joint Surg [Am]* 58: 400–407, 1976.

75 Fielding JW, Hensinger RN, Hawkins RJ. Os odontoideum. *J Bone Joint Surg [Am]* **62**: 376–383, 1980.

76 Fielding JW, Stillwee WT, Spyropoulos EC. Use of computed tomography for the diagnosis of atlanto-axial rotatory fixation. *J Bone Joint Surg [Am]* **60**: 1102–1104, 1978.

77 Fowler JL, Sandhu A, Fraser RD. A review of fractures of the atlas vertebra. *J Spinal Disord* **3**: 19–24, 1990.

78 Francis WR, Fielding JW, Hawkins RJ, Pepin J, Hensinger RN. Traumatic spondylolisthesis of the axis. *J Bone Joint Surg [Br]* **63**: 313–318, 1981.

79 Fujii E, Kabayashi K, Hirabayashi K. Treatment in fractures of the odontoid process. *Spine* **13**: 604–609, 1988.

80 Gabrielsen TO, Maxwell JA. Traumatic atlanto-occipital dislocation. *AJR Am J Roentgenol* **97**: 624–629, 1966.

81 Gallie WE. Fractures and dislocations of the cervical spine. *Am J Surg* **46**: 495–501, 1939.

82 Garber JN. Abnormalities of the atlas and axis vertebrae: Congenital and traumatic. *J Bone Joint Surg [Am]* **46**: 1782–1791, 1964.

83 Garfin SR, Rothman RH. Traumatic spondylolisthesis of the axis (hangman's fracture). In Sherk HH, Dunn EJ, Eismont FJ, et al (eds) *The Cervical Spine*, 2nd ed, 344–354. Cervical Spine Research Society. Philadelphia: JB Lippincott, 1989.

84 Gehweiler JA, Osborne RL Jr, Becker RF. *The Radiology of Vertebral Trauma*. Philadelphia: WB Saunders, 1980.

85 Geisler FH, Cheng C, Poka A, Brumback RJ. Anterior screw fixation of posteriorly displaced Type II odontoid fractures. *Neurosurgery* **25**: 30–38, 1989.

86 Gerhart TN, White AA III. An impacted dens fracture in an elderly woman. *Clin Orthop* **167**: 173–175, 1982.

87 Goldstein SJ, Woodring JA, Young AB. Occipital condyle fracture associated with cervical spine injury. *Surg Neurol* **17**: 350–352, 1982.

88 Grantham SA, Dick HM, Thompson RC, Stinchfield FE. Occipitocervical arthrodesis: Indications, technique, and results. *Clin Orthop* **65**: 118–129, 1969.

89 Grantham SA, Lipson SJ. Rheumatoid arthritis of the cervical spine. In Sherk HH, Dunn EJ, Eismont FJ, et al. (eds) *The Cervical Spine*, 2nd ed, 564–572. Cervical Spine Research Society. Philadelphia: JB Lippincott, 1989.

90 Griswold DM, Albright JA, Schiffman E, Johnson R, Southwick WO. Atlanto-axial fusion for instability. *J Bone Joint Surg [Am]* **60**: 285–292, 1978.
91 Hadley MN, Browner CM, Liv SS, Sonntag VKH. New subtype of acute odontoid fractures (Type IIA). *Neurosurgery* **22**: 67–71, 1988.
92 Hadley MN, Dickman CA, Browner CM, Sonntag VKH. Acute traumatic atlas fractures: Management and long-term outcome. *Neurosurgery* **23**: 31–35, 1988.
93 Hadley MN, Dickman CA, Browner CM, Sonntag VKH. Acute axis fractures: A review of 229 cases. *J Neurosurg* **71**: 642–647, 1989.
94 Hall JE, Denis F, Murray J. Exposure of the upper cervical spine for spinal decompression by a mandible and tongue splitting approach. *J Bone Joint Surg [Am]* **59**: 121–123, 1977.
95 Harding-Smith J, MacIntosh PK, Sherbon KJ. Fracture of the occipital condyle. *J Bone Joint Surg [Am]* **63**: 1170–1171, 1981.
96 Harris JH, Edeiken-Monroe B (eds). *The Radiology of Acute Cervical Spine Trauma*, 2nd ed. Baltimore: Williams & Wilkins, 1987.
97 Haughton S. On hanging, considered from a mechanical and physiological point of view. *London, Edinburgh, and Dublin Philosophical Magazine and Journal of Science* **92**: 23–34, 1866.
98 Henry AK. *Extensile Exposure*, 2nd ed, 53–80. Edinburgh: E. and S. Livingstone, 1957.
99 Hensinger RN. Congenital anomalies of the cervical spine. In Rothman RH, Simeone FA, et al. (eds) *The Spine*, 3rd ed, 261–314. Philadelphia: WB Saunders, 1992.
100 Hinchey JJ, Bickel WH. Fractures of the atlas. Review and presentation of data on eight cases. *Ann Surg* **121**: 826–832, 1945.
101 Hohl M, Baker HR. The atlanto-axial joint radiographic and anatomical study of normal and abnormal motion. *J Bone Joint Surg [Am]* **46**: 1739–1752, 1964.
102 Holness RO, Heustis WS, Howes WJ, Langille RA. Posterior stabilization with an interlaminar clamp in cervical injuries: Technical note and review of the long term experience with the method. *Neurosurgery* **14**: 318–322, 1984.
103 Husby J, Sorensen KH. Fracture of the odontoid process of the axis. *Acta Orthop Scand* **45**: 182–192, 1974.
104 Itoh T, Tsuji H, Katoh Y, Yonezawat T, Kitagawa H. Occipitocervical fusion reinforced by Luque's segmental spinal instrumentation for rheumatoid diseases. *Spine* **13**: 1234–1238, 1988.
105 Jefferson E. Fracture of the atlas vertebra. Report of four cases and a review of those previously recorded. *Br J Surg* **7**: 407–422, 1920.
106 Jofe MH, White AA, Panjabi MM. Clinically relevant kinematics of the cervical spine. In Sherk HH, Dunn EJ, Eismont FJ, et al. (eds) *The Cervical Spine*, 2nd ed, 57–69. Cervical Spine Research Society. Philadelphia: JB Lippincott, 1989.
107 Johnson RM, Hart DL, Simmon EF, Romsby ER, Southwick WO. Cervical orthosis: A study comparing the effectiveness in restricting cervical motion in normal subjects. *J Bone Joint Surg [Am]* **59**: 332–339, 1977.
108 Johnson RM, Murphy MJ, Southwick WO. Surgical approaches to the spine. In Rothman RH, Simeone FA, et al. (eds) *The Spine*, 3rd ed, 1634–1696. Philadelphia: WB Saunders, 1992.
109 Kahanavitz N, Mehringer MC, Johanson PH. Intracranial entrapment of the atlas complicating an untreated fracture of the posterior arch of the atlas. A case report. *J Bone Joint Surg [Am]* **63**: 831, 1981.
110 Kanavel AB. Bullet located between the atlas and the base of the skull: Technique for removal through the mouth. *Surg Clin* **1**: 361–6, 1919.
111 Keterson L, Benzel E, Orrison W, Coleman J. Evaluation and treatment of atlas burst fractures (Jefferson fractures). *J Neurosurg* **75**: 213–220, 1991.
112 Knoringer P. Double threaded compression screws in osteosyntheses of acute fractures of the odontoid process. In Voth D, Glees O (eds) *Diseases of the Cranio-Cervical Junction*, 217. Berlin–New York: De Gruyter, 1987.
113 Koch RA, Nickel VL. The halo vest. An evaluation of motion and forces across the neck. *Spine* **3**: 103–7, 1978.
114 Landells CD, Peteghem PKV. Fractures of the atlas: Classification, treatment and morbidity. *Spine* **13**: 450–452, 1987.
115 Lesoin F, Autricque A, Jomin M. Use of C-D instrumentation for cranio-cervical junction osteosyntheses. *Proceedings of the Sixth International Congress on C-D Instrumentation*, 249. Montpellier, France: Sauramps Medical, 1989.
116 Levine AM, Edwards CC. The management of traumatic spondylolisthesis of the axis. *J Bone Joint Surg [Am]* **67**: 217–226, 1985.
117 Levine AM, Edwards CC. Treatment of injuries in the C1–C2 complex. *Orthop Clin North Am* **17**: 31–44, 1986.
118 Levine AM, Edwards CC. Traumatic lesions of occipito-atlanto-axial complex. *Clin Orthop* **239**: 53–68, 1989.
119 Levine AM, Edwards CC. Fractures of the atlas. *J Bone Joint Surg [Am]* **73**: 680–691, 1991.
120 Levine AM, Rhyne AL. Traumatic spondylolisthesis of the axis. *Semin Spine Surg* **3**: 47–60, 1991.
121 Lewallen RP, Morrey BF, Cabanela ME. Respiratory arrest following displaced odontoid fractures. *Clin Orthop* **188**: 187–190, 1984.
122 Libson SJ. Fractures of the atlas associated with fractures of the odontoid process and transverse ligament ruptures. *J Bone Joint Surg [Am]* **59**: 940–943, 1977.
123 Magerl F, Seeman PS. Stable posterior fusion of the atlas and axis by transarticular screw fixation. In Kehr P, Weidner A (eds) *The Cervical Spine*, 322–7. New York, Vienna: Springer-Verlag, 1987.
124 Mariani PJ. Occipital condyle fracture presenting as retropharyngeal hematoma. *Ann Emerg Med* **19**: 1447–9, 1990.
125 McAfee PC. Cervical spine trauma. In Frymoyer JW (ed) *The Adult Spine: Principles and Practice*, 1063–1106. New York: Raven Press, 1991.
126 McAfee PC, Bohlman HH, Riley LH, Robinson RA, Southwick WO, Nachlas NE. The anterior retropharyngeal approach to the upper part of the cervical spine. *J Bone Joint Surg [Am]* **69**: 1371–1383, 1987.
127 McAfee PC, Cassidy JR, Davis RF, North RB, Ducker TB. Fusion of the occiput to the upper cervical spine. A review of 37 cases. *Spine* **16S**: 490–494, 1991.
128 McGraw RW, Rusch RM. Atlanto-axial arthrodesis. *J Bone Joint Surg [Br]* **55**: 482–488, 1973.
129 McGregor M. The significance of certain measurements of the skull in the diagnosis of basilar impression. *Br J Radiol* **21**: 171–181, 1948.

130 Menezes AH, VanGilder JC. Trans-oral retropharyngeal approach to the anterior craniocervical junction. Ten-year experience with 72 patients. *J Neurosurg* **69**: 895–903, 1988.
131 Meyer PR Jr, Cotler HB. Fusion techniques for traumatic injuries. In Cotler JM, Cotler HB (eds) *Spine Fusion: Science and Techniques*, 189–246. New York: Springer-Verlag, 1990.
132 Meyer PR Jr, Heim S. Surgical stabilization of the cervical spine. In Meyer PR Jr (ed) *Surgery of Spine Trauma*. New York: Churchill Livingstone, 397–523, 1989.
133 Meyer PR Jr, Rusin JJ, Haak MH. Anterior instrumentation of the cervical spine. In An HS, Cotler JM (eds) *Spinal Instrumentation*, 61–6. Baltimore: Williams & Wilkins, 1992.
134 Miller MD, Gehweiler JA, Martinez S, Charlton OP., Daffner RH. Significant new observations on cervical spine trauma. *AJR Am J Roentgenol* **130**: 659–663, 1978.
135 Miz G. Cervical spine instability and biomechanics of treatment. In Errico TJ, Bauer RD, Waugh T. (eds) *Spinal Trauma*, 2nd ed, 123–140. Philadelphia: JB Lippincott, 1991.
136 Montane I, Eismont FJ, Green BA. Traumatic occipitoatlantal dislocation. *Spine* **16**: 112–116, 1991.
137 Montesano PX, Anderson PA, Schlehr F, Thalgott JS, Lowrey G. Odontoid fractures treated by anterior odontoid screw fixation. *Spine* **16S**: 33–37, 1991.
138 Moskovich R, Crockard HA. Post-traumatic atlanto-axial subluxation and myelopathy. Efficacy of anterior decompression. *Spine* **15**: 442–447, 1990.
139 Mouradian WH, Fietti VG Jr, Cochran GVB, Fielding JW, Young J. Fractures of the odontoid. A laboratory and clinical study of mechanism. *Orthop Clin North Am* **9**: 985–1001, 1978.
140 Muller ME, Allgower M, Schneider R, Willenegger H. (eds) *Manual of Internal Fixation*, 627–682. Berlin, New York: Springer-Verlag, 1990.
141 Murphy MJ, Southwick WO. Surgical approaches and techniques. In Sherk HH, Dunn EJ, Eismont FJ, et al (eds) *The Cervical Spine*, 2nd ed, 775–791. Cervical Spine Research Society. Philadelphia: JB Lippincott, 1989.
142 Murphy MJ, Wu JC, Southwick WO. Complications of halo fixation. *Orthop Trans* **3**: 126, 1979.
143 Nakanishi T, Sasaki T, Tokita N, Hirabayashi K. Internal fixation of the odontoid fracture. *Orthop Trans* **6**: 176, 1982.
144 Newman P, Sweetnam R. Occipitocervical fusion. An operative technique and its indications. *J Bone Joint Surg [Br]* **51**: 423–431, 1969.
145 Nordt JC, Stauffer ES. Sequelae of atlantoaxial subluxation in two patients with Down syndrome. *Spine* **6**: 437–440, 1981.
146 Norrell HA. Fractures and dislocations of the spine. In Rothman RH, Simeone FA, et al. (eds) *The Spine*, 1st ed, 529–66. Philadephia: WB Saunders, 1975.
147 Oda T, Panjabi MM, Crisco JJ, Oxland TR, Katz L, Nolte LP. Experimental study of atlas injuries II. Relevance to clinical diagnosis and treatment. *Spine* **16S**: 466–473, 1991.
148 Osgood RB, Lund CC. Fractures of the odontoid process. *New Engl J Med* **198**: 61–72, 1928.
149 Panjabi MM, Oda T, Crisco JJ, Oxland TR, Katz L, Nolte LP. Experimental study of atlas injuries I. Biomechanical analysis of their mechanism and fracture patterns. *Spine* **16S**: 460–465, 1991.
150 Paradis GR, Jones JM. Post traumatic atlantoaxial instability: The fate of the odontoid process fracture in 46 cases. *J Trauma* **13**: 359–366, 1973.
151 Parke WW. The vascular relations of the upper cervical vertebrae. *Orthop Clin North Am* **9**: 879–889, 1978.
152 Parke WW, Rothman RH, Brown MD. The pharyngovertebral veins: An anatomical rationale for Grisel's syndrome. *J Bone Joint Surg [Am]* **60**: 568–574, 1984.
153 Penning L. *Functional Pathology of the Cervical Spine*. Baltimore: Williams & Wilkins, 1968.
154 Penning L. Normal movements of the cervical spine. *AJR Am J Roentgenol* **130**: 317–326, 1978.
155 Pepin JW, Bourne RB, Hawkins RJ. Odontoid fractures with special reference to the elderly patient. *Clin Orthop* **193**: 178–183, 1985.
156 Pierce DS, Barr JS. Use of the halo in cervical spine problems. *Orthop Trans* **3**: 125, 1979.
157 Pierce DS, Barr JS. Fractures and dislocations at the base of the skull and upper cervical spine. In Sherk HH, Dunn EJ, Eismont FJ, et al. (eds) *The Cervical Spine*, 2nd ed, 312–24. Cervical Spine Research Society. Philadelphia: JB Lippincott, 1989.
158 Powers B. Traumatic anterior-occipital dislocations. *Neurosurgery* **4**: 12–17, 1979.
159 Price AE. Unique aspects of pediatric spine injuries. In Errico TJ, Bauer RD, Waugh T (eds) *Spinal Trauma*, 2nd ed, 581–625. Philadelphia: JB Lippincott, 1991.
160 Ranawat CS, O'Leary P, Pellicci P, Tsairis P, Marchisello P, Dorr L. Cervical fusion in rheumatoid arthritis. *J Bone Joint Surg [Am]* 1979; **61**: 1003–10.
161 Ransford AO, Crockard HA, Pozo JL et al. Craniocervical instability treated by contoured loop fixation. *J Bone Joint Surg [Am]* 68: 193–197, 1986.
162 Redlund-Johnell I, Patterson H. Radiographic measurements of the cranio-vertebral region. *Acta Radiol Diag* **25**: 23–28, 1984
163 Riley LH Jr. Surgical approaches to the anterior structures of the cervical spine. *Clin Orthop* **91**: 16–20, 1973.
164 Roberts A, Wickstrom J. Prognosis of odontoid fractures. *J Bone Joint Surg [Am]* **54**: 1353, 1972.
165 Robinson RA. Approaches to the cervical spine C1–T1. In Schmedek HH, Sweet WH (eds) *Operative Neurosurgical Techniques*. New York: Grune & Stratton, 1982.
166 Rogers WA. Fractures and dislocations of the cervical spine. An end result study. *J Bone Joint Surg [Am]* **39**: 341–376, 1957.
167 Roy-Camille R, Mazel C, Saillant G, Benazet JP. Rationale and techniques of internal fixation in trauma of the cervical spine. In Errico TJ, Bauer RD, Waugh T (eds) *Spinal Trauma*, 2nd ed, 163–191. Philadelphia: JB Lippincott, 1991.
168 Roy-Camille R, Saillant G, Berteaux D, Marie-Anne S. Early management of spinal injuries. In McKibbin B (ed) *Recent Advances in Orthopaedics*, 57. Edinburgh: Churchill Livingstone, 1979.
169 Ryan MD, Taylor TKF. Odontoid fractures, a rational approach to treatment. *J Bone Joint Surg [Br]* **64**: 416–21, 1982;
170 Sassard WR, Heinig CF, Pitts WR. Posterior atlanto-axial dislocation without fracture. Case report with successful conservative treatment. *J Bone Joint Surg [Am]* **56**: 625–8, 1974.
171 Schatzker J, Rorabeck CH, Waddell JP. Fractures of the dens (odontoid process). An analysis of thirty-seven cases. *J Bone Joint Surg [Br]* **53**: 392–405, 1971.

172 Schatzker J, Rorabeck CH, Waddell JP. Non-union of the odontoid process: An experimental investigation. *Clin Orthop* **108**: 127–37, 1975.
173 Schiff DCM, Parke WW. The arterial supply of the odontoid process. *J Bone Joint Surg [Am]* **55**: 1450–1456, 1973.
174 Schneider RC, Livingston KE, Cave AJE, Hamilton G. Hangman's fracture of the cervical spine. *J Neurosurg* **22**: 141–154, 1965.
175 Schwartz GA, Wigton RS. Fracture-dislocation in the region of the atlas and axis, with consideration of delayed neurologic manifestations and some roentgenographic features. *Radiology* **28**: 601–607, 1937.
176 Scott EW, Haid RW, Peace D. Type I fractures of the odontoid process: Implications for atlanto-occipital instability. *J Neurosurg* **72**: 488–492, 1990.
177 Segal LS, Grimm JO, Stauffer SE. Non-union of fractures of the atlas. *J Bone Joint Surg [Am]* **69**: 1423–1433, 1987.
178 Shah JP, Shaha AR. Transmandibular approach to the upper cervical spine. In Sundaresan N, Schmidek H, Schiller A, Rosenthal D (eds) *Tumors of the Spine: Diagnosis and Clinical Management*, 329–336. Philadephia: WB Saunders, 1990.
179 Sherk HH. Lesions of the atlas and axis. *Clin Orthop* **109**: 33–41, 1975.
180 Sherk HH. Fractures of the atlas and odontoid process. *Orthop Clin North Am* **9**: 973–983, 1978.
181 Sherk HH, Nicholson JT. Fracture of the atlas. *J Bone Joint Surg [Am]* **52**: 1017–1024, 1970.
182 Sherk HH, Snyder BJ. An exceptional case analysis of upper posterior neck fusion. *Orthop Trans* **3**: 125, 1979.
183 Simmons EH. Surgery of the spine in rheumatoid arthritis and ankylosing spondylitis. In Evarts CM (ed) *Surgery of the Musculoskeletal System*, Vol. 2, 85. New York: Churchill Livingstone, 1983.
184 Simmons EH, duToit G. Lateral atlanto-axial arthrodesis. *Orthop Clin North Am* **9**: 1101–1115, 1978.
185 Skold G. Fractures of the neural arch and odontoid process of the axis. A study of their causation. *Zeitschr Rechtsmed* **82**: 89–103, 1978.
186 Smith GW, Robinson RA. The treatment of certain cervical spine disorders by anterior removal of the intervertebral disc and interbody fusion. *J Bone Joint Surg [Am]* **40**: 607–624, 1958.
187 Smith MD, Phillips WA, Hensinger RN. Complications of fusions to the upper cervical spine. *Spine* **16**: 702–705, 1991.
188 Sonntag VKH, Hadley MN, Spetzler RF. The transoral–transclival approach to the upper cervical spine. In Sundaresan N, Schmidek H, Schiller A, Rosenthal D (eds) *Tumors of the Spine: Diagnosis and Clinical Management*, 319–329. Philadephia: WB Saunders, 1990.
189 Southwick WO. Current concept review: Management of fractures of the dens (odontoid process). *J Bone Joint Surg [Am]* **62**: 482–486, 1980.
190 Southwick WO, Robinson RA. Surgical approaches to the vertebral bodies in the cervical and lumbar regions. *J Bone Joint Surg [Am]* **39**: 631–644, 1957.
191 Spence KF, Decker S, Sell KW. Bursting atlantal fracture associated with rupture of the transverse ligament. *J Bone Joint Surg [Am]* **52**: 543–549, 1970.
192 Spencer JA, Yeakley JW, Kaufman HH. Fracture of the occipital condyle. *J Neurosurg* **15**: 101–103, 1984.
193 Stauffer ES. Direct transoral anterior approaches to the upper cervical spine. In Sherk HH, Dunn EJ, Eismont FJ et al. (eds) *The Cervical Spine*, 2nd ed, 805–822. Cervical Spine Research Society. Philadelphia: JB Lippincott, 1989.
194 Steel HH. Anatomical and mechanical considerations of the atlanto-axial articulations. *J Bone Joint Surg [Am]* **50**: 1481–1482, 1968.
195 Steib JP, Kehr P, Mitteau M. C1–C2 instrumentation with CD pediatric material. *Proceedings of the Sixth International Congress on C-D Instrumentation*, 245. Montpellier, France: Sauramps Medical, 1989.
196 Stewart, G. Horizontal fracture of the anterior arch of the atlas. *Radiology* **122**: 349–352, 1977.
197 Traynelis VC, Marano GD, Dunker RO, Kaufman HH. Traumatic atlanto-occipital dislocation. Case report. *J Neurosurg* **65**: 863–70, 1986.
198 VanGilder JC. *The Craniovertebral Junction and its Abnormalities*, 9–27. Mt Kisco, New York: Futura Publishing, 1987.
199 Verbiest H. A lateral approach to the cervical spine. Technique and indications. *J Neurosurg* **28**: 191–203, 1968.
200 Wackenheim A. *Roentgen Diagnosis of the Craniovertebral Region*. Berlin: Springer-Verlag, 1974.
201 Washington ER. Non-traumatic atlanto-occipital and atlanto-axial dislocation. *J Bone Joint Surg [Am]* **41**: 341–344, 1959.
202 Weidner A. Internal fixation with metal plates and screws. In Sherk HH, Dunn EJ, Eismont FJ et al (eds) *The Cervical Spine*, 2nd ed, 404–421. Cervical Spine Research Society. Philadelphia: JB Lippincott, 1989.
203 Werne S. Studies in spontaneous atlas dislocation. *Acta Orthop Scand (Suppl.)* **23**: 1–28, 1957.
204 Wertheim SB, Bohlman HH. Occipitocervical fusion. Indications, techniques, and long-term results in thirteen patients. *J Bone Joint Surg [Am]* **69**: 833–836, 1987.
205 White A, Panjabi M. *Clinical Biomechanics of the Spine*. Philadelphia/Toronto: JB Lippincott, 1978.
206 Whitesides TE. Lateral retropharyngeal approach to the upper cervical spine. In Sherk HH, Dunn EJ, Eismont FJ et al (eds) *The Cervical Spine*, 2nd ed, 517–527. Cervical Spine Research Society. Philadelphia: JB Lippincott, 1989.
207 Whitesides TE, McDonald AP. Lateral retropharyngeal approach to the upper cervical spine. *Orthop Clin North Am* **9**: 1115–1127, 1978.
208 Wilber RG, Peters JG, Likaver MJ. Surgical techniques in cervical spine surgery. In Errico TJ, Bauer RD, Waugh T (eds) *Spinal Trauma*, 2nd ed, 145–158.. Philadelphia: JB Lippincott, 1991
209 Wong DA, Mack RP, Craigmile TK. Traumatic atlanto-axial dislocation without fracture of the odontoid. *Spine* **16**: 587–589, 1991.
210 Wood-Jones F. The ideal lesion produced by judicial hanging. *Lancet* **1**: 53, 1913.
211 Zigler JE, Waters RL, Nelson RW, Capen DA, Perry J. Occipito-cervical-thoracic spine fusion in a patient with occipitocervical dislocation and survival. *Spine* **11**: 645–646, 1986.

12 Traumatic injuries to the adult lower cervical spine

J. Michael Simpson, Douglas Sutton, Steven J. Rizzolo and Jerome M. Cotler

Cervical spine injuries are a major cause of disability in today's society. The goals of management for patients with unstable cervical spine injuries include: (1) preservation of life; (2) treatment of associated injuries and prevention of complications; (3) preservation of intact neurologic function; (4) enhancement of neurologic recovery; (5) restoration of spinal stability and prevention of spinal deformity; and (6) maximization of functional recovery. This chapter strives to present an overview of the protocols used for the evaluation and treatment of cervical spine injuries at the authors' institution. The principles presented are derived from many years of experience at the Regional Spinal Cord Injury Center of Delaware Valley (RSCICDV), and represent the knowledge accumulated during treatment of approximately 3000 patients.

EMERGENCY EVALUATION

Evaluation and management of known or suspected cervical spine injury comprise a staged process. Proper management of unstable spine injuries begins with the evaluation and treatment of patients by emergency personnel in the field and continues with proper patient immobilization and transport to the emergency center. A high index of suspicion is the key to prevention of further neurologic injury during transport. All patients with head or high energy trauma, neurologic deficit, or complaints of neck pain must be assumed to have a cervical spine injury. Particular attention must be given to the unconscious patient, who may lack protective reflex muscle tone. The most effective method of cervical spine immobilization for transport is through supine positioning of the patient on a spine board, combined with use of a hard cervical collar and sandbags taped on either side of the head.[58] A hard collar alone provides adequate control of flexion and extension, but fails to control cervical rotation. The Philadelphia collar has been demonstrated to be significantly better in preventing sagittal and translational rotation when compared to other semi-rigid cervical orthoses, and is an excellent choice for the acute stabilization and transport of patients with suspected cervical spine injuries.[87]

When feasible, a cursory neurologic examination is advisable before moving any patient suspected of having cervical injury. Once this is completed, a cervical collar is placed on the patient. Log-rolling is the preferred method of patient mobilization onto the spine board, during which care is taken to maintain the head and neck in line with the body. Once the patient is placed on the spine board, the cervical region is additionally bolstered with sandbags. The rest of the patient is then secured to the spine board in the event of thoracic or lumbar spinal injury. The patient should be prevented from further movement of the spine until the patient is evaluated by a physician and radiographs obtained in the emergency room.[97,109]

Advanced trauma life support (ATLS) guidelines mandate an awareness of potential cervical spine injuries during primary and secondary resuscitative measures. During the primary patient survey, which is completed in the field, any manipulation of the patient's airway must be accompanied by in-line manual traction to prevent inadvertent motion of the spine. Patients with high cervical spinal cord injury may require ventilator and/or circulatory support. A detailed neurologic examination is delayed until secondary survey, but initial neurologic assessment should be included in the primary survey. Prompt and accurate diagnosis of cervical injuries in the emergency room demands a continuing high index of suspicion. Frequently, cervical spine injuries are missed during trauma resuscitation because attention is focused on more obvious or life-threatening injuries. In a review of 300 cervical spine fractures, Bohlman[18] reported that 100 were initially missed in the emergency room. The most common causes for missed cervical spine injuries in the emergency room include multiple trauma, multiple non-contiguous fractures, and altered consciousness (coma, intoxication).[20] Diagnostic delay ranged from one day to over one year. As many as 3–16% of patients with evidence of cervical fracture will also have a non-contiguous spine fracture, the most common cervical pattern being a fracture of the C1–C2 complex and a second remote subaxial cervical spine fracture.[68,88,124] In an analogous fashion, those patients who present for evaluation with known or obvious cervical spine injuries require a thorough screening for associated injuries.[108] Almost 50% of patients with acute spinal cord injury have other significant skeletal or visceral injuries.[23,67,80,115,120]

Soderstrom et al[115] reviewed records of 288 patients sustaining blunt cervical spine injuries, and found that 4.2% had sustained significant intra-abdominal injuries. All of these injuries were occult and detected by peritoneal lavage, which is a useful diagnostic aide, especially in patients whose physical examination is difficult. The procedure is highly sensitive in detecting injuries, can be done quickly, and has low morbidity.[115] Computed tomography (CT), which may be used in evaluation of the cervical spine, is less sensitive than peritoneal lavage in determination of intra-abdominal injury.

In the emergency room, ATLS protocols prevail.[1] Airway management remains the first priority in the care of these patients. If intubation is required at this stage, a lateral radiograph of the cervical spine is first recommended. However, this is not always feasible, depending on the patient's status. If no radiograph is available, nasotracheal intubation with the head and neck stabilized in a neutral position is recommended. If a contraindication to nasotracheal intubation exists, a cricothyroidotomy should be performed. Fiberoptic intubation may also be a helpful technique in these situations, minimizing the need for cervical manipulation.

An assessment of the patient's circulatory status then follows. Sites of obvious hemorrhage must be identified and controlled, while secondary assessment for occult blood loss is completed. Hemodynamic data may be difficult to interpret, especially in the presence of spinal shock. Adequate support through administration of fluid, blood, volume expanders, or vasoconstrictors may be required, depending on the source and degree of decompensation.

Throughout the emergency room process, these patients are best managed through a team approach. The resuscitation is supervised by a member of the trauma service, whereas evaluation and treatment of any spine injury are carried out by a three-member spinal cord team composed of members of the orthopedic, neurosurgical, and physical medicine and rehabilitation services. Each member of this team is responsible for evaluating the patient. Detailed neurologic examination by all members is required and is documented. Detailed and precise neurologic examination is critical in the assessment of initial and follow-up patient status, with accurate documentation being essential; whenever possible, serial examinations should be performed by one or more determined examiners. Motor and sensory evaluation should be conducted and level of function determined in a standardized fashion. The most popular and established guidelines are those of the American Spinal Cord Injury Association (ASIA).[6] In brief, those patients lacking motor power distal to the level of injury (ASIA level A,B) have a poor prognosis, and those patients with trace (ASIA level C) or functional motor power (ASIA level D) have a better prognosis. The presence or absence of distal motor function cannot be determined accurately until spinal shock has been reversed, and this is heralded by the return of the bulbocavernosus reflex. The details of neurologic evaluation are reviewed in Chapter 4, whereas various spinal cord syndromes and associated complications are reviewed in Chapter 6.

RADIOGRAPHIC EVALUATION

The initial radiographic assessment of the cervical spine consists of a mandatory cross-table lateral radiograph demonstrating the base of the skull, all seven cervical vertebrae, and the superior end-plates of T1. Although the cross-table lateral radiograph is an excellent screening tool which, by itself, will diagnose 70–79% of all cervical spine injuries, a full cervical spine series is indicated in all patients suspected of cervical injury.[41] A complete cervical spine series consists of lateral, anteroposterior, and open-mouth views, which will diagnose 90–95% of all cervical spine injuries.[49,73,90,119] In patients with large shoulders and/or short necks, it is often difficult to visualize the C7–T1 junction on a lateral film, and it may be necessary either to apply traction through the arms or to obtain a swimmer's view.[52,77,111] Unconscious or uncooperative patients, and those with upper extremity fractures, may require computed or conventional tomography to evaluate the cervicothoracic junction fully.

In evaluating the lateral radiograph, four lines are drawn or visualized to ensure normal anatomic relationships, including the anterior spinal line, posterior spinal line, spinolaminar line, and basilar line of Wackenstein (Fig. 12.1). The anterior and posterior spinal lines course along the anterior and posterior aspects of the vertebral bodies respectively, forming continuous smooth lines. The overall contour should be a gently sloping lordosis. The spinolaminar line is drawn, connecting the posterior aspect of the foramen magnum to the anterior cortex of each spinous process, and should also be a smooth lordotic curve. There is one normal variation in this line, of which the interpreter must be aware. The spinolaminar line of C2 may lie 2–3 mm posterior to that of C3, but is normal. The basilar line of

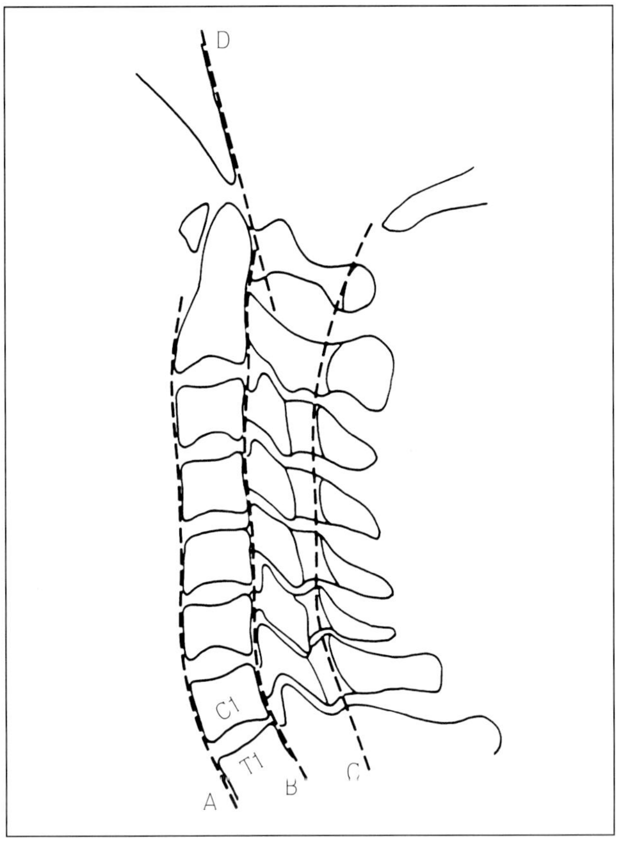

Figure 12.1
Lateral view of the cervical spine with four lines drawn, demonstrating normal bony cervical relationships. Line A is the anterior spinal line that starts at the anterior aspect of C2, and continues inferiorly along the anterior surface of each vertebral body. This should be a smooth, uninterrupted line to C7. Line B is the posterior spinal line, which follows the posterior vertebral body surfaces, and this should also be smooth and uninterrupted. Line C represents the spinolaminar line, which connects the posterior aspect of the foramen magnum to the anterior cortex of each cervical spinous process. This should be a continuous, smooth, lordotic curve, with one possible exception: the spinolaminar line of C2 may lie 2–3 mm posterior to this curve, which is a normal variant. Line D is the basilar line of Wackenstein, which lies along the posterior surface of the clivus and is at a tangent to the posterior cortex of the odontoid tip. This is important in defining craniovertebral relationships

Wackenstein lies along the posterior surface of the clivus, and is at a tangent to the posterior cortex of the odontoid tip. This relationship is important in evaluating craniovertebral relationships.

Additionally, lateral radiograph evaluation should include scrutiny of vertebral body height, articular pillars, alignment of articular facets, interspinous widening, and spinous process fracture. The articular pillars are rhomboid in shape, and the two pillars of any one vertebra should be superimposed on a true lateral radiograph. With an absence of this normal relationship, the observer should be alert to the possibility of fracture or facet dislocation. The interspinous distances below the level of C3 should be almost equal. An increased distance usually indicates posterior ligamentous injury. Translations >3.5 mm and angulations >11° are regarded as unstable.[126]

The prevertebral (retropharyngeal) soft tissues should also be evaluated on the lateral radiograph. A prevertebral soft-tissue space measuring between 7 and 10 mm at C2 indicates a possible abnormality and additional studies should be considered. When this soft-tissue space is >10 mm, the patient must be considered to have a cervical injury and further work-up is required.[123]

The role of flexion–extension lateral radiographs in an emergency setting remains controversial. They may be useful in the alert, cooperative patient without neurologic deficit who complains of neck pain. In this setting, a positive flexion–extension study has obvious clinical implications, but a negative film does not rule out acute injury. Patients with acute cervical spine injury may have muscle spasm which masks cervical instability for up to 2–3 weeks[59] Therefore, in spite of a negative study, for any patient in whom the index of suspicion is sufficiently high to obtain flexion–extension films, immobilization in a rigid cervical orthosis is recommended, and follow-up films are taken in 2–3 weeks.

The spinous processes may also be viewed on the anteroposterior radiograph for evidence of rotation or interspinous widening. An abrupt shift in position of any one spinous process may indicate a fracture of the articular pillar or facet dislocation. A widened interspinous distance 1.5 times that above or below the questionably injured segment indicates an anterior dislocation.[92] The lateral border of the cervical spine normally has an uninterrupted, wavy appearance. The facet joints themselves should not be seen on an anteroposterior projection. If a space is identified on this view, fracture of the pedicle or articular mass with subsequent rotation must be suspected. Open-mouth views are used in evaluation of the upper cervical spine. Characteristic abnormalities of the upper cervical spine are reviewed in Chapter 11.

Oblique views at 45° provide excellent visualization of the intervertebral foramina, pedicles, and facet joints. The pillar view is obtained with the head rotated 45–50° toward the unaffected side with the central X-ray beam directed at C7 with 30–40° caudal angulation. This view is particularly useful in visualizing the articular pillars and for patients suspected of hyperextension injuries.[88]

Computed tomography is an excellent method of evaluating patients with cervical spine injuries. Its advantages include speed, availability, supine positioning, axial imaging,

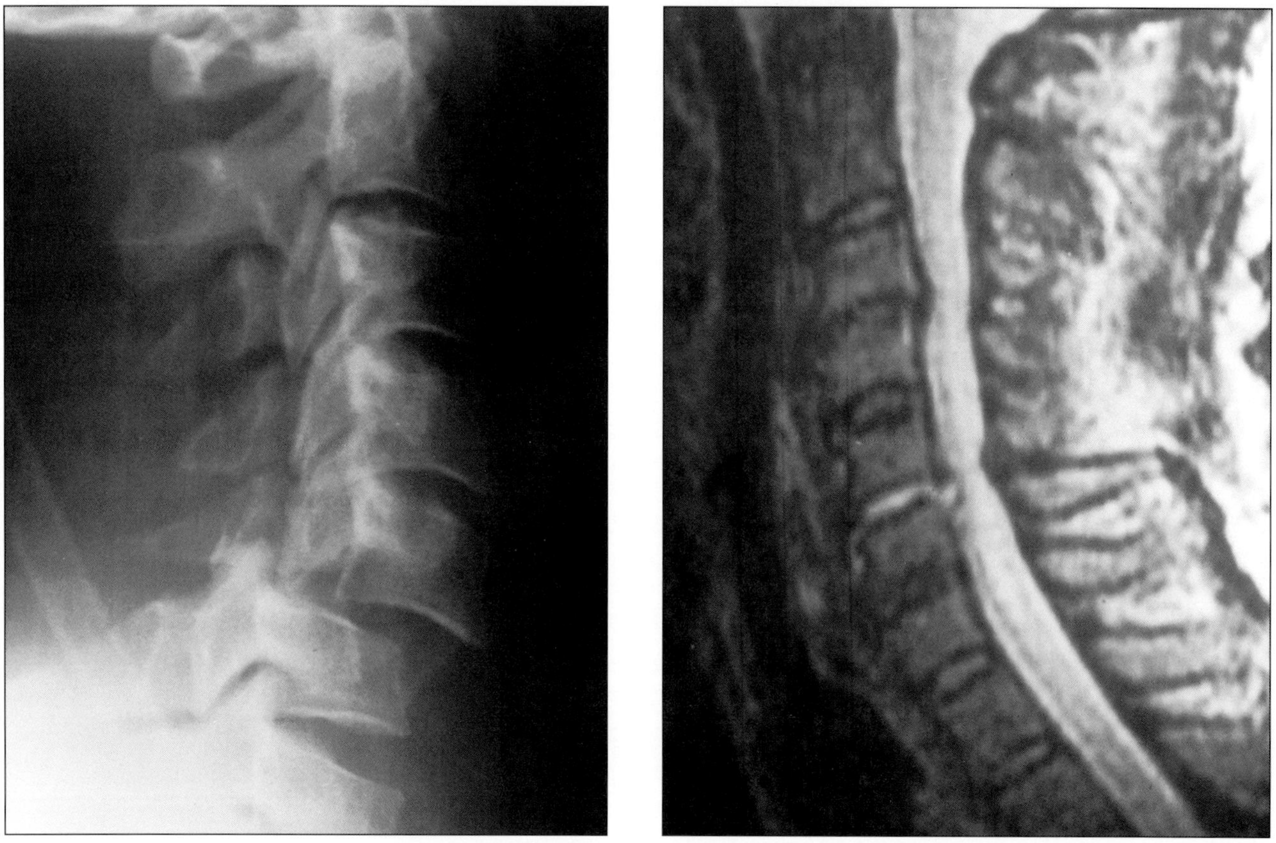

a

b

Figure 12.2
(a) Lateral radiograph demonstrating a bilateral facet dislocation. This patient underwent a successful, physician-monitored, closed reduction. (b) Post-reduction MRI scan clearly demonstrating the presence of a disc herniation at the injured segment. This patient required anterior decompression and interbody arthrodesis, followed by a posterior cervical fusion

and excellent cortical detail. As a result of the cost and relatively high dose of radiation, it should not, however, be used as a screening modality. Rather, computed tomography should be reserved to delineate the bony anatomy of fractures seen or suspected on plain radiographs, and for cases in which the lower cervical spine cannot be adequately visualized. Scanning should consist of 2- to 3-mm consecutive images and include at least one vertebra above and below the suspected level of injury. In patients with cervical neurologic deficit and no obvious fracture on plain radiograph, computed tomography scanning can be used, and should include one level above and below the level of neurologic deficit.

Conventional tomography, for the most part, has been replaced by computerized scanning for the diagnosis of cervical spine fractures. However, plain tomography is useful in the diagnosis of minimally displaced horizontal fractures. Horizontal fracture of the odontoid or facets may be missed on axially oriented computed tomograms and sagittal reconstructions, but are often well delineated on anteroposterior and lateral tomograms. Furthermore, tomograms are useful in the evaluation of the cervicothoracic junction and in the postoperative evaluation of graft healing.

Magnetic resonance imaging (MRI) has become a popular modality in evaluating cervical trauma patients and, in many ways, has revolutionized our ability to determine the extent of cervical spine and spinal cord injury.[33,53,72] It has generally replaced myelography as a diagnostic tool in cervical trauma. Advantages of MRI include its lack of ionizing radiation, direct multiplane imaging capabilities, ability to detect non-contiguous fractures, and, most importantly, its ability to determine the degree of soft-tissue injury, including the intervertebral disc, spinal cord, and ligamentous structures. Recent studies have demonstrated that the incidence of disc injury complicating cervical spine trauma is significantly higher than initially thought, and is more than 50% in some injury patterns (Fig. 12.2).[57,96,99,100] Magnetic resonance imaging is not only capable of accurately depicting the presence of injury to these structures, but is able to quantitate the degree of injury to these structures as well.[12,36,66,110] T2-weighted images are best for visualizing the spinal cord.[36,110] Imaging signals, consisting of intramedullary hematoma and/or spinal cord contusion associated with edema, encompassing more than one spinal segment, have been shown to be associated with more severe neurologic deficits.[36,110] Less severe injuries have been correlated with normal spinal cord signal and edema encompassing one segment or less.[110] Whether this will be a useful modality to establish long-term prognosis remains uncertain. Magnetic resonance imaging is indicated in the following: (1) all patients with complete or incomplete neurologic deficits to search for and quantify the degree of spinal cord compression; (2) any patient in whom the neurologic status deteriorates; and (3) cases in which there is suspicion of posterior ligamentous injury in spite of negative plain radiographs. Currently, computed tomography provides greater detail of bony anatomy and, therefore, patients may require both computed tomograms and MRI scans. In the future, MRI may provide cortical detail equivalent to computed tomography, and therefore obviate the need for a second study. The disadvantages of MRI include its relatively long acquisition time, limited availability in some institutions, and contraindications. MRI is contraindicated in patients with pacemakers, aneurysm clips, metallic fragments in the eye or spinal cord, and severe claustrophobia. Furthermore, ventilator support and cardiac monitoring of patients during MRI scanning must be accomplished with non-ferromagnetic equipment.

EARLY MANAGEMENT CONSIDERATIONS IN CERVICAL SPINE INJURIES

There are many aspects of patient care that require early consideration in cervical injury. Once the patient's medical status is secured, and diagnostic radiographic studies obtained, the stability or instability of the injury must be recognized, deformity and subluxation reduced and immobilized, and complications associated with cervical injury averted. These topics, the understanding of which is imperative to proper and successful management, are now reviewed.

Stability

The concept of stability, in many respects, is vague. Radiographic measurements of translation and angulatory abnormalities are helpful, but are limited in the ability to recognize potential for neurologic injury in many fracture patterns. Spinal stability has been defined as 'the ability of the spine under physiologic loads to maintain the relationship between vertebrae in such a way that there is neither initial nor subsequent damage to the spinal cord or nerve roots'.[16] Based on multifactorial considerations which, in fact, determine stability, White et al[126] suggest that a checklist of dynamic and static radiographic criteria and neurologic findings be used (Table 12.1). These criteria are particularly helpful in equivocal cases of instability, but are not required in the vast majority of presenting cervical injuries. In brief, any of the following situations must be considered to represent an unstable injury of the cervical spine:

- anterior and posterior column injury;
- any structural injury associated with injury to the spinal cord;
- gross deformity of the cervical spine with or without neurologic involvement.

The classification schemes described by Holdsworth,[60] Allen et al[5] and Denis[43] help us in our ability to determine the applied forces responsible for injury and the extent of structural damage to the spine. These classifications, which are reviewed in detail later, may help the clinician in determining stability, but are most helpful in determining treatment options.

Reduction and Immobilization of Cervical Injury

Cervical immobilization is required for any patient suspected of being injured. A rigid cervical orthosis is required while diagnostic studies are completed. When radiographs reveal significant osseous or ligamentous injury, it is preferable to immobilize the cervical spine through application of cervical traction. For most injuries, the authors prefer application of MRI-compatible Gardner–Wells tongs, with pins placed neutral or 1 cm behind the external auditory canal, and just above the pinna. Pins placed in front of this point will exert an extension moment on the spine, whereas those placed behind will impart a flexion moment. In the emergency room, patients are placed on a manual turning frame (Stryker), and on admission to the ward are transferred to an automatic rotating bed. The weight required for immobilization of cervical spine injuries must be tailored to the individual injury, but, in most cases, 4.50–6.75 kg of weight is sufficient. The post-traction alignment of the spine should

Table 12.1 Checklist for the diagnosis of clinical instability in the middle and lower cervical spine*

Element	*Point value*
Anterior elements destroyed or unable to function	2
Posterior elements destroyed or unable to function	2
Positive stretch test	2
Radiographic criteria†	4
A Flexion–extension radiographs:	
(1) Sagittal plane translation > 3.5 mm or 20% (2 pts)	
(2) Sagittal plane rotation > 20° (2 pts)	
or	
B Resting radiographs:	
(1) Sagittal plane displacement > 3.5 mm or 20% (2 pts)	
(2) Relative sagittal plane angulation > 11° (2 pts)	
Abnormal disc narrowing	1
Developmentally narrow spinal canal:	1
1 Sagittal diameter < 13 mm	
or	
2 Pavlov's ratio < 0.8†	
Spinal cord damage	2
Nerve root damage	1
Dangerous loading anticipated	1
Total of 5 or more = unstable	

*Reproduced from White AA, Panjabi MM. The problem of clinical instability in the human spine: A systematic approach. In: *Clinical Biomechanics of the Spine*. Philadelphia: JB Lippincott, 1978: 314.
†See Figures 5.35 and 5.36 in White AA, Panjabi MM, above, for information on making these measurements.

always be checked after application of weight with plain radiographs as well as neuromuscular assessment. In those cases where timing or logistics of a trauma resuscitation preclude thorough evaluation or application of traction, the patient should be maintained in a rigid cervical orthosis.

Spinal deformity resulting from cervical spine injury is not only capable of causing the initial spinal cord injury, but may also be responsible for ongoing neurologic compromise via a destructive cycle of vascular compromise and edema.[54] Therefore, attempted closed reduction is indicated in all cases of cervical spine injury demonstrating shortening, angulation, and/or translation. The goal of closed reduction is restoration of normal spinal alignment, which may result in decompression of the spinal canal, enhance neurologic recovery, restore the stability of intact bony elements, and prevent further neurologic injury. Many animal and several recent clinical studies demonstrate that the extent of neurologic recovery is influenced by the duration and degree of neurologic compression.[2,31,40,44,75,106,122]

Closed reduction should be attempted as rapidly as possible upon admission to the hospital. Closed reduction must always be attempted in a closely supervised setting, with vigilant radiographic and neurologic monitoring. Patients should be awake, alert, and cooperative during attempted closed reduction in order to provide feedback during the procedure.[100] Reduction is accomplished via a combination of skeletal traction, patient positioning, and postural bumps.[38,40] Patients should be placed on a Stryker frame and Gardner–Wells tongs applied as previously described. Reduction begins with 4.5 kg of applied traction, and is increased by 4.5 kg in a sequential fashion at 10- to 20-minute intervals until an acceptable reduction is achieved. Evaluation of vertebral distraction is performed after each incremental change in the traction weight. A lateral cervical spine radiograph is taken 5–10 minutes after the weight change. The patient's neurologic status is also evaluated after each weight change through either the patient's ability to perform an established motor function or a change in sensory level. After reduction is achieved, the weight is reduced to 4.5–9.0 kg, and repeat lateral radiographs obtained to confirm maintenance of reduction. MRI-compatible tongs are preferred, unless a high weight (approximately 30 kg or 70 pounds) reduction is anticipated, in which case stronger stainless steel tip tongs should be used. The role of manipulation during closed reduction is controversial and should be reserved for those familiar with its indications and technique.[37] The weight required for reduction of an individual cervical spine injury is quite variable, and the maximum amount of weight which can be safely applied is not known.[88] Attempted closed reduction should be discontinued when (1) the spine is reduced, (2) >1 cm distraction occurs at the zone of injury and/or another location, (3) the patient's neurologic status deteriorates, or (4) the physician believes additional attempts have little or no chance of success. Closed reduction has been successfully achieved in up to 90–95% of cases.[116] Following successful closed reduction, preoperative alignment of the spine can usually be maintained with 4.5–6.75 kg of axial traction, but dictates that the patient remain in a supine position.

In selected injury patterns, preoperative immobilization of unstable fractures in a halo vest is a safe and effective technique in maintaining reduction while facilitating patient mobilization, nursing care, and pulmonary toilet. However, close patient monitoring with serial radiographs is necessary to recognize displacement.[98] MRI-compatible halo-vest orthoses allow for any further diagnostic intervention that may be required. Open reduction is indicated if acceptable alignment cannot be achieved closed.

Since the 1960s, the halo-vest orthosis has been used to stabilize the cervical spine in cases of fracture–dislocation, infectious disease, and neoplasm. The halo vest has been shown to be more effective in restricting cervical motion when compared with more conventional cervical orthoses.[64,70] However, up to 30% of normal cervical spine motion has been reported even after stabilization with a halo device.[69] The advantages of using a halo in patients with lower cervical spine injuries include both the physical and psychological benefits of early mobilization. Avoidance of complications is associated with prolonged bedrest, shorter hospital and rehabilitation stays, and less interference with mandibular motion and eating. The halo also has the advantage of being able to position the neck more precisely in the preferred alignment to counteract the direction of instability. These advantages make the halo attractive for use in both non-surgical and post-surgical management of lower cervical spine injuries. Non-surgical management of cervical injuries in a halo vest does require careful follow-up, because failure rates may range from 10% to 40%, depending on the specific injury pattern.[29,30,35,62,76]

Complications associated with the use of the halo vest are also frequent, most of them being related to pin loosening and pin tract infection.[50,76] These complications can be minimized if attention is paid to application and maintenance of the halo. The initial application should be performed using a sterile technique. The ring should be positioned 'below the equator' or below the greatest circumference of the patient's skull, so that any pressure on the ring will not cause the halo to shift cephalad and out of position. The pins should be initially torqued to 0.7 to 0.9 joules (6 to 8 inch-pounds), and re-torqued to the same level after 24–48 hours of application.[50] The anterior pins should be placed in the 'safe zone' just superior to the middle or lateral third of the orbit, thereby protecting the supraorbital nerve.[50] If pins loosen, they should be re-torqued to the original application torque, assuming that bony resistance is felt within one to two turns. If no resistance is met, the pin site should be changed. Careful molding and fitting of the vest are also important to eliminate accessory motion. Careful follow-up for change in spinal alignment and maintenance of the halo are necessary to minimize associated complications.

Prevention of Perioperative Complications

Patient immobilization, which is required for many cervical injuries, predisposes the patient to a host of medical complications before surgical stabilization. These include pulmonary dysfunction, peptic ulcer disease, deep venous thrombosis, and skin breakdown. As is the case with most trauma patients, complication rates are most effectively reduced through rapid intervention and mobilization. In addition, prophylactic measures initiated on admission minimize patient risk. Prophylaxis of pulmonary complications includes prevention of aspiration and aggressive pulmonary toilet. Gastrointestinal bleeding, usually the result of developing peptic ulcer disease, is reported to occur in up to 9–40% of patients, and is most common 10–14 days after injury.[3,18,24,74] The risk of ulceration may be aggravated by the use of steroids and can be combatted through the use of H_2-receptor blockers and early enteral feeding. The incidence of deep vein thrombosis in spinal cord injury patients has been reported to be as high as 25–95%, and is clinically relevant in 25–35% of patients.[55,79] Although ongoing research continues at the authors' institution, the current prophylaxis protocol calls for adjusted low-dose heparin and compression boots. Skin breakdown is best treated through prevention with vigilant nursing care and use of rotating beds. Established skin ulcers must be aggressively treated with débridement, local wound care, and pressure relief.

Corticosteroids

The theoretical benefit of steroids in patients with acute spinal cord injury is to decrease inflammation and minimize neural tissue damage and dysfunction at the cellular level. The theoretical disadvantages are the undesirable systemic consequences of steroids, including, but not limited to, immunosuppression and gastrointestinal bleeding. Initial studies, using relatively low doses of steroids administered over the course of several weeks, resulted in significant increases in infection and gastrointestinal bleeding rates with little or no improvement in neurologic function.[25–27] In a recent multi-center randomized study, Bracken et al[26] evaluated the safety and efficacy of large doses of methylprednisolone started within 8 hours of admission and administered over the first 24 hours. The authors reported a significant improvement of motor scores in patients with motor incomplete lesions who were treated with methylprednisolone as opposed to a placebo or naloxone. Infection rates of 7.9% versus 3.6%, and gastrointestinal bleeding rates of 4.5% versus 3%, were noted in the steroid and placebo groups, respectively. The shortcomings of the study include a lack of control over subsequent operative intervention between the study groups as well as no mention of the degree of functional motor improvement associated with increased motor scores. It must be reiterated that the study included only those patients treated within 8 hours of blunt spinal cord injury, and did not include penetrating spinal cord injuries. The ultimate role of steroids in the acute treatment of spinal cord injury thus remains unclear. Based on the relatively modest increase in complication rates noted in more recent studies, the recommended bolus of methylprednisolone 30 mg/kg body weight is administered by the authors to all patients with acute (<8 hours) blunt spinal cord injury, followed by an infusion of 5.4 mg/kg per hour over 23 hours.

SURGICAL TREATMENT OF UNSTABLE CERVICAL SPINE INJURIES

General Principles

Surgical decompression must be considered in all cases of radiographically demonstrable neurologic compression after realignment of the spine.[7,11,14,15,21] Decompression is mandatory in cases of incomplete neurologic injury to promote recovery. When complete neurologic injury occurs, decompression may facilitate root recovery which, in cervical cord injuries, may significantly improve functional status.[13,18,19,127] With a normal neurologic examination, decompression is not mandatory, although if the injury resulting in neural compression also predisposes the spine to late deformity, it may be indicated as part of a procedure designed to reconstruct structural integrity.

The approach for surgical decompression should be dictated by the anatomic location of neurologic compression. Because the overwhelming majority of compression is caused by either vertebral body retropulsion or herniated disc material (anterior structures), most cervical decompressions are performed anteriorly. Laminectomy as a means of spinal cord decompression is contraindicated in cervical trauma; it has been shown to be of little therapeutic value, and predisposes the patient to late kyphotic deformity and poor results.[60,61,91,103,112,118] It is reserved for the few patients with depressed laminar fractures causing posterior compression of the cord, and for the rare patient with ankylosing spondylitis and epidural hematoma formation. In those cases that require posterior stabilization following anterior cervical decompression, the authors' preference has been to perform these procedures at the same surgical sitting, whenever medically feasible.

In most surgical cases, regardless of the planned surgical approach, the Stryker frame is used as the operative table; this frame incorporates a pulley to facilitate cervical traction. In those cases in which the patient has been immobilized before surgery in a halo-vest orthosis, traction can be applied through a halo bail. Alternatively, either anterior or posterior bars of the halo can be taped to the frame and the opposite vest and bars removed, allowing unrestricted access to the neck.

The indications for use of spinal cord monitoring during surgery for acute cervical spine injuries are not well delineated. Somatic sensory evoked potential monitoring is probably of most use in those patients with intact neurologic function below the level of injury in whom significant intraoperative manipulation of the spinal column is anticipated. Evidence of significant signal deformity is checked with a wake-up test.

Almost universally, all patients at the authors' institution who undergo surgical stabilization for acute cervical spine trauma are immobilized in a halo vest after surgery. Although it is recognized that this may represent a certain degree of over-treatment, the authors have found that the halo vest is well tolerated by most patients, and carries a low complication rate.[101] In fact, the authors feel that the potential for catastrophic neurologic complications accompanying a loss of spinal alignment warrants aggressive postoperative immobilization. Once early signs of healing are visible, patients are often switched to a rigid cervical orthosis until healing is complete.

Timing of Surgery

Initial studies of early surgical intervention (<3–5 days) in patients with acute spinal cord injury reported increased mortality and neurologic deterioration, leading many to recommend a delay in operative intervention for 1–2 weeks.[78,94] However, the degree of neurologic damage following experimental spinal cord injury in animals is affected not only by the degree, but also by the duration, of cord compression, leading other authors to recommend urgent decompression.[2,31,40,44,45,75,106,122]

There can be no doubt that early decompression and stabilization of unstable spine injuries offer the benefits of patient mobilization as it does in all trauma patients. Furthermore, in recent studies where spinal cord monitoring and improved anesthetic and surgical techniques have been employed, no increase in morbidity or mortality has been demonstrated following early surgical intervention.[2,71,73,75] The authors therefore proceed with operative decompression and stabilization of patients with acute spinal cord injury in a medically expedient manner.

Classification and Treatment Options for Adult Subaxial Cervical Spine Fractures

Plain radiographs, computed tomography, and magnetic resonance imaging allow accurate definition of the extent of structural injury. With this knowledge, these injuries can be appropriately classified and treated, thereby avoiding or minimizing complications of treatment. Classification schemes have been universally applied to all fractures of the body and serve several functions. With reference to the cervical spine, a classification system should ideally serve to describe the cervical injury accurately and efficiently, to define the force vectors responsible for production of injury (which will subsequently facilitate reduction and restoration of spinal alignment), and to determine the structural stability of the injury.

Holdsworth[60] was the first to attempt classification of spinal injuries. With his system, the spinal column is divided into anterior and posterior columns. The anterior column is composed of the anterior longitudinal ligament, vertebral bodies, intervertebral discs, and posterior longitudinal ligament. The posterior column is inclusive of the pedicles, lamina, spinous processes, ligamentum flavum, capsular ligaments, and the supraspinous and interspinous ligaments. He subsequently classified all spinal injuries into six categories, including simple wedge compression fractures, dislocations, extension injuries, burst fractures, rotational fracture–dislocations, and shear injuries. For each injury type, a particular mode of failure is implied. This system, however, fails in its ability to determine stability accurately, and its clinical applicability is thereby limited.

The classification system described by Allen et al[5] represents a mechanistic approach to spine injury analysis, and is based on the position of the neck at the time of injury and or applied force vectors. In this scheme, six categories or phylogenies of injury are described. Each phylogeny is then subdivided into stages that are descriptive of injury severity. The higher numbered stages represent more severe forms of structural injury and imply a greater potential for neurologic injury. Injury designation can usually be accomplished based on the mechanism of injury and review of plain radiographs. Crucial to the differentiation of injury patterns is recognition that compressive loads result in shortening of the vertebral elements whereas distraction results in lengthening.

Although this mechanistic classification is the most useful, it is not without limitations. It cannot be universally applied to all injuries, because some injuries appear to represent a combination of patterns and may fail to fit well into any one phylogeny. Nevertheless, this system does provide our most comprehensive understanding of injury production and therefore facilitates our ability to treat them properly. There is a broad spectrum of acceptable treatment modalities for these various fracture patterns. There is much controversy about the need and type of surgery for a particular injury. The purpose here is not to labor over the advantages and disadvantages of every option, but simply to present the treatment plan preferred by the authors for each category of injury, based on their experience at RSCICDV (Fig. 12.3).

A two-column concept is used in the work of both Holdsworth[60] and Allen et al.[5] Denis[43] has described three columns in the thoracolumbar spine, which are equally helpful in the cervical region. With this concept, the anterior column is composed of the anterior longitudinal ligament and the anterior tw0-thirds of the intervertebral disc and vertebral body. The middle column includes the posterior longitudinal ligament and the posterior one-third of the intervertebral disc and vertebral body. The posterior column includes the vertebral arches, and the supporting ligamentous and capsular structures. In this scheme, any injury that involves the middle column must be considered unstable.

Compressive Flexion Injury

The most common mechanism that results in compressive flexion injuries is motor vehicle accidents and shallow dives, and the most common levels of injury are C4–C5 and C5–C6. Compressive loads applied to the flexed spine result in compression of the anterior column of the spine and distraction of the posterior column. The resultant shortening of the anterior column and lengthening of the posterior column can be graded into five stages (Fig. 12.4). In compressive flexion stages 1 (CFS1) and 2 (CFS2) (vertebral body blunting and beaking), the structural integrity of the anterior column is partially intact and ligamentous failure of the middle and posterior elements has not occurred. Neurologic injury is uncommon in stages 1 and 2. Although there is risk of late kyphotic deformity, most patients can be managed successfully in a rigid cervical orthosis or halo-vest orthosis for 8–12 weeks.

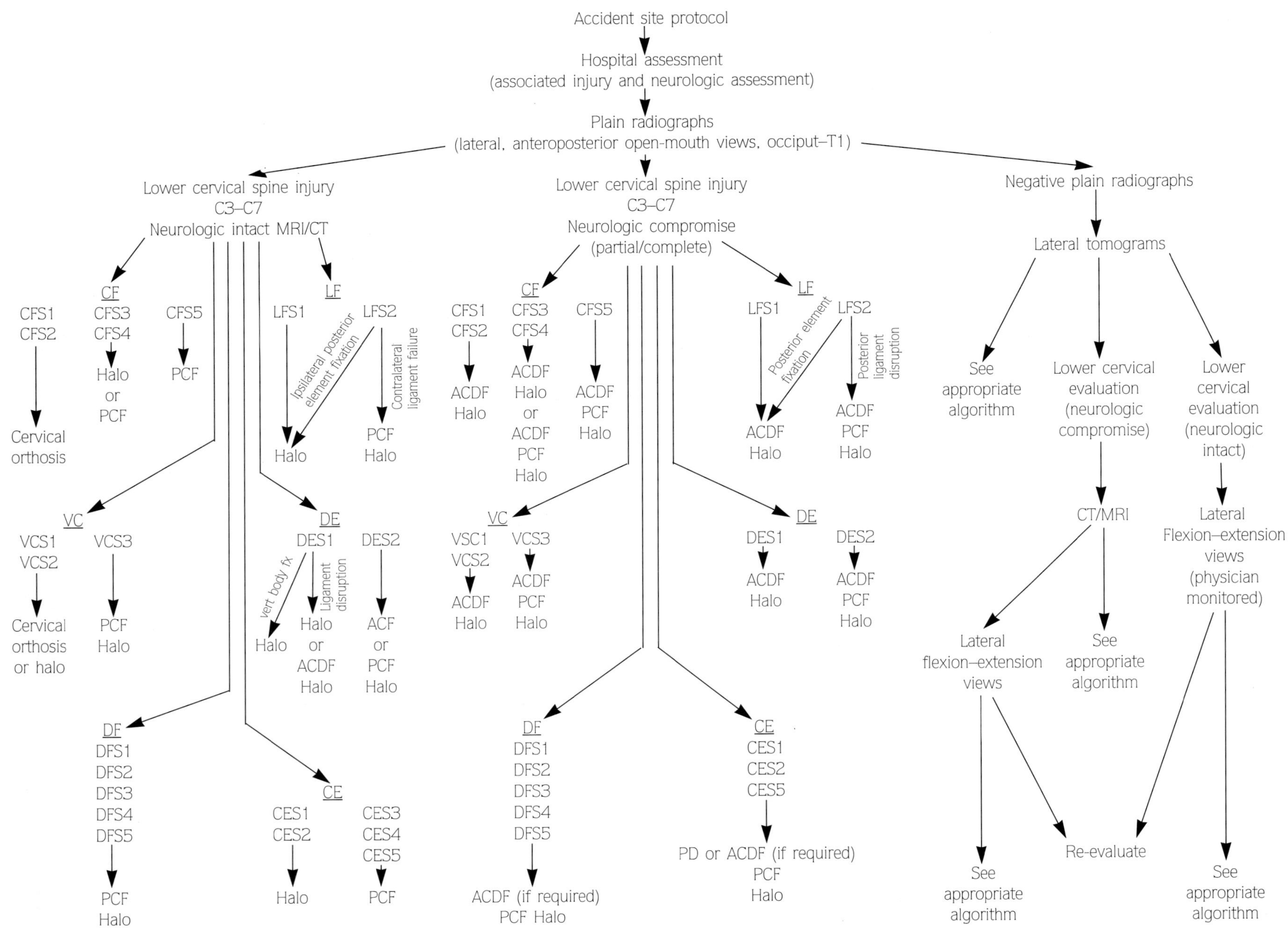
Accident site protocol
Hospital assessment
(associated injury and neurologic assessment)
Plain radiographs
(lateral, anteroposterior open-mouth views, occiput–T1)
Lower cervical spine injury
C3–C7
Neurologic intact MRI/CT
CF
CFS1
CFS2
Cervical orthosis
CFS3
CFS4
Halo or PCF
CFS5
PCF
LF
LFS1
LFS2
Ipsilateral posterior element fixation
Contralateral ligament failure
Halo
PCF Halo
VC
VCS1
VCS2
Cervical orthosis or halo
VCS3
PCF Halo
DE
DES1
vert body fx
Ligament disruption
Halo
Halo or ACDF Halo
DES2
ACF or PCF Halo
DF
DFS1
DFS2
DFS3
DFS4
DFS5
PCF Halo
CE
CES1
CES2
Halo
CES3
CES4
CES5
PCF
Lower cervical spine injury
C3–C7
Neurologic compromise
(partial/complete)
CF
CFS1
CFS2
ACDF Halo
CFS3
CFS4
ACDF Halo or ACDF PCF Halo
CFS5
ACDF PCF Halo
LF
LFS1
LFS2
Posterior element fixation
Posterior ligament disruption
ACDF Halo
ACDF PCF Halo
VC
VSC1
VCS2
ACDF Halo
VCS3
ACDF PCF Halo
DE
DES1
ACDF Halo
DES2
ACDF PCF Halo
DF
DFS1
DFS2
DFS3
DFS4
DFS5
ACDF (if required)
PCF Halo
CE
CES1
CES2
CES5
PD or ACDF (if required)
PCF
Halo
Negative plain radiographs
Lateral tomograms
See appropriate algorithm
Lower cervical evaluation (neurologic compromise)
CT/MRI
Lateral flexion–extension views
See appropriate algorithm
Lower cervical evaluation (neurologic intact)
Lateral Flexion–extension views (physician monitored)
Re-evaluate
See appropriate algorithm
See appropriate algorithm

In stages 3 and 4 (fracture of the vertebral body without displacement, and <3 mm displacement, respectively), complete posterior ligamentous disruption is possible (Fig. 12.5). These patients require evaluation by MRI to rule out posterior ligamentous disruption. A halo-vest orthosis is sufficient for patients with an intact posterior column. However, for those patients with ligamentous disruption, the risk of late kyphotic deformity is high, and posterior cervical fusion and postoperative halo immobilization recommended. Again, neurologic compromise is not common.

Patients with stage 5 lesions (posterior displacement of the vertebral body) have complete failure of the anterior, middle, and posterior columns of the spine. Axial traction, applied through cranial tongs, combined with extension rolls under the upper thoracic spine often results in only partial realignment of the spine. In cases involving lower energy trauma, posterior cervical fusion with postoperative halo immobilization may be all that is required. In cases involving higher energy trauma with significant comminution and collapse of the vertebral body, and for patients with evidence of anterior cord compression, anterior decompression (corpectomy) and anterior strut graft reconstruction may be necessary. In most of these cases, the authors prefer to augment this construct with a posterior fusion and postoperative halo immobilization to minimize graft complications and late kyphotic deformity. The role of anterior cervical internal fixation remains controversial, but may limit the need for a second surgical approach.

For patients presenting with stage 1–4 injuries and either partial or complete neurologic injury, an MRI scan is required to evaluate the compressive pathology. In most cases of neurologic compromise, disc herniation accounts for neurologic compression and requires anterior decompression and interbody arthrodesis. For injuries with incomplete or complete spinal cord injury and evidence of posterior stage 3 ligament disruption, a concomitant posterior arthrodesis is recommended. Others may prefer isolated anterior decompression and plate fixation.

Figure 12.3

Management algorithm of suspected cervical spine injuries. Accident site and hospital assessment protocols are discussed fully in the text. If plain radiographs reveal obvious cervical injury, they are then classified according to the classification scheme of Allen et al. With this classification scheme, all injuries are placed into one of six phylogenies, including compressive flexion (CF), vertical compression (VC), distractive flexion (DF), lateral flexion (LF), distractive extension (DE), and compressive extension (CE) injuries. Each phylogeny is subsequently divided into various stages, with the higher numbered stages representative of more severe structural injury to the spine, and greater potential for neurologic injury. For each of the diagnosed injuries, there are subdivided into categories based on neurologic function. This is an important distinction, because for those patients with any evidence of neurologic compromise or evidence of neurocompressive lesions, some form of decompression is required to enhance neurologic recovery. For each of these scenarios, treatment options, based on the authors' experience at the Regional Spinal Cord Injury Center of the Delaware Valley (RSCICDV), is given. Although many of these recommendations may be the source of controversy and discussion, the authors feel that management complications have been minimized, neurologic recovery enhanced, and structural stability obtained. For those patients with complaints of neck pain and negative plain radiographs, an algorithm for further evaluation is also offered – see text for discussion. ACDF, anterior cervical decompression and fusion; PCF, posterior cervical fusion; PD, posterior decompression; ACF, anterior cervical fusion

Vertical Compression Injury

Vertical compression injuries are most common following motor vehicle accidents, diving accidents, and direct blows to the top of the skull. The most common levels of injury are C6 and C7. These injuries are the result of compressive forces applied to a neutrally aligned spine, and lead to shortening of both the anterior and middle columns of the spine. This injury pattern occurs in three stages (Fig. 12.6). Vertical compression stage 1 and 2 (VCS1 and VCS2) injuries involve cupping of one or both end-plates of the vertebral body, and represent partial failure of the anterior column. The posterior ligamentous structures are usually uninjured, and late kyphotic deformities unusual. Therefore, patients who are neurologically intact can be managed for 6–8 weeks in a rigid cervical orthosis or halo vest. Patients with neurologic involvement will require MRI evaluation followed by anterior cervical discectomy and fusion with postoperative halo immobilization.

Vertical compression stage 3 (VCS3) injuries usually involve fragmentation and displacement of the vertebral body, and are sometimes referred to as 'burst fractures' (Fig. 12.7). Occasionally, VCS3 may involve bony failure in the anterior column followed by ligamentous failure of the middle and posterior columns with subsequent posterior translation and cord impingement. An important distinction between VCS3 and CFS5 injuries must be realized. In most VCS3 injuries, the neural canal is narrowed by retropulsed vertebral bone, which is an exception to the generalization that most cervical cord injuries are a result of translation. Axial traction may result in reduction of the fracture, but not consistently. Patients without neurologic injury may simply require posterior fusion with postoperative halo immobilization. However, many of these patients will

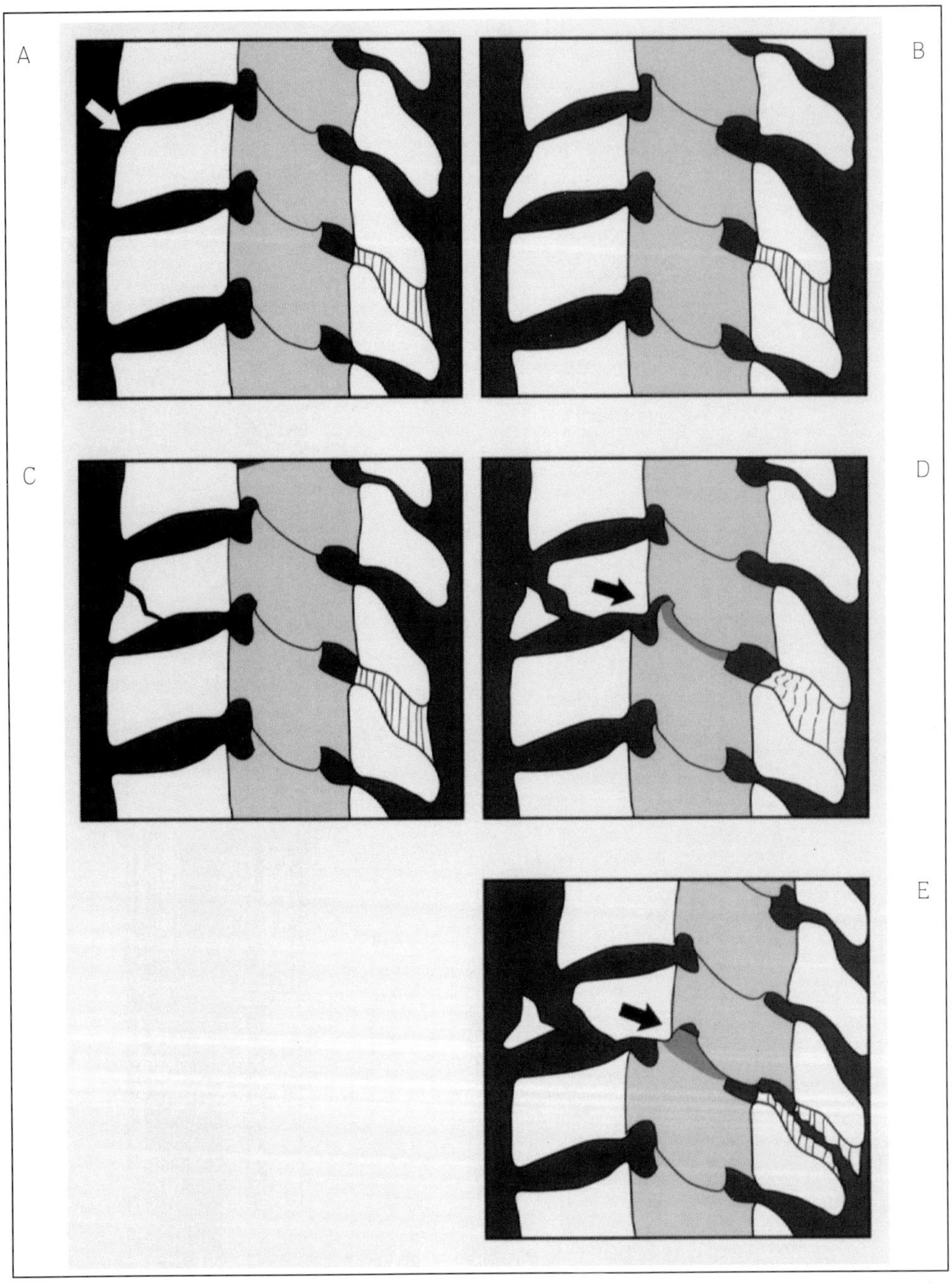

Figure 12.4
(A) Compression flexion stage 1 (CFS1): this represents the most minor injury as a result of a compressive load applied to the spine when held in a flexed position, and the lesion consists simply of rounding of the anterosuperior aspect of the vertebral body. There is no disruption of the posterior ligamentous structures. The middle and posterior columns are completely intact. (B) Compressive flexion stage 2 (CFS2): there is now an obliquity to the anterior surface of the vertebral body, and concomitant loss of anterior column height. This results in a 'beaked' appearance of the anteroinferior surface of the vertebral body. Again, ligamentous structures remain intact posteriorly. (C) Compressive flexion stage 3 (CFS3): in this stage, a fracture line clearly passes obliquely from the anterior surface of the vertebral body, and extends through the inferior subchondral plate. In this diagram, the posterior ligamentous structures are shown to be intact, although they may be injured and require examination through MRI. (D) Compressive flexion stage 4 (CFS4): in addition to the fracture line seen in CFS3, this lesion includes translation of the inferoposterior vertebral margin into the neural canal at the involved motion segment. This is indicative of early ligamentous failure through the middle and posterior ligamentous complexes. The amount of posterior translation is, however, <3 mm. (E) Compressive flexion stage 5 (CFS5): this lesion represents full ligamentous disruption of all columns with marked posterior translation in excess of 3 mm. It is a grossly unstable lesion

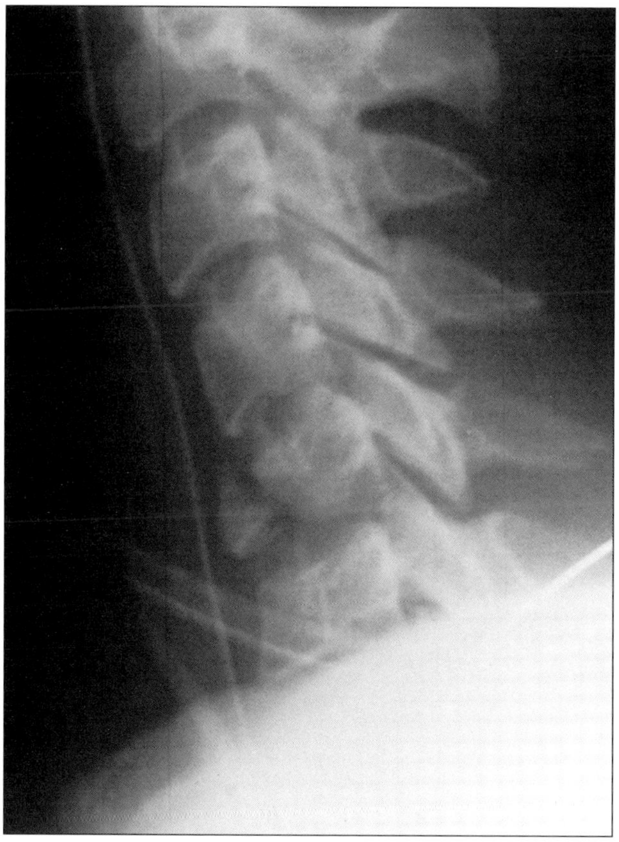

Figure 12.5
Lateral radiograph of a compressive flexion stage 4 injury with mild posterior subluxation of the inferoposterior vertebral margin into the neural canal, measuring approximately 2–3 mm. MRI of this patient did show interspinous ligament injury. This patient was neurologically intact; a posterior cervical fusion was advised and completed

present with neurologic injury, and will therefore require some form of anterior decompression and reconstruction augmented with posterior arthrodesis and halo-vest orthosis. Most commonly, vertebral corpectomy followed by strut graft reconstruction is required.

Distractive Flexion Injury

Distractive flexion represents the most common injury pattern and is most often caused by motor vehicle accidents and falls from a height. Injury is most common between C5–C6 and C6–C7. Distractive loads applied to the spine in a flexed position cause tensile failure (ligamentous or bony) and lengthening of the posterior column in the early stages, and associated failure of the anterior and middle columns during the latter stages. In early stage lesions, radiographs may reveal an anterior compressive element of failure usually in the lower-most vertebrae in the injury motion segment. This should not be confused with the compression flexion phylogeny, the distinguishing characteristics of distractive flexion injuries being early posterior column ligamentous disruption. In late-stage distractive flexion injury, middle and anterior column ligamentous disruption, secondary to tensile forces, is seen. Shear forces generated by this injury pattern result in variable degrees of anterior translation of the superior vertebra of the involved motion segment.[9] The amount of anterior displacement is dependent upon the degree of posterior element failure (Fig. 12.8). In general, less than 25% anterior subluxation is indicative of facet subluxation (distractive flexion stage 1, DFS1), 25–50% subluxation indicative of unilateral facet dislocation (DFS2), and 50% or greater subluxation indicative of bilateral facet dislocation (DFS3). Full body displacement is defined as a DFS4 injury. All stages of flexion distraction injury may be associated with facet fractures as well.

Closed reduction should be attempted for all stages of distractive flexion injuries as soon as the patient is medically stable. Recent evidence from our spinal cord injury unit indicates that greater recovery of neurologic deficits is obtained in patients who were successfully reduced within 8 hours of injury.[40] Several authors have offered formulas for determining the weight required for reduction of cervical spine dislocations, but none has proved effective. Some authors recommend using no more than 22.5 kg of weight for fear of overdistraction.[22,117] High weight reduction has been reported with significantly higher success rates of attempted closed reduction.[37,38,116] In a recent report of 81 consecutive attempted closed reductions using weights of up to 54 kg (average 29 kg), the reduction success rate was 91%.[116] Following reduction, an MRI is completed to evaluate for compressive pathology.

Following successful closed reduction, patients with distractive flexion injuries treated by non-surgical methods in the halo-vest orthosis have up to a 64% incidence of late instability. Failure to achieve an adequate reduction or maintain reduction may be the result of a fracture dislocation with loss of the normal bony restraint against anterior displacement; this is normally provided by the articular processes. Primary posterior cervical fusion is preferred for patients in all stages of distractive flexion injuries when neurologically intact. Unsuccessful closed reduction requires open reduction and posterior cervical fusion. Patients with neurologic deficits usually require anterior decompression, discectomy, and fusion before posterior stabilization.

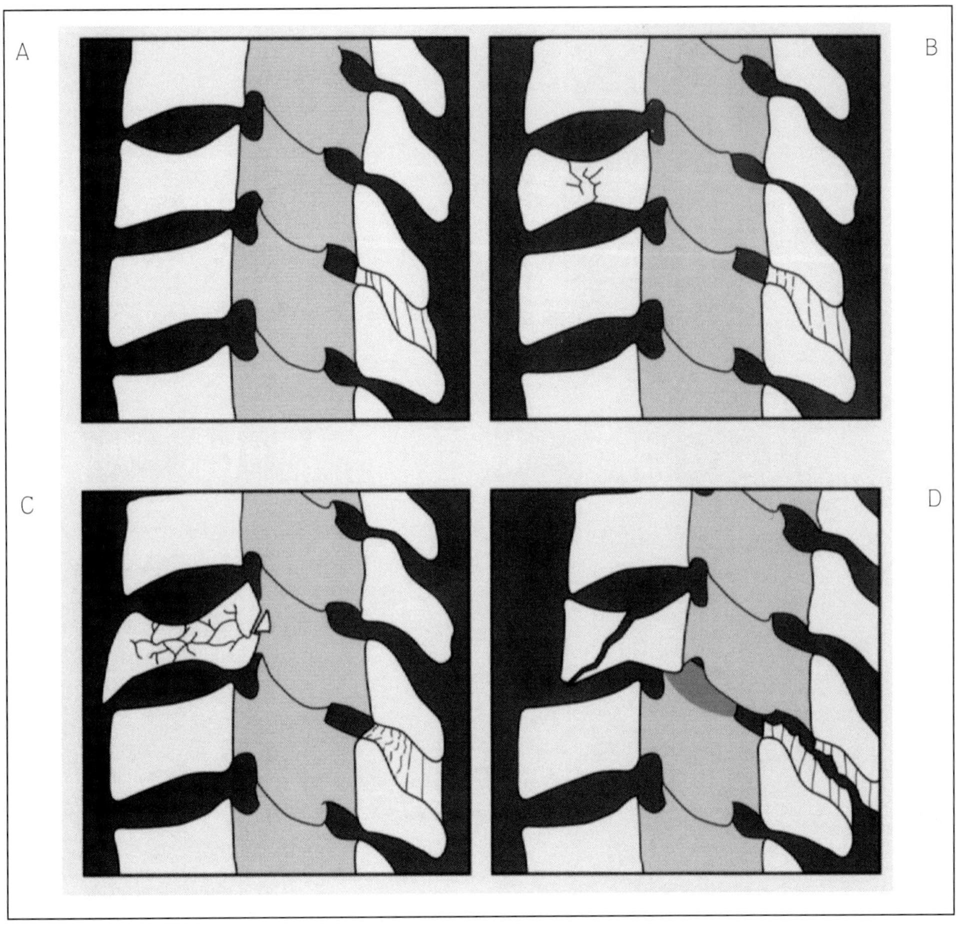

Figure 12.6
(A) Vertical compression stage 1 (VCS1): this lesion consists simply of a fracture of either the superior or inferior vertebral end-plate, resulting in a 'cup-like' deformity. The stage 1 lesion usually involves both the anterior and middle columns, but does not result in ligamentous failure. (B) Vertical compression stage 2 (VCS2): both vertebral end-plates are involved in a VCS2 lesion. Fracture lines may be demonstrated through the vertebral body, but displacement is minimal. Ligamentous structures remain intact. The spinal canal remains patent. (C) Vertical compression stage 3 (VCS3): this lesion represents simply a progression of the vertebral body damage as seen in a VCS2 lesion. The vertebral body has become fragmented, and residual pieces displace peripherally in multiple directions. The posterior portion of the vertebral body bulges into the neural canal, potentially compressing the spinal cord. This lesion occurs without significant ligamentous disruption. (D) VCS3 injury with ligamentous disruption through the anterior, middle, and posterior ligamentous columns, narrowing the neural canal by two mechanisms. Bone is retropulsed from the vertebral body, and approaches the lamina at the injured segment. Additionally, there is posterior translation through the motion segment, usually resulting in a complete neurologic injury

It has been recently recognized that 54–80% of patients with distractive flexion injuries have associated acute disc herniations at the level of injury.[57,96,99,100] Several authors have reported catastrophic neurological damage following closed reduction of this injury complex.[10,47,97,125] Careful review of these studies, however, indicates that many of these patients underwent closed reduction under general anesthesia. No case of neurologic deterioration caused by herniated nucleus pulposus during a conscious closed reduction has been reported. In a recent study, a 54% incidence of herniated nucleus pulposus, diagnosed by MRI, was seen in 50 consecutive cases of unilateral or bilateral facet dislocation.[102] All patients in this study underwent emergency attempted closed reduction with a

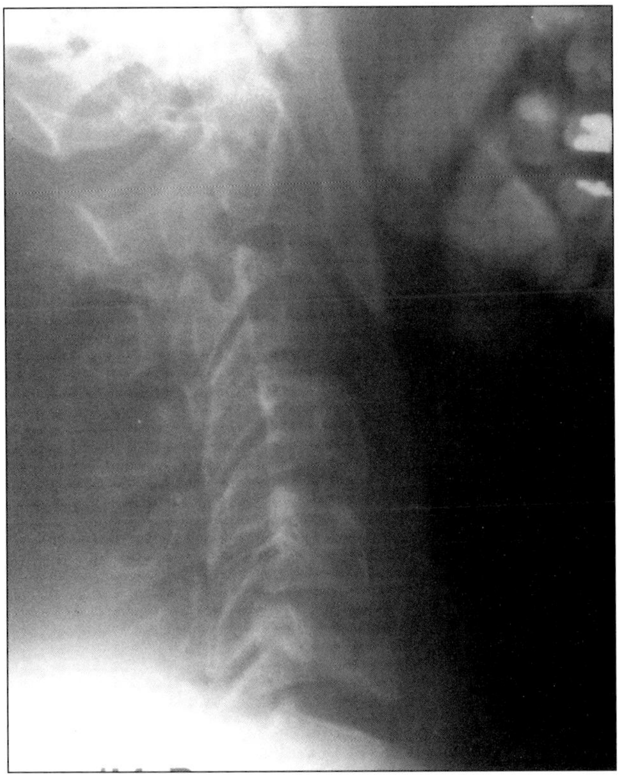

Figure 12.7
A lateral radiograph of a VCS3 injury with posterior vertebral body displacement and comminution. This patient sustained an incomplete injury requiring an anterior vertebrectomy and reconstruction followed by a posterior arthrodesis with a triple-wire technique

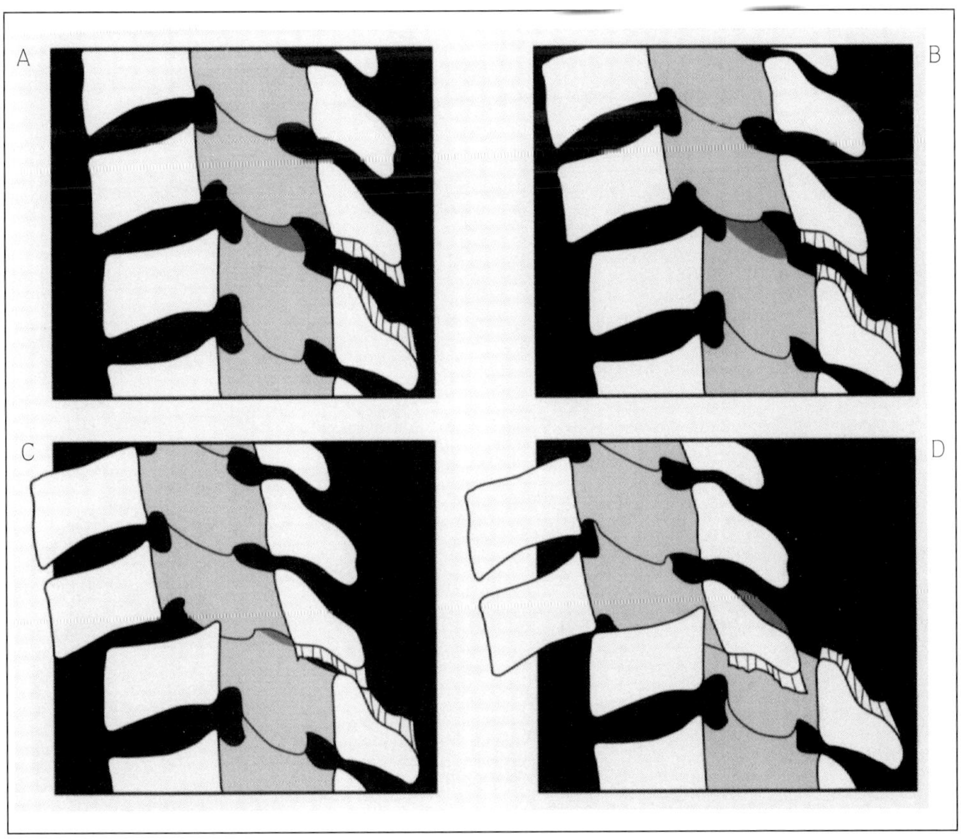

Figure 12.8
(A) Distractive flexion stage 1 (DFS1): with failure of the posterior ligamentous complex, subluxation of the facet joint occurs with interspinous widening and mild kyphosis. In the early stages, there may be a concomitant compressive failure of the anterior elements of the lower most vertebrae in the injured motion segment. This may, in fact, resemble the initial stages of a compressive flexion phylogeny. (D) Distractive flexion stage 2 (DFS2): this lesion represents a unilateral facet dislocation. Vertebral body translation with a unilateral facet dislocation is no more than 25%. Posterior and middle column disruption is complete. Anterior column ligamentous structures may remain intact. (C) Distractive flexion stage 3 (DFS3): this lesion represents a bilateral facet dislocation with approximately 50% vertebral body width translation anteriorly. The posterior surfaces of the superior vertebral articular process lie against the anterior surfaces of the inferior articular processes. (D) Distractive flexion stage 4 (DFS4): in the DFS4 injury, full vertebral body width translation occurs with injury to all ligamentous complexes

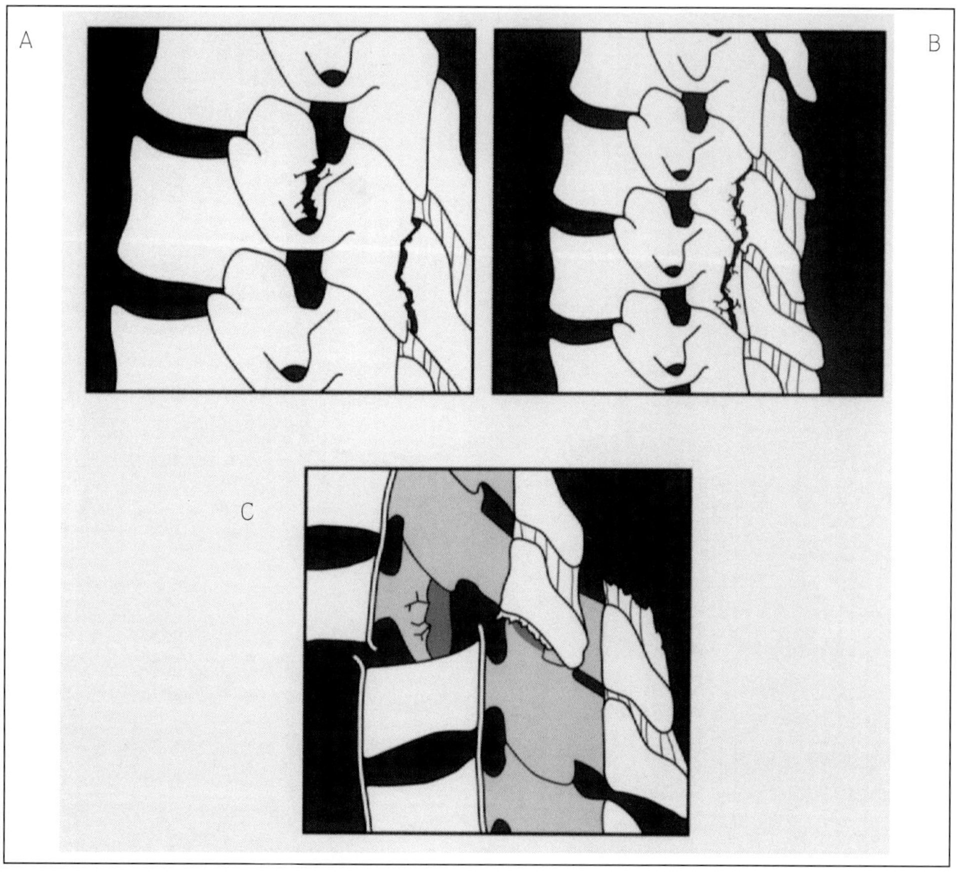

Figure 12.9
(A) Compressive extension stage 1 (CES1): this oblique view of the cervical spine demonstrates fracture through the pedicle and lamina of the injured vertebrae. The CES1 lesion consists of such fractures with or without rotatory vertebral body displacement. Laminar fractures are often difficult to see on plain radiographs. Oblique and pillar views will most reliably reveal CES1-type injuries. (B) Compressive extension stage 2 (CES2): oblique projection demonstrating bilaminar fractures, which most commonly occur at contiguous multiple levels. There is no evidence of other soft-tissue failure in the cervical motion segment. (C) Compressive extension stage 5 (CES5): this lesion consists of bilateral vertebral arch fractures and ligamentous failure of all three columns. With such an injury, vertebral body translation is seen, and often results in a complete spinal cord injury

success rate of 80%. The presence of a herniated disc had no effect upon the anatomic and neurologic outcome of attempted closed reduction in those 27 patients with herniated discs. Neurologically, four patients improved, and none worsened during the closed reduction attempt. Based on the results of this study, the authors continue to recommend conscious closed reduction of all cervical spine dislocations and severely comminuted fractures. Magnetic resonance imaging is not indicated before routine reduction, because the delay associated with obtaining an MRI may compromise neurologic recovery. For patients in which closed reduction fails, MRI is a prerequisite to open reduction. Patients with herniated discs should have anterior cervical discectomy before reduction and fusion. The authors recommend concomitant posterior arthrodesis and halo-vest immobilization.

Compressive Extension Injury

The most common mechanism responsible for compressive extension injuries includes motor vehicle accidents,

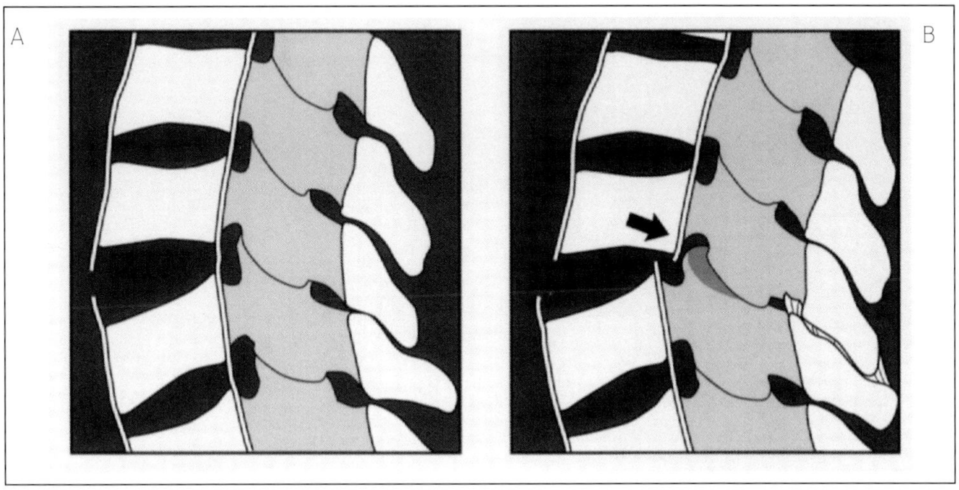

Figure 12.10
(A) Distractive extension stage 1 (DES1): this injury, alternatively, can occur through the anterior ligamentous complex or result from a transverse fracture through the vertebral body. Radiographically, there will be a widening of the disc space anteriorly at the injured segment without posterior vertebral body displacement. (B) Distractive extension stage 2 (DES2): this lesion is characterized by failure of all three ligamentous complexes through the involved motion segment with posterior vertebral body displacement into the neural canal. As this lesion often reduces with the head held in flexion, plain radiographic features may be subtle. However, MRI will delineate a significant three-column injury to the spine

falls, and diving accidents. Compressive extension injuries occur at all levels of the subaxial spine, and may be associated with C1–C2 injuries. Compression forces applied to the spine in extension result in early failure of the posterior column of the spine followed by failure of the anterior column. The injury may not be evident on the initial lateral radiograph. Oblique views or computed tomograms may be necessary to establish a diagnosis (Fig. 12.9). Stages 1 and 2 of compressive extension injuries result in single- or multi-level posterior element fractures without vertebral body displacement, which are best managed with a rigid cervical orthosis or halo-vest orthosis. Later stages are relatively uncommon, and were originally thought to be hypothetical in the original classification. Later stages are more unstable, and may require stabilization. Posterior cervical fusion using standard wire techniques may be difficult to perform with the multiple contiguous fractures at adjacent levels. Plate–screw constructs may be useful in these situations. If neurologic injury exists, preoperative MRI should be obtained, followed by appropriate decompression and stabilization. Neurologic compression may occur posteriorly or anteriorly with this mechanism. Decompression must obviously be directed toward the pathology, followed by appropriate stabilization procedures.

Distractive Extension Injury

Distractive extension injuries are most frequently caused by motor vehicle accidents and falls. The distractive forces applied to the spine in extension cause tensile failure and lengthening of both the anterior and posterior columns of the spine (Fig. 12.10). Failure can be either bony or ligamentous, and MRI is often helpful in determining the extent of soft-tissue injury. The injuries without evidence of vertebral body displacement on static and flexion–extension films (distractive extension stage 1 or DES1) can be treated in a rigid orthosis or halo as spontaneous ankylosis may occur. Alternatively, for anterior ligamentous injury, a primary anterior arthrodesis may be considered. Vertebral body displacement (DES2) mandates fusion. Anterior fusion with plate fixation is most often successful. Posterior fusion can be added in extremely unstable cases.

Lateral Flexion Injury

Lateral flexion injuries most frequently occur during motor vehicle accidents and blows to the side of the head. The asymmetric nature of force loading in the coronal plane results in tensile failure of one side of the spine, and

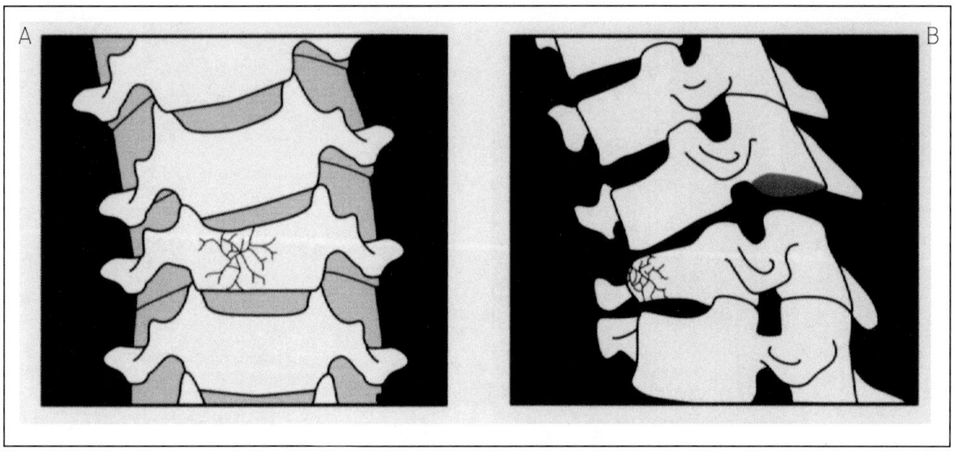

Figure 12.11
(A) Lateral flexion stage 1 (LFS1): this lesion simply consists of an asymmetric compression fracture of the vertebral body, and is often associated with an ipsilateral vertebral arch fracture. The asymmetric compression is most evident on the anteroposterior view. (B) Lateral flexion stage 2 (LFS2): lateral asymmetric compression of the vertebral body occurs with contralateral ligamentous failure or vertebral arch fracture with displacement as seen on the anteroposterior radiograph

compressive failure of the opposite side (Fig. 12.11). Once again, injuries without displacement (stage 1) can often be managed without surgery, whereas displaced injuries (stage 2) most frequently require surgical stabilization and fusion. Preoperative MRI may help to define the extent of soft-tissue injury.

Summary of Treatment Options for Cervical Spine Injuries

An algorithm of surgical decision making is given in Fig. 12.3 for each phylogeny and stage of injury. Certainly, debate and controversy exist concerning the need and type of surgical intervention. However, the authors feel strongly that aggressive management facilitates recovery and rehabilitative measures with minimal associated complications. The threshold for performing combined anterior and posterior procedures for decompression and stabilization is low, because the benefits of obtaining a well decompressed and stabilized cervical spine outweigh the risk for deformity, pseudoarthrosis, neurologic loss, and delayed rehabilitation. These recommendations are not iron-clad, but must be tailored to the specific needs and requirements of the individual case. However, adherence to these principles should minimize complication and maximize both the rehabilitative process and functional outcome.

Posterior Fusion Techniques

Posterior surgical stabilization of unstable lower cervical spine injuries represents an alternative to non-operative management and prolonged recumbency. Hadra, in 1891, reported the first case of posterior wiring for a fracture of the lower cervical spine.[56] Since then, numerous techniques for internal fixation and fusion of the cervical spine have been reported, and include wires, plates and screws, and laminar clamps.

One of the more popular procedures is the posterior spinous process wire technique, which is a modification of the Roger technique.[80,81,93,104,105] Patients are maintained in Gardner–Wells tongs traction on a Stryker frame and positioned prone. Alternatively, if a halo-vest orthosis has been placed before the operation, the anterior struts may be taped to the Stryker frame to secure the patient. For any patient being considered for surgery, an open C-shaped halo ring is used by the authors which permits posterior surgical access. In addition a halo composed of MRI-compatible material is preferred, in case postoperative studies are required. Tape is used to pull the shoulders toward the foot of the bed providing longitudinal traction. Once the patient is positioned, a lateral radiograph should be taken to verify maintenance of alignment.

A standard posterior surgical approach is used. Subperiosteal dissection is completed with electrocautery to minimize blunt trauma across the injured segment and, potentially, to underlying neurologic structures. A Cobb elevator is used only for retraction of soft tissues during subperiosteal dissection. The dissection is carried to the lateral edge of the lateral masses and self-retaining retractors placed. Care is taken not to disrupt the facet capsule of uninvolved segments. A lateral radiograph is repeated at any time there is uncertainty about the operative level.

Regardless of the particular wire technique, involved drill holes must be placed through the base of the spinous process. Ideally, a right-angled, 2-mm burr is used at the junction of the spinous process and lamina. Often, the surgeon is able to pass the burr safely to the opposite side of the spinous process. Alternatively, the cortex of the opposite side can be drilled separately and the holes then connected with a towel clip.

In the cephalad vertebra, the hole should be placed in the cephalad portion of the base of the spinous processes to prevent the wire cutting through as a result of the caudal-directed force when tightened. Likewise, the hole placed in the caudad vertebra should be placed in the caudal portion of the base of the spinous process to prevent cephalad cutting through. A stainless steel wire (16 or 18 gauge) is then passed through the holes, and a corticocancellous bone graft harvested from the iliac crest and fashioned to the appropriate size. Holes are then made in the graft for passage of the wires. The wires on the right and left sides are tightened together with compression of the graft onto the decorticated surface of the posterior elements. Such simultaneous twisting is important to achieve symmetric tension across the involved vertebral levels. If interspace widening is present, a third wire may be passed through the hole in cephalad vertebrae, and then around the caudal spinous process and tightened to augment stability. If used, this third wire should be placed before securing the bone graft.

Bone graft harvesting is a relatively simple and safe procedure, although it warrants a few comments. For isolated posterior cervical fusions, a curvilinear incision, based at the posterior superior iliac spine and extending anteriorly along the crest, is made. Then an oscillating saw is used to remove a tricortical graft of appropriate length. Ideally the width of the graft is 2.0 cm. Following this, the saw is used to split the graft in half, creating two unicortical slabs of bone, into which drill holes are placed at appropriate levels to allow passage of wires. Positioning of the grafts is also important. The graft is slid down the spinous process wires, contacting the decorticated spinous process and laminar surfaces. The cortical edge of the graft is placed under the bulbous portion of the spinous process, maximizing bony contact and securing the graft during the tightening process. The posterior elements are routinely decorticated at each level to be fused using a high-speed burr; other authors have reported, however, good results without decortication.[14]

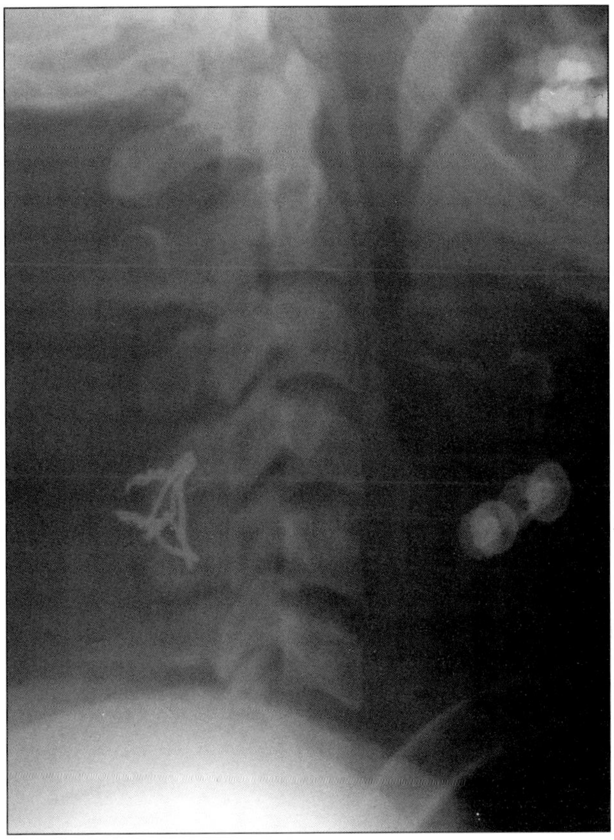

Figure 12.12
Postoperative lateral radiograph of a posterior cervical arthrodesis performed with a triple-wire technique. The cephalad wires are placed through a drill hole, which was placed in the most cephalad portion of the cephalad spinous process. The inferior wires are placed through the most inferior aspect of the spinous process. This construct is extremely stable, as shown through biomechanical testing

Bohlman's triple-wire technique is a popular approach to posterior fusion, and is the technique preferred by the authors.[82,83] One midline tethering wire of 20–22 gauge stainless steel is passed through and around the involved spinous processes; this is then passed through and around the most superior and the most inferior spinous processes. Placing the wire in this way prevents a 'cheese-cutter' effect of the wire cutting through the bone. Once this is completed, two additional 16- or 18-gauge wires are placed through the graft as described previously and tightened simultaneously (Fig. 12.12). It is the authors' belief that patients should be maintained in a halo-vest orthosis after surgery until union occurs. This technique is described in further detail in Chapter 19.

Another described technique of posterior cervical fusion is known as the Dewar procedure.[32,42,113] Following a standard posterior approach and light decortication of the spinous processes and laminae, corticocancellous grafts are laid on the base of the spinous process and lamina, with the cancellous surfaces opposing. Drill holes are first placed through the graft at the level of the spinous process. Kirschner wires are then introduced percutaneously and successively through the paraspinal muscles, the pre-drilled graft, the base of the spinous process, and then out through the second pre-drilled graft. The K wires are then cut off within 1 cm of the grafts, and 18-gauge wire looped around the inferior spinous process, brought cephalad around the K wires, and tied in front of the distal spinous process. Several series have reported excellent fusion rates using this technique.[17,32,42]

Lateral mass screws and plates were introduced as an alternative to posterior wiring techniques. Several screw-insertion techniques have been proposed. The most popular techniques employed are those of Magerl, Anderson, and Roy-Camille;[8,63,107] these techniques share the common goal of achieving purchase in the lateral articular mass. Magerl's[63] described starting point is 2–3 mm medial and cephalad to the intersection of the lines bisecting the exposed lateral mass, whereas Roy-Camille's[107] starting point is at the intersection of these two lines. Magerl then angles the drill 25° laterally, parallel to the surface of the superior articular process, whereas Roy-Camille screws are angled 10° laterally, perpendicular to the posterior vertebral cortex.[63,107] Anderson recommended placing the screws 1 mm medial to the center of the lateral mass, parallel to the facet joints and directed 10° laterally.[62] The methods of Magerl and Roy-Camille both attempt to avoid the central area ventral to the articular mass, where the exiting nerve root can be found. Finally the plates are secured, followed by bone grafting. When one motion segment (two vertebrae) is to be stabilized, holes are drilled bilaterally in the articular pillars of the two vertebrae. Likewise, if two motion segments are to be stabilized, then holes are drilled bilaterally in the pillars of the three vertebrae involved.

There are several factors that may help increase the safety margin of screw insertion. First, a thorough understanding of the anatomy is crucial, and care must be taken to expose the entire lateral mass fully, including clearance of all osteophytes to define its borders. Second, the use of an image intensifier will help guide placement. Third, smooth-tipped screws are preferred over pointed self-tapping screws to prevent injury to the nerve root or vertebral artery. Using a drill with a stop to prevent inadvertent penetration or, alternatively, drilling the hole manually is safe and provides better proprioceptive feedback to the surgeon. Last, bicortical purchase of the screws adds to the strength of the construct; however, care must be exercised not to allow excessive penetration beyond the ventral cortex. The procedure is more technically demanding than wire-fixation techniques, with theoretical risk of injury to the spinal nerves and vertebral arteries. Several biomechanical studies have demonstrated no significant difference in strength when compared to other posterior fusion techniques, leading some to recommend its use only as an alternative procedure.[34,121] Extension injury patterns with the associated spinous process fractures and/or laminar fractures may, however, preclude the use of standard posterior wiring techniques. It is this type of injury pattern with associated posterior element disruption that may constitute a good indication for posterior plating. Additionally, patients with post-laminectomy instability or significant rotational instability may benefit from posterior plate fixation.

The Halifax clamp has been reported as an alternative method of posterior cervical fixation. A stainless steel clamp is applied to the laminae of the segments to be fused. Holness reported satisfactory results in 51 patients over a 10-year period.[62] The authors believe, however, that this technique offers inferior stability compared to the described wiring and plating techniques. It offers support or resistance to flexion, but is limited in its resistance to rotation or extension.

Anterior Fusion Techniques

The anterior approach to the cervical spine is useful for both fusion and surgical decompression of the anterior spinal cord. The Smith–Robinson[114] surgical approach, described in 1959, has been the cornerstone of treatment for patients at the authors' institution with partial and complete neurologic involvement. The authors prefer a right-sided surgical approach. Care must be taken not to injure the recurrent laryngeal nerve as it crosses the C6 level from the tracheoesophageal groove. The patient is placed in cervical traction through Gardner–Wells tongs or the traction bail of the halo ring. A transverse incision generally suffices for two- and three-level exposure. An oblique incision along the medial border of the sternocleidomastoid is made for more than three-level exposures. The platysma muscle is sharply divided, and the deep cervical fascia encountered as it surrounds the sternocleidomastoid muscle; this fascia is divided just anterior to the border of the muscle. The dissection is directed medial to the carotid sheath through the pre-tracheal fascia. A plane is developed between the carotid sheath and the trachea with further medial dissection, allowing medial retraction of the esophagus; the anterior surface of the spinal column can then be visualized. The prevertebral fascia, which overlies the anterior cervical column, is highly vascular and should be incised with bipolar electrocautery. Subperiosteal dissection is carried medially and laterally, allowing placement of a self-retaining retractor underneath the periosteal edges and longus colli muscles, thereby avoiding direct traction on the esophagus, trachea, sympathetic chain, and contents of the carotid sheath. Intraoperative radiographs with a marker in the intervertebral disc are used to confirm the appropriate level. The annulus is incised sharply, and the disc material removed in a piecemeal fashion with pituitary rongeurs and curettes. Every attempt should be made to preserve the posterior longitudinal ligament and posterior osteophytes.[65] Measurements of the disc space are made and a tricortical iliac crest graft used that measures approximately 1 cm in depth and 6–8 mm in height. Before placement of the graft, the end-plates are lightly decorticated with a high-speed burr. The burr is then used to create a transverse groove in the superior end-plate, effectively creating a notch to help lock in the graft which is gently placed in the intervertebral space using a tamp. The graft is recessed 1–2 mm posterior to the anterior edge of the vertebra, and a probe used to verify that there is no posterior impingement of the graft into the spinal canal. Traction is removed, and the wounds are irrigated and closed over suction drains.

In cases involving severe vertebral body comminution and/or collapse, a corpectomy may be indicated. When performing a fusion in conjunction with a vertebral corpectomy, the superior and inferior vertebrae should be fashioned to create a peg and slot or two slots. The space spanning the superior and inferior vertebrae is filled by an appropriately sized, tricortical iliac crest strut graft; it is important to make sure that the graft spans the superior end-plate of the proximal uninvolved vertebra to the inferior end-plate of the distal uninvolved vertebra. Again, caution must be used when placing the graft to prevent posterior impingement into the spinal canal or kyphosis. If any suspicion of posterior instability exists, then the patient is turned, and posterior fusion performed (Fig. 12.13). Posterior instability is a relative contraindication to performing an anterior fusion as the primary treatment. Long-term results using one-stage anterior decompression and posterior stabilization with circumferential arthrodesis have been reported recently with low morbidity, and 93% improvement in patients with incomplete neurologic injuries.[86]

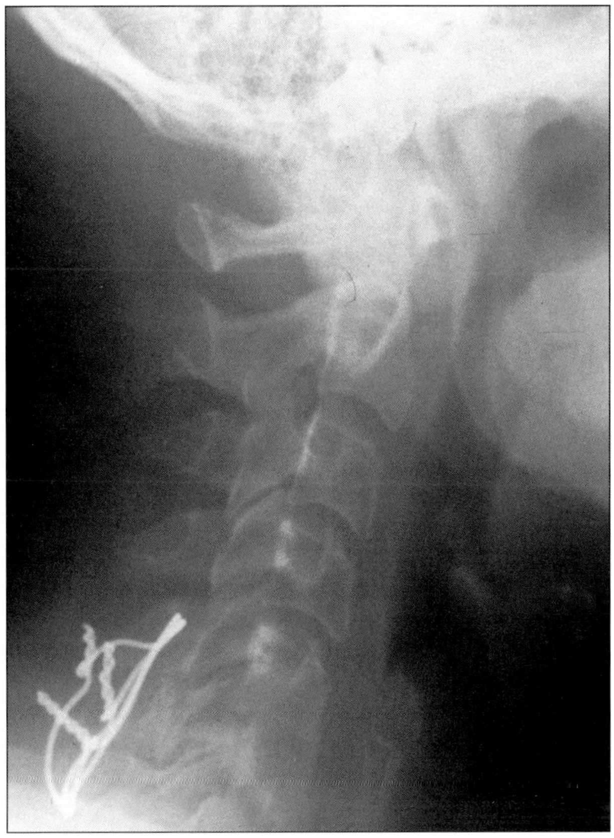

Figure 12.13
Lateral radiograph of a patient requiring combined anterior decompression and reconstruction followed by a posterior arthrodesis. An iliac crest strut graft is well seated. A posterior arthrodesis is used to enhance the stability of the construct and promote early healing

The role of anterior plate fixation following anterior decompression and fusion remains controversial. In vitro biomechanical studies have demonstrated that combined anterior and posterior stabilization procedures are significantly stronger than isolated anterior or posterior constructs. One recently reported series (15 patients) had a high rate of union (93%) using anterior plating following anterior decompression and fusion.[84] Two screws are placed in each vertebral body. The issue of bicortical versus unicortical screws remains controversial. Bicortical screws provide increased stability, but, if inserted, caution must be used to avoid entering the spinal canal. This complication can be minimized by using fluoroscopic control as well as a drill-stop technique to palpate for decreased resistance as it enters the spinal canal. Proper alignment of the spine should be achieved before inserting the plates and the screws because they must not be directed into the disc space. Complication rates as high as 40% have been reported, although this value appears to be decreasing as familiarity with the technique increases. If there is any evidence of screw loosening, the implant should be removed immediately to prevent late complications associated with erosion into adjacent structures. As stated, the precise indications for anterior plating remain controversial. Biomechanically, these plates serve as a tension band and, therefore, the anterior plate is most effective in extension injuries, preventing cervical spinal distraction or tension across the intervertebral disc. Plates placed anteriorly are at a biomechanical disadvantage in controlling widening of the facet joints and posterior structures. As most injuries in the cervical spine involve distraction flexion patterns, most patients would be better managed with one-stage anterior decompression and fusion with sequential posterior wiring, rather than augmenting an anterior fusion with anterior internal fixation alone.

This type of postoperative immobilization continues to be controversial, although the authors' preference has been to immobilize these patients in a halo-vest orthosis until union occurs, regardless of surgical approach or technique.

The biomechanics of the different cervical fixation devices have been studied by a number of authors.[3,51,121] Several studies have compared fixation techniques (Roger's wire technique, Bohlman's triple-wire technique, sublaminar wires, Magerl posterior hook plate, Roy-Camille posterior plate, and Caspar anterior plate), and found that, with cyclical testing, the anterior cervical plate instrumentation proved inadequate and was the least rigid of all those tested. There were no significant differences among any of the posterior stabilization methods tested. The authors concluded that there is no place for sublaminar wire fixation, because of the increased risks associated with their placement. They also felt that posterior plating offered no additional advantage over posterior wiring techniques, especially given the greater technical challenge associated with their insertion. Finally, the use of methyl methacrylate has been condemned by a number of the authors in the treatment of acute or chronic traumatic injuries.[49,85] Its use has only been justified in cases of pathologic cervical spine fractures.[46]

REFERENCES

1 *Advanced Trauma Life Support Course by Committee on Trauma*, 3rd ed, 9–24. American College of Surgeons, 1991.

2 Aebi M, Mohler J, Zach GA, Morscher E. Indication, surgical technique and results of 100 surgically treated fractures and fracture-dislocations of the cervical spine. *Clin Orthop* **203**: 244–257, 1980.

3 Albert TJ, Levine MJ, Balderston RA, Cotler JM. GI complications in spinal cord injury. *Spine* **16**(suppl.): S522–S525, 1991.

4 Allen BL, Anderson LD, Barr JS, *et al.* Fractures and dislocations. In Sherk HH, Dunn EJ, Eismont FJ, *et al.* (eds), *The Cervical Spine*, 2nd ed., Chapter 6, 286–463. Cervical Spine Research Society. Philadelphia: JB Lippincott, 1989.

5 Allen BL, Ferguson RL, Lehmann TR, O'Brien RP. A mechanistic classification of closed, indirect fractures and dislocations of the lower cervical spine. *Spine* **7**: 1–27, 1982.

6 American Spinal Injury Association. *Standard for Neurologic and Functional Class of Spinal Cord Injury.* Chicago: American Spinal Injury Association, 1992.

7 Anderson PA, Bohlman HH. Anterior decompression and arthrodesis in patients with motor complete cervical spinal cord injury: Long-term neurologic recovery in 52 patients. Part II. *J Bone Joint Surg [Am]* **74**: 683–692, 1992.

8 Anderson PA, Henley MB, Grady MS, Montesano PX, Winn GR. Posterior cervical arthrodesis with AO reconstruction plates and bone graft. *Spine* **16**: 72–79, 1991.

9 Annertz M, Persson L, et al. Posterior wiring without bony fusion in traumatic distractive flexion injuries of the mid to lower cervical spine. Long-term follow-up in 30 patient. *Spine* **16**: 467–472, 1991.

10 Apple DF, McDonald AR, Smith RA. Identification of herniated nucleus pulposus in spinal cord injury. *Paraplegia* **25**: 78–85, 1987.

11 Bailey RW, Badgley CE. Stabilization of the cervical spine by anterior fusion. *J Bone Joint Surg [Am]* **42**: 565–594, 1992.

12 Beers JG, Raque GH, Wagner GG, et al. MR imaging in acute cervical spine trauma. *J Comput Assist Tomogr* **12**: 755–761, 1988.

13 Benzel EC, Larson SJ. Functional recovery after decompressive operation for thoracic and lumbar spine fractures. *Neurosurgery* **19**: 772–778, 1986.

14 Benzel EC, Larson SJ. Recovery of nerve root function after complete quadriplegia from cervical spine fractures. *Neurosurgery* **19**: 809–812, 1986.

15 Benzel EC, Larson SJ. Functional recovery after decompressive spine operation for cervical spine fractures. *Neurosurgery* **20**: 742–746, 1987.

16 Bernhardt M, White AA, Panjabi MM, McGowan DP. Biomechanical considerations of spinal stability. In Rothman RH, Simeone FA (eds), *The Spine*, 3rd ed, 1167–1195. Philadelphia: WB Saunders, 1992.

17 Bernstein AJ, Simmons EH, Capicotto WN, Simmons ED, Delahunt SP, Graziano GP. The Dewar posterior cervical fusion: Description and comparative results. Presented at the Annual Meeting of the Cervical Spine Research Society, Palm Desert, California, December 1992.

18 Bohlman HH. Acute fractures and dislocations of the cervical spine: An analysis of 300 hospitalized patients and review of the literature. *J Bone Joint Surg [Am]* **61**: 1119–1142, 1979.

19 Bohlman HH. Late anterior decompression and fusion for spinal cord injuries: Review of 100 cases with long term results. *Orthop Trans* **4**: 42–43, 1980.

20 Bohlman HH, Anderson PA. The Neck. In D'Ambrosia RD (ed.) *Musculoskeletal Disorders, Regional Examination, Differential Diagnosis*, 2nd ed, 219–86. Philadelphia: JB Lippincott, 1985.

21 Bohlman HH, Anderson PA. Anterior decompression and arthrodesis in patients with incomplete cervical spinal cord injury: Long-term results of neurologic recovery in 58 patients. Part I. *J Bone Joint Surg [Am]* **74**: 671–682, 1992.

22 Bohlman HH, Ducker TB, Levine AM, McAfee PC. Spine trauma in adults. In Rothman RH, Simeone FA (eds), *The Spine*, 3rd Ed. Philadelphia: WB Saunders, 973–1166, 1992.

23 Bohlman HH, Freehafer A, Dejak J. The results of treatment of acute injury of the upper thoracic spine with paralysis. *J Bone Joint Surg [Am]* **67**: 360–369, 1985.

24 Bohlman HH, Zdeblick TA. Complications of treatment of fractures and dislocations of the cervical spine. In Epps C (ed.), *Complications of Orthopaedic Surgery*, 897–918. Philadelphia: JB Lippincott, 1985.

25 Bracken MB, Collins WF, Frieman DF, et al. Efficacy of methylprednisolone in acute spinal cord injury. *JAMA* **251**: 45–52, 1984.

26 Bracken MB, Shepard MJ, Collins WF, *et al.* A randomized, controlled trial of methylprednisolone or naloxone in the treatment of acute spinal cord injury. Results of the second national acute spinal cord injury study. *N Engl J Med* **322**: 1405–1411, 1990;

27 Bracken MB, Shepard MJ, Hefenbrand KG, et al. Methylprednisolone and neurologic function one year post spinal cord injury. *J Neurosurg* **63**: 704–713, 1985.

28 Brodkey JS, Miller CF Jr, Harmody RM. The syndrome of acute central cervical spinal cord injury revisited. *Surg Neurol* **14**: 251–257, 1980.

29 Bucci MN, Dauser RC, Maynard FA, Hoff JT. Management of post-traumatic cervical spine instability: Operative fusion versus halo-vest immobilization. Analysis of 49 cases. *J Trauma* **28**: 1001–1006, 1988.

30 Bucholz RD, Cheung KC. Halo-vest versus spinal fusion for cervical injury: Evidence from an outcome study. *J Neurosurg* **70**: 884–892, 1989.

31 Burke DC, Berryman D. The place of closed manipulation in the management of flexion-rotation dislocations of the cervical spine. *J Bone Joint Surg [Am]* **53**: 165–182, 1971.

32 Capicotto WN, Simmons EH, Graziano G. The Dewar fusion in traumatic injuries to the cervical spine. *Orthop Trans* **13**: 206, 1989.

33 Chakeres DW, Flickinger F, Bresnahan JC, et al. MR imaging of acute spinal cord trauma. *Am J Neurol Res* **8**: 5, 1987.

34 Coe JD, Warden KE. Biomechanical evaluation of cervical spinal stabilization methods in a human cadaveric model. *Spine* **14**: 1122–1131, 1989.

35 Cooper PR, Maravilla KR, Sklar FH, Moody SF, Clark WK. Halo immobilization of cervical spine fractures: Indications and results. *J Neurosurg* **50**: 603–610, 1979.

36 Cotler HB, Kulkarni MV, Bondurant FJ. Magnetic resonance imaging of acute spinal cord trauma: Preliminary report. *J Orthop Trauma* **2**: 1–4, 1988.

37 Cotler HB, Miller LS, DeLucia FA, Cotler JM, Davne SH. Closed reduction of cervical spine dislocations. *Clin Orthop* **214**: 185–199, 1987.

38 Cotler JM, Hervison GJ, Nasuti JF, Ditunno JF, An HS. Closed reduction of traumatic cervical spine dislocations using traction weights up to 140 pounds. Presented at the Annual Meeting of the Cervical Spine Research Society, Philadelphia, Pennsylvania, December 1991.

39 Cotler JM, Hussey RW. Spinal injuries. In Dee R (ed.), *Principles of Orthopaedic Practice*, 907–931. New York: McGraw-Hill, 1989.

40 Cotler JM, Nasuti J, Ditunno JF, An HS. Improvement of motor index score after rapid closed reduction of traumatic cervical spine dislocation using traction weights up to 130 pounds. Presented at the Annual Meeting of American Spinal Injury Association, Toronto, Ontario, Canada, 1992.

41 Daffner RH, Deeb ZL, Rothfus WE. The posterior vertebral body line: Importance in the detection of burst fractures. *Am J Roentgenol Radium Ther Nucl Med* **148**: 93–96, 1987.

42 Davey JR, Rorabeck CH, Bailey SI, Bourne RB, Dewar FP. A technique of posterior cervical fusion for instability of the cervical spine. *Spine* **10**: 722–728, 1985.

43 Denis F. The three column spine and its significance in the classification of acute thoracolumbar spinal injuries. *Spine* **8**: 817–831, 1983.

44 Dolan EJ, Tator CH, Endrenyi L. The value of decompression for acute experimental spinal cord injury. *J Neurosurg* **53**: 749–755, 1980.

45 Ducker TB, Lucas JT, Walleck CA. Recovery from spinal cord injury. *Clin Neurosurg* **30**: 495–513, 1983.

46 Dunn EJ. The role of methylmethacrylate in the stabilization and replacement of tumors of the cervical spine. A project of the Cervical Spine Research Society. *Spine* **2**: 15–24, 1977.

47 Eismont FJ, Arena MJ, Green BA. Extrusion of an intervertebral disc associated with traumatic subluxation or dislocation of facets. *J Bone Joint Surg [Am]* **73**: 1555–1560, 1991.

48 Eismont FJ, Bohlman HH. Posterior methylmethacrylate fixation for cervical trauma. *Spine* **6**: 347–353, 1981.

49 Galli RL, Spaite DW, Simmon RR. The cervical spine. In *Emergency Orthopaedics*, 96–99. East Norwalk, CT: Appleton and Lange, 1989.

50 Garfin SR, Botte MJ, Waters RL, Nickel VL. Complications in the use of the halo fixation device. *J Bone Joint Surg [Am]* **68**: 320–325, 1986.

51 Gill K, Paschal S, Corin J, Ashman R, Bucholz RW. Posterior plating of the cervical spine. A biomechanical comparison of different posterior fusion techniques. *Spine* **13**: 813–816, 1988.

52 Gisbert VL, Hollerman JJ, Ney AL, et al. Incidence and diagnosis of C7–T1 fractures and subluxations in multiple-trauma patients: Evaluation of the advanced trauma life support guidelines. *Surgery* **106**: 702–709, 1989,

53 Goldberg AL, Rothfus WE, Deeb ZL, *et al.* The impact of magnetic resonance on the diagnostic evaluation of acute cervicothoracic spinal trauma. *Skeletal Radiol* **17**: 89, 1988.

54 Gooding MR, Wilson CB, Hoff JT. Experimental cervical myelopathy. Effects of ischemia and compression of the canine cervical spine. *Neurosurgery* **43**: 9–12, 1975.

55 Green D, Lee MY, Ito V, et al. Fixed versus adjusted dose heparin in prophylaxis of thromboembolism in spinal cord injury. *JAMA* **260**: 1255–1258, 1988.

56 Hadra BE. The Classic: Wiring the vertebrae as a means of immobilization in fractures and Pott's disease. *Clin Orthop* **112**: 4–8, 1975.

57 Harrington JF, Likavel MJ, Smith AS. Disc herniation in cervical fracture subluxation. *Neurosurgery* **29**: 374–379, 1991.

58 Heckman JD (ed.), *Emergency Care and Transportation of the Sick and Injured*, 5th ed, 334–349. Chicago: American Academy of Orthopaedic Surgeons, 1992.

59 Herkowitz HR, Rothman RH. Subacute instability of the cervical spine. *Spine* **9**: 348–352, 1984.

60 Holdsworth FW. Fractures, dislocations, and fracture-dislocations of the spine. *J Bone Joint Surg [Am]* **52**: 1534–1551, 1970.

61 Holdsworth FW, Hardy A. Early treatment of paraplegia from fractures of the thoracolumbar spine. *J Bone Joint Surg [Br]* **35**: 540–550, 1953.

62 Holness RO, Huestis WS, Howes WJ, Langille RA. Posterior stabilization with an interlaminar clamp in cervical injuries: Technical note and review of the long-term experience with the method. *Neurosurgery* **14**: 318–322, 1984.

63 Jeanneret B, Magerl F, Ward EW, Ward JCH. Posterior stabilization of the cervical spine with hook plates. *Spine* **16**: 56–63, 1991.

64 Johnson RM, Hart DL, Simmons EF, Ramshy GR, Southwick WO. Cervical orthoses. *J Bone Joint Surg [Am]* **59**: 332–339, 1977.

65 Jones AA, Rothman RH, Balderston RA. Fusion techniques for degenerative disease. In Cotler JM, Cotler HB (eds), *Spinal Fusion: Science and Technique*, 139–168. New York: Springer-Verlag, 1990.

66 Kalfas I, Wilberger J, Goldberg A, Prostko R. Magnetic resonance imaging in acute spinal cord trauma. *Neurosurgery* **23**: 295–299, 1988.

67 Kauffer H, Hayes JT. Lumbar fracture-dislocations: A study of 21 cases. *J Bone Joint Surg [Am]* **48**: 712–730, 1966.

68 Keenen TL, Antony J, Benson DR. Non-contiguous spinal fractures. *J Trauma* **30**: 489–491, 1990.

69 Koch RA, Nickel VL. The halo-vest: An evaluation of motion and forces across the neck. *Spine* **3**: 103–107, 1978.

70 Kostuick JP. Indications for use of halo immobilization. *Clin Orthop* **154**: 46–50, 1981.

71 Krengel WF, Anderson PA, Hansen Y, Ayley JC. Early versus delayed stabilization after cervical spinal cord injury. Presented at the Annual Meeting of the North American Spine Society, Boston, Massachusetts, 1992.

72 Kulkarni MV, McArdle CB, Kopanicky D, et al. Acute spinal cord injury: MR imaging at 1.5 T. *Radiology* **164**: 837, 1987.

73 Lahd WH. Efficacy of the post-traumatic cross table lateral view of the cervical spine. *Emerg Med* **2**: 243, 1985.

74 Leramo OB, Tator CH, Hudson AR. Massive gastroduodenal hemorrhage and perforation in acute spinal cord injury. *Surg Neurol* **17**: 186–190, 1982.

75 Levi L, Wolf A, Rigamonti D, Ragheb J, Mirvis S, Robinson WL. Anterior decompression of cervical spine trauma. Does timing of surgery affect outcome? *Neurosurgery* **29**: 216–222, 1987.

76 Lind B, Sihlbom H, Nordwall A. Halo-vest treatment of unstable traumatic cervical spine injuries. *Spine* **13**: 425–432, 1988.

77 Lodge T, Higgenbottom E. Fractures and dislocations of the cervical spine. *X-Ray Focus* **7**: 2, 1966.

78 Marshall FM, Reynolds GG, Fountains S, Wilmot C, Hamilton R. Neurologic prognosis after traumatic quadriplegia. *J Neurosurg* **50**: 611–616, 1979.

79 Merli GJ, Herbison GJ, Ditunno JF, et al. Deep venous thrombosis prophylaxis in acute spinal cord injury patients. *Arch Phys Med Rehabil* **69**: 661–664, 1988.

80 Meyer PR. *Surgery of Spine Trauma*. New York: Churchill Livingstone, 1989.

81 Meyer PR Jr, Cotler HB. Fusion Techniques for Traumatic Injuries. In Cotler JM, Cotler HB (eds), *Spinal Fusion: Science and Technique*, 189–247. New York: Springer-Verlag, 1990.

82 McAfee PC, Bohlman HH. The triple wire fixation technique for stabilization. *Orthop Trans* **9**: 142, 1985.

83 McAfee PC, Bohlman HH. The triple wire fixation technique for stabilization. *Orthop Trans* **10**: 455, 1986.

84 McAfee PC, Bohlman HH. One stage anterior cervical decompression and posterior stabilization with circumferential arthrodesis. A study of 24 patients who had a traumatic or a neoplastic lesion. *J Bone Joint Surg [Am]* **71**: 78–88, 1989.

85 McAfee PC, Bohlman HH, Ducker T, Eismont FJ. Failure of stabilization of the spine with methylmethacrylate. *J Bone Joint Surg [Am]* **68**: 1145–157, 1986.

86 McAfee PC, Zeidman SM, Ducker TB, Bohlman HH. Combined anterior cervical decompression and posterior stabilization: Review of 75 cases. Presented at the Annual Meeting of the Cervical Spine Research Society, Palm Desert, California, December 1992.

87 McGuire RA, Degnan G, Amundson GM. Evaluation of current extrication orthoses in immobilization of the unstable cervical spine. *Spine* **15**: 1064–1067, 1990.

88 Miller LS, Cotler HB, DeLucia FA, Cotler JM, Hume EL. Biomechanical analysis of cervical distraction. *Spine* **12**: 831–837, 1987.

89 Miller MP, Gehweiler JA, Martinez S, et al. Significant new observations on cervical spine trauma. *Am J Roentgenol Radium Ther Nucl Med* **130**: 659–663., 1978.

90 .More SE. Emergency evaluation of cervical spine injuries: CT versus radiographs. *Ann Emerg Med* **14**: 973, 1985.

91 Morgan TH, Wharton GW, Austin GN. The results of laminectomy in patients with incomplete spinal cord injuries. *Paraplegia* **9**: 14–23, 1971.

92 Naidich JB, Naidich TP, Garein C, et al. Interspinous distance: A useful sign of anterior cervical dislocation in the spinal frontal projection. *Radiology* **123**: 113–116, 1977.

93 Norrell HA. Fractures and dislocations of the spine. In Rothman RH, Simeone FA (eds), *The Spine*, 3rd ed, 529–566. Philadelphia: WB Saunders, 1952.

94 Osterholm JL. *The Pathophysiology of Spinal Cord Trauma*. Springfield, IL: Thomas, 1978.

95 Piazza MR, Balderston RA, Cotler JM. Complications in cervical spine injury. In Balderston RA, An HS (eds) *Complications in Spinal Injury*, 105–136. Philadelphia: WB Saunders, 1991.

96 Pratt ES, Green DA, Spengler DM. Herniated intervertebral discs associated with unstable spinal injuries. *Spine* **15**: 662–665, 1990.

97 Raflin G, Jenneret B, Magerl F. Tetraplegia following cervical spine fusion. Presented at the Annual Meeting of the Cervical Spine Research Society, European Section, St Gallen, Switzerland, 1989.

98 Ramsey M, Rizzolo SJ, Cotler JM, Balderston RA, Solit R. Temporary immobilization of unstable cervical spine injuries in the halo-vest orthosis. Presented at the Annual Meeting of the Cervical Spine Research Society, Palm Desert, California, December 1992.

99 Raynor RB. Cervical cord compression secondary to acute disc protrusion in trauma. *Spine* **2**: 39–43, 1977.

100 Rizzolo SJ, Piazza MR, Cotler JM, Balderston RA, Schaefer D, Flanders A. Intervertebral disc injury complicating cervical spine trauma. *Spine* **16**(suppl.): S187–S189, 1991.

101 Rizzolo SJ, Piazza MR, Cotler JM, Hume EL, Cautilli GA, O'Neill D. The effect of torque pressure on halo pin complication rates: A randomized prospective study. *Spine* (in press).

102 Rizzolo SJ, Vaccaro AR, Cotler JM, Balderston RA, Ergener J, Dailey S. Incidence and clinical implications of disc injury in patients with acute cervical spine dislocations. Presented at the Annual Meeting of the American Academy of Orthopaedic Surgeons, San Francisco, California, February 1993.

103 Roberts JB, Curis PH. Stability of the thoracic and lumbar spine in traumatic paraplegia following fracture of fracture-dislocations. *J Bone Joint Surg [Am]* **52**: 1115–1130, 1970.

104 Rogers WA. Treatment of fracture-dislocation of the cervical spine. *J Bone Joint Surg [Am]* **24**: 245–258, 1942.

105 Rogers WA. Fractures and dislocations of the cervical spine. An end-result study. *J Bone Joint Surg [Am]* **39**: 341–376, 1957.

106 Rorabeck CH, Rock GM, Hawkins RL, Bourne RB. Unilateral facet dislocation of the cervical spine. An analysis of results in 26 patients. *Spine* **12**: 23–27, 1987.
107 Roy-Camille R, Saillant G, Berteaux D, Serge MA. Early management of spinal injuries. In McKibbin B (ed.), *Recent Advances in Orthopaedics*, 57–87. Edinburgh: Churchill Livingstone, 1989.
108 Saboe LA, Reid DC, David LA, Warren SA, Grace MG. Spine trauma and associated injuries. *J Trauma* **31**: 43–48, 1991.
109 Saul TG, Ducker TB. The spine and spinal cord. In Watt J et al. (eds), *American College of Surgeons: Early Care of the Injured Patient*, 3rd ed, 196–205. Philadelphia: WB Saunders, 1982.
110 Schaefer DM, Flanders A, Northrup BE, Doan HT, Osterholm JL. Magnetic resonance imaging of acute cervical spine trauma: Correlation with severity of neurologic injury. *Spine* **14**: 1090–1095, 1989.
111 Scher A, Vambeck V. An approach to radiological examination of the cervicodorsal junction following injury. *Clin Radiol* **28**: 24–43, 1977.
112 Schneider RC, Cherry G, Pantek H. The syndrome of acute central cervical spinal cord injury: Special reference to the mechanisms involved in hypertension injuries of the cervical spine. *J Neurosurg* **11**: 546–577, 1954.
113 Segal D, Whitelaw FP, Gumps V, Pick RY. Tension band fixation of acute cervical spine fractures. *Clin Orthop* **159**: 211–222, 1981.
114 Smith GW, Robinson RA. The treatment of certain cervical spine disorders by the anterior removal of the intervertebral disc and interbody fusion. *J Bone Joint Surg [Am]* **40**: 607–624, 1958.
115 Soderstrom CA, McArdle DQ, Ducker TB, Militello PR. The diagnosis of intra-abdominal injury in patients with cervical cord trauma. *J Trauma* **23**: 1061–1065, 1983.
116 Star AM, Jones AA, Cotler JM, Balderston RA, Sinha R. Immediate closed reduction of cervical spine dislocations using traction. *Spine* **15**: 1068–1072, 1990.
117 Stauffer ES, Kaufer H, Kling TF. Fractures and dislocations of the spine. In Rockwood CA, Green DP (eds), *Fractures in Adults*. Philadelphia: JB Lippincott, 987–1093, 1984.
118 Stauffer ES, Wood W, Kelly EG. Gunshot wounds of the spine: The effects of laminectomy. *J Bone Joint Surg [Am]* **61**: 389–392, 1979.
119 Stover SC. *Spinal Cord Injury: The Facts and Figures*. Birmingham, Alabama: University of Alabama, 1986.
120 Streitweiser DR, Knopp R, Wales LR et al. Accuracy of standard radiographic views in detecting cervical spine fractures. *Ann Emerg Med* **12**: 538, 1983.
121 Sutterlin CE, McAfee PC, Warden YE. A biomechanical evaluation of cervical spinal stabilization methods in a bovine model, static and cyclical loading. *Spine* **13**: 795–802, 1988.
122 Tarlov IM. Spinal cord compression studies. Time limits for recovery after gradual compression in dogs. *Arch Neurol Neurosurg Psychol* **71**: 588–597, 1954.
123 Templeton PA, Young JWR, Mirvis SE, Buddemeyer EV. The value of retropharyngeal soft tissue measurement in trauma of the adult cervical spine. *Skeletal Radiol* **16**: 98–104, 1987.
124 Vaccaro AR, An HS, Lin SS, Sun S, Balderston RA, Cotler JM. Noncontiguous injuries of the spine. *J Spinal Disorders* **5**: 320–329, 1992.
125 Walters RN, Adkins RH, Nelson R, Garland D. Cervical spinal cord trauma: Evaluation and nonoperative treatment in halo immobilization. *Contemp Orthop* **14**: 35–45, 1987.
126 White AA, Southwick WO, Panjabi MM. Clinical instability in the lower cervical spine. A review of past and current concepts. *Spine* **1**: 15–27, 1970.
127 Whitehill R, Richman JA, Glaser JA. Failure of immobilization of the cervical spine by the halo-vest. *J Bone Joint Surg [Am]* **68**: 326–332, 1986.

13 Cervical spine injury in the skeletally immature patient

Brian E. Black,
Howard S. An and
J. Michael Simpson

Injuries to the cervical spine in the skeletally immature patient are uncommon, accounting for only 1.9% of all cervical spine injuries.[19] It is extremely important that the differences in cervical spine injury patterns between the child and adult are understood, so that there is appropriate recognition of potential or actual injuries, and management of injuries is provided with reduced risk for complications. In smaller children, the upper cervical spine is most commonly injured, and the literature has shown that, as the child's age increases, the incidence of lower cervical spine injury increases. This changing pattern of spine injury relates to changes in cervical anatomy with maturation.

CERVICAL SPINE ANATOMY IN THE SKELETALLY IMMATURE PATIENT

From birth to skeletal maturity, based on cartilaginous models the cervical vertebrae continue to ossify. In the case of the first cervical vertebra, separate ossification centers are present in the lateral masses at birth. A third center of ossification for the anterior arch is present in only about 20% of neonates and is not generally seen until the child is 1 year of age. After birth, the process of ossification proceeds from the lateral masses posteriorly into the posterior arches, usually completing closure of the posterior atlantal ring by the third year of life. The ossific nucleus of the anterior arch fuses with the lateral masses by 6–9 years of age. The diameters of the spinal canal actually reach adult size by the age of 4 years, with thereafter little potential for further growth of C1.

Morphologic development of the axis includes centers of ossification in the dens, centrum, and neural arches. In the neonate, the dens begins with two longitudinal primary ossification centers, which are usually fused at birth. The odontoid develops an apical epiphysis which appears when the child reaches 6 or 7 years of age. This ossiculum terminale fuses with the rest of the dens by the twelfth year.

The odontoid is separated from the body of C2 by growth cartilage which disappears by the age of 7 years, and which allows for longitudinal growth of both the dens and centrum. This growth center is actually within the eventual body of C2, and is histologically continuous with the neurocentral synchondroses of the centrum and posterior elements. In the skeletally immature patient, this represents important information, because dens fractures will occur along this growth mechanism, and thus are partially within the body of C2 and have a significantly enhanced chance of healing. This is in contrast to adult odontoid fractures, which usually occur much higher.

In a skeletally immature child blood supply to the dens also varies from that of the adult. In the child, there are soft-tissue attachments near the ossiculum terminale which allow penetration of vessels. Furthermore, the distal end of the dens is supplied by vessels entering just medial to the facet joints, which go toward the dentocentral synchondrosis before entering the main portion of the dens. This circulation is usually uninjured in childhood fractures, and is responsible for the high rate of union.

The third to seventh cervical vertebrae have similar patterns of ossification of the vertebral bodies and posterior arches. One ossification center develops in each of the two neural arch cartilage centers, whereas one ossification center forms in the vertebral centrum. Each posterior arch ossific nucleus spreads from its point of origin at the base of the transverse process dorsally into the arch and ventrally into the pedicle. The ossified portions of each neural arch fuse with each other posteriorly by the age of

2–4 years. Before fusion of these nuclei, radiolucent lines on frontal anteroposterior radiographs of the spine should not be confused with congenital abnormalities.

Secondary ossification centers develop, in late childhood, in the cartilaginous ring apophysis about the margin of the vertebral bodies; they consist of hard cortical bone when completely formed. They also fuse to the primary centers at about 15–16 years of age. In addition, secondary centers of ossification develop at the tips of the spinous processes during early adolescence. They generally fuse to the underlying ossific nuclei at the end of vertebral growth.

EPIDEMIOLOGY

Five percent of cases of traumatic paraplegia occur in children.[28] Motor vehicle accidents are the main cause of pediatric traumatic paraplegia;[1] below 2 years of age, child abuse is a common etiology.[9] In Rang's study[28] of 450 paraplegic children aged over 12 years, treated at the Ontario Crippled Children's Center, 12% of these patients had traumatic paraplegia, 2% of paraplegias developed secondary to acquired disease, and 86% were due to myelomeningocele. The most common birth injury to the spine is thought to be a Salter type I end-plate separation.

SPECIAL CONSIDERATIONS IN PEDIATRIC CERVICAL TRAUMA

Increased Elasticity

One of the major differences in the infant, child or adolescent compared to the adult is that of increased elasticity. Leventhal has shown that the pediatric bony and ligamentous spine tolerates four times as much stretch as the spinal cord.[21] This explains why pediatric cervical injuries may present with severe cord injury and normal radiographs in as many as 20% of cases. This pattern of neurologic injury with no radiographic findings is known as 'spinal cord injury without radiographic abnormality' (SCIWORA).[27]

Multiple contiguous or near-contiguous fractures are also much more common in the pediatric population.[5,21] This is due to the increased elasticity of the pediatric spine, which allows for dissipation of the energy of injury over multiple segments.

Transport of Children with Suspected Cervical Injury

Infants and small children up to the age of 5 years who are suspected of having cervical injuries need to be transported in a different manner to the transport of an adult.[20] Suspicion of cervical spine injury in the child should be raised if there is loss of consciousness and/or lacerations about the head, face, or chest. In the field, small children with these findings should have their neurologic examination documented before being moved. In transport, the child's position should not be changed, and the child should be moved as a unit.

Flexion of the neck in the small child and infant is contraindicated in transport, because the most common level of injury in the small child involves the occiput–C1–C2 complex. If the odontoid process is intact, but the atlantoaxial ligaments have been disrupted, spinal cord compression may occur if the child's head and neck are held in a flexed position. When compared to the adult, small children have a disproportionately large head compared to their torso. Therefore, if a small child is transported positioned on a flat spine board, flexion of the neck will result, and to prevent this flexion special precaution must be taken to place the shoulders of the small child or infant on bolsters. Alternatively, a specially made pediatric spine board, designed to account for these differences in small children, may be used.

Radiographic Differences

Radiographic evaluation[3,18,26] of the spine must be carefully and systematically accomplished to rule out cervical spine injury. Knowledge of normal radiographic parameters of the pediatric cervical spine prevents over-treatment. In performing all radiographic tests, the cervical spine must be adequately immobilized to prevent iatrogenic injury during transport or patient positioning. Anteroposterior (AP), lateral, and open-mouth radiographs should be obtained and include views from the occiput to T1. On the lateral radiograph, the vertebral body height, anterior and posterior spinal lines, spinolaminar lines, alignment of spinous processes, and sagittal plane contours should be evaluated. On the AP radiograph, the pedicle width and alignment, body height, body alignment, spinous process alignment, and transverse processes should be evaluated. Oblique radiographs, and anteroposterior and lateral tomography may also be helpful. In addition, computed tomography (CT) or magnetic resonance imaging (MRI) may be indicated.

The pediatric cervical spine has distinct radiographic differences from that of the adult; many of these are directly attributed to multiple primary and secondary centers of ossification, and their intervening synchondroses. It is obviously important not to mistake these normal findings as evidence of fracture. Normal findings in the pediatric spine include the persistence of a lucent zone in the anterior region of the atlas called the 'neurocentral synchondrosis' which, as indicated earlier, fuses by the seventh year. The odontoid synchrondrosis is seen as a lucent area in the waist of the dens and is known to fuse at 3–6 years of age. Before closure, these lucencies can be mistaken for a fracture. The atlantodental interval is also increased in children compared to adults, with up to 4 mm being considered normal.

Pediatric vertebral bodies are more rounded in appearance than in the adult, and can be mistaken for compression fractures. Notching of the anterior and posterior vertebral body is normal, resulting from localized vascularity of these regions. These changes can also be mistaken for fractures. In the child, the retropharyngeal space can be up to 8 mm in width, particularly when the child is crying. In the adult, this space should be less than 3 mm.

Pseudosubluxation of C2 onto C3 of up to 4 mm is common and seen in 20% of the normal pediatric population. Marked anterior displacement on a lateral cervical flexion radiograph can be seen from 1 to 8 years of age. Similar pseudosubluxation of C3 onto C4 may also be seen and is considered normal. In children under the age of 8 years, the C2–C3 articulation is the normal fulcrum of the cervical spine movement and accounts for this appearance. This is in contrast to the normal fulcrum of movement in the adult, which occurs at the C5–C6 level.

Pseudosubluxation can be differentiated from true instability in the pediatric age group. In cases of pseudosubluxation, the spinal laminar line remains uninterrupted on the lateral radiograph, whereas in true subluxation, this landmark is not contiguous. Furthermore, pseudosubluxation reduces on lateral extension views, whereas true instability will not reduce completely and is usually associated with a history of traumatic injury and pain.

Absence of cervical lordosis is another common, normal finding seen in 15% of the pediatric population. Furthermore, the facets of the upper cervical vertebrae are more horizontal than those of the lower cervical vertebrae, particularly in the younger child.

Increased Healing Potential of the Cervical Spine of Small Children

Cervical dislocations in children below the age of 9 years have a high potential for healing, without development of instability, after closed reduction. The reason for this potential may be inferred from Aufdermaur's study of cadavers, where dislocations apparent on radiographs were found to actually be unossified fractures at autopsy.[2] This author (BEB) has reported further on fracture-type healing seen after closed reduction of apparent dislocations in small children.[5] Therefore, the potential for healing of cervical dislocations in small children may be due to the fact that many of these apparent dislocations are, in fact, fractures that heal by bony union.

Other Differences

In children, some vertebral body reconstitution may occur if the growth plates are not badly damaged after cervical spine injury.[8,13] Long-term bracing can play a role in the attempt to improve deformity in these cases.

Children tolerate immobilization better than adults,[6,11] and traction and bedrest may therefore be used for a prolonged period of time with very low risk of complications.

The incidence of post-paralytic neuromuscular spinal deformity is 100% after pediatric cervical quadriplegia and paraplegia.[22] These deformities should be braced when apparent. Typically, such post-traumatic conditions eventually require surgical correction and stabilization.

Child abuse should always be considered in the differential diagnosis when considering etiology of pediatric cervical injuries. The whiplash/shaken child syndrome is a strong indicator of child abuse. In these children, intracranial and intraocular hemorrhages, spinal cord injury, cerebral palsy, paralysis, and even death may be associated with the cervical injury. Other stigmata of child abuse should be sought on physical examination and radiographic assessment.

Children with skeletal anomalies may be at risk of cervical injury. For example, extensive subaxial Klippel–Feil fusions may also result in excessive atlantoaxial motion and potential for instability with subsequent acute injury.

PATTERNS OF PEDIATRIC CERVICAL INJURY

SCIWORA

Spinal cord injury without radiographic abnormality (SCIWORA) can occur in the pediatric age group[14,27,34] and result from either spinal cord concussion, contusion, or infarction. The most probable mechanism responsible for such injury patterns is related to the elasticity of the pediatric spine. Hyperextension or hyperflexion of the spine may fail to produce bony or ligamentous injury, but result in significant stretch of the less pliable spinal cord. It has been suggested additionally that a transiently displaced Salter I-type fracture of the vertebral cartilaginous end-plate may induce spinal cord injury while producing no radiographic abnormality. Melzak[23] reported on 29 cases of pediatric spinal cord trauma in patients under 13 years of age. Sixteen of these patients failed to demonstrate any evidence of fracture. Fortunately, most cases of SCIWORA represent a concussion of the spinal cord, which results in only transient loss of spinal cord function. Recovery is complete in most cases. Contusions of the spinal cord represent the next level of injury severity. These injuries will have varying degrees of recovery with potential for residual spasticity. The most severe form of SCIWORA is that of spinal cord infarction, which fortunately is rare. When infarction occurs, the result is a complete and permanent flaccid paralysis. Many reports of a delayed onset paralysis have been noted in children with SCIWORA. Magnetic resonance imaging is extremely useful in the diagnostic work-up of suspected SCIWORA,[14] and, in many respects, delineates the extent of spinal cord injury.

As mentioned earlier, the incidence of spinal deformity, that is, scoliosis, kyphosis, or lordosis, is high in complete spinal cord injuries. The incidence of such deformities in cervical cord lesions is approximately 100%. Patients who sustain such spinal cord lesions must undergo periodic clinical and radiographic evaluation. When the lesions occur, bracing must be tried, although it usually fails. Early surgical intervention is usually required.

Atlanto-occipital Dislocation

The anatomy of the atlanto-occipital articulation in children has little inherent bony stability and is essentially reliant on ligamentous integrity.[8,15,16] In adults, the steep inclination of the joint affords considerable bony stability. In the skeletally immature patient, however, the relatively small size of the occipital condyles and the relatively horizontal plane of the atlanto-occipital articulations make these joints less stable, particularly when extension-type forces are applied. Dislocation without fracture is possible (Fig. 13.1). Subluxation or dislocation of this articulation is also possible through any inflammatory process which may lead to ligamentous laxity.

The incidence of atlanto-occipital subluxation or dislocation in the pediatric patient is unknown. Total dislocation is a rare finding and generally results in fatality secondary to transection of the medulla oblongata or spinal–medullary junction. Radiographically, there will be evidence of significant retropharyngeal swelling and loss of the normal relationship between the odontoid and basiocciput. Plain radiographs may suffice in the diagnosis. CT scan with axial images and reformatted sagittal reconstructions may be helpful.

Surviving pediatric patients with injury to the atlanto-occipital articulation demonstrate variable clinical manifestations. Susceptible areas of neurologic dysfunction include the brain stem, the caudal cranial nerves, the proximal portion of the spinal cord, and the upper two to three cranial nerves. Many surviving patients, unfortunately, are ventilator-dependent quadriplegics.

Treatment of this disorder depends on the degree of subluxation or dislocation and evidence of neurologic compromise. For all patients, initial cervical immobilization and adherence to standard resuscitative measures, including airway maintenance and possible intubation, are required. The injuries are very unstable and, at a minimum, require prolonged immobilization in either a cervical halo vest or cranial tong traction. Lightweight traction with close physician supervision, sequential lateral radiographs, and neurologic assessment is advised. Care must be taken not to distract the occiput–C1 region excessively. Once reduction is obtained traction may be reduced to maintenance levels.

In the infant and young child, conservative management has been successful. In the older child, however, posterior occipitocervical arthrodesis may be required because of the difficulty in obtaining and maintaining reduction.

For patients with symptomatic subluxation of the atlanto-occipital articulation secondary to inflammatory processes, a period of immobilization is all that is required. A short period of cranial tong traction or cervical orthosis generally suffices. It is necessary to monitor the atlanto-occipital relationship with serial lateral radiographs.

Posterior surgical stabilization in the young child is best performed simply as onlay graft supplemented with external immobilization through a halo vest. More standard wiring techniques, as described in Chapter 19, can be used in older children and adolescents. The use of a halo device in the child can present unique problems. Halo pins should be placed anterolaterally and posterolaterally where the bones are thickest. The temporal fossa region is quite thin and should be avoided.

Atlas Fractures

Atlas fractures are uncommon in the pediatric literature.[4,7,24] When seen, they are usually the result of axially applied, compression forces, with the secondary consequence of forcing the occipital condyles downward into the lateral masses of the atlas. The result is a centrifugal displacement of the lateral masses in a typical 'burst'-type fracture pattern. In most of these injuries, the displacement is minimal, although with more severely applied axial forces, the spread of the lateral masses may result in rupture of the transverse atlantal ligament, which serves as the primary stabilizer of the C1–C2 articulation. Axial compression coupled with hyperextension may result in an associated fracture of the posterior arch of C1 where it is grooved by the vertebral arteries. Most patients will have evidence of anterior and posterior ring disruption, possibly occurring through the neurocentral synchondroses.

Neurologic compromise is uncommon with these injuries. At this level the already capacious spinal canal is usually further decompressed by centrifugal spreading of bony fragments. Spinal cord damage, however, may occur with more significant levels of initially applied force.

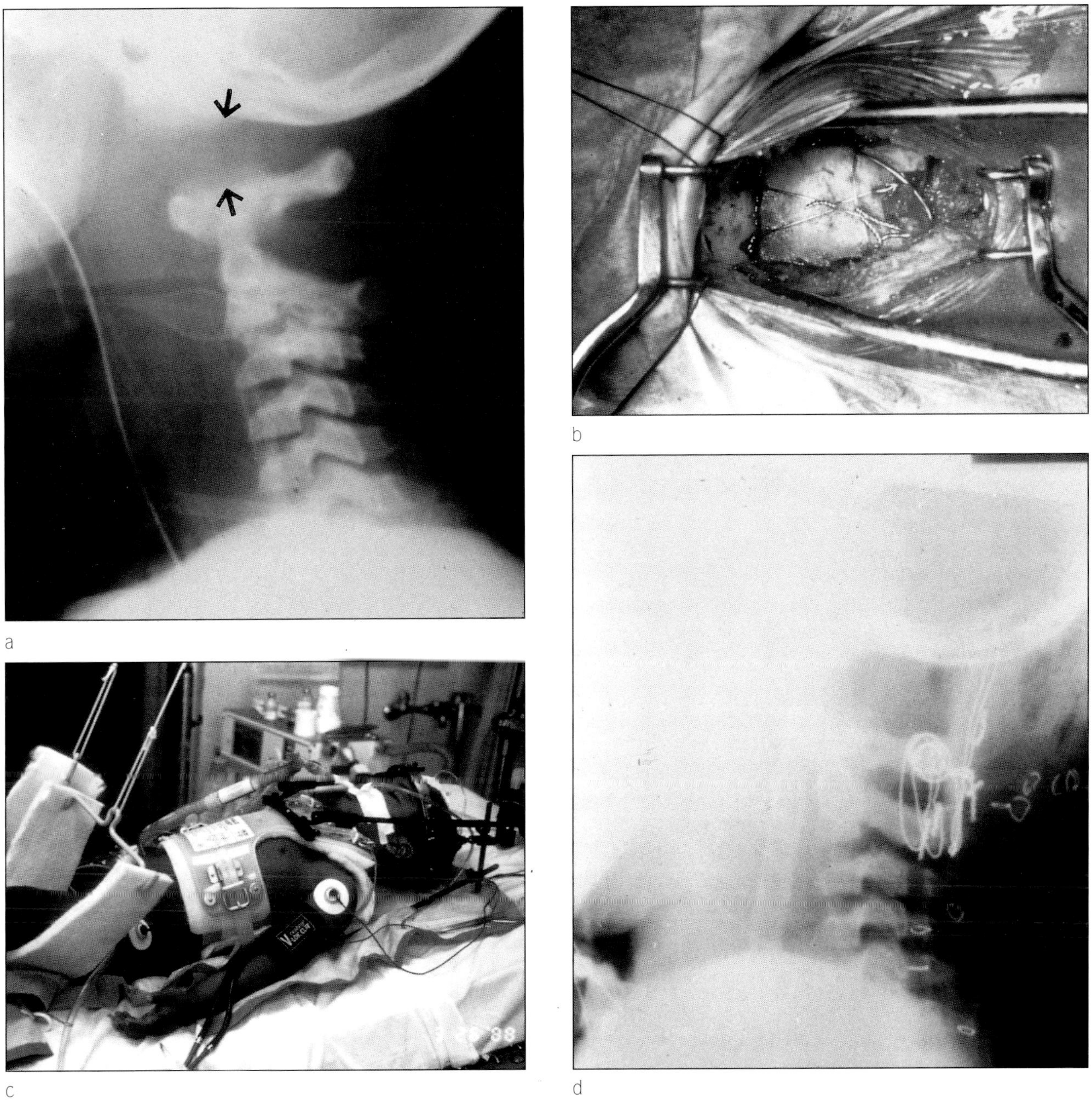

Figure 13.1
Case 1: 4½-year-old black male, pedestrian motor vehicle accident, who sustained occiput–C1–C2 dislocations, is ventilator dependent and quadriplegic. (a) Increased occiput-to-C1 distance (arrows); (b) intraoperative photograph of posterior occiput–C2 wiring with bone grafting; (c) halo vest and ventilator in the intensive care unit; (d) lateral radiograph showing occiput-to-C2 wiring

Identification of these fractures may be difficult by plain radiographs. Anteroposterior open-mouth views are helpful, but often difficult to obtain in younger children as a result of poor cooperation. Computed tomography offers the most precise imaging of these fractures. However, it is imperative that the plane of imaging is parallel to the horizontal plane of the atlas. Improper gantry alignment can lead to missed fractures.

Conservative treatment measures are in order for all atlas fractures. As in adults, most fractures heal without incident, given proper immobilization in a Minerva cast or halo brace. Healing of the fracture may be assessed with serial CT. Lateral flexion and extension radiographs should be obtained once bony union is apparent to assess if there is any residual ligamentous instability.

Atlantoaxial Subluxation

Essentially there are four lesions that involve the atlantoaxial articulation in the pediatric population which require discussion: traumatic ligamentous disruption, ligamentous laxity secondary to local inflammation, rotatory subluxation or dislocation, and odontoid epiphyseal separation.[12,13,17] In the atlantoaxial region, Steele's rule of thirds is an important anatomic principle to bear in mind.[31] This principle states that the odontoid, spinal cord, and free space each occupy one-third of the available space. Therefore, atlantoaxial instability is more dangerous in the presence of an intact odontoid process. As a child with atlantoaxial instability flexes forward, the intact dens encroaches on the free space and spinal cord. Chronic, developmental, ligamentous instability is associated with Down's syndrome and may result in spinal cord compression. For this reason, Down's syndrome children require lateral flexion/extension screening radiographs before any vigorous athletic participation.

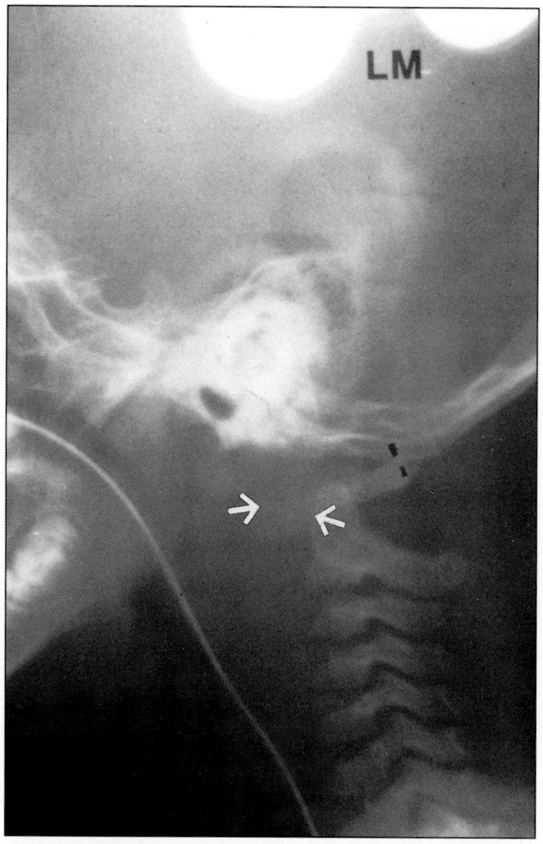

Figure 13.2
Case 2: 2 year old, motor vehicle accident, who sustained C1–C2 subluxation and transverse ligament rupture with an 8-mm atlantodental interval (ADI) (arrows), was neurologically intact. Patient was placed in a halo for 2 months, but still had an ADI of 5 mm. A fusion C1–C2 was performed with excellent results

Traumatic Atlantoaxial Ligamentous Disruption

Traumatic atlantoaxial ligamentous disruption[12] is rare, as the more susceptible odontoid tends to fail before the ligament (Fig. 13.2). With an incompetent ligament, the atlantodental interval is increased as the atlas subluxates anterior to the odontoid, which obviously leads to a diminished canal space for the spinal cord. The normal atlantodental interval in the child in the neutral or flexed position is 3 mm, and diminishes to 2 mm at skeletal maturity.

Atlantoaxial subluxation secondary to inflammation, also known as 'Grisel's syndrome', is caused by inflammation from an upper respiratory retropharyngeal infection, tuberculosis, osteomyelitis, tumor, or rheumatoid arthritis. Capsular distension and ligamentous softening, caused by these inflammatory processes, results in the instability and an increase in the atlantoaxial interval. Quadriparesis has been reported. These patients should have the displacement reduced in extension, followed by placement into a halo vest or Minerva cast for 8 weeks. If radiographic evidence of instability persists at that time, a posterior spinal fusion from C1 to C2 is indicated.

Treatment of the uncommon traumatic disruption of the transverse ligament in the child consists of reduction through extension, and placement of the child in a Minerva cast, halo cast, or halo vest. Immobilization is maintained for a period of 8–12 weeks, followed by awake, active, physician-supervised lateral flexion and extension radiographs, to determine if any residual instability exists. If there is no evidence of instability, the child is then placed in a cervical collar for a few weeks. To ensure stability it is probably important to obtain serial radiographs at 3-month intervals for 1 year. With a persistent or recurrent increase in the atlantodental interval, a posterior C1–C2 arthrodesis is advised.

In performing an isolated posterior C1–C2 arthrodesis in the child, it is imperative that attention to detail be given in surgical dissection. A standard longitudinal incision may

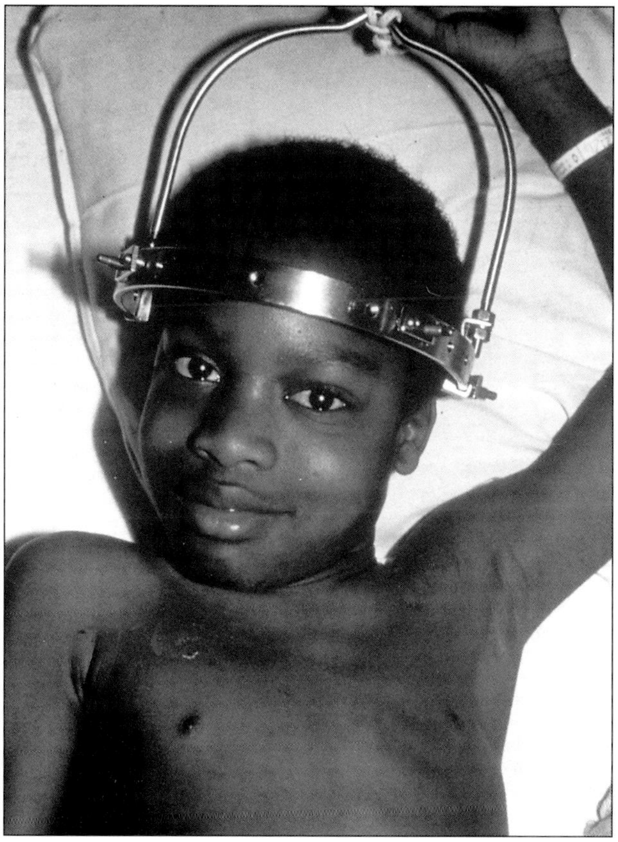

Figure 13.3
Case 3: Clinical 'cock Robin' appearance of atlantoaxial rotatory dislocation in halo traction

be used. Alternatively, however, a transverse incision at the C1–C2 level can be used, limiting bony dissection only to the involved segments and giving improved cosmetic results. It is important to limit exposure proximal and distal to the C1–C2 articulation because undesired extension of the fusion mass can easily occur in children, further limiting motion. Posterior exposure of the posterior arch of C1 should also be limited to approximately 1 cm from the midline to prevent inadvertent injury to the vertebral arteries.

Once the exposure is completed, surgical options include simply an onlay graft followed by halo immobilization, or use of some form of wire fixation, that is, a Gallie or Brooks technique. In the young child, the inherent risks of wire placement make it ill-advisable, and healing of these fusions is almost universal anyway. Careful decortication of the posterior arch of C1 and C2, meticulous placement of bone graft, and proper immobilization lead to successful fusion in most patients. In the older child and adolescent, Gallie or Brooks-type wire fixation is a reasonable alternative followed by immobilization in a halo vest or Minerva-type orthosis.

Atlantoaxial Rotatory Subluxation and Dislocation

Atlantoaxial rotatory subluxation or dislocation may be caused by trauma or inflammatory processes; it can also be spontaneous and of uncertain etiology. Fortunately, these conditions are usually mild and on the whole resolve spontaneously. Most patients present with an acute onset of pain and torticollis, and some history of mild trauma, although in some cases the process develops gradually and is associated with little or no discomfort. A few patients may present with a fixed deformity secondary to rotatory C1–C2 subluxation and have been described as having a 'cock-robin' appearance (Fig. 13.3). Compensatory rotation of other portions of the cervical spine can, however, mask these abnormalities. Neurologic deficit, vertebral artery compromise, and possibly death can occur and have been reported, although they are extremely rare.

Routine anteroposterior, lateral, and open-mouth odontoid radiographs are required in cases of suspected atlantoaxial rotatory subluxation. The open-mouth odontoid radiograph will demonstrate the asymmetric placement of the dens between the lateral articular masses of the atlas (Fig. 13.4a). On the lateral radiograph, the atlas may appear to be wedge shaped. Any increase in the atlantodental interval should be noted. Axial CT imaging can also be of help in determining the extent of subluxation and, in addition, may determine the integrity of the transverse ligament (Fig. 13.4b).

Fielding has described four types of atlantoaxial rotatory displacement.[13] Type I is the most common, and involves pure rotation of the atlas about the dens with no displacement. In type I rotatory subluxation, complete resolution of the disorder can be expected without specific intervention. Typically, complaints from the child are mild. Use of a soft collar and analgesics allow the condition to resolve spontaneously. In protracted cases, reduction can usually be obtained through use of halter traction and analgesics for a few days.

In type II and III atlantoaxial rotatory subluxation, mild-to-significant anterior displacement of the atlas occurs in addition to the rotatory deformity. In these cases, halter traction is required for reduction, followed by immobilization for 6 weeks, during which use of a Minerva cast or brace is required. After 6 weeks of immobilization, the paent is evaluated for any residual instability is evaluated by taking

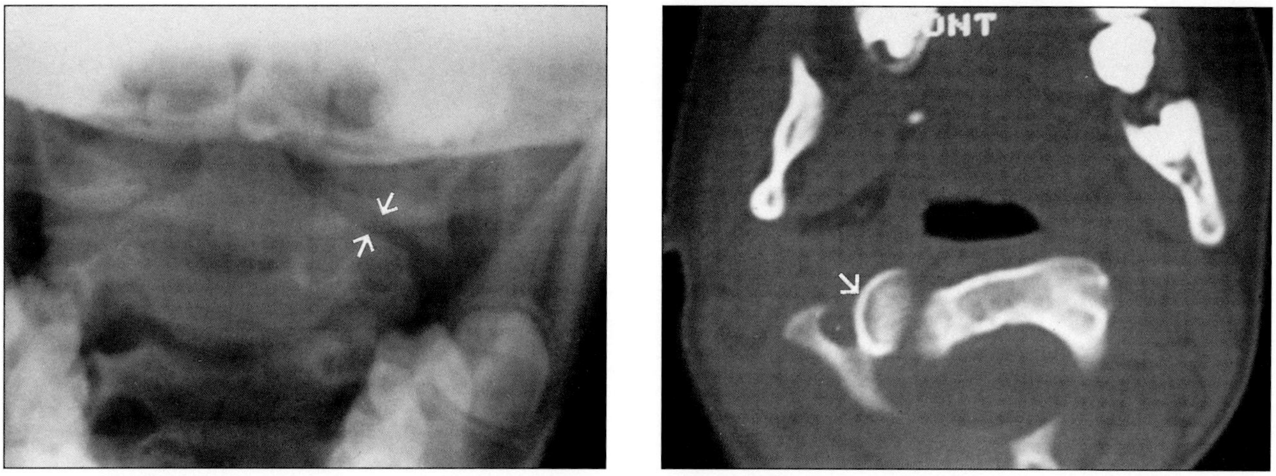

a b

Figure 13.4
Case 4: 8-year-old who fell off a TV and sustained C1–C2 traumatic rotatory subluxation; neurologically normal. (a) Widening of C1–C2 joint is shown by arrows; (b) computed tomogram showing inferior facet joint of C1 and asymmetry between the left and right sides. The patient was treated by closed reduction in halter traction, then a Philadelphia collar. Complete resolution was obtained

lateral flexion and extension radiographs under active conditions supervised by the physician. With no evidence of instability, these children are initially placed in a soft cervical collar for a few weeks and followed with serial radiographs to ensure stability. Patients with types II and III atlantoaxial rotatory displacement are at risk of recalcitrant atlantoaxial instability, and may require posterior C1–C2 arthrodesis.

Type IV atlantoaxial rotatory displacement involves posterior displacement of the atlas secondary to hypoplasia or aplasia of the odontoid. This may be an unstable condition, and require C1–C2 arthrodesis. Isolated, congenital aplasia of the dens is usually a stable condition, although it may present with instability following acute trauma.

In general, the indications for C1–C2 arthrodesis for atlantoaxial rotary displacement include the following: neurologic involvement, residual anterior displacement, failure to achieve and maintain correction (particularly common if the deformity is more than 3 weeks old at presentation), and/or recurrent deformity after 6–8 weeks of adequate non-surgical treatment.

Dens Fractures

Fracture of the dens represents an uncommon injury in the child, and is rare in children under the age of 3 years. In most cases of odontoid fracture, there is a history of significant trauma. Most of these injuries can be readily diagnosed on plain radiographs. Evidence of fracture may be subtle and include only swelling or widening of the retropharyngeal soft-tissue space. In more obvious cases, a fracture line with displacement can be demonstrated through the odontoid epiphyses. The physician should be careful not to misinterpret the closing dentocentral synchondrosis as an odontoid fracture. In the conscious patient with an acute fracture, there will be complaints of pain and possibly a subjective sense of instability. Many of these children will actually hold their head with two hands to prevent motion.

There is some controversy in the literature regarding the odontoid epiphysis. Earlier authors concluded that the cartilage plate in the immature odontoid was a synchondrosis, and not a true growth plate. This conclusion was simply based on their observation that no growth arrests occurred following odontoid epiphyseal separations. However, more recent anatomic studies have shown that the odontoid cartilage plate represents a true physis.[26] As these fractures propagate through this epiphysis, the fracture line is seen well into the body of the axis.

In contrast to the high incidence of odontoid non-union and potential for neurologic sequelae in adults, children typically experience a good result after conservative management. In Sherk's series of 24 cases of pediatric odontoid fractures treated by closed means, 23 of these went on to heal, and only one patient required atlantoaxial fusion.[30] All of Sherk's patients had good results. In general, odontoid epiphyseal fractures are easily reducible, stable in plaster, form callous, and heal rapidly. In the older child and adolescent, the synchondrosis at the base of the dens is fused with the body of the axis. Treatment of these fractures with a closed synchondrosis is no different to the treatment in an adult. Basilar fractures (adult type III) heal well when reduced and stabilized. Apical odontoid fractures (adult type I) are generally benign injuries and can be treated with symptomatic immobilization. These fractures may be associated with injury to the atlanto-occipital complex, which should be ruled out. Displaced fractures of the dens above the level of the atlantoaxial articular facets (type II) have a high rate of non-union. Closed reduction is attempted followed by halo immobilization. For fractures that fail to reduce adequately, or those that go on to non-union, a posterior C1–C2 arthrodesis is recommended (Fig. 13.5).

The most common neurologic complication associated with odontoid fractures in the child is damage to the greater occipital nerve, giving referred pain to the occiput. The most serious potential complication is spinal cord injury.

Pediatric odontoid fractures are treated by closed reduction and followed by halo vest or Minerva casting for 12 weeks. Children tolerate prolonged skeletal traction much better than adults and, as such, traction is a viable form of treatment for refractory cases until early callus is seen. At 12 weeks after the injury, flexion/extension lateral cervical radiographs are obtained. If no abnormal motion occurs, the fracture is well healed and a soft collar is worn temporarily. If motion persists at the fracture site, posterior C1–C2 arthrodesis is recommended.

Os odontoideum of the adult is thought possibly to be the result of a non-union of a previously undiagnosed pediatric odontoid fracture. Development of late atlantoaxial instability may complicate even a minimally displaced odontoid fracture; therefore, follow-up must be performed at least until skeletal maturity. In cases of hypermobility accompanying an os odontoideum, posterior stabilization is also recommended.

Pediatric Hangman's Fracture

C2 hangman's fractures,[4,7] or pedicle fractures, are uncommon in childhood (Fig. 13.6). The mechanism of injury can be acute flexion or extension. When they occur, these fractures typically represent isolated lesions, which should undergo closed reduction and be maintained in a halo or Minerva cast in extension for 8 weeks. Non-union is unusual in these injuries. If non-union occurs, posterior C2–C3 arthrodesis is indicated. Familial congenital pseudoarthrosis with potential instability after acute trauma has been reported.[25,32]

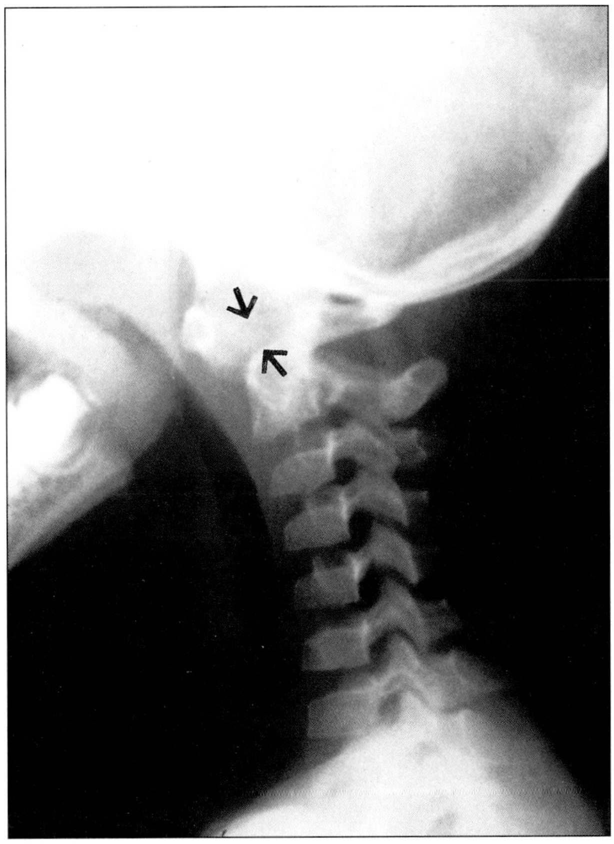

Figure 13.5
Case 5: 6 year old who fell off bike and presented with an unstable fracture of odontoid (vertical migration of the odontoid shown by arrows). The patient was neurologically intact, and underwent successful C1–C2 posterior fusion

C2–C3 Subluxation and Dislocation

Pediatric C2–C3 subluxation and dislocation[4,9,10,29] must be differentiated from pseudosubluxation (Fig. 13.7a). True injury is usually associated with a significant history of pain and trauma, with injuries about the head, face, neck, and chest noted on physical examination. Pseudosubluxation reduces when the spine is simply extended; however, true injury at this level will not reduce on extension. When true subluxation or dislocation is identified or suspected, other associated fractures of the cervical and thoracolumbar spine should be sought. Magnetic resonance imaging is useful in assessing soft-tissue swelling and hemorrhage in the region, and aid in the assessment of spinal cord injury. As mentioned previously, the spinal laminar line is undisturbed in pseudosubluxation, but disrupted in true dislocation or subluxation.

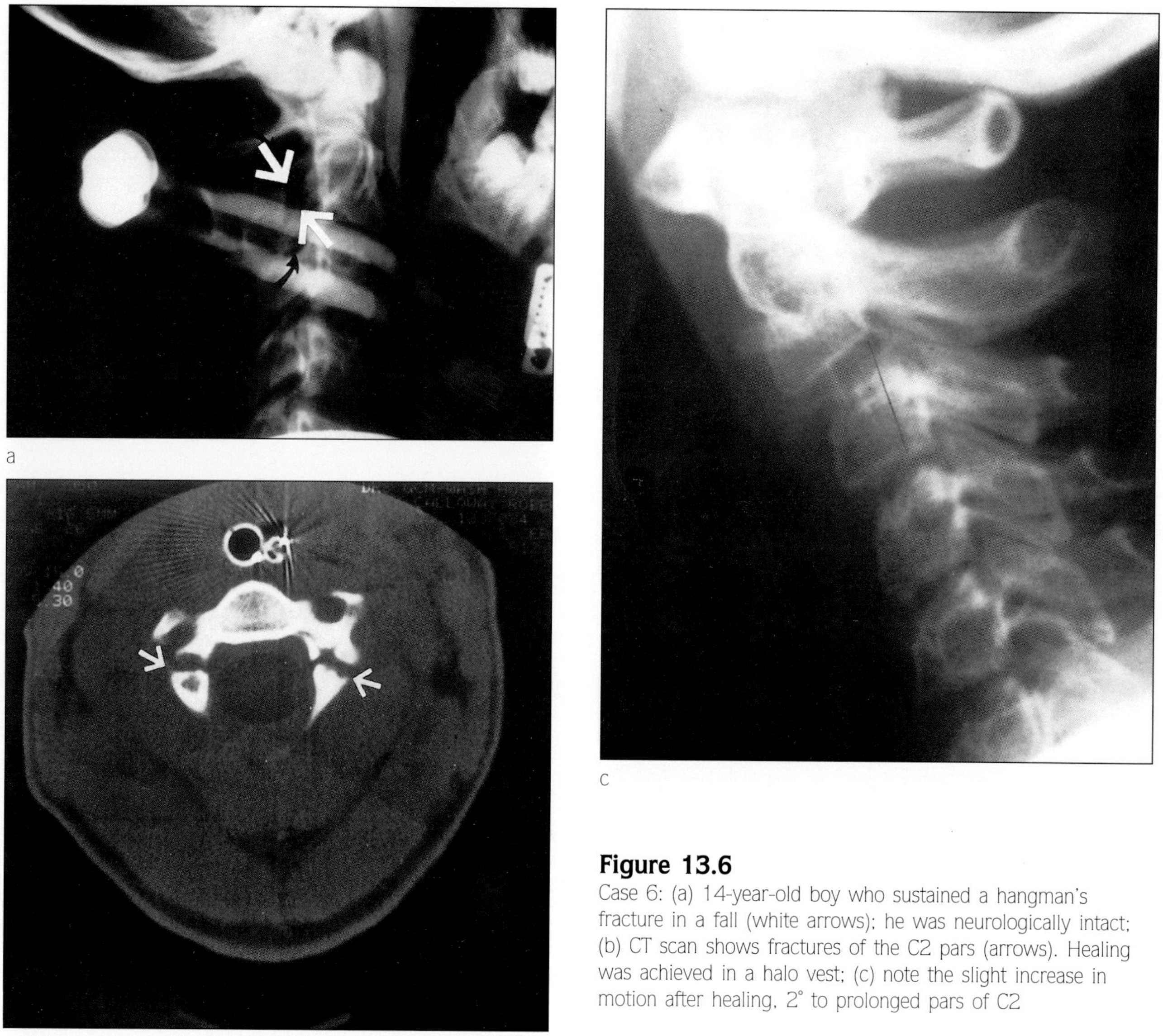

Figure 13.6
Case 6: (a) 14-year-old boy who sustained a hangman's fracture in a fall (white arrows); he was neurologically intact; (b) CT scan shows fractures of the C2 pars (arrows). Healing was achieved in a halo vest; (c) note the slight increase in motion after healing, 2° to prolonged pars of C2

In small children up to the age of 8 true C2–C3 subluxation or dislocation is likely to heal after reduction by closed means. After the age of 8 years, healing potential is not as good and fusion is generally required. However, the present authors believe that a trial of closed reduction and immobilization is reasonable for 8–12 weeks followed by flexion and extension radiographs to assess instability. Pseudosubluxation can also occur at the C3–C4 level.

Mid-to-lower Pediatric Cervical Spine Injuries

Pediatric mid-to-lower cervical spine injuries[4,9,10,29,33] tend to be seen in the older child (Fig. 13.8). As the age of the child increases into the late juvenile age group and adolescence, upper cervical spine injuries become less frequent

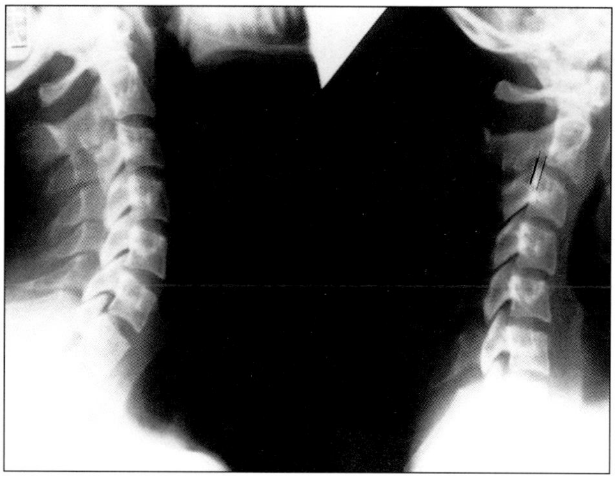

a

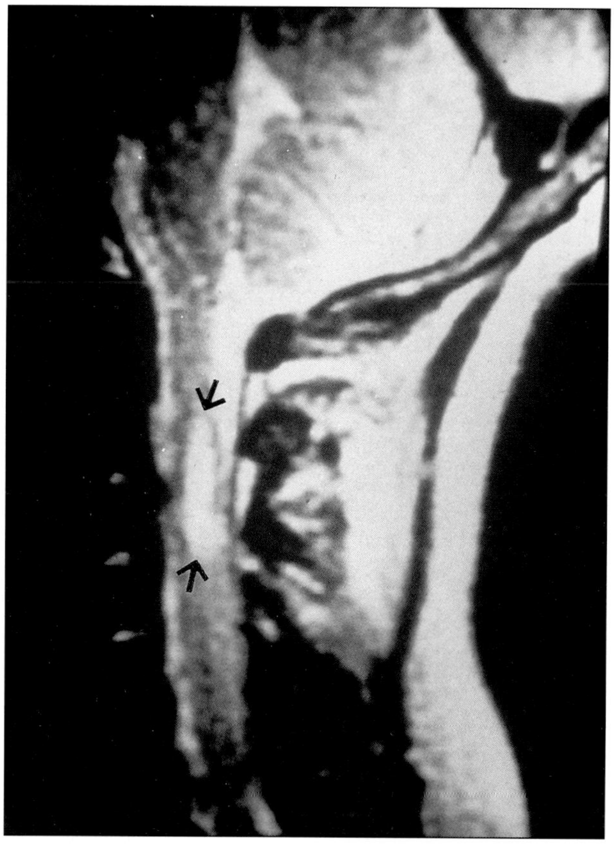

b

Figure 13.7
Case 7: (a) 9 year old who sustained C2–C3 subluxation after a motor vehicle accident with Brown–Séquard syndrome at presentation; (b) MRI scan shows cord edema (arrows). The patient was treated in a Philadelphia collar. Normal allignment returned with full resolution of neurological deficits

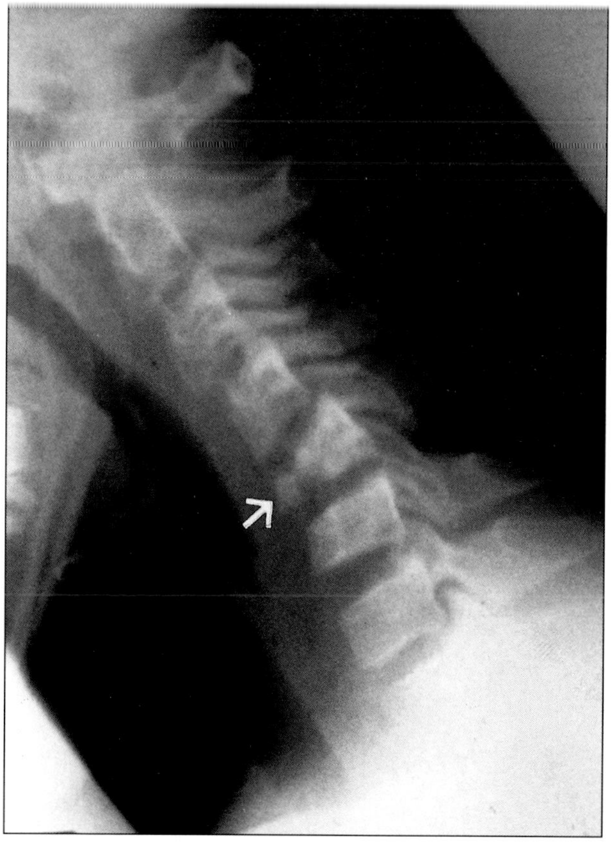

Figure 13.8
Case 8: 12-year-old boy who fell off bike and sustained quadrilateral fracture of C5 (arrow). The patient was neurologically intact. Initial treatment in a Minerva cast resulted in residual chronic instability requiring posterior fusion at C4–C5–C6

and lower cervical spine injuries become prevalent. Mid-to-lower cervical spine injuries in the older pediatric age group follow similar patterns to those in the adult.

The age at which the pediatric spine injury and healing become more biomechanically adult-like is 8–11 years. However, in younger children with mid-to-lower cervical spine subluxations or dislocations, a trial of immobilization following closed reduction should be attempted because of the high healing rate and potential for autofusion in this age group. As mentioned earlier, at age 8 years and older, these injuries typically will not heal adequately without surgical fusion. From age 9 onwards, the usual fracture pattern and fracture dislocation pattern of the adult is seen in the pediatric population.

The neurologic status of the child with a lower cervical spine injury must be kept in mind when considering treatment options. Post-reduction MRI of the cervical spine is advised to rule out compressive pathology. With evidence of cord compression and neurologic deficit, consideration should be given to surgical decompression and stabilization. Operative intervention under the circumstances may allow for nerve root or spinal cord recovery in incomplete injuries. Decisions concerning anterior or posterior approaches are dependent on the anatomic location of cord compression.

In intact patients who are 8 years or older, primary posterior stabilization is generally advocated. The present authors prefer the triple wire technique by Bohlman[7] with autogenous iliac crest bone. Again, it must be emphasized that surgical dissection should be limited only to the involved levels, otherwise propagation of the fusion to undesired levels may occur. Anterior stabilization procedures are generally contraindicated in the intact, young child, because they damage the superior and inferior end-plates. Furthermore, the anterior longitudinal ligament is quite thick and strong, and in most cases represents the only remaining stabilizing structure.

Decompressive laminectomy is also not generally advised to relieve pressure on the damaged spinal cord or neurologic compromise. Such procedures may add to the traumatically induced instability. Multi-level laminectomy also has potential for long-term development of kyphosis or the swan-neck type of deformities. If laminectomy is required for post-reduction evidence of posterior spinal cord compression, concomitant posterior facet arthrodesis followed by halo immobilization is required. Arthrodesis may be performed by simple grafting, facet wiring or, in the older child, lateral mass plate fixation.

In the unusual case of a lower cervical fracture–dislocation in an infant or young child, closed reduction and immobilization usually suffice, with 6–8 weeks of skeletal traction followed by bracing as the recommended treatment. Such fractures usually heal by bony union and become stable. In the young adolescent and older patient, spontaneous fusion is unlikely, and surgical fusion is usually required. As young adolescents have good tolerance of immobilization, an attempt at postural reduction and closed treatment is reasonable. Abnormal motion after 6–8 weeks of closed treatment is an indication for fusion in these younger adolescents.

Compression fractures of the cervical spine involving the centrum are uncommon in children. If growth disturbance occurs in the anterior centrum and is associated with posterior ligamentous disruption, chronic instability or development of progressive cervical kyphosis is possible. Early identification of this process is important so that appropriate early surgical intervention can be undertaken before there is significant deformity or cord compression. Anterior fusion is to be avoided.

Use of allograft has been shown to result in poor fusions or pseudoarthrosis. Autogenous iliac crest bone graft is favored even in this pediatric population. Attempts at anterior fusion are generally successful, however, if the posterior fusion does not occur; a rapidly progressive kyphosis and spinal cord compression may result.

Cervical End-plate Injury

Injury to the physeal end-plate of the pediatric cervical vertebrae is uncommon, and is usually the result of hyperextension forces from motor vehicle accidents, falls, or child abuse. Injury at this level usually occurs at the inferior end-plate, because the uncinate processes are thought to protect the superior end-plate.

Most of these reported physeal injuries were thought to occur in the adolescent population, and suggested a susceptibility of this region during physeal closure. Others feel, however, that this injury is often unrecognized in the younger patient radiographically. These injuries may occur at any level in the cervical spine.

Many of these injuries involve significant neurologic compromise, and most commonly represent transection-type injuries of the spine and neurologic structures. For the intact patient, any application of traction may lead to overdistraction and development of quadriplegia.

There are many special considerations involved in the diagnosis and management of suspected cervical spine injury in the pediatric population. Many of these considerations are rooted in an understanding of the anatomic differences from the adult, and the propensity for many of these injuries to self-stabilize with sufficient external support and immobilization. Strict adherence to treatment protocols, coupled with this knowledge, will help prevent inadvertent neurologic injury and iatrogenic catastrophes, and maximize outcomes.

REFERENCES

1 Anderson JM, Schmitt AH. Spinal injury in children: a review of 156 cases seen from 1950 through 1978. *Mayo Clin Proc* **55**: 499–504, 1980.

2 Aufdermaur HR. Spinal injuries in juveniles. Necropsy findings in twelve cases. *J Bone Joint Surg [Br]* **56**: 513–519, 1974.

3 Bailey DK. The normal cervical spine in infants and children. *Radiology* **59**: 712–718, 1952.

4 Birney TJ, Hanley EN Jr. Traumatic cervical spine injuries in childhood and adolescence. *Spine* **14**: 1277–1282, 1989.

5 Black BE. Thoracic and Lumbar Spine Injuries: Different than the Adult. Sixtieth annual meeting of the American Academy of Orthopaedic Surgeons, San Francisco, February 1993.

6 Blockey NJ, Purser DW. Fractures of the odontoid process of the axis. *J Bone Joint Surg [Br]* **38**: 794, 1956.

7 Bohlman HH. Acute fractures and dislocations of the cervical spine. *J Bone Joint Surg [Am]* **61**: 1119–1142, 1979.

8 Bucholz RW, Burkhead WZ. The pathologic anatomy of fatal atlanto-occipital dislocations. *J Bone Joint Surg [Am]* **61**: 248, 1979.

9 Cattell HS, Filtzter DL. Pseudosubluxation and other variations in the cervical spine in children. *J Bone Joint Surg [Am]* **47**: 1295–1309, 1965.

10 Crawford AH. Operative treatment of spine fractures. *Orthop Clin North Am* **21(2)**: 325–339, 1990.

11 Evans DL, Bethem DL. Cervical spine injury. *J Pediatr Orthop* **9**: 563–568, 1989.

12 Fielding JW, Green R. Cervical spine injury in children. In *The Cervical Spine*, 268–281. Philadelphia; JB Lippincott, **1983**.

13 Fielding JW, Hawkins BJ. Atlanto-axial rotatory fractures. *J Bone Joint Surg [Am]* **59A**: 37, 1977.

14 Flanders AE, Schaefer DM, Dvan HT, et al. Acute cervical spine trauma: correlation of MR imaging findings with degree of neurologic deficit. *Radiology* **177(1)**: 25–33, 1990.

15 Gabrielson TO, Maxwell JA. Traumatic atlanto-occipital dislocation. *AJR Am J Roentgenol* **97**: 67, 1966.

16 Goergopoulos G, Pizzutillo PD, Lee MS. Occipital atlantal instability in children. *J Bone Joint Surg [Am]* **69**: 429, 1987.

17 Gwen JD, Harle TS, Harris H Jr. Anterior subluxation of the cervical spine. Hyperflexion sprain. *AJR Am J Roentgenol* **2**: 243–250, 1981.

18 Hegenbarth R, Ebel KD. Roentgenogram findings in fractures of the vertebral column in childhood: examination of 35 patients and its results. *Pediatr Radiol* **5**: 34, 1976.

19 Henrys SP, Lyne ED, Lifton C, Salciccioli G. Clinical review of cervical spine injuries in children. *Clin Orthop* **129**: 172, 1977.

20 Herzenberg JE, Hensenger RN, Dedrick DK. Emergency transfer and positioning of young children who have an injury of the cervical spine. *J Bone Joint Surg [Am]* **71**: 15–22, 1989.

21 Leventhal HR. Birth injuries of the spinal cord. *J Pediatr* **56**: 557–563, 1960.

22 Mayfield JC, Eberlie JC, Winter RB. Spine deformity subsequent to acquired childhood spinal cord injury. *J Bone Joint Surg [Am]* **63**: 1401–1411, 1981.

23 Melzak J. Paraplegia among children. *Lancet* **ii**: 45, 1969.

24 Mikane Y, Watanabe R, Yamano Y, Ishii K. Fracture through a synchondrosis of the anterior arch of the atlas. *J Bone Joint Surg [Br]* **69**: 483, 1987.

25 Nordstrom REA, Ludenranta TV, Kaitila II, Laasonen EMI. Familial spondylolisthesis of the axis vertebra. *J Bone Joint Surg [Br]* **68**: 704, 1986.

26 Ogden JA. *Skeletal Injury in the Child.* Philadelphia, Lea and Febiger, 1982.

27 Pang D, Wilberge JE. Spinal cord injury without radiographic abnormalities in children. *J Neurosurg* **57**: 114–129, 1982.

28 Rang M. *Children's Fractures.* Philadelphia, JB Lippincott, 1974.

29 Rathbone D, Johnson G, Letts M. Spinal cord concussion in pediatric athletes. *J Pediatr Orthop* **12**: 616–620, 1992.

30 Sherk HH, Schmit L, Lane JM. Fracture and dislocation of the cervical spine in children. *Orthop Clin North Am* **7**: 593–604, 1977.

31 Steel HH. Anatomic and mechanical considerations of the atlanto-axial articulations. *J Bone Joint Surg [Am]* **50**: 1481–1482, 1968.

32 Swirschurk L. Anterior dysplasia of C2 in children. *Physiologie* **122**. 759–765, 1977.

33 Torg JS, Pavolv H, Genuario SE, Sennett B, Wisarksi RJ, Pobre BH, Johre C. Neuropraxia of the cervical spine with transient paraplegia. *J Bone Joint Surg [Am]* **68**: 1354–1370, 1986.

34 Yngve DA, Harris WO, Herndon WA, et al. Spinal cord injury without osseous spine fracture. *J Pediatr Orthop* **8**: 53, 1988.

14 Tumors of the cervical spine

Daniel A. Green and
Steven R. Garfin

Tumors of the cervical spine present a significant treatment challenge for the spine surgeon. Whether primary or metastatic, these tumors can be difficult to diagnose as well as to manage. Although many cervical tumors are best treated non-surgically, surgery is frequently indicated, because bony stability and neurologic integrity may be threatened by bone destruction and tumor mass. Neurologic compromise at the cervical level can be catastrophic and, although the risks of surgery may be significant, the results can provide a greatly improved quality of life for the patient.

CLINICAL SYMPTOMS OF CERVICAL TUMORS

Both benign and malignant tumors almost always present with pain as the initial symptom.[43] Tumor pain is often persistent and not necessarily associated with activity. It may, in fact, be more noticeable at night when other stimuli are less. This is one of the hallmarks of pain related to tumors, and helps to distinguish it from pain secondary to mechanical or degenerative processes. Pain may remain localized to the cervical region or be referred to the midscapular or shoulder regions. When a tumor involves the upper cervical spine, motion may be decreased, particularly rotation.[19] If the tumor causes irritation or compression of a nerve root, radicular symptoms may be present. In a patient with metastatic disease to the spine, radicular pain is felt to be the most useful warning sign of impending spinal cord or nerve compression.[2]

Neurologic deficits usually present after pain; however, in 8% of patients with metastatic spread to the spine, symptoms of cord compression will be the presenting symptom.[46] Neurologic deficits may be manifested as myelopathy, radiculopathy, or myeloradiculopathy. Tumors at the cervicothoracic junction may involve the lower roots of the brachial plexus or result in a Horner's syndrome if the superior sympathetic ganglion is involved.[46]

LABORATORY, RADIOGRAPHIC, AND TISSUE EVALUATION OF CERVICAL SPINE TUMORS

When a lesion of the spine is first suspected or discovered, a differential diagnosis must be made. Fracture, infection, primary tumors (both benign and malignant), as well as metastatic disease must be considered.

Blood studies, including a complete blood count with white cell differential count and erythrocyte sedimentation rate, should be carried out. Other helpful blood tests include serum protein electrophoresis to screen for myeloma, acid phosphatase or prostate-specific antigen in males to help rule out prostate cancer, and serum calcium which may be increased in some malignant lesions such as lung or breast carcinoma as well as lymphoma.[18] Additionally, renal and liver function tests should be ordered to assess involvement of these organs.

Urinalysis for Bence-Jones proteins may be ordered together with the serum protein electrophoresis to diagnose multiple myeloma and plasmacytoma. Urinalysis also detects red blood cells, which if present, may be the result of a hypernephroma. Additional tests of the urinary tract would then be indicated.

If there is any suspicion of a tumor to the spine, the first radiographic study ordered should be plain radiographs. Although the lesion is usually visible on these radiographs, there are cases when, due to location or early presentation, these will be negative. In the upper cervical spine, tumors are not seen on plain radiographs about half of the time.[37] A bone scan may show abnormal uptake in a lesion

Table 14.1 Location of cervical tumors

Anterior	*Posterior*
Giant cell tumor	Osteoid osteoma
Fibrous dysplasia	Osteoblastoma
Eosinophilic granuloma	Osteochondroma
Hemangioma	Aneurysmal bone cyst
Intraosseous neurilemoma	
Metastatic lesions	
Most malignant primary tumors	
Myeloma/plasmacytoma	
Lymphoma/leukemia	

before it is demonstrable using plain radiographs. Additionally, it is an excellent screening examination to look for other areas of bone involvement in metastatic disease. Although technetium bone scans are quite sensitive, lesions may be missed. This is most common in multiple myeloma where bone turnover is low, and therefore radioactive isotope uptake is limited. If a patient has received recent chemotherapy, the bone turnover may also be decreased, and therefore produce a false-negative bone scan.[48]

Computed tomography (CT) of a tumor lesion is an excellent way to assess bone involvement. When a neurologic deficit is present, myelography combined with CT can be used to evaluate cord compression. In cases of complete myelographic dye block, only a portion of the cervical spine neurologic structures will be assessed with myelography. As it is important to know the extent of neural compression to plan treatment, a second myelographic injection may be required above the block to demonstrate the opposite end of compression. It is imperative that the physician involved realizes the potential for multiple areas of spinal involvement, especially in metastatic disease. Because of this, Levine recommends that patients who are to have surgery for metastatic tumor should have a myelogram of the cervical, thoracic, and lumbar spine to evaluate whether there are other areas of compression.[26] However, myelography has been associated with sudden neurologic deterioration, particularly when dye is introduced from below the lesion, which is most probably related to a 'release of pressure' distal to the lesion and the sudden expansion of the tumor mass into the surrounding dorsal space. Fortunately, as magnetic resonance imaging (MRI) has improved, the requirement for myelography has decreased.

In many respects, MRI represents the study of choice in evaluating tumors of the cervical spine; it demonstrates soft tissue masses within and outside the canal without the need for contrast. In most situations, MRI can give the same information regarding cord compression as CT enhanced with myelographic dye. In addition, MRI can demonstrate abnormal signals in bone marrow, which may represent metastatic bony deposits that would be missed on plain radiographs or technetium bone scanning. Gadolinium-enhanced MRI further increases the ability to evaluate a soft tissue mass and helps distinguish tumor from such entities as an abscess or hematoma. Unfortunately, MRI does not currently demonstrate details of bone involvement as well as CT, and therefore CT still has an important role and should be considered complementary, not supplementary, to MRI in assessment of bone involvement and stability.

Arteriography is useful in the evaluation and preoperative planning for cervical tumors. Some tumors, such as metastatic renal cell carcinoma and aneurysmal bone cysts, may be quite vascular. Angiography can demonstrate this and, if desired, embolization used to decrease vascularity prior to excision.[9] Bohlman et al[3] recommend that all patients who are to have tumor resection in the cervical spine undergo preoperative arteriography. In the cervical spine, where tumor resection may be close to the vertebral arteries, it is useful to have an arteriogram to help plan the surgical resection and reconstruction. In rare cases, where one vertebral artery may have to be embolized or sacrificed as part of the resection, an arteriogram can demonstrate whether this artery is the dominant artery to the brain stem – a contraindication to surgical sacrifice.[43]

When a tumor of the cervical spine is discovered, rapid diagnosis is mandatory for timely and appropriate treatment. In the case of metastatic disease, the tumor type can often be inferred. Some primary tumors have characteristics that are classic, pre-empting the need for biopsy, such as eosinophilic granuloma or osteoid osteoma. When diagnosis of the lesion is not absolutely certain, biopsy is a requirement.

Before biopsy of a cervical lesion, a bone scan can be of benefit to look for more accessible lesions. A platelet count and coagulation profile should also be obtained before biopsy. With a prolonged coagulation time, or a platelet count of less than 40 000–50 000 per microliter (40×10^9–50×10^9 per liter), biopsy should be delayed.[23] A pre-biopsy urinalysis can be used to search for red blood cells in the urine which are an indicator of a hypernephroma. If red cells are seen, an intravenous pyelogram may be used to make a better evaluation of the kidneys, because these lesions can be extremely vascular and biopsy may result in significant bleeding.

Biopsies can be performed percutaneously or by formal, open procedures, the latter being able to retrieve large amounts of tissue for diagnosis. Certain tumors, such as Ewing's sarcoma, plasmacytoma, and eosinophilic granuloma, as well as metastatic lesions without bony instability, are frequently treated without surgery and, therefore, it is advantageous to avoid an open biopsy, if possible. Many other primary tumors require surgical excision. In such cases, open biopsy with a frozen section can be performed. If the pathologic diagnosis is made, surgical excision and reconstruction can then be completed during the same operative sitting.

Percutaneous needle techniques using fluoroscopic control or CT-directed biopsy can often confirm a diagnosis without the associated morbidity of open surgery. These should be done under local anesthesia, so that the patient can alert the physician to any neurologic changes that occur during the procedure.

The success of a closed biopsy is dependent on many factors, in particular, the location of the tumor, the type of tumor, and the type of biopsy needle used. With sclerotic tumors, such as prostate metastases, it may be difficult to obtain sufficient tissue for histologic diagnosis. Fyfe and coworkers have demonstrated that in certain tumor types, particularly metastatic tumors, where a larger sample is often required for diagnosis, a biopsy needle with a diameter of 2 mm or greater more gives the most accurate results. Smaller gauge biopsy needles may be sufficient in infectious processes and myeloma.[14,21]

In the cervical region, needle biopsy is more difficult than in other areas of the spine. The vertebral bodies are smaller in the cervical spine, and multiple neurovascular structures become potential targets for injury, including the spinal cord, nerve roots, and carotid or vertebral arteries. All such structures are present within a relatively small area. Approach to the anterior vertebral body involves avoidance of the trachea, esophagus, and carotid sheath structures. For these reasons, CT-directed biopsy, as opposed to biopsy using fluoroscopy, is advantageous for percutaneous biopsy in the cervical spine.[23]

A transoral approach can be used to biopsy the vertebral bodies of the upper three cervical vertebrae. Before biopsy, broad-spectrum antibiotics should be used to cover any potential contamination by oral flora. Care must be taken to stay in the midline, because lateral deviation may result in inadvertent injury to the vertebral arteries.[21]

When approaching the lower cervical vertebral bodies, a standard anterior approach, employing the interval between the carotid sheath structures laterally and the esophagus and trachea medially, may be used. A lateral approach has also been described which approaches the vertebral bodies posterior to the sternocleidomastoid muscle. The carotid sheath structures may be safer with this approach as they are anterior to the path of the needle.[33]

PRIMARY TUMORS

Primary tumors located in the spine are rare. Primary tumors of the appendicular skeleton occur much more frequently. In a large series of primary spinal tumors identified over a 50-year period, only 82 cases were found, of which only 6 (7%) represented primary cervical lesions.[49] Metastatic tumors represent the most common form of tumor to the cervical spine.[49]

Primary tumors may be either benign or malignant. Fortunately, primary benign tumors occur more frequently than primary malignant tumors. Children and adolescents with a spinal tumor have a much greater chance than adults of the tumor being benign.[3,21] In a series of 23 patients with primary cervical spine tumors reported by Bohlman et al[3] all patients under 21 years of age had benign lesions.

Benign Primary Tumors

Although tumors in the cervical spine may be benign, they may cause sufficient destruction to the bone for instability to result. Neurologic compromise may be related to vertebral body collapse or compression from an expansile bone lesion and/or soft tissue mass. Surgical treatment may require extensive decompression and reconstruction for these 'benign' lesions.

Benign tumors usually present with pain. By the time pain is present, most tumors will be apparent on plain radiographs. Rarely, such as in the case of an osteoid osteoma, the tumor will not be detected on plain radiographs. In these cases, a bone scan, MRI, or CT scan may be required to localize the lesion. MRI and CT, as well as myelography and angiography, may help with planning surgical therapy.

The treatment of most benign tumors consists of complete excision or curettage. Reconstruction should be with bone rather than methylmethacrylate, because the patient is usually expected to have a normal life expectancy. Some of the more common benign tumors which affect the cervical spine will be discussed below.

Aneurysmal Bone Cyst

Aneurysmal bone cysts are rare lesions, usually found in young adults and children. They are most frequently seen in the posterior elements of the spine and can be found at any level of the vertebral column. In a large series of spinal aneurysmal bone cysts, 20 of 92 lesions (22%) were located within the cervical spine.[20]

These lesions appear cystic on radiographs, with a thin, expanded cortex. Such expansion can result in compression of the spinal cord or cervical nerve roots. As these tumors increase in size, compression may become severe.

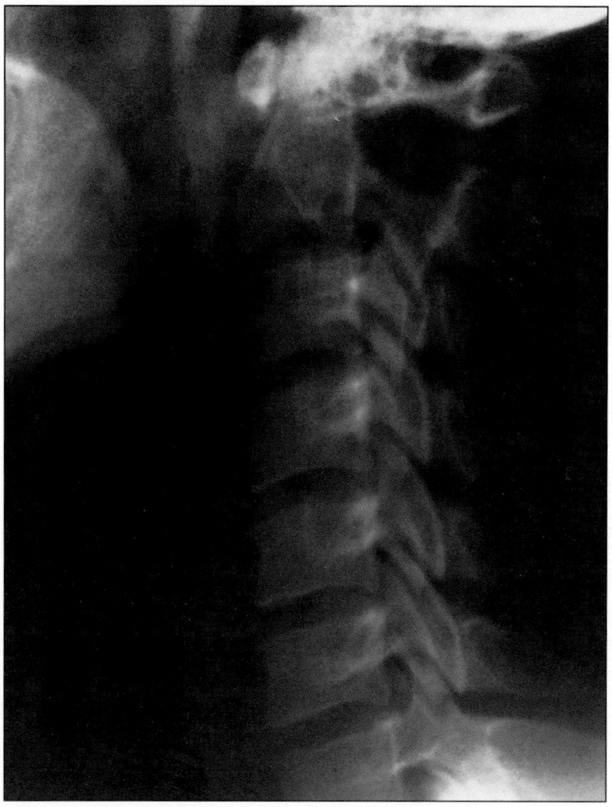

a

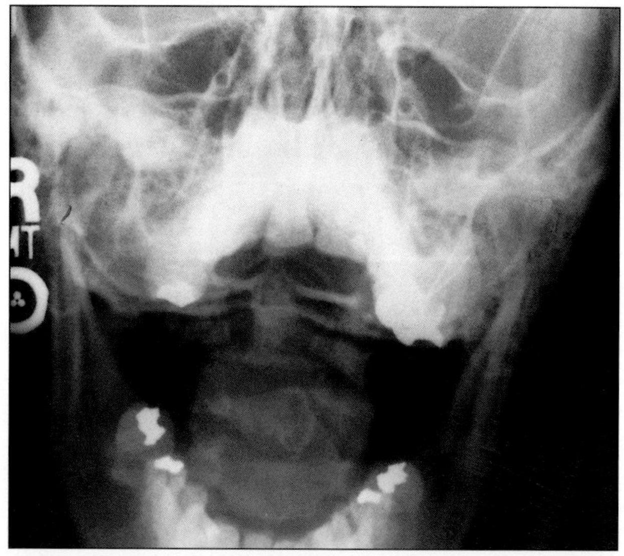

b

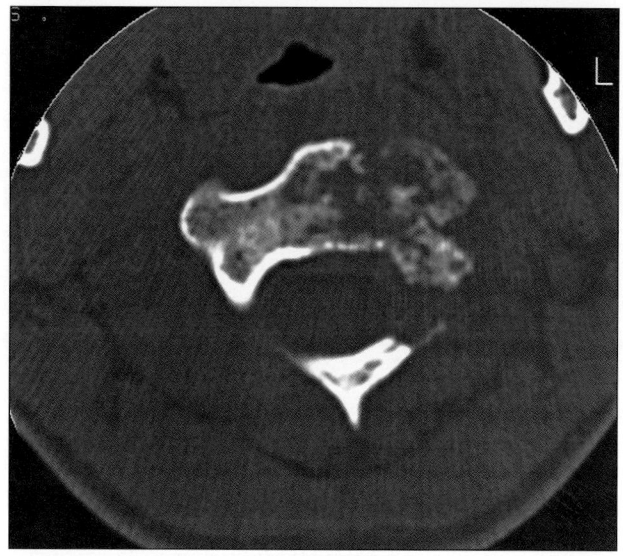

c

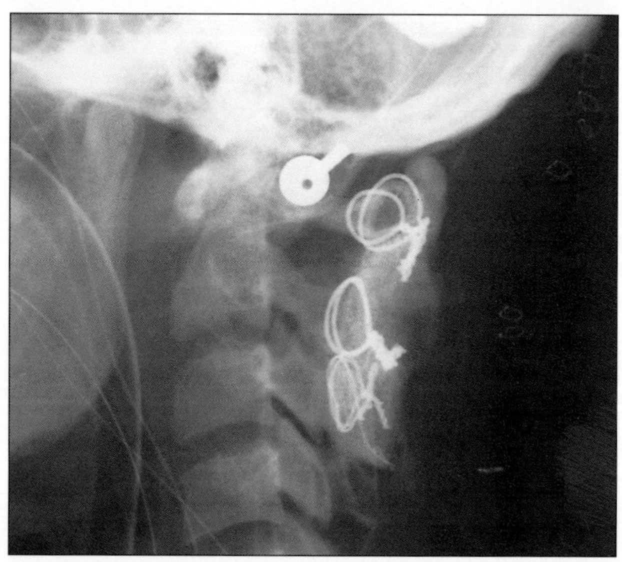

d

Figure 14.1
Thirty-four-year-old with metastatic breast carcinoma. The patient was neurologically intact, but had severe neck pain and headaches. She had previously been treated with chemotherapy and maximum radiation therapy to the cervical lesions. (a) Lateral radiograph demonstrating normal alignment and no obvious lesion; (b) open-mouth odontoid view shows asymmetry of the lateral mass of C1 and C2; (c) computed tomogram through the body of C2 demonstrates destruction of body. This destructive lesion involved the C1–C2 facet on the left; (d) Post-operative lateral radiograph shows a construct consisting of titanium mesh wired to the lamina of C1–C3 and methylmethacrylate. Bone graft was also sandwiched laterally between the mesh and bone. Sublaminar wires were used at C2 and C3 because the spinous processes were too small at these levels to use interspinous wiring

For this reason, surgical treatment is generally required and includes total excision of the lesion with reconstruction and fusion as indicated. If complete excision is not possible, curettage and bone grafting should be performed.[20] These lesions are frequently highly vascular and an arteriogram is helpful in demonstrating the pattern of vascularization before surgical treatment in order to decrease the vascularity.[43] DeRosa et al[5] have reported on the successful treatment of aneurysmal bone cysts in the lumbar spine with vascular embolization only. Excision and curettage were not needed. There are no similar reports in the cervical spine.

Eosinophilic Granuloma

Eosinophilic granuloma is most commonly seen in children before the age of 10 years. It is a benign, self-limiting condition occurring in the vertebral body which may present alone or as part of histiocytosis X syndrome – this includes other diseases, such as Hand–Schueller–Christian disease and Letterer–Siwe disease. Eosinophilic granuloma may present anywhere in the spinal column, but is less common in the cervical spine than in thoracic or lumbar areas.[42] Eosinophilic granuloma in the spine is commonly referred to as vertebra plana, because the involved level may become compressed and appear flattened on plain radiographs. This appearance is felt by some to be so diagnostic as to make biopsy unnecessary. Other lesions, however, can result in a similar 'coin on edge appearance'.[51] Infection and Ewing's sarcoma can present with a similar radiographic appearance.[16,31,35] Infection, however, will often have a narrowing of the adjacent disc space, whereas with eosinophilic granulomata, disc height is maintained.[31] O'Donnell and colleagues believe that biopsy is indicated for patients over 20 years of age at presentation, and those with radiating pain, neurologic deficit or compression, constitutional symptoms, hepatosplenomegaly, adenopathy, elevated liver enzymes, multiple bony lesions, elevated urinary catecholamines, neural arch lesions, asymmetric irregular end-plates, or the presence of a soft tissue mass.[31]

Histologically these lesions have eosinophils, histiocytes, and plasma cells. To assure the diagnosis, Langerhans' cells from the reticuloendothelial system must be present.

Treatment for eosinophilic granuloma is usually nonoperative. Immobilization and observation give good results in most cases. The cartilaginous end-plate is generally spared as the lesion resolves; reconstitution of vertebral body height occurs.[16,31,42] If a neurologic deficit occurs, radiation therapy may be indicated in order to decrease the tumor mass compressing the spinal cord or cervical nerves. Low-dose radiation is usually all that is required.[16]

Osteochondroma

Osteochondromas of the spine most commonly arise from the posterior elements, particularly the spinous processes.[28] Of symptomatic spinal osteochondromas, 60% arise in the cervical region. They may involve the lamina and result in neurocompressive symptoms.

When a patient has multiple osteochondromatosis, the diagnosis can be inferred. Vertebral involvement occurs in approximately 7% of patients with osteochondromatosis, but neurologic involvement is rarely observed. In an isolated osteochondroma, the diagnosis may be more difficult. Osteochondromas in the spine are similar to those found in other areas of the axial skeleton.[28] They are generally larger than they appear on plain radiographs because the cartilaginous cap may not be seen unless the hyaline cartilage has calcified. Computed tomography with myelography or MRI will document the extent of neural compression and may be helpful in planning therapy.

Malignant degeneration of spinal osteochondromas is rare, though possible, and is seen in approximately 1% of cases. Benign osteochondromas stop growing at the end of skeletal growth. Documentation of growth after the end of skeletal growth may be a sign of malignant degeneration.

Treatment of a neurocompressive lesion is excision. Reconstruction and fusion will depend on the extent of the resection. If the osteochondroma does not result in neurologic compression, removal is generally unnecessary unless there are symptoms of irritation of the soft tissues produced by the mass.

Osteoid Osteoma and Osteoblastoma

Osteoid osteomas and osteoblastomas are benign lesions with identical histologic features.[38] Traditionally, a lesion larger than 1.5 cm in diameter has been called an osteoblastoma, and a lesion smaller than this an osteoid osteoma. A recent study has demonstrated that osteoblastomas frequently invade the epidural space and have a soft tissue component which may be adherent to the dura. These authors feel that if there is invasion of the neural foramen or epidural space, then the lesion should be called an osteoblastoma regardless of size.[38] Both osteoid osteomas and osteoblastomas can be found throughout the spine including the cervical region. In one series, 29% of spinal osteoid osteomas and osteoblastomas were located in the cervical region.[36] Both lesions are usually located in the posterior elements of the spine.

Osteoid osteomas and osteoblastomas of the spine usually present with significant pain and torticollis.[38] Pain is generally unrelated to activity and frequently occurs during sleep. The pain may be decreased with the use of aspirin or non-steroidal anti-inflammatory medications. However, despite the classic description of pain relief with anti-inflammatory use, only 10% of patients report significant relief with these drugs.

An osteoid osteoma often presents with pain before radiographic changes are seen.[36] If a patient has complaints consistent with, or suspicious of, an osteoid osteoma, and radiographs are negative, a bone scan should be obtained. With the exception of one case report, bone scans are reported to have no false negatives in demonstrating osteoid osteomas.[12] If the bone scan is positive, a CT scan of the area can be obtained to demonstrate the exact location and size of the nidus.

Traditionally, treatment for osteoid osteomas and osteoblastomas has been surgical. For successful surgical treatment, the entire nidus must be resected. Persistent pain after surgery generally indicates incomplete removal of the tumor.[36] The presence or absence of an epidural mass should be determined, if possible, before excision of the lesion. MRI or a myelographically enhanced CT scan is recommended for this purpose.

Non-operative treatment of osteoid osteomas throughout the skeleton using long-term non-steroidal anti-inflammatory medications has been described. Kniesl and Simon[24] reported on 9 of 24 patients with osteoid osteomas who were treated in this manner. All nine obtained relief of their symptoms by an average of 33 months. In follow-up studies, the patients were able to discontinue their medication and the nidus was seen to have ossified or become encased in thickened bone.[24] In areas that are difficult to approach surgically, or when excision would lead to a complex spinal reconstruction, this may be considered as a treatment alternative.

Giant Cell Tumor

As in other regions of the skeleton, giant cell tumors are benign, but aggressive, lesions. They are usually found in the vertebral body. An extensive lesion can result in collapse of the body leading to instability and neural compromise.[13] Plain radiographs usually demonstrate an area of focal rarefaction, though some present with a more geographic, lytic appearance with marginal sclerosis. CT is very important in the preoperative evaluation of these tumors because complete excision is the key to eradication of the lesion. CT is also useful in early identification of recurrences and should be used in postoperative follow-up on a routine basis. Treatment is through surgical excision and bone grafting. Radiotherapy may be required when only subtotal resection is possible, to destroy remaining tumor cells. Local recurrence of giant cell tumors is not uncommon and is felt to be a consequence of incomplete resection. As a result of the invasive nature of giant cell tumors, they tend to have a poorer prognosis, although many feel that they are less invasive than those in the extremities. Prolonged disease-free survival periods have been reported following resection or curettage with radiation. There are other benign processes which are seen in the cervical spine. These include hemangiomas, intraosseous neurilemomas, and fibrous dysplasia.

PRIMARY MALIGNANT TUMORS

Multiple Myeloma and Solitary Plasmacytoma

The most common primary malignant tumor of the spine is multiple myeloma or solitary plasmacytoma. Multiple myeloma implies more than one area of tumor deposit and plasmacytoma usually has only a single focus. Myeloma is generally seen in older patients and plasmacytoma in younger individuals. The natural history of these two lesions differs significantly, and therefore the clinical distinction between the two remains pertinent.

Solitary plasmacytoma is rare, comprising only 3% of all plasma cell neoplasms. Although the course of multiple myeloma is usually rapidly progressive and lethal, patients with solitary plasmacytoma may have prolonged survival rates despite eventually progressing. Seventy-five percent of patients with multiple myeloma die within 1 year of diagnosis, and almost all within 4 years. The 5-year survival rate for solitary plasmacytoma is approximately 60%. The radiographic picture of plasmacytoma or multiple myeloma of the cervical spine is one of a lytic vertebral body or multiple vertebral bodies. The body may collapse, resulting in instability or neural compression. Biopsy can determine the diagnosis, although Bence-Jones protein in the urine or a monoclonal spike seen on serum protein electrophoresis provides the diagnosis of myeloma. An iliac crest bone marrow biopsy may also reveal the diagnosis, making biopsy of the cervical spine lesion unnecessary.

If there is no cervical instability, radiotherapy and systemic chemotherapy represent the treatment of choice for multiple myeloma. If potential instability exists, the patient should be placed in a halo vest while undergoing chemotherapy and radiotherapy. If there is a good response, with significant reconstitution of the vertebral bodies, the halo may be removed, and the patient can avoid surgical stabilization.[1]

If stability or neurologic compromise secondary to bone collapse is an issue, posterior stabilization and/or corpectomy and reconstruction may be required. As myeloma patients often survive for long periods of time, reconstruction should include bone fusion rather than depend on instrumentation or methylmethacrylate alone.

Osteosarcoma

Only 2% of all primary osteogenic sarcomas arise in the spine. Treatment of such lesions of the spine is particularly difficult, and outcomes poor. The average survival upon diagnosis of a spinal osteosarcoma is 6–10 months.

Vertebral osteosarcoma generally arises in the anterior elements in 95% of cases. The radiographic appearance is one of cortical destruction, soft tissue calcification, and collapse of the vertebrae in advanced cases. CT or MRI can generally demonstrate intraspinal and paraspinal soft tissue masses clearly, allowing for accurate preoperative planning. Surgical treatment has generally been limited to local tumor excision followed by radiotherapy. However, some physicians are now advising a more aggressive surgical approach with wide resection followed by reconstruction and radiotherapy. The results of such an aggressive approach have not, however, been well delineated.

Ewing's Sarcoma

Approximately 3.5% of all Ewing's sarcomas arise in the spinal column. Prognosis is generally poor for spinal lesions compared to extremity lesions. Ewing's sarcoma is a small round-cell tumor and is most commonly seen in adolescent patients. When present in the cervical spine, it is located in the vertebral body. It can result in a vertebra plana-type lesion with collapse of the vertebral body, and may therefore resemble an eosinophilic granuloma.[16,31,35] It is generally radiosensitive and treatment of choice includes immobilization and radiotherapy combined with chemotherapy.[45] Surgical treatment is indicated for decompression of neural elements and stabilization of the vertebral column.

Chordomas

Chordomas arise from vertebral remnants of embryonic notochord and can be found throughout the spine, although they most often present at the extremes (upper cervical or sacral spine). This is a relatively rare malignancy found in patients in the fifth or sixth decade of life. The appearance is that of an expansile lesion with a soft tissue mass.[8] Chordomas usually start in the vertebral body but can extend locally, and are capable of distant metastases. Chordomas may reach considerable size before metastasizing, and symptoms of constipation, urinary frequency, or nerve root compression may appear before patients present to their physicians.

Surgical extirpation of the tumor is the only curative procedure. A wide surgical margin must be obtained in such cases. A biopsy of the tumor should not be performed until all appropriate staging studies have been evaluated, after which an open biopsy through a direct posterior approach is generally preferred. The biopsy incision tract must be excised *en block* with the tumor at the time of the definitive resection procedure. Any local recurrence of the chordoma represents a grim prognostic sign, reducing the likelihood of cure.

Chondrosarcoma

Chondrosarcomas are slow growing and relatively resistant to radio- and chemotherapy. These lesions have a tendency to recur locally and, as such, have a relatively poor prognosis. Approximately 10% of all chondrosarcomas arise in the spinal column.

Radiographs of such tumors generally demonstrate bone destruction, and may have an associated soft tissue mass with calcifications. CT of the tumor is valuable in preoperative planning, and can demonstrate the extent of the lesion and degree of spinal cord compression. Surgical treatment includes wide surgical excision in attempts to cure the patient, but is rarely possible. Postoperative high-dose radiotherapy may improve survival in these patients.

Other less common primary malignant tumors of the cervical spine include fibrosarcoma, malignant fibrous histiocytoma, and lymphoma.

METASTATIC TUMORS

Regardless of the type of malignant tumor, the spine represents the most common area for skeletal metastases. This is probably related to the red marrow which persists in adult vertebral bodies. This marrow is more vascular than that in the peripheral skeleton and has a sinusoidal system which allows cancer cells to leave the general circulation and lodge within the cancellous bone.[18]

Metastatic tumors in the cervical spine are much more common than primary tumors. However, only 15% of metastatic lesions to the spine are located in the cervical area with far more seen in the thoracic and lumbar spine.[26] Most metastases are located in the vertebral bodies, as opposed to the posterior elements. Bone destruction and spinal compression therefore usually occur anteriorly. Neural compression may be from bone or tumor. The dura itself is rarely penetrated by tumor, although it may respond to tumor by reactive thickening.[18]

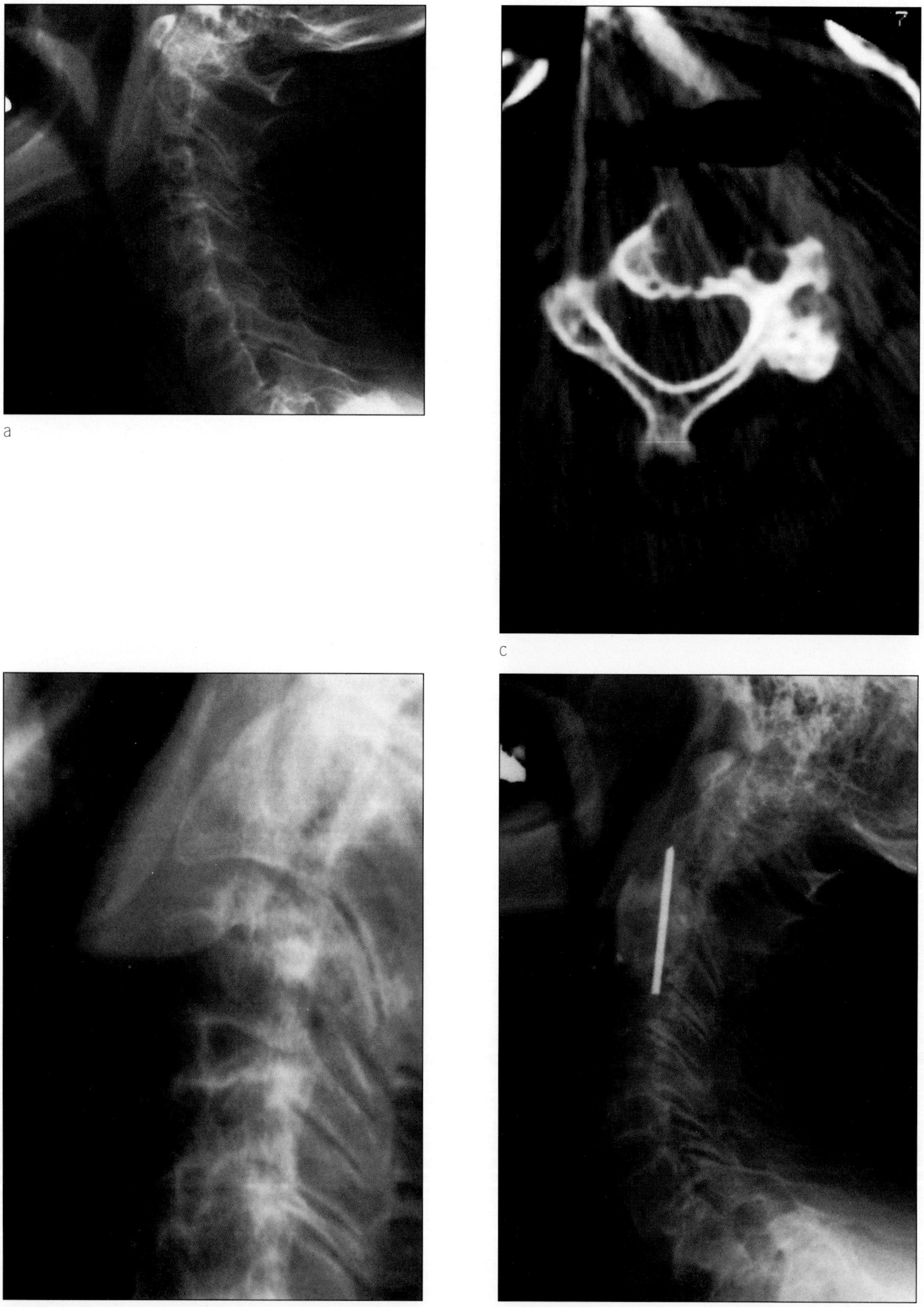

a

c

b

d

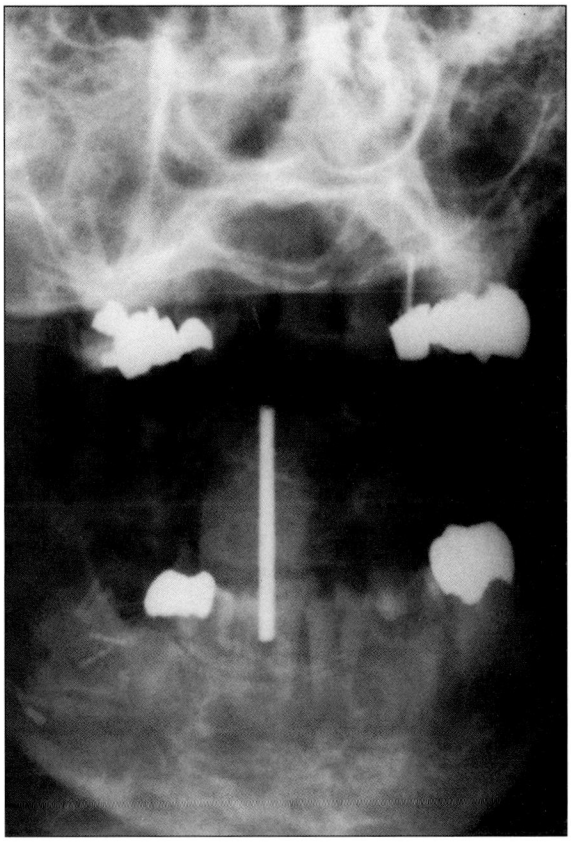

e

Figure 14.2
Sixty-seven-year-old with a history of metastatic poorly differentiated lung adenocarcinoma 6 years before presentation. The patient had severe neck pain and difficulty swallowing, but was neurologically intact. A closed biopsy of C3 done at an outside facility was negative for tumor. (a) Lateral radiograph which was read as demonstrating spondylosis with no evidence of tumor. Note the poor cortical margin anteriorly at C3. (b) Coned-down view of the upper cervical spine demonstrating a lesion within the body of C3. (c) Computed tomography of C3 with large lytic lesion within the body of C3. The posterior wall appears intact. (d) Although this is considered to be a Harrington class II lesion, with bone involvement without instability or neurologic compromise, it is a potentially highly unstable lesion should the remaining posterior cortex of the body of C3 fail. As the patient also required an open biopsy and had dysphagia, a debulking of the tumor mass was performed as well as a C3 corpectomy and strut graft using methylmethacrylate with a Steinmann pin. (e) Open-mouth odontoid view. The patient had significant relief of her pain and underwent postoperative radiotherapy after the wound had healed

The most frequent tumors to spread to the spine are breast, lung, prostate, and kidney.[15] Others, such as thyroid and uterine tumors, occur less frequently. Nine percent of tumors in the spine arise from an indeterminate primary source.[2] In a series of 130 metastatic extradural spinal tumors, lung cancer, followed equally by breast and prostate cancer, were the most frequent tumors to metastasize to the cervical spine.[15]

Occasionally, a metastatic spinal tumor may be an incidental finding during a metastatic work-up for a known primary tumor. Pain is almost always the first symptom of metastasis to the spine,[18] with neurologic deficit usually presenting after pain. In approximately 8% of patients, cord compression will be the first symptom or sign of spinal metastases.[15]

Diagnosis must be made by biopsy if the primary tumor is not known. If another bone lesion exists in addition to the cervical spine lesion, it may be easier to biopsy this other site. A bone scan can be used to look for other areas of skeletal tumor deposit.

Treatment is based on the tumor type, the extent of bony involvement, and the presence of neural compromise, as well as the overall condition of the patient and the patient's wishes. Treatment of metastatic disease to the spine could consist of combined hormonal and chemotherapy, radiotherapy, and surgical therapy. A multi-team approach, including an oncologist, radiotherapist, and spine surgeon, is necessary when planning the course of therapies. Family members, and often psychologists or psychiatrists and nurse specialists, can be helpful to the patient in making difficult decisions regarding his or her treatment.

Harrington's classification of metastatic disease to the spine is quite useful as a general guideline to surgical treatment, with its description of five classes.[18]

- Class I: there is no significant neurologic involvement and no bony destruction although tumor is present within the vertebral body.
- Class II: some destruction of bone is present, although there is no collapse or instability. There is no significant neurologic involvement. In class I and II lesions, depending on the tumor type, the lesion can often be treated with hormonal manipulation and/or chemotherapy. Treatment does not necessarily require radiotherapy. Should hormonal therapy and chemotherapy fail to decrease pain or stop tumor progression, radiation therapy may then be indicated.[18]
- Class III: major neurologic compromise without significant bony destruction. This includes epidural metastasis without evidence of bone involvement. These tumors are generally treated with radiotherapy. Steroids may be added to the treatment of those receiving radiotherapy to minimize edema, which may further neurologic compromise.[18] If there is significant and rapid neurologic deterioration, urgent surgical decompression should be considered.

- Class IV: vertebral collapse with pain or instability, but without significant neurologic compression.
- Class V: collapse or instability with major neurologic compromise. Class IV and V lesions require surgical decompression and reconstruction if the patient is healthy enough to withstand the operation.[18]

Indications for surgery, according to Harrington, include progression of cord impingement by radio-resistant tumor, recurrent tumor after maximum radiotherapy, bone detritus compressing neural tissue, progressive kyphotic deformity with intractable pain, and/or progressive kyphotic deformity associated with disruption of the posterior elements.[18]

The patient's overall condition and immune status should be considered before making the decision to intervene surgically. Chemotherapy and debilitation can result in immunocompromise, which is a relative contraindication to surgery. DeWald found that results of surgical treatment were compromised when the white blood cell count was less than 1000 per microliter (1×10^9 per liter), the platelet count less than 80 000 per microliter (80×10^9 per liter) and when paralysis had been present for more than 3 weeks.[6] Life expectancy also plays a role in the decision to operate. The time required for surgery and recovery, coupled with increased risks in a weakened patient, means that there are relative contraindications to surgery in a patient with less than 2–3 months left to live.[26,43]

When a neurologic deficit exists, the prognosis for recovery of neurologic function appears to be dependent on the pre-treatment neurologic status, as well as the rapidity of onset of the neurologic compromise. The worse the pre-treatment neurologic status, the less the likelihood of significant improvement. Similarly, with rapid onset of neurologic deficit, i.e. within 24 hours, the prognosis for improvement decreases.[2] This is true whether surgery is required for treatment, as in a Harrington class V lesion, or whether radiotherapy is the treatment of choice, as in a Harrington class III lesion.

Radiation Therapy

Radiotherapy may be indicated as the primary treatment for metastatic deposits within bone in patients with no neurologic compromise (Harrington class I or II), as well as with neurologic compromise (Harrington class III). Radiotherapy can greatly reduce pain caused by tumor infiltration into bone and can shrink the tumor mass which compresses neural tissue.[2,15,18,26,52] The success of radiotherapy is dependent on the radiosensitivity of the tumor. Tumors such as lymphoma, myeloma, Ewing's sarcoma, neuroblastoma, and seminoma are quite radiosensitive,[15,45] whereas breast and prostate carcinomas are of intermediate radiosensitivity. Lung, renal, thyroid, melanoma, and soft tissue sarcomas are relatively radioresistant.[15,26,45] In a review of the literature examining the effectiveness of radiotherapy for metastatic neurologic compression, multiple series have shown significant neurologic improvement in 34–50% of patients.[2] In some benign tumors, radiotherapy may be used with or without surgical excision to decrease the chance of recurrence and decrease tumor activity, for example, eosinophilic granuloma and giant cell tumors.[16,45] Unfortunately, in the spine, the amount of radiation that can be delivered safely is limited by the amount of radiation that the spinal cord can receive. A common dose is approximately 35–40 grays (Gy) delivered over 1–2 weeks. If tumor recurs, further radiation may not be possible because the risk of transverse myelopathy may be extremely high. As new techniques develop, such as high-energy proton beam irradiation, a dose of radiation can be delivered to the tumor with greater accuracy and less scatter to non-tumorous tissue. This should make radiotherapy safer and more effective.[45]

SURGICAL CONSIDERATIONS

Surgical treatment of metastatic spread to the cervical spine is performed for stabilization and/or decompression of the involved vertebral segments. Anterior surgery, posterior surgery, or combined anterior and posterior surgery may be necessary to achieve these goals.

There are several factors that must be considered when contemplating surgical intervention. Such factors include extent and localization of tumor, presence or absence of neurologic deficit, deformity, and development of instability. As most metastatic lesions are found in the vertebral body rather than in the posterior elements, collapse and/or neural compression usually occurs anteriorly. Approximately 75% of all cases of neural compression secondary to metastatic disease occur as a result of anterior compression from tumor in the vertebral body, whereas only 15% of cases of dural compression result from tumor in the posterior elements, and 10% from lateral compression.[2] For this reason, in the majority of destructive and neural compressive lesions, anterior surgery with decompression and stabilization is required.[18]

The preoperative evaluation is critical in patients with metastatic lesions to the spine. Magnetic resonance imaging is an excellent modality for identifying metastatic lesions within the spine and demonstrating dural compression. However, computed tomography provides a more exact and thorough evaluation of the bone architecture, quality of remaining bone, and feasibility of spinal fixation. Levine recommends preoperative evaluation of all patients with a complete cervical-to-lumbar myelogram,[26] because he believes that patients with evidence of epidural compression at two non-contiguous sites are not reasonable surgical candidates – they have a high rate of associated operative morbidity and short life expectancy. Myelography can also effectively demonstrate the extent of a block in those patients with neurologic involvement. A C1–C2 puncture should be done in any patient with a complete block from below for full evaluation of the extent of the lesion. Follow-up CT evaluation of any involved area is recommended, and also in regions of the spine where placement of hardware is considered.

Finally, some consideration must be given to life expectancy. For patients with a life expectancy of 3 months or less, surgery is often not considered a viable option. It must be remembered that, for any surgical interventions, the question of the patient's quality of life is being addressed.

For surgical candidates with metastatic disease of the spine, it is desirable to limit the amount (duration/extent) of postoperative immobilization. Immediate stabilization using hardware and/or methylmethacrylate offers immediate postoperative stabilization and may obviate the need for bracing. Harrington recommends that, if survival is judged as less than 2 years, then methylmethacrylate should be used. Supplemental bone grafting of remaining exposed bone can be added in an attempt to achieve bony fusion – in the hope that the patient will outlive the methylmethacrylate fixation.[18] Bone grafting requires time for healing; and brace immobilization is usually required during this period unless rigid internal fixation (i.e. methylmethacrylate) is used. If radiotherapy is used within 2 months of surgery, incorporation of bone grafts is hindered dramatically.[10,17,18] Chemotherapy also seems to have this effect on bone healing.[17,18] If the success of surgery relies on a bony fusion, radiotherapy and probably chemotherapy should be delayed until at least 2 months after surgery. If this is not possible, methylmethacrylate should be considered.

SURGICAL ALTERNATIVES FOR METASTATIC DISEASE OF THE CERVICAL SPINE

Once the preoperative evaluation is complete, the actual method of surgical intervention is chosen. Basically there are three surgical approaches which can be chosen in completing decompression of the neural elements and/or stabilization of the cervical spine for metastatic disease: an anterior approach, posterior approach, or combined anterior–posterior approaches.

Anterior approach

As mentioned earlier, most metastatic lesions in the cervical spine involve the vertebral body and can result in anterior dural compression. Currently available data clearly demonstrate superior results when anterior decompressive and stabilizing procedures are performed for anterior compressive lesions, when compared to posterior decompressive procedures for anterior pathology.[18,47]

The decompressive portion of the procedure is performed as described in Chapter 9. Once the decompression is complete, the spine requires stabilization. For patients who have not had previous laminectomy and have no posterior tumor, a single anterior approach should suffice.[26] Several surgical alternatives and controversy exist. Strut grafting with tricortical iliac crest, fibular strut, or rib may be used. Alternatively, methylmethacrylate may be used as an anterior spacer, especially in cases with relatively short life expectancy. The use of bone grafts is often unacceptable because of problems with bone healing (especially when adjunct chemotherapy or radiotherapy is contemplated), prolonged immobilization, and possibility of tumor recurrence. However, in patients with long or normal life expectancy, use of such grafts is advocated. The specific techniques for graft implantation with iliac crest or fibular strut are described in Chapter 2. These grafting techniques may be augmented with anterior fixation devices such as the Caspar or AO plate-screw systems when the grafts are inadequately secured through compression. The routine use of hardware is not advocated by the authors.

For patients requiring postoperative radiotherapy and/or chemotherapy to the operative site, prolonged immobilization, and with a life expectancy of less than 6 months, or with poor bone quality, the use of a methylmethacrylate spacer block for surgical reconstruction is advocated. Employment of such a spacer can provide immediate and secure fixation, and allow for rapid rehabilitation and return to a more functional and enjoyable lifestyle. Ono and coworkers have described a ceramic prosthesis which is secured to the superior and inferior uninvolved vertebrae via anchor holes and cement.[32] However, we do not feel that this construct provides optimal fixation.

When stabilization of the cervical spine with methylmethacrylate is deemed appropriate, the following techniques are preferred by the authors. The integrity of a posterior wall which will prevent inadvertent extrusion of methylmethacrylate must first be evaluated. Many feel that, if the posterior longitudinal ligament remains intact, no additional barrier is required to protect the dura and spinal cord. In cases where the integrity of the ligament is violated, titanium mesh should be placed into the posterior aspect of the defect. A U-shaped piece of this mesh is placed posteriorly and along the lateral walls of the decompressed segment. After this placement, short segments of

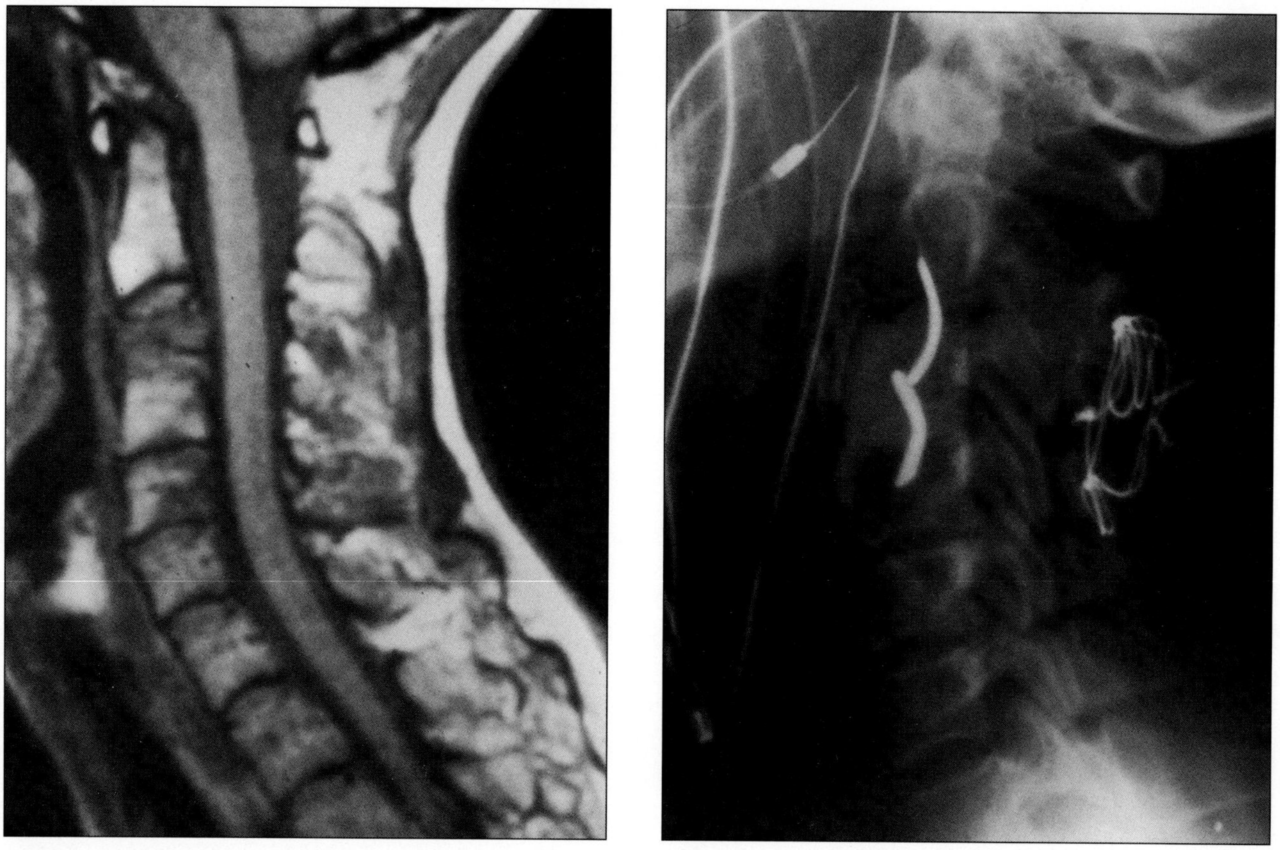

a b

Figure 14.3
Sixty-year-old with metastatic lung adenocarcinoma. The patient was neurologically intact. This would, therefore, be considered a Harrington class IV lesion. (a) Lateral magnetic resonance image demonstrates involvement of the entire body of C3 as well as collapse and mild kyphotic deformity. (b) Lateral radiograph demonstrates the reconstruction which consists of an anterior corpectomy and strut with methylmethacrylate and wires and posterior interspinous wiring

small diameter Kirshner wires are drilled into the adjacent vertebral bodies, with three or four such pins usually being placed in each vertebra. Low-viscosity methylmethacrylate is then injected into the defect using a syringe. This is preferred to manual packing of the cement to prevent posterior extrusion. It is advisable to prepare the cement in a cool environment (iced saline bath) to limit the exothermic reaction during the curing process. This method provides excellent stabilization.

Alternatively, the surgeon may use a right-angled burr to go through the end-plate of the vertebral body, and above and below the lesion, and partially hollow out these vertebral bodies. Titanium mesh is placed along the posterolateral walls of the decompressed segment, and 3.5-mm cortical screws are then placed bicortically, through the hollowed out vertebral bodies. As the methacrylate is introduced into the corpectomy site, it is manually compressed into the vertebral bodies, embedding the screws and mesh in the cement.

In most cases, either of these constructs will suffice. If, however, there is significant, concomitant destruction of posterior elements or significant posterior cord compression, posterior stabilization and/or decompression may be needed.

Posterior approach

Spinal cord decompression may be attempted posteriorly through laminectomy, but is controversial. As noted earlier, the vast majority of compressive lesions occur anterior to the spinal cord and, as such, require an anterior procedure. Laminectomy should be reserved only for those with posterior or posterolateral dural compression. Use of laminectomy for routine decompression of metastatic tumors of the cervical spine has failed to improve the neurologic status of patients in a high percentage of cases.[17] Additionally, there is a potential for progressive deformity (kyphosis, translation) and continuation or worsening of pain. Laminectomy with radiotherapy for neurologic compromise secondary to anterior compression by tumor has been shown to be no better than radiotherapy alone.[15,52] However, in the carefully selected and properly identified patient, posterior decompression coupled with appropriate stabilization can give rewarding results. The technique of posterior laminectomy is described in Chapters 2 and 10.

On occasion, patients with metastatic disease to the cervical spine without neurologic deficit may require cervical stabilization for instability and pain.[26,37] Such instability may occur in either the upper or lower cervical spine, and can generally be addressed by an isolated posterior stabilization procedure with excellent results. From a Cervical Spine Research Society survey, Fielding et al[13] have recommended extending a posterior fusion at least two levels above and below the original lesion. However, no specific indications were discussed as to when a posterior fusion should be added to supplement an anterior decompression and stabilization.[13] The triple wire technique described by Bohlman, and reviewed in Chapter 19, is advocated. Adjunct use of methylmethacrylate and wire mesh for any of the techniques may enhance short-term stability (3 months) while the bone grafts heal. However, the use of methylmethacrylate should be limited. This is due to the fact that when stressed in tension, methylmethacrylate fails early. Panjabi et al[34] demonstrated that cement used posteriorly is relatively weak and that it may fail with as small a force as that created by physiological flexion of the neck. In a case report, failure occurred at the ends of the construct, where the methacrylate attached to the bone.[10,34]

When methacrylate is used posteriorly, it should be supplemented with wires, wire mesh, and/or other instrumentation. Lipson[27] has described a helpful technique when using methylmethacrylate as well as cortical and cancellous bone grafts. Fixation wires, either sublaminar, interspinous, and/or facet, are first placed at the levels to be fused. Exposed bone is then decorticated and cancellous bone graft applied over the decorticated surface. This is followed by the application of a structural cortical graft which has an area cut out for the spinous processes. The fixation wires are passed through holes made in the cortical graft and then threaded through the wire mesh which also has holes cut out for the spinous processes. The fixation wires are then tightened over the wire mesh compressing the underlying bone graft. Methylmethacrylate is placed on the mesh, embedding the wires and spinous processes.[17] This technique has the advantages of using graft for a bony fusion and methacrylate for immediate stability, and of embedding the methacrylate into wires which improves fixation of the cement and increases its fracture strength in tension and rotation. Problems with this technique are that the mesh, bone graft, and methacrylate result in a large posterior mass over which closure may be difficult. As stated earlier, if radiation is used in the early postoperative period, the bone graft has a significant chance of not healing.[17,18] Levine has reported good results using this technique in cancer patients.[26,37]

Dunn,[7] reporting for the Cervical Spine Research Society, reviewed 24 cases in which methylmethacrylate was used either anteriorly or posteriorly. Only two patients developed late instability, one secondary to local recurrence. Harrington[17] reported on 14 patients, all of whom had methylmethacrylate as part of their stabilization. All patients received radiotherapy, averaging 43.75 Gy after the operation. There were no cases of local recurrence and only one failure of fixation. Harrington felt that with this amount of radiation, bone graft incorporation would not be successful. There appear to be no adverse effects of radiotherapy on methylmethacrylate and no adverse effects of methylmethacrylate on the response of a lesion to radiotherapy.[17]

When laminectomy is complicated by deformity or potential for instability, a posterolateral arthrodesis should be completed. Facet wiring or lateral mass plating techniques are reasonable if bone stock is of sufficient quality. For osteoporotic patients or patients with significant tumor involvement of the lateral mass, a cervical orthosis, halo device, or anterior stabilization procedure may be required.

Combined anterior–posterior approach

Combined anterior–posterior surgical techniques for metastatic disease may be required in some cases. For primarily anterior compressive lesions, anterior reconstruction and stabilization is generally adequate. However, if anterior fixation and stability are suboptimal, a concomitant posterior arthrodesis may facilitate patient recovery, minimize the need for external cervical support, and minimize the potential for complication. The authors have a low threshold for the decision to augment procedures with a posterior arthrodesis. If any question of adequacy exists over anterior stabilization, the posterior fusion is carried out. Anterior and posterior procedures may also be required for anterior and posterior spinal cord compression. Under these circumstances, a combined approach may be needed to provide adequate cord decompression and special stabilization. Finally, pathologic fracture–dislocations of the cervical spine, although rare, will generally require both anterior and posterior stabilization techniques.

Sherk et al[43] recommend using a posterior fusion for metastatic tumors when both the anterior and posterior columns are involved with tumor or when more than one level is involved anteriorly or posteriorly. Surgery, in these cases, should include a long posterior fusion using methylmethacrylate and wiring of the posterior elements from C1 to C6, C7 or T1 using Lipson's technique as described earlier. After posterior surgery, anterior corpectomy with stabilization using methylmethacrylate can then be performed. The authors believe that the increased length of the posterior fusion protects against late instability resulting from tumor progression above or below the anterior fusion and stabilization.[43]

SURGICAL TECHNIQUES FOR METASTATIC DISEASE OF THE UPPER CERVICAL SPINE

The upper cervical spine (C1 and C2) is different from the lower cervical spine. Neurologic compromise is rare in this region because there is more space available for the spinal cord compared to the lower (C3–C7) cervical spine. The neurologic damage that does occur is usually the result of bony instability, not direct tumor compression.[41] Anterior surgery is, therefore, much less commonly required in the upper cervical spine. Rare cases in which anterior surgery may be required include cases of neurologic compromise secondary to bony compression which cannot be adequately relieved through realignment and posterior stabilization, or the case of tumor compression of the cord which is non-responsive to radiotherapy.

There are three main patterns of upper cervical involvement:[37] (1) involvement of the lateral mass of C1; (2) involvement of the posterior elements of C2; and (3) involvement of the body of C2, with or without odontoid fracture.

When the lateral mass of C1 is destroyed, rotatory instability often results. An occiput-to-C2 fusion will stabilize the spine and decrease pain.[37] Radiotherapy can be used to treat the tumor within the lateral mass.

When there is involvement of the posterior elements of C2, a cervical orthosis and radiotherapy is again indicated.[37] Posterior fusion may help with pain control, if necessary.

When the body of C2 is involved without neurologic compression, immobilization in an orthosis with radiotherapy is indicated. Immobilization is required until there is restoration of the body or stability is felt to exist.[37] When the body of C2 is involved, and neurologic deficit or gross destruction is present, treatment depends on the patient's overall condition, on the presence and degree of neurologic compromise, and on bony stability. If cord compression results from a kyphotic deformity at C2, realignment with traction, followed by posterior stabilization, can decompress and stabilize the spine. For patients with neural compression secondary to collapse of the C2 body or tumor, a combined anterior decompression and posterior procedure may be required. If the patient has a limited life expectancy, realignment with traction followed by use of a halo vest and radiotherapy may achieve pain control and offer stability.[37]

SURGICAL APPROACHES

Most cervical tumors that require surgery can be approached through either the standard Smith–Robinson anterior approach to the spine or a midline posterior approach. Chapter 2 describes these approaches. However, there are tumors that require less commonly used approaches for surgical management, and upper cervical spine tumors and tumors at the cervicothoracic junction that require anterior decompression and stabilization are examples.

The upper cervical spine can be approached anteriorly in two distinct ways: a transmucosal approach through the oral cavity, or an extramucosal, retropharyngeal approach. The transmucosal approaches include the mandible- and tongue-splitting approach,[22,29,39] the mandibular swing approach,[39,40] and the transoral approach.[4,11,44]

The mandible- and tongue-splitting approach requires initial tracheotomy for airway control. The mandible is osteotomized in the midline between the front incisors. The tongue is also split straight in the midline, down to the root of the tongue and the vallecula of the epiglottis. With each side of the dissection retracted laterally, the posterior pharynx is adequately exposed. The mucosa of the pharynx is incised in the midline and the mucosal and muscular layers dissected together laterally, exposing the upper cervical spine. Closure requires plating or wiring the mandible. After the operation, meticulous oral hygiene is essential, including rinsing the mouth every 3 hours with antibiotics and spraying the oral cavity with saline or hydrogen peroxide.[22,39]

The mandibular swing approach is similar to the mandible- and tongue-splitting approach except that the tongue is retracted to one side and the mucosal incision is made in the lingual gingiva at the floor of the mouth,

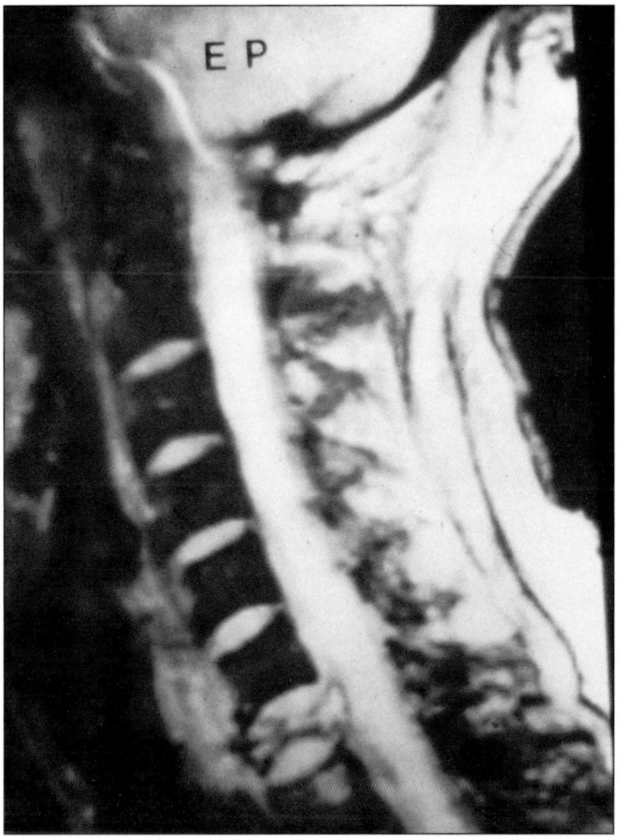

a

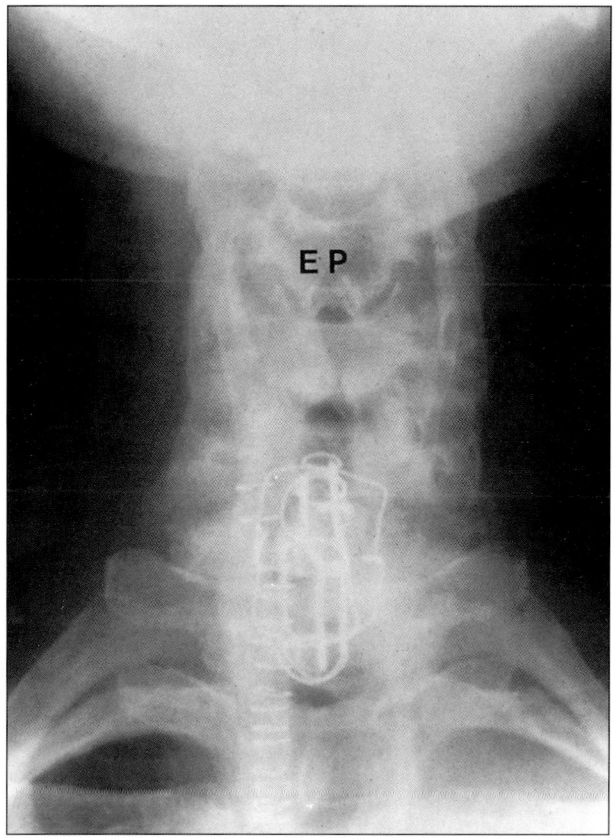

c

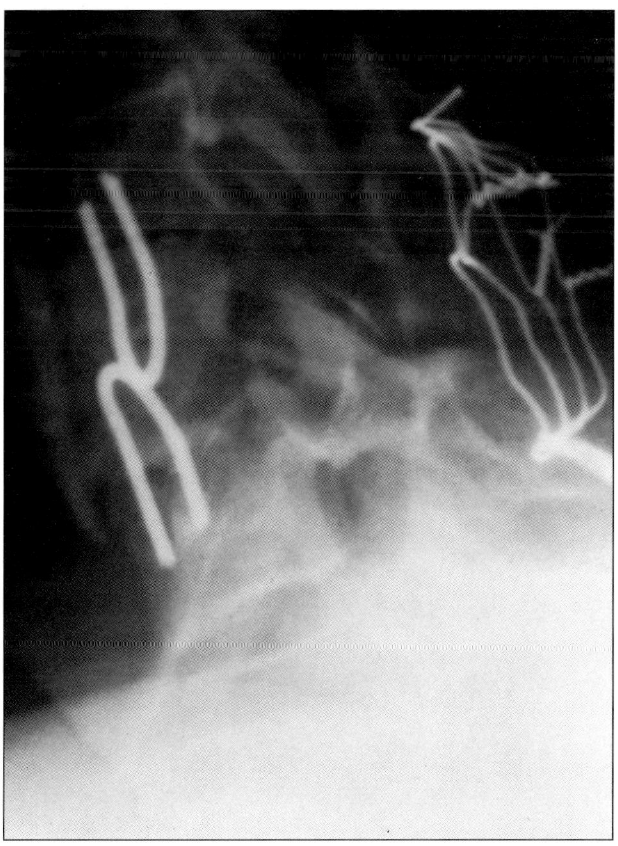

b

Figure 14.4
Patient with metastatic glioblastoma multiform to C7. The patient had myelopathy. (a) Magnetic resonance image demonstrating collapse of C7 with canal compromise; (b) postoperative lateral radiograph: posterior instrumentation was added to the anterior corpectomy and methacrylate reconstruction in order to increase stability and decrease the risk of anterior failure; (c) post-operative anterior radiograph: the patient had significant improvement of his myelopathy following surgery and was ambulatory until his death. (Courtesy of Dr R Chesnut, Department of Neurosurgery, University of California, San Diego Medical Center)

thereby avoiding splitting of the tongue. Both approaches allow visualization from the clivus to C4.[39]

A common approach for anterior exposure and removal of the odontoid peg is the transoral approach directly through the posterior pharyngeal wall, and is relatively common for removal of the odontoid process in patients with rheumatoid arthritis. It does not require tracheotomy. Rubber catheters are placed through the nose, their ends are sewn to the soft palate, and they are used to retract the soft palate into the nasopharynx. A self-retaining retraction apparatus is then used to expose the posterior oropharynx adequately. After sterile preparation of the oropharynx has been completed, a longitudinal incision is made, centered on the tubercle of the atlas which can be palpated through the posterior mucosal wall.[22,39] Sonntag et al[44] recommend the use of an operating microscope with a 300-mm lens, along with intraoperative fluoroscopy, to assist with decompression.[44]

The transoral approach is limited in its exposure. The mandible-splitting approach offers increased access to the upper cervical spine which is necessary if an anterior fusion is to be performed. When a transoral approach is used for decompression, a posterior fusion may also be necessary for stabilization purposes.

Early reports demonstrated an infection rate when using the transoral approach of as high as 50%.[11] However, Sonntag et al,[44] in a series of 29 patients treated over a 10-year period, reported no wound infections, although there were two cases of meningitis which may have been unrelated to this approach.[44] Crockard et al,[4] in a series of 22 rheumatoid patients who underwent a transoral approach for odontoid resection, reported no infections.[4]

A retropharyngeal approach to the upper cervical spine can also be used for upper cervical spine tumors. Its proponents feel that it allows adequate exposure for tumor excision and reconstruction from the clivus to C3. It is a cranial extension of the familiar Smith–Robinson approach to the anterior cervical spine and is entirely extramucosal.[30,47]

The anterior retropharyngeal approach is performed by first placing the patient in Gardner–Wells tongs with approximately 10 pounds (4.5 kg) of weight. Awake nasotracheal intubation is performed and (while still awake) the neck is extended. A transverse submental incision is made and the platysma opened in line with the incision. The retromandibular veins are ligated as necessary and the mandibular branch of the facial nerve is identified and protected. It is helpful to have a sterile nerve stimulator available for use during this approach to identify nerves. The submandibular salivary gland must be dissected out and removed, and the salivary duct securely ligated. The digastric and stylohyoid muscles are then identified and divided after the digastric has been tagged for later repair. The hyoid should then be mobile, allowing it to be retracted medially along with the hypopharynx. The hypoglossal nerve is identified and then protected and retracted superiorly. The prevertebral fascia is seen in the plane between the medially retracted hypopharynx and the laterally retracted carotid sheath. The longus colli muscles are identified and retracted laterally, revealing the upper cervical vertebrae. Branches of the carotid artery and internal jugular vein require ligation to increase the cephalad exposure. As the dissection proceeds in the caudad direction, the superior thyroid vessels (care should be taken to isolate and protect the superior laryngeal nerve), followed by the lingual, ascending pharyngeal and facial vessels, will require ligation, in that order.[30,47]

Postoperative palsies may occur from excessive traction. The facial nerve is particularly susceptible because superior retraction may injure this nerve as it exits from the stylomastoid foramen in the skull.

A lateral retropharyngeal approach to the spine posterior to the carotid sheath can also be used in the upper cervical spine.[50] This approach does not offer the same exposure as the procedures described above for decompression and strut grafting.[30]

Tumors at the cervicothoracic junction are also difficult to approach anteriorly. Posterolateral thoracotomy is often required for large invasive lung carcinomas as most of these tumors have an extensive paraspinous tumor mass.[46]

The trans-sternal approach to the cervicothoracic junction allows adequate exposure of the upper two thoracic vertebrae.[25,46] This approach is performed through a T-shaped incision. The horizontal component is made 1 cm above the clavicle from the lateral border of the sternocleidomastoid muscle on one side to the lateral border on the other. The longitudinal portion of the incision is made in the midline. The sternal and clavicular heads of the sternocleidomastoid muscle are detached at their origins. The sternohyoid and sternothyroid muscles are sectioned above the sternal notch and clavicle. The origin of the pectoralis major must be dissected laterally off the sternum and medial half of the clavicle. The medial third of the clavicle on the side of the spine to be approached is removed by disarticulation from the manubrium after a lateral cut in the clavicle has been made with a saw. The manubrium is then removed using a power drill and heavy scissors. This exposes the underlying brachiocephalic artery and vein. Branches off the brachiocephalic vessels may have to be ligated to allow the brachiocephalic vessels to be retracted inferiorly. The plane between the carotid sheath laterally and the esophagus and trachea medially is then identified. The recurrent laryngeal nerve should be identified and retracted with the medial structures. The longus colli muscles are then stripped laterally, revealing the vertebral bodies. After decompression, strut grafting with bone or methylmethacrylate spacer placement can be performed through this approach.[25,46]

CONCLUSION

Treatment of tumors of the cervical spine can be extremely challenging. Primary benign tumors often require extensive surgery for resection, even though the tumor itself is benign. With good surgical technique and proper reconstruction, surgical morbidity can be diminished, and the tumor can often be completely removed.

Primary malignant tumors and metastatic tumors require a multi-specialty approach. Surgery is only one treatment option and, often, non-surgical treatment with radiotherapy, hormonal therapy, or chemotherapy is indicated and can give good results. The surgeon should not look at surgical excision as the only means of palliation or cure in these patients, nor should other physicians feel that surgery in patients with malignant tumors is futile. Appropriate indications, with the appropriate use of radiotherapy, chemotherapy, and hormonal therapy, surgical fusion, instrumentation, and decompression can significantly improve the quality of life for those suffering from malignant cervical tumors.

REFERENCES

1 Abitbol JJ, Botte MJ, Garfin SR, Akeson W. The treatment of multiple myeloma of the cervical spine with a halo vest. *J Spinal Dis* **2**: 263–267, 1989.

2 Black P. Spinal metastasis: Current status and recommended guidelines for management. *Neurosurgery* **5**: 726–746, 1979.

3 Bohlman HH, Sachs BL, Carter JR, et al. Primary neoplasms of the cervical spine. *J Bone Joint Surg [Am]* **68**: 483–494, 1986.

4 Crockard HA, Pozo JL, Ransford AO, et al. Trans-oral decompression and posterior fusion for rheumatoid atlanto-axial subluxation. *J Bone Joint Surg [Br]* **68**: 350–356, 1986.

5 DeRosa GP, Graziano GP, Scott J. Arterial embolization of an aneurysmal bone cyst of the lumbar spine: A report of two cases. *J Bone Joint Surg [Am]* **72**: 777–780, 1990.

6 DeWald RL, Bridwell KH, Prodromas C, et al. Reconstructive spinal surgery as palliation for metastatic malignancies of the spine. *Spine* **10**: 21–26, 1985.

7 Dunn EJ. The role of methylmethacrylate in the stabilization and replacement of tumors of the cervical spine. *Spine* **2**: 15–24, 1977.

8 Dunn EJ, Davidson RI, Desai S. Chapter 12. Tumors involving the cervical spine – Diagnosis and management of the cervical spine. In Sherk HH, Dunn EJ, Eismont FJ, *et al* (eds) *The Cervical Spine*, 2nd ed, 693–722. (The Cervical Spine Research Society) Philadelphia: JB Lippincott 1989.

9 Dysart SH, Swengel MD, van Dam BE. Aneurysmal bone cyst of a thoracic vertebra. *Spine* **17**: 846–848, 1992.

10 Emery SC, Brazinski MS, Kok A, et al. The biological and biomechanical effects of irradiation on anterior spinal bone grafts – a canine model (Abstract). *North American Spine Society Proceedings*, 1992: **19**.

11 Fang HSY, Ong GB. Direct anterior approach to the upper cervical spine. *J Bone Joint Surg [Am]* **44**: 565–594, 1960.

12 Fehring TK, Green NE. Negative radionuclide scan in osteoid osteoma: A case report. *Clin Orthop* **185**: 245–249, 1984.

13 Fielding JW, Pyle RN, Fietti VG. Anterior cervical vertebral body resection and bone grafting for benign and malignant tumors. *J Bone Joint Surg [Am]* **61**: 251–253, 1979.

14 Fyfe SI, Henry APJ, Mulholland RC. Closed vertebral biopsy. *J Bone Joint Surg [Br]* **65**: 140–143, 1983.

15 Gilbert RW, Kim J, Posner JB. Epidural compression from metastatic tumor: Diagnosis and treatment. *Ann Neurol* **3**: 40–51, 1978.

16 Green NE, Robertson WW, Kilroy AW. Eosinophilic granuloma of the spine with associated neural deficit. *J Bone Joint Surg [Am]* **62**: 1198–1202, 1980.

17 Harrington KD. The use of methylmethacrylate for vertebra body replacement and anterior stabilization of pathological fracture dislocations of the spine due to metastatic disease. *J Bone Joint Surg [Am]* **63**: 36–46, 1981.

18 Harrington KD. Metastatic disease of the spine, current concepts review. *J Bone Joint Surg [Am]* **68**: 1110–1115, 1986.

19 Hastings DE, MacNab I. Neoplasms of the atlas and axis. *Can J Surg* **11**: 290, 1968.

20 Hay MC, Patterson D, Taylor TKF. Aneurysmal bone cysts of the spine. *J Bone Joint Surg [Am]* **60**: 406–411, 1978.

21 Herkowitz HN, Weslowski DP. Percutaneous biopsy of the spine: Techniques, results, and complications. In Garfin SR (ed), *Complications of Spine Surgery*, Chap. 18. Baltimore Williams & Wilkins 1989.

22 Honma G, Murota K, Shiba R, et al. Mandible and tongue-splitting approach for giant cell tumor of axis. *Spine* **14**: 1204–1210, 1989.

23 Kattapuram SV, Rosenthal DI. Percutaneous needle biopsy of the spine. In Sundaresan N, Schmidek H, Schiller A, Rosenthal D (eds) *Tumors of the Spine: Diagnosis and Clinical Management*, 46–51. Philadelphia, WB Saunders 1990.

24 Kneisl JS, Simon MA. Medical management compared with operative treatment for osteoid osteoma. *J Bone Joint Surg [Am]* **74**: 179–185, 1992.

25 Kurz LT, Pursel SG, Herkowitz HH. Modified anterior approach to the cervico-thoracic junction. *Spine* **165**: 5542, 1991.

26 Levine AM. Operative techniques for treatment of metastatic disease of the spine. *Semin Spine Surg* **2**: 210–227, 1990.

27 Lipson SJ. Cervical myelopathy and posterior atlanto–axial subluxation in patients with rheumatoid arthritis. *J Bone Joint Surg [Am]* **67**: 593–597, 1985.

28 Malat J, Virapongse C, Levine A. Solitary osteochondroma of the spine. *Spine* **11**: 625–628, 1986.

29 Martin H, Tollefsen HR, Gerold FP. Median labiomandibular glossotomy. *Am J Surg* **102**: 753–759, 1961.

30 McAfee PC, Bohlman HH, Riley LH, et al. The anterior retropharyngeal approach to the upper part of the cervical spine. *J Bone Joint Surg [Am]* **69**: 1371–1383, 1987.

31 O'Donnell J, Brown L, Herkowitz H. Vertebra plana-like lesions in children: Case report with special emphasis on the differential diagnosis and indications for biopsy. *J Spinal Dis* **4**: 480–485, 1991.

32 Ono K, Tada K. Cited in Dunn EJ, Davidson RI, Desai S. Tumors involving the cervical spine: Diagnosis and management of tumors of the cervical spine. In Sherk HH, Dunn EJ, Eismont FJ, et al (eds), *The Cervical Spine,* 2nd ed, 711. (The Cervical Spine Research Society) Philadelphia: JB Lippincott 1989.

33 Ottolenghi LE, Schajowicz F, DeSchantt DA, et al. Aspiration biopsy of the cervical spine. *J Bone Joint Surg [Am]* **46**: 715–733, 1964.

34 Panjabi MM, Hopper W, White AA, et al. Posterior spine stabilization using methylmethacrylate. *Spine* **2**: 241–247, 1977.

35 Paulsen JO, Jensen JT, Thommesen P. Ewing's sarcoma simulating vertebra plana. *Acta Orthop Scand* **46**: 211–215, 1975.

36 Pettine KA, Klassen RA. Osteoid osteoma and osteoblastoma of the spine. *J Bone Joint Surg [Am]* **68**: 354–361, 1986.

37 Phillips E, Levine LM. Metastatic lesions of the upper cervical spine. *Spine* **14**: 1071–1077, 1989.

38 Raskas DS, Graziano GP, Herzenberg JE, et al. Osteoid osteoma and osteoblastoma of the spine. *J Spinal Dis* **5**: 204–211, 1992.

39 Shah JP, Shaha AR. Transmandibular approaches to the upper cervical spine. In Sundaresan N, Schmidek H, Schiller A, Rosenthal D (eds) *Tumors of the Spine: Diagnosis and Clinical Management,* 329–335. Philadelphia: WB Saunders 1990.

40 Shah JP, Shemen L, Strong EW. Surgical therapy of oral cavity tumors. In Thawley SE, Panje WR (eds) *Comprehensive Management of Head and Neck Tumors,* 551–562. Philadelphia: WB Saunders 1986.

41 Sherk HH. Tumors of the atlas and axis. *Clin Orthop* **109**: 33–41, 1975.

42 Sherk HH, Nicholson J, Nixon JE. Vertebra plana and eosinophilic granuloma of the cervical spine in children. *Spine* **3**: 116–121, 1978.

43 Sherk HH, Nolan JP, Mooar PA. Treatment of tumors of the cervical spine. *Clin Orthop* **233**: 163–167, 1988.

44 Sonntag VKH, Hadley MN, Spetzler, RF. The transoral–transclival approach to the upper cervical spine. In Sundaresan N, Schmidek H, Schiller A, Rosenthal D (eds), *Tumors of the Spine: Diagnosis and Clinical Management.* Philadelphia, WB Saunders, 1990: 319–28.

45 Suit HD, Austin-Seymour M. The role of radiation therapy. In Sundaresan N, Schmidek H, Schiller A, Rosenthal D (eds) *Tumors of the Spine: Diagnosis and Clinical Management,* 86–91. Philadelphia: WB Saunders 1990.

46 Sundaresan N, DiGiacinto GV. Surgical approaches to the cervicothoracic junction. In Sundaresan N, Schmidek H, Schiller A, Rosenthal D (eds) *Tumors of the Spine: Diagnosis and Clinical Management,* 358–368. Philadelphia: WB Saunders 1990.

47 Sundaresan N, Sachdev VP. Anterior approaches to the cervical spine. In Sundaresan N, Schmidek H, Schiller A, Rosenthal D (eds) *Tumors of the Spine: Diagnosis and Clinical Management,* 349–357. Philadelphia: WB Saunders 1990.

48 Van Zantzen TGM, Tevle GJ, Golding RP, et al. CT and nuclear imaging in vertebral metastasis. *Clin Nucl Med* **11**: 334, 1986.

49 Weinstein JN, McLain RF. Primary tumors of the spine. *Spine* **12**: 843–851, 1987.

50 Whitesides TI. Surgical approaches and techniques – lateral retropharyngeal approach to the upper cervical spine. In Sherk HH, Dunn EJ, Eismont FJ, et al (eds) *The Cervical Spine,* 2nd ed Chapter 13, 796–804. (The Cervical Spine Research Society) Philadelphia: JB Lippincott 1989.

51 Wickenhauser J, Sunder-Plassman AM, Zaunbauer F, et al. Vertebra plana calve. *Neuroradiology* **18**: 221–225, 1975.

52 Young RF, Post EM, King GA. Treatment of spinal epidural metastases. *J Neurosurg* **53**: 741–748, 1980.

15 Intradural lesions of the cervical spine

William R. White

In comparison to the wide range of pathology which affects the cervical spine, intradural lesions are a somewhat rare, but important, group of spinal disorders which require discussion. Neoplastic, vascular, congenital, and degenerative diseases can all occur within the cervical spine. Appropriate treatment can improve life expectancy and reduce associated morbidity. Many of these lesions are potentially curable. Symptoms associated with intradural lesions are often subtle and slowly progressive. The illness can actually be at an advanced stage when a diagnosis is made. Finally, those lesions that occur in the cervical spine may also occur caudally in the thoracic and lumbar spine. This chapter is devoted to the cervical spine. Table 15.1 gives a brief outline of the common lesions.

PHYSICAL SIGNS AND SYMPTOMS

Physical signs and symptoms are usually a reflection of the anatomic position of the lesion and its relationship to the spinal cord, nerve roots, dura, and blood vessels, and its cephalocaudal location in the spine. Figure 15.1 shows the important anatomic features of the spinal cord.

Motor fibers arise from the precentral gyrus and form the pyramidal tract. About 80% of these fibers cross to the opposite side in the pyramidal decussation in the lower medulla, creating the lateral corticospinal tract.[8] This tract is located in the posterolateral portion of the cord. Fibers synapse with second-order anterior horn cells which form the motor root.

Sensory fibers are both crossed and uncrossed. Fibers that convey pain, temperature, and some tactile sensation enter the cord through the dorsal root, and synapse over several segments with second-order neurons, which cross to the opposite side. These then ascend in the anterolateral segment of the cord as the lateral spinothalamic tract. Fibers which convey position, vibration, some touch, and discriminative sensibility, ascend in the ipsilateral dorsal column, and synapse with their second-order neurons in the nuclei cuneatus and gracilis before crossing to the opposite side.

Most of the blood supply of the spinal cord is derived from the anterior spinal artery. In the upper cervical region, ventral branches of the vertebral artery form the anterior spinal artery with contributions from the radicular arteries. The lower segments of the cervical cord are supplied by radicular vessels from the inferior thyroid artery and the costocervical trunk. There are two dorsal arteries on the posterior surface of the cord.

Intramedullary lesions expand from the central portion of the spinal cord. These tumors progress insidiously, causing neurologic signs and symptoms through internal compression and involvement of fiber tracts and cell bodies. Pain and dysesthesia are common. Fibers that cross the central portion of the canal (pain and temperature) are affected earlier than those that are uncrossed (touch). This produces a dissociated, suspended, sensory loss (diminished pain and temperature with preserved touch) over the shoulders, arms, and chest. The cell bodies of the anterior horn cells can be destroyed with resultant wasting of the musculature of the upper extremities. If the lesion extends up into the brain stem, lower cranial nerve nuclei can be involved. As the lesion enlarges, the surrounding long fiber tracts become involved, causing weakness of the lower extremities, gait imbalance, spasticity, hyperreflexia, and urinary incontinence. Loss of bowel or bladder function is an uncommon presenting symptom of spinal cord tumors, because the degree of compression necessary to produce these symptoms will have already produced pain and dysesthesia. Persistent pain is seen in almost all intramedullary tumors, and typically is described as a deep aching that fails to subside. Upper cervical cord lesions may involve the respiratory pathways, affecting the diaphragm, and can be associated with sleep apnea (Ondine's curse).

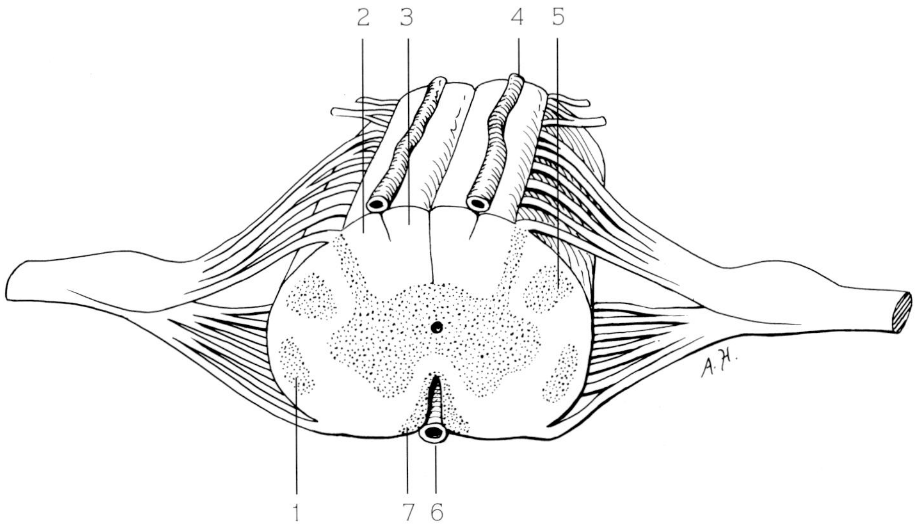

1. Lateral spinothalamic
2. Fasciculus cuneatus
3. Fasciculus gracilis
4. Posterior spinal artery
5. Lateral corticospinal
6. Anterior spinal artery
7. Ventral corticospinal

Figure 15.1
Illustration of important anatomic features of the spinal cord. Fasciculus gracilis and cuneatus compose the posterior columns, conveying position and vibration. The lateral spinothalamic tracts convey pain, temperature, and tactile sensation. Anterior and lateral corticospinal tracts represent descending motor fibers

Table 15.1 Intradural lesions of the cervical spine

Neoplastic
Intramedullary
Astrocytoma
Ependymoma
Hemangioblastoma
Metastatic
Extramedullary
Meningioma
Schwannoma (neurilemmoma), neurofibroma
Dermoid, epidermoid
Lipoma
Metastatic
Congenital
Syringomyelia
Vascular
Arteriovenous malformation
Degenerative
Amyotrophic lateral sclerosis
Vitamin B_{12} deficiency
Other
Multiple sclerosis

Intradural extramedullary lesions produce pain and neurologic deficits. Pain occurs from involvement of the dura mater and pia arachnoid, and crowding of the intraspinal contents. This can produce local pain and limitation of neck motion. If spinal nerve roots are affected, radicular pain, sensory loss, and weakness may ensue. Pain under these circumstances is sharp and more knife-like compared to intramedullary lesions. The pain is often intensified by any Valsalva maneuver. Mass effect on the spinal cord will affect the long fiber tracts. Laterally placed lesions affecting one side of the cord may produce a Brown–Séquard syndrome. Unilateral compression of the corticospinal tract and the lateral spinothalamic tract result in ipsilateral weakness and contralateral numbness. Anterior lesions produce bilateral weakness and sensory loss, depending on the extent of the cord compression.

Lesions of the foramen magnum present in unusual ways. Pain in the occipital area and postauricular area is common. If the lesion extends into the posterior cranial fossa, the lower cranial nerves are involved. Nystagmus may be seen, and the forearms and hands may be wasted, presumably from compression of the anterior spinal artery or its tributaries from the vertebral artery. Respiratory embarrassment may also occur.

Intradural lesions in children may cause an unexplained scoliosis, i.e. one that does not seem to fit the usual age or anatomic distribution.

RADIOGRAPHIC AND IMAGING STUDIES

The most effective work-up for intradural lesions is accomplished with routine cervical spinal radiographs and magnetic resonance imaging (MRI).

Cervical spinal radiographs are simple to do, inexpensive, and can provide valuable information. The diameter of the spinal canal may be widened, as can be seen in a long-standing intramedullary tumor. There may be scalloping of the vertebral bodies from dural ectasia, and enlargement of one or many intervertebral foramina, both associated with neurofibromatosis. In addition, underlying cervical spondylosis, kyphosis, swan neck deformity, and congenital defects are seen.

Magnetic resonance imaging is the diagnostic test of choice for intradural lesions. It permits visualization of the spinal cord and spine, without the radiation or invasiveness associated with myelography. The author's preference is a scanner with a high-field strength magnet of 1–1.5 tesla. This gives the finest detail and minimizes motion artifact. Contrast enhancement with gadolinium or newer agents is essential. A scan of the head and complete spinal canal may be necessary to see the full extent of the lesion and any associated anomalies, such as hydrocephalus or craniocervical anomalies, such as platybasia. Sagittal, axial, and sometimes coronal scans are done. T1-, T2-, and T1-weighted images with contrast enhancement are necessary.

Intramedullary lesions are well seen on MRI. Ependymomas and astrocytomas occur centrally within the spinal cord, expand the spinal cord, and enhance with contrast. Cysts are associated with these tumors about 40–50% of the time; they can be small or extend for long distances throughout the spinal cord. Hemangioblastomas are also intramedullary tumors. They are highly vascular, enhance intensely, and often have associated cysts. Multiple sclerosis, not uncommonly, is a diagnostic problem when evaluating the possibility of intramedullary tumor. Acute and subacute plaques can enhance with contrast and even expand the spinal cord somewhat. Generally, they do not expand the cord greatly, and the clinical situation often provides a clue to the diagnosis. With time, these lesions should fade, and a judicious period of follow-up will help with the diagnosis. Syringomyelia, often associated with a Chiari type I malformation, is well demonstrated. Tonsilar ectopy is seen on the lateral scan, and the syrinx, often with multiple septa, is very dramatic.

Extramedullary lesions are also well displayed. Meningiomas are solid and sometimes hard to see without contrast, but they usually enhance with contrast. They may be dorsal, lateral, or ventral to the cord. Calcified tumors may not enhance. Computer tomography can be useful in this situation. Schwannomas (neurilemmomas) enhance with contrast, may be cystic, can be intradural as well as extradural, or both, and can enlarge the neural foramen. Lipomas, dermoids, and intradural metastatic tumors (carcinomatous meningitis) are well seen. Multiple enhancing lesions attached to roots make a diagnosis of carcinomatous meningitis highly likely in the appropriate clinical setting. These can be very extensive.

Computed tomography is less valuable than MRI, but is much better for bone detail. Enlarged neural foramina and scalloped vertebral bodies are clearly demonstrated.

Myelography still can play an important role in the diagnosis of small extramedullary tumors, particularly when followed by computed tomography. There is some risk of worsening a patient's neurologic deficit when there is a high-grade obstruction, as seen with larger tumors. It is particularly useful in the diagnosis of arteriovenous malformations which may be hard to see with MRI. Spinal angiography is essential for evaluation of arteriovenous malformations and hemangioblastoma.

INTRAMEDULLARY TUMORS

Intradural intramedullary tumors constitute approximately 30% of all intradural spinal tumors.[2,14] The most common of these originate from the glia of the spinal cord and its derivatives. Ependymoma and astrocytoma are the most frequently encountered of such tumors in the adult.[5,6] Hemangioblastoma and other rare tumors, such as intramedullary neurofibromas and metastatic tumors, can be seen. In adults, intramedullary tumors have their highest incidence in midlife and affect males and females equally. Astrocytomas are the most common intradural intramedullary tumor of childhood.

Ependymomas occur throughout the whole spinal cord. In the cervical region, local and radicular pain are common complaints, and weakness in the extremities is also commonly seen. They generally have a benign pathology, arising from the ependyma of the central spinal canal, and are more common in the thoracic region than the cervical area. They seem to have a special predilection for the conus medullaris, and often arise from the filum terminale. Subarachnoid seeding may occur. As ependymomas are not infiltrating tumors, they displace and expand the spinal cord from the center and, therefore, usually have a fairly clear demarcation from the normal cord and can be totally resected.

Intramedullary tumors are usually not well detected on plain radiographs. Occasionally, widening of the spinal canal will be seen. However, myelography will demonstrate a pisiform thickening of the cord, although MRI is generally considered the test of choice for these tumors, with the tumor being isotense with the spinal cord on T1-weighted images, whereas T2 images give a radicular appearance. Gadolinium-enhanced images demonstrate sharp tumor margins.

Surgical excision is the treatment of choice. Ependymomas are radiosensitive, but postoperative radiation is not usually recommended, except for malignant ependymomas or when a total excision could not be accomplished. Radiation extends the time of recurrence from 3 to 8 years after subtotal excision.[2]

Astrocytomas are usually low-grade tumors analogous to the cerebellar astrocytoma in children. Well-differentiated astrocytomas predominantly affect males, whereas malignant astrocytomas have an equal sex distribution. Astrocytomas have a peak incidence in the fourth and fifth decades, and are twice as common as ependymomas in children. The tumor arises eccentrically in the cord. Physical findings are similar to those for ependymomas, but may be more one-sided. Associated cysts are common; these can extend for long lengths throughout the spinal cord. In some cases, a well-defined demarcation can be seen between the tumor and cord; in the remainder of cases, this does not happen. Malignant astrocytomas also occur and have a very poor prognosis. They are relentlessly progressive in spite of all modalities of treatment.

Plain radiographs may reveal interpedicular widening at the level of the tumor. Spinal deformity, namely kyphosis or kyphoscoliosis, may be seen in association with this tumor in nearly one-third of cases, especially children. Again MRI is the diagnostic tool of choice for astrocytomas. The tumor will be hypointense on T1-weighted images, and hyperintense but poorly demarcated on T2 images. Gadolinium enhancement is irregular. In general, it is difficult to differentiate astrocytoma from ependymoma on MRI appearance.

Treatment is surgical exploration and attempted resection. It may be possible to accomplish a near-total removal in cases where there is a good plane of demarcation. Barring this, an attempt may be made to remove most of the tumor, decompressing the spinal cord. However, attempts to perform an extensive tumor resection with poor margins will often result in neurologic deficit. In such infiltrative cases, a posterior myelotomy may be done allowing further expansion of the tumor outside the cord and prolonging neurologic function. Dural closure is best completed with a fascial patch graft which allows for maximal cord decompression. Radiation is generally used for recurring tumor, but may be used in infiltrative tumors with subtotal resection, once the wound is sufficiently healed; it appears to be of benefit in delaying recurrence and should be considered when the surgeon is unable to decompress the cord adequately by surgery or if the pathology was malignant. Half of the patients develop recurrence in about 4 years.[2] Some centers recommend routine postoperative radiation for adults with astrocytomas.[4]

Hemangioblastomas are rare; they are of obscure pathologic origin, containing endothelial and stromal cells, and pericytes with numerous large vascular channels. They occur more often in the cerebellum and brain stem, but are found in the cervical and thoracic spinal cord. In cases with multiple central nervous system tumors, or if associated with at least one visceral lesion (pheochromocytoma, abdominal cysts, renal cell carcinoma), the patient is felt to have the Von Hippel–Lindau complex, which is an autosomal dominant, inherited disorder.[11]

Plain radiographs are usually not helpful. Lesions in the spinal cord are clearly seen on MRI, and are often associated with cysts that are not lined with neoplastic cells. Spinal angiography is necessary for full preoperative evaluation of hemangioblastomas and to delineate the vascular supply to such tumors.

These tumors have a distinct capsule surrounding them and, as such, can generally be completely resected. Surgery of these vascular lesions is best completed at the tumor margins to minimize bleeding complications. Postoperative radiotherapy has not been shown to be of value.

Dermoids, epidermoids, teratomas, and neurofibromas can all occur within the cord substance. Surgical excision is usually curative if total removal is possible. Intramedullary metastatic tumors also occur. In the author's experience, small cell carcinoma of the lung has been associated with intramedullary metastatic tumors, but can occur in association with other primary tumors.

SURGICAL CONSIDERATIONS IN INTRAMEDULLARY CERVICAL SPINAL CORD TUMORS

Surgical excision of intramedullary neoplasms is always challenging. The author prefers the prone position with the patient fixed in a Mayfield pin-holder headrest. The head of the table is elevated until the neck is level and parallel to the floor. This minimizes escape of spinal fluid and is less tiring than the sitting position; there is also less chance of air embolus. A posterior approach to the cervical spine is completed over the affected area, and a wide laminectomy completed over the full length of the lesion, preserving the facet joints. If the tumor is associated with a large cyst and small area of enhancement, the laminectomy may be limited to this area alone. It is wise to prep the whole extent of the lesion in case some unexpected finding is encountered during the course of the surgery. In children, laminoplasty may be considered in an effort to prevent swan neck defor-

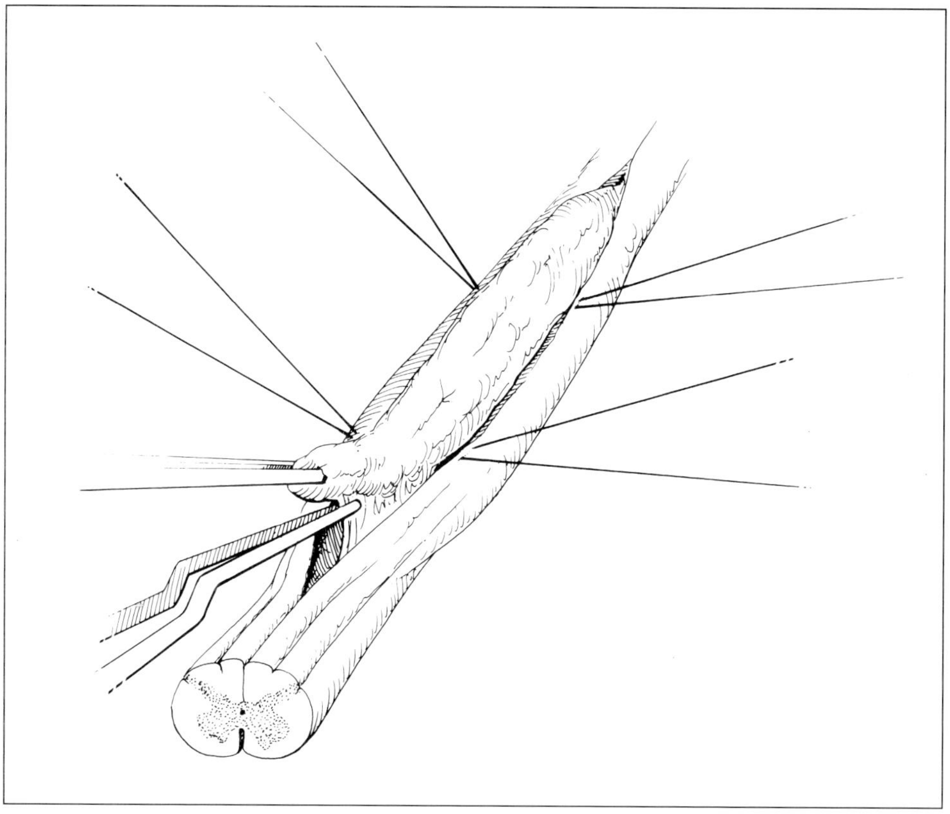

Figure 15.2
Surgical excision of intramedullary ependymoma. This represents a non-infiltrative lesion which can usually be completely resected. After the myelotomy, the cord is retracted with stay sutures placed in the pia. The edge of the tumor is elevated, and small vessels feeding the tumor are coagulated

mity.[10] Intraoperative ultrasonography is very helpful in determining the length of required laminectomy and demonstration of lesions within the spinal cord. Intraoperative spinal evoked responses are being used by many surgeons, but it is not clear if the outcome is affected. The delay in time required to acquire the information seems to limit its usefulness, in addition to the fact that many of the impulses are transmitted in the dorsal columns, which may already be impaired by the tumor. Refinements in technology and newer techniques, such as motor evoked responses, will undoubtedly become useful.[4,15]

The operating microscope is absolutely essential. The dura mater is opened in the midline and sewn up to the muscles. The tumor may present on the surface in a localized region. A midline myelotomy is usually done, but if there is loss of function of one dorsal column, it may help to complete the myelotomy there. The author has found both the carbon dioxide and KTP lasers to be very helpful in making a clean myelotomy. Fine stay sutures in the pia will hold the cord open. Myelotomy should be completed over the full length of the solid portion of the tumor; if there is a large cyst, it may be limited to the area of enhancement alone.

Large neoplasms are usually first debulked with the ultrasonic aspirator; then an effort is made to find a plane of demarcation between the tumor and the normal cord. This is usually possible with ependymomas – the edge of the tumor is elevated, and the small vessels feeding the tumor coagulated. In this way, the ependymoma can be lifted from the cord completely (Fig. 15.2). Astrocytomas are more infiltrating and it is better to work within the confines of the tumor, thinning it out to more normal appearing tissue from inside out. The judgment of where to stop is not an easy one. Hemangioblastomas are completely removable, and often present on the surface with a large arterial feeder. Dissecting on the surface of the lesion allows complete removal without entering the normal cord. If there is a cyst, it does not need to be resected. If the cord has been well decompressed, the dura is closed in water-tight fashion with interrupted or interlocking sutures. If there is not much room for the cord, the author prefers a fascia lata graft. Freeze-dried dura, pericardium, and silicone grafts have been used. After surgery, the surgeon must watch for cerebrospinal fluid leak, respiratory difficulties, urinary disturbances, and deep vein thrombophlebitis.

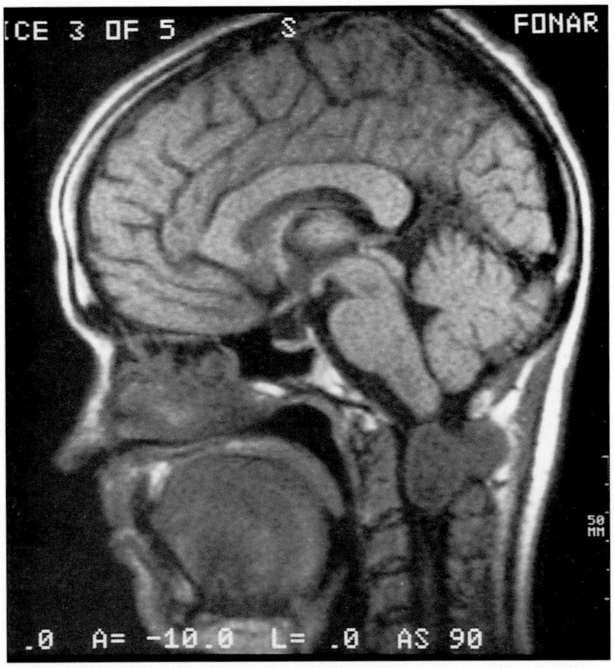

Figure 15.3
MRI, lateral unenhanced scan of a malignant schwannoma at C1–C2 in a 29-year-old female with neurofibromatosis

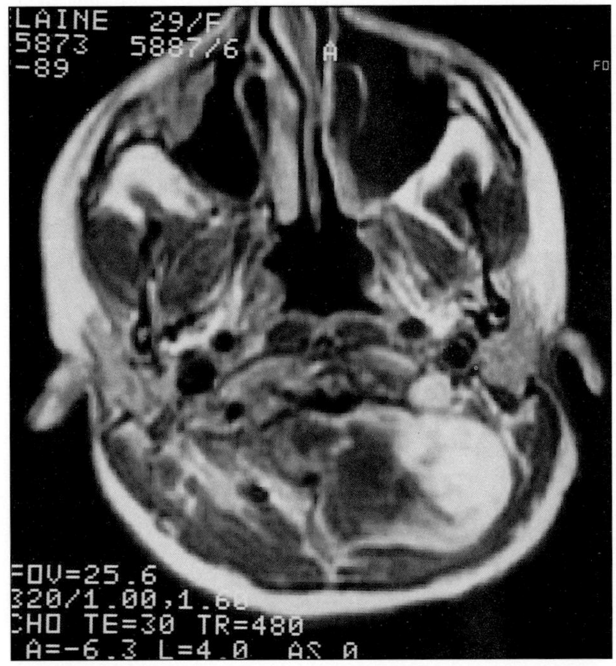

Figure 15.4
Axial enhanced MRI of the patient in Fig. 15.3

INTRADURAL EXTRAMEDULLARY TUMORS

Extramedullary tumors are more common than intramedullary tumors, being about twice as common. Such tumors schwannomas, meningiomas, dermoids and epidermoids, and lipomas.[12]

Schwannomas (sometimes called neurilemmomas) are the most common extra-axial tumor. They arise from Schwann cells, which invest the axons after they leave the spinal cord, and tend to arise from the sensory portion of the nerve. Neurofibromas are a diffuse enlargement of the whole nerve. Both may be associated with neurofibromatosis, although schwannomas are far more common. These tumors are generally benign, although malignant forms are seen (Figs 15.3 and 15.4). They can be intradural, extradural, or both.

Patients with schwannomas typically give a long history of symptoms. Cervical schwannomas are symptomatic for an average of 7 years before diagnosis. Radicular pain is the primary symptom and is seen in 75% of patients. This pain is generally progressive and most bothersome at night. Weakness is less common and, when seen, is discrete. For smaller tumors, weakness may be demonstrated in those muscles supplied by a single nerve root. With larger tumors, however, cord displacement and myelopathy may occur. As they develop on the side of the canal, symptoms are more often lateralized, such as those seen with a Brown–Séquard syndrome. Multiple tumors can be seen in association with neurofibromatosis.

Plain radiographs may demonstrate widening of the neural foramen on oblique projections. The study of choice, however, remains MRI. Schwannomas will appear hypointense on T1 images and hyperintense on T2 images. These tumors enhance well with gadolinium and can be cystic. These findings are similar to those seen in meningiomas and, therefore, MRI cannot always differentiate between the two lesions (Figs 15.3 and 15.4).

Treatment is surgical excision, which is usually curative. Postoperative radiotherapy may be considered for malignant schwannomas. The effective dose is high, and does present some risk of affecting the spinal cord.

Meningiomas are more common in the thoracic than the cervical spine, and are much more common in women. In the cervical spine, 80% are found anteriorly, whereas those

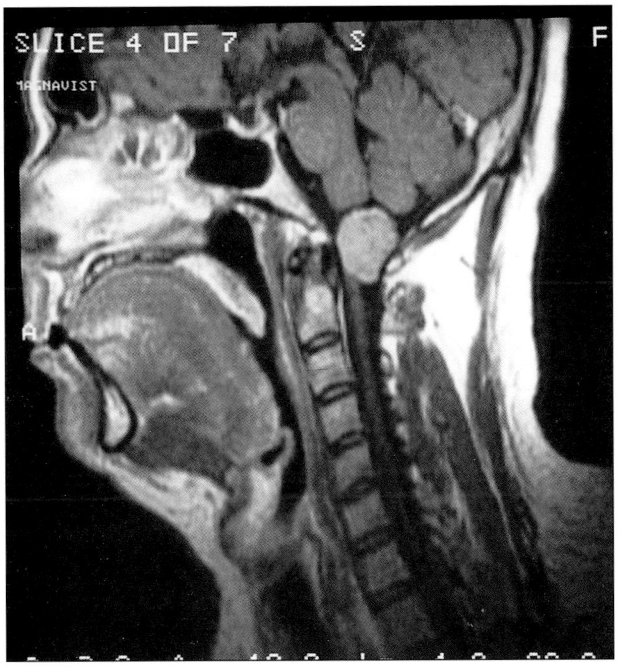

Figure 15.5
Lateral enhanced MRI of meningioma at the foramen magnum in a 46-year-old male

tumors arising in the thoracic spine tend to arise posteriorly. In the region of the foramen magnum, they may arise at the entrance of the vertebral artery intradurally (Fig. 15.5). In such cases, preoperative angiography may be helpful.

Meningiomas grow slowly, causing local and radicular pain and cord compression; symptoms can be present for months or years before detection. Most patients will have significant weakness at the time of diagnosis, with only 20% demonstrating normal motor function.

Plain radiographs are normal in 80% of cases. MRI scan is the most helpful radiologic examination. These tumors have homogeneous signal characteristics, and are hypointense on T1-weighted images; they also uniformly enhance with gadolinium (Fig. 15.5).

Treatment is surgical excision and even patients with severe deficits can make significant recovery. In cases where the entire tumor is successfully resected, recurrence is uncommon. However, for resection to be complete, the sites of dural attachment must also be removed. For patients with incomplete resection, radiotherapy should be considered.

Dermoids, epidermoids, teratomas, and intradural lipomas are all found in an extramedullary location. Some lipomas are subpial in location and can achieve a significant size, producing neurologic deficits. Treatment is surgical excision.

Metastatic tumors may seed the subarachnoid space, attaching to individual nerve roots, causing multifocal root and cranial nerve deficits (carcinomatous meningitis). Diagnosis is made with contrast-enhanced MRI and lumbar puncture.

Treatment is radiotherapy or intrathecal chemotherapeutic agents or both. Except for leukemia and lymphoma, the prognosis is poor.

SURGICAL CONSIDERATIONS FOR INTRADURAL EXTRAMEDULLARY TUMORS

Most extramedullary tumors can be approached with a standard laminectomy, if the tumor is dorsal or lateral to the cord. Ultrasonography is helpful in determining if adequate bone has been removed. Sometimes the tumor can be a bit difficult to see before the arachnoid is opened, particularly if it is below the dentate ligaments, so sectioning the dentate is helpful to gain exposure. Debulking of the tumor with an ultrasonic aspirator or laser greatly facilitates the operative procedure, with the KTP laser being quite maneuverable in the confined space available. After thinning to the point where it is not necessary to retract the cord to any great degree the tumor is carefully dissected from the spinal cord. It is usually necessary to section the dorsal root from which a schwannoma can arise and, sometimes, sectioning of more than one dorsal root will be necessary. Heavily calcified meningiomas can defy the best laid surgical plans, and have a propensity to be associated with postoperative neurologic deficit. For anteriorly situated tumors, the surgeon should consider a lateral approach to the lesion, removing the facets and some of the pedicles to gain access to the mass without retracting the cord. In the upper cervical spine, the vertebral artery can be skeletonized and part of the occipital condyle removed. Dural defects, which occur when the dural base of a meningioma is excised, should be repaired to provide water-tight closure. If the attachment cannot be excised, it is coagulated with the bipolar forceps or laser.

Dermoids, epidermoids, and lipomas are removed wherever possible. Leaving small amounts, which may be intimately adherent to the cord, does not seem to preclude a favorable long-term outcome.

The results of surgery for all extramedullary tumors are usually gratifying. Many patients will make remarkable recoveries with physical therapy and time, in spite of severe preoperative neurologic deficits.

SYRINGOMYELIA

Syringomyelia (hydromyelia) is a dilatation of the central canal of the spinal cord. It is usually mid–cervical, and extends down into the thoracic spine, but can extend up into the upper cervical region, and even into the brain stem (syringobulbia). It is most commonly associated with a Chiari type I malformation (Fig. 15.6), or hydrocephalus, and is sometimes seen with an Arnold–Chiari malformation. Occasionally, there is no other associated anomaly. The exact etiology of this entity has been the subject of much discussion over the years. Generally, it is felt that the syrinx develops when there is an increase in the pressure of the cerebrospinal fluid, which enters the central canal of the spinal cord. The Chiari type I malformation is an elongation of the cerebellar tonsils; the latter extend into the upper cervical canal, obstructing the opening of the fourth ventricle, and allowing the undampened pressure of the cerebrospinal fluid to be transmitted onto the central canal. Symptoms are similar to those of intramedullary cord tumors with pain, wasting of the arms and hands, and sensory aberrations with a cape-like, dissociated sensory loss over the shoulders and arms.

Treatment is somewhat uncertain. There is no evidence that asymptomatic, incidentally found lesions will necessarily progress. However, most physicians agree that symptomatic lesions should be treated, and certainly those with neurologic deficits require decompression. Patients with hydrocephalus should be shunted. Decompression of the foramen magnum seems to be a reasonable first step, if a Chiari type I malformation is found. A limited (1–2 cm) suboccipital craniectomy, and a C1, and possibly C2, laminectomy are completed. Once the dura is widely opened, there are several options. Some surgeons explore the opening of the fourth ventricle and lyse adhesions, some prefer placement of a shunt in the fourth ventricle to ensure persistent drainage from the fourth ventricle, whereas others do neither. All sew in a sizable dural graft in order to leave adequate room for the tonsils and medulla.[3,9] Over a period of weeks to months, a gradual reduction in the size of the syrinx may be seen. If the syrinx is very large, the symptoms and findings are severe, or symptoms progress after decompression of the foramen magnum, exploration of the syrinx is indicated. Exposure is completed over the widest portion of the cyst or below the cervical cord to minimize the risks. The syrinx will usually be visible through the thinned fiber tracts. The cyst is then fenestrated and a Silastic T tube inserted and left in the subarachnoid space. Shunting of the syrinx in this fashi[illegible] the peritoneum or pleura has become more commonplace. Each of these modalities can decompress the cord, and arrest the symptoms. However, the long-term outlook is uncertain at this time. It appears that overall improvement or stabilization occurs about 75–90% of the time.[7,13] Some patients require multiple procedures.

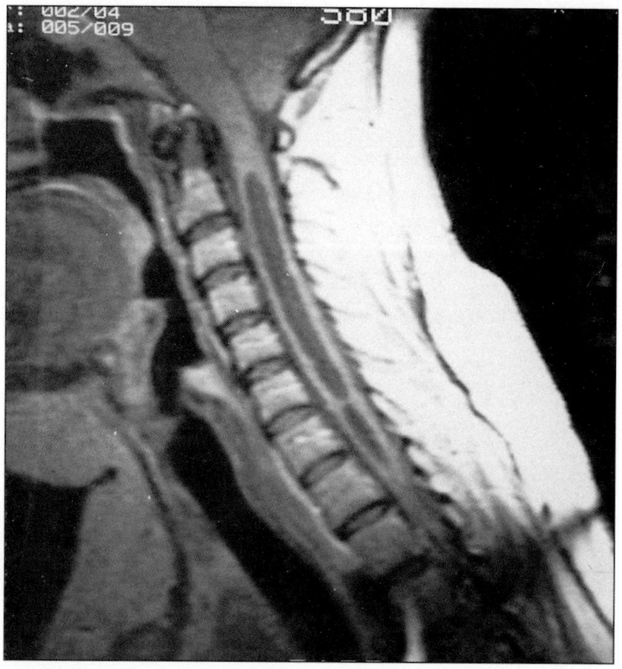

Figure 15.6
Lateral MRI of a 55-year-old patient with syringomyelia and a Chiari type I malformation

ARTERIOVENOUS MALFORMATIONS

Arteriovenous malformations of the spinal cord are rare. They are more often found in the thoracic cord and conus medullaris than in the cervical cord. Myelography and spinal angiography demonstrate these lesions better than MRI (Figs 15.7 and 15.8). They are divided into four types.[1]

Type I is a dural arteriovenous fistula located in the dura or just intradurally, surrounding the nerve root. It is fed most often by one radicular artery, although more than one feeder vessel can be seen. Drainage of type I fistulas is into the veins on the dorsal surface of the spinal cord which can cause congestion and intramedullary ischemia. Patients present with progressive spastic paraparesis, and these lesions are successfully treated by surgical obliteration of the fistula. It is not necessary to remove the distended vein from the dorsal surface of the cord. Embolization has also been effective, but there is a higher rate of recanalization of the fistula.

Type II arteriovenous malformations represent true ones, with a nidus within the cord, fed by branches of the anterior and posterior spinal arteries. They have a high flow

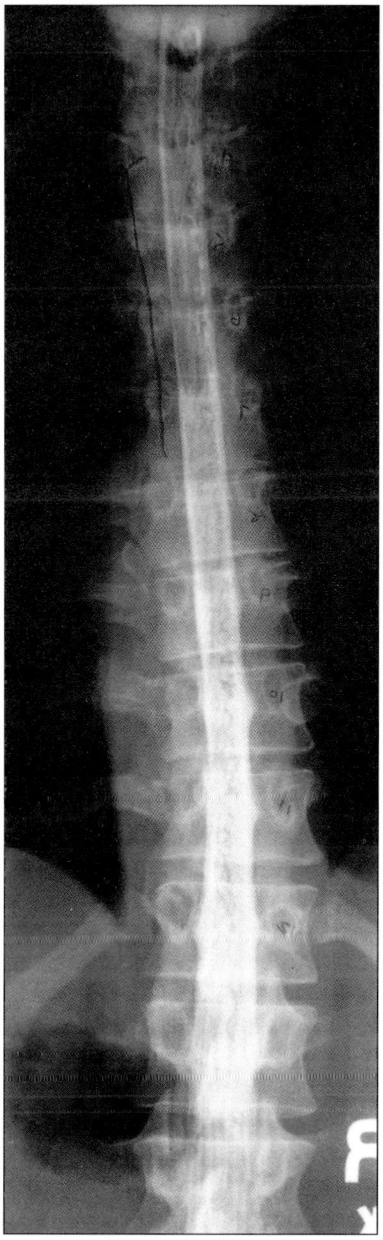

Figure 15.7
Myelogram of 41-year-old man with a type I arteriovenous malformation of the thoracic cord

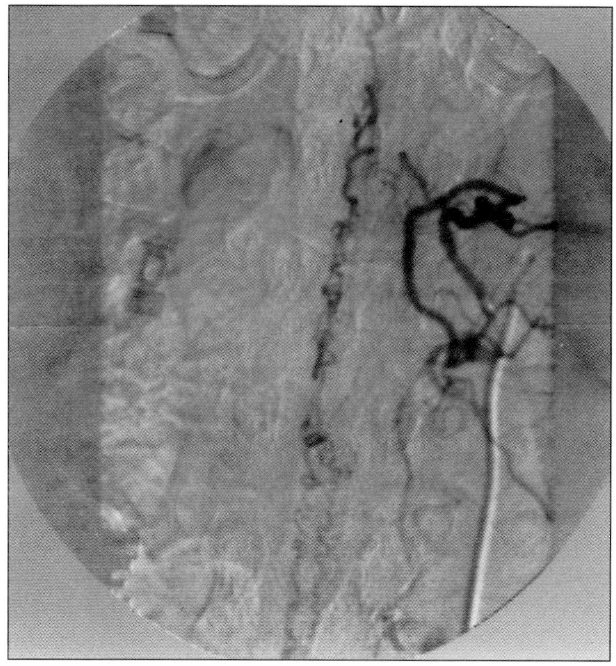

Figure 15.8
Spinal angiogram of the patient in Fig. 15.7

rate, and present either with acute hemorrhage or progressive myelopathy. They are treated by either surgery or embolization, or both. Occasionally, there is a successful outcome.

Type III arteriovenous malformations are extensive complex malformations which involve the cord (intra- and extramedullary), and extend into the bone and soft tissue. Treatment is rarely successful. Embolization, partial resection, and feeder ligation have been attempted with mixed success.

Type IV arteriovenous malformation is a direct fistula between the anterior spinal artery and adjacent venous structures. The size of the fistula is variable. Smaller ones are best treated surgically through an anterior approach; larger ones are embolized.

SUMMARY

In this chapter, an attempt has been made to present a brief overview of the most important intradural lesions. The portion on surgical techniques represents certain personal preferences, and is not intended to discount other methods in dealing with these lesions. As a whole, these are illnesses that are fascinating to work up and treat, and the results can be very gratifying. Except for malignant astrocytomas and some arteriovenous malformation, treatment can result in permanent cure of the illness or significant prolongation of life, and improvement in neurologic deficits.

REFERENCES

1 Anson J, Spetzler R. Classification of spinal arteriovenous malformations and implications for treatment. *Barrow Neurological Institute Quarterly* **8**(2): 2–8, 1992.
2 Barba D, Marshall I. Intradural tumors. *Semin in Spine Surg* **2**: 228–242, 1990.
3 Batzdorf U. Chiari malformations and syringomyelia. In Apuzzo M (ed), *Brain Surgery: Complications and Avoidance*, 1985–2001. New York: Churchill Livingstone, 1993.
4 Cooper P. Intramedullary spinal cord tumors. In Camins M, O'Leary P. (eds) *Disorders of the Cervical Spine*, 507–518. Baltimore, MA: Williams & Wilkins, 1992.
5 Epstein F, Farmer J, Freed D. Adult intramedullary spinal cord ependymomas: The results of surgery in 38 patients. *J Neurosurg* **79**: 204–209, 1993.
6 Epstein F. Epstein N. Surgical management of holocord intramedullary spinal cord astrocytomas in children. Report of three cases. *J Neurosurg* **54**: 829–832, 1981.
7 Garcia–Uria J, Leunda G, Carillo R, Bravo G. Syringomyelia: Long–term results after posterior fossa decompression. *J Neurosurg* **54**: 380–382, 1981.
8 Haymaker W. *Bing's Local Diagnosis in Neurological Diseases*, 15th ed, 1–22. St Louis, MO: CV Mosby, 1969.
9 Morawetz R. Surgical management of Chiari I malformations and syringomyelia. In Rengachary S, Wilkins R (eds) *Neurosurgical Operative Atlas*, vol. 3, 99–108. Baltimore, MA: Williams & Wilkins, 1993.
10 Raimondi A, Gutierrez F, Di Rocco C. Laminotomy and total reconstruction of the spinal arch for spinal canal surgery in childhood. *J Neurosurg* **45**: 555–560, 1976.
11 Rengachary S. Hemangioblastomas. In Wilkins R,. Rengachary S. (eds) *Neurosurgery*, 772–782 New York, St Louis: McGraw–Hill, 1985.
12 Rogers H, Long D, Chou S, French L. Lipomas of the spinal cord and cauda equina. *J Neurosurg* **34**: 349–354, 1971.
13 Tator C, Kotoo M, Rowed D. Favorable results with syringo-subarachnoid shunts for treatment of syringomyelia. *J Neurosurg* **56**: 517–523, 1982.
14 Stein B. Spinal intradural tumors. In Wilkins R, Rengachary S. (eds) *Neurosurgery*, 1048–1061. New York, St Louis: McGraw-Hill, 1985.
15 Stone J. Evoked potentials in neurosurgery. *Contemp Neurosurg* **15**(13): 1–6, 1993.

16 Infections of the cervical spine

John G. Heller

PYOGENIC CERVICAL VERTEBRAL OSTEOMYELITIS

The incidence of osteomyelitis in the cervical spine varies from 3% to 27% of all cases of vertebral osteomyelitis. If intravenous drug abusers are excluded, the range narrows to 3–15%. An appropriate mean incidence can probably be drawn from the data of Malawski and Lukawski,[62] because they have reported the largest contemporary series. Among 442 patients with vertebral osteomyelitis, cervical involvement was found in only 6% of cases. Intravenous drug use apparently imposes an increased probability of cervical involvement. Sapico found that 27% of cases of vertebral osteomyelitis associated with intravenous drug abuse involved the cervical spine. The incidence of thoracic disease was, in turn, surprisingly low in these hosts, 4.5%, and the relative incidence of lumbar disease was largely unaffected by intravenous drug abuse.[28,88,89,98] The predisposition toward cervical disease has been attributed to the use of central venous injection sites, especially the jugular veins.[28]

Clinical History and Physical Findings

The clinical presentation is consistently non-specific. Of patients ≥90% complain primarily of neck pain.[89] The pain can vary widely in intensity and distribution, and radiation to the trapezial and shoulder areas is common. In a few patients, the primary symptoms will be radicular or myelopathic. It can be difficult to distinguish these patients from those in the population with non-specific neck complaints caused by degenerative processes. A small group of patients present with atypical symptoms such as headaches, chest pain, dysphagia or asphyxia. Swallowing or respiratory difficulties are noted in varying degrees in 11%,[89] and usually prompt a search for causes of obstruction. Rarely, a patient may present with respiratory insufficiency and altered mental status resulting from either overwhelming sepsis or a high spinal cord lesion.[6]

The initial physical findings vary widely, but are generally unremarkable. Almost all patients will demonstrate evidence of local cervical tenderness, but muscular spasm is noted far less frequently. Limited motion is evident in 15%. Of all vertebral osteomyelitis cases 17% are associated with neurologic deficits, but the frequency is higher among cervical cases. Stone et al[98] found that over half of their patients with cervical osteomyelitis had evidence of neurologic deficits. Eismont et al[26] noted paralysis in 82% of their cervical cases, and felt that cervical involvement was a specific risk factor for paralysis in vertebral osteomyelitis. It is noteworthy that intravenous drug abusers tend to exhibit a lower incidence of neurologic deficits than other hosts. Sapico and Montgomerie[88] attributed this difference to a tendency to seek treatment earlier in the process. This may be a result of a lower tolerance to pain or the individual's drug-seeking behavior patterns.

Fevers are evident in half the patients, and leukocytosis is present in only 40%. However, the erythrocyte sedimentation rate is almost universally elevated. In general, laboratory studies are not terribly helpful in making the diagnosis of vertebral osteomyelitis.

Delayed diagnosis is the rule, which is not surprising given the non-specific nature of the presentations. However, historical information, when sought, may provide a clue to the diagnosis. Recent events associated with bacteremias, sources of direct inoculation, or blunt trauma should be sought through detailed interrogation. Any intravenous drug abuser with complaints of progressive axial pain should be considered to have vertebral osteomyelitis until proved otherwise (Fig. 16.1). Recent diagnostic or therapeutic procedures may have caused transient bacteremias and seeding of vertebral foci; genitourinary procedures, especially in the presence of infection, are frequently associated with vertebral osteomyelitis. In some series, as many as half of the reported cases of vertebral osteomyelitis are associated with urinary tract sources. Procedures about the head and

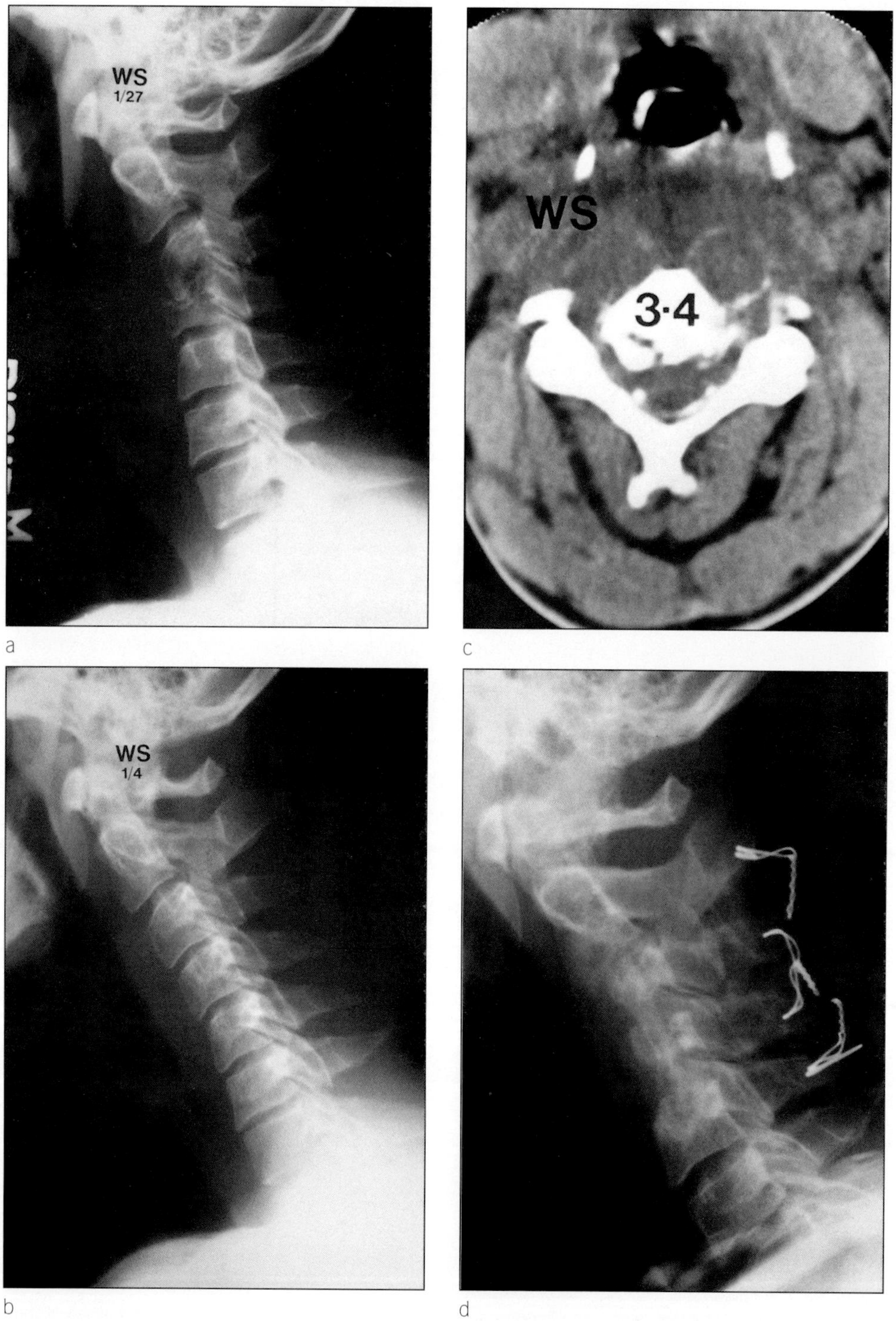

Figure 16.1
(a) Lateral radiograph of a 35-year-old male (WS) intravenous drug abuser, who presented with severe neck pain, advancing quadriparesis, fever, and dehydration. Note the advanced destruction of the C3–C4 disc space with vertebral collapse and kyphosis. He had been seen one week earlier with complaints of neck pain. (b) The lateral radiograph from that initial evaluation was read as normal. Closer inspection revealed early disc height loss with increased prevertebral soft-tissue width. (c) Emergency myelography–computed tomography documented ventral cord compression from a combination of an epidural abscess and his kyphosis. He was treated with skeletal traction and emergency anterior decompression and reconstruction with an iliac crest autograft. The patient attempted halo removal numerous times during the next 3 months. (d) A posterior fusion was done for a delayed union. He recovered normal neurologic function

neck may carry a particular risk for cervical involvement. Cases of osteomyelitis have been reported following dental extractions, tonsillectomy, head and neck surgery, esophageal dilatation, and carotid angiography.[26,55,73,79,100,106,111] Bacteremias may also be due to remote sites of infection, such as cutaneous ulcers (especially with intravenous drug abusers), decubitus ulcers, pneumonia, intra-abdominal or biliary sepsis, infected orthopaedic implants[122] (Fig. 16.2), bacterial endocarditis, and the like.

Direct inoculation may occur with penetrating trauma, contiguous spread from local infections, or diagnostic and therapeutic procedures. A history of new or increasing

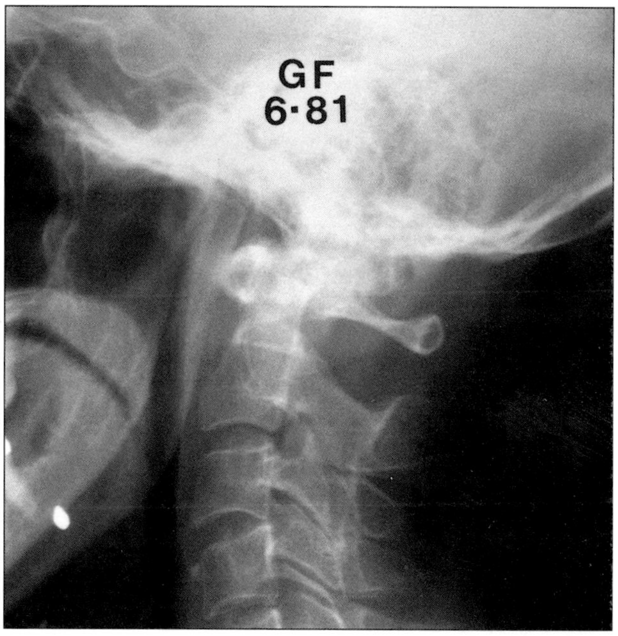

a

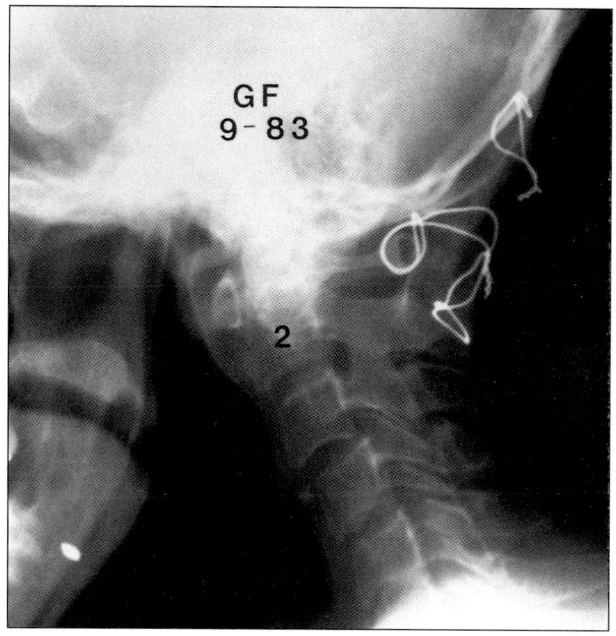

c

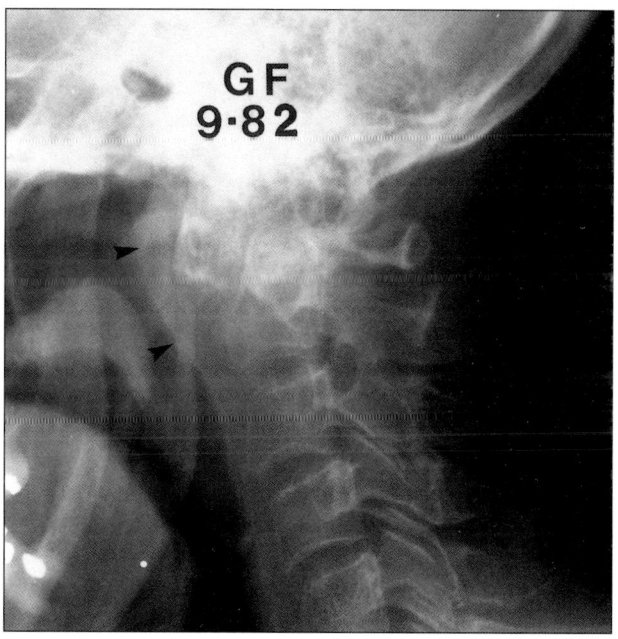

b

Figure 16.2
Patient GF developed progressive neck pain while being treated for a total knee arthroplasty infected with *Pasteurella multocida*. Baseline plain radiographs demonstrated normal cervicocranial alignment (a). Atlantoaxial infection with *P. multocida* lead to anterior C1–C2 subluxation, and superior migration of the odontoid (b). After reduction in skeletal traction, an occipitocervical fusion was performed (c). (Reproduced from Zigler et al[122] by courtesy of HH Bohlman)

neck pain in the setting of any of the above should raise the question of spinal infection. This is particularly true in the case of patients whose physiology might tend to mask their symptoms. For instance, a steroid-dependent rheumatoid patient who complains of increasing neck pain, and seems to be exhibiting decreased functional capacities should be regarded with particular suspicion.[68] A diligent effort should be made to diagnose an evolving infection and/or instability that has been masked by a patient's debilitated condition; this is also important for other immunosuppressed patients, including diabetics and the elderly.[6,12,26,68,89]

Radiographic Studies

The diagnosis of osteomyelitis may be supported by imaging studies. Plain radiographs, including anteroposterior, lateral, obliques, and open-mouth views, should first be taken. If the symptoms indicate recent onset, the radiographic features may not have evolved. Within the first 3 weeks of onset, disc space narrowing or abnormal prevertebral soft-tissue contours may be seen (Fig. 16.1).[62] In evaluation of the lateral cervical radiograph, it is not possible to depend on the absolute dimensions of the prevertebral tissues alone, but is important to compare the suspicious areas to adjacent segments which should have the same dimensions. For example, if an infection is present at C5 and C6, and the prevertebral tissues measure only 18 mm, the radiograph should not yet be declared normal. As the soft tissues anterior to C7 and T1 are the same as those in front of C5 and C6, the retrotracheal space should have the same dimensions along this interval. In this hypothetical patient, if the prevertebral tissues at the subjacent levels measure only 10 mm, then the radiograph is abnormal, and further evaluation is essential.

After the first 3 weeks, the plain radiographic features of vertebral osteomyelitis become more obvious. Loss of disc space height is followed by erosive changes in the associated vertebral end-plates, and then by reactive bone formation. More advanced changes may include fracture and collapse of the vertebral bodies and progressive kyphosis (see Fig. 16.1). Enlargement of any developing paraspinal abscess may lead to distortion of prevertebral soft-tissue contours, as noted earlier. Extension to adjacent levels is common. Malawski and Lukawski[62] reported involvement of at least two vertebrae in 79% of patients in their series. Such changes may mimic those seen in metastatic disease; involvement of the disc space, however, favors the diagnosis of infection. When carefully scrutinized, plain radiographs alone may give an overall accuracy approaching 74%.[70] Unfortunately, diagnostic changes present on plain radiographs are often missed, ignored, or misinterpreted, leading to delayed or inappropriate treatment in some cases.[12] It is important to be particularly careful not to mistake destructive cervical spondyloarthropathy or 'pseudodiscitis', which may be seen in renal dialysis patients, for infectious intervertebral discitis or osteomyelitis. This entity has been described in up to 9% of patients on long-term hemodialysis. Although the plain radiographic and scintigraphic features may be identical, magnetic resonance imaging (MRI) characteristics will exclude the possibility of infection by the low signal intensity on T2-weighted images.[64,84]

Radionuclide scans may be more helpful than plain radiographs early in the disease process. Technetium bone scans are quite sensitive within a short time from the onset of symptoms, but they lack specificity. Gallium and indium scans are more specific for inflammatory processes, but they suffer from decreased sensitivity, especially if the patient has already received antibiotics. Furthermore, these tests require a long time for completion. They have the additional advantage of providing a survey of the entire body so that synchronous sites of infection may be identified. Multiple sites of vertebral osteomyelitis can be expected in 4% of cases.[62]

Computed tomography is helpful in defining the extent and type of bone involvement, and intraosseous abscesses and sequestra are readily identified. In addition, the paravertebral soft tissues are well demonstrated. The size and location of associated abscesses can be well delineated. The addition of intrathecal contrast material provides further information about spinal canal encroachment by bone debris, granulation tissue, or epidural abscesses. Samples of cerebrospinal fluid (CSF) may also be sent for analysis at the time of contrast instillation to determine whether an associated meningitis is present. This may prove particularly useful in cases of cervical osteomyelitis, because the clinical manifestations overlap significantly with meningitis and epidural abscess formation. Indeed, all three conditions may coexist.

Magnetic resonance imaging is uniquely helpful in the diagnosis of spinal infections. It provides excellent, multiplanar delineation of the pathologic process and regional anatomy; involved vertebrae and discs show a characteristic pattern of decreased signal intensity on T1-weighted images, and increased signal intensity on the corresponding T2-weighted images.[70,71,81,89,93] It can also detect associated epidural abscesses or other causes of spinal cord compromise. The addition of gadolinium-enhanced images further potentiates the diagnostic sensitivity and specificity of MRI. Post et al[81] reported that gadolinium-enhanced images provided better definition of spinal cord compression than non-enhanced MRI. They also felt that enhanced images allowed localization of optimal sites for percutaneous biopsy, and distinction between active infections and those that had responded to treatment.

In choosing among the available imaging modalities, it is helpful to know the relative sensitivity, specificity, and accuracy of each test. Modic et al[70] have reported comparative data for plain radiographs, technetium bone scans, combined technetium and gallium scans, and non-enhanced MRI. Their results are summarized in Table 16.1. The overall accuracy in diagnosing vertebral osteomyelitis was 94% for MRI and 94% for combined technetium and gallium scans. The latter suffer in the clinical setting because of their inherent delays in imaging, lack of regional anatomic definition, and sensitivity to previous antibiotic administration. Furthermore, the accuracy of MRI was probably underestimated because their work preceded the advent of gadolinium.

It is the obligation of the treating physician to be efficient and cost-effective in the choice of diagnostic technology. If the history and physical examination are suggestive of a

Table 16.1 Comparative analysis of spinal imaging techniques for vertebral osteomyelitis

Technique	*Sensitivity (%)*	*Specificity (%)*	*Accuracy (%)*
Radiography	82	57	73
Technetium-99 (^{99m}Tc)	90	78	86
Gallium (Ga)	92	100	95
^{99m}Tc–Ga combined	92	100	94
MRI*	96	93	94

*Magnetic resonance imaging without paramagnetic contrast material.
Adapted from Modic et al.[70]

spinal infection, and spinal stability or the neurologic status does not mandate emergency treatment, then the work-up should start with plain radiographs and basic screening blood work. The results of an SMA-18, urinalysis, cell blood count with differential, platelet count, and erythrocyte sedimentation rate, together with the radiographic findings, should help identify the vast majority of infections. This basic information also helps to sort out most infections from the other disease processes in the differential diagnosis – primarily tumors. If the picture remains suspicious but not diagnostic, particularly if the symptoms are of recent onset, a bone scan should be completed. It is readily available, highly sensitive, and inexpensive. Definitive treatment may await diagnostic confirmation through appropriate cultures and definition of the affected regional anatomy using MRI. The latter may also facilitate the determination of optimal biopsy sites to maximize the yield of cultures.[81]

In the presence of a significant or progressive neurologic deficit, time is of the essence. When cervical instability is present, the patient must be protected from further harm while the work-up proceeds. Skeletal traction should be instituted with MRI-compatible tongs, if available. Emergent gadolinium-enhanced MRI would be the imaging modality of choice to identify the location, type, and extent of infection, and to differentiate it from neoplastic processes. Myelography and computed tomography would be the second choice of imaging. It may not be as specific, but it is highly sensitive and provides good anatomic definition. A lateral C1–C2 puncture should be completed in the event that a high-grade block exists at the level of the lesion. A sample of cerebrospinal fluid must be sent for culture, Gram stain, cell count and differential, and glucose and protein determinations.

Microbiology of Pyogenic Vertebral Osteomyelitis

The spectrum of organisms in vertebral osteomyelitis varies considerably. Certain hosts are more likely to be infected with certain patterns of organisms. *Staphylococcus aureus* remains the most probable organism, possibly accounting for up to 75% of all positive cultures.[12,28,62,69,122] Virtually any other organism has been reported to cause vertebral osteomyelitis, including tuberculous, fungal, and anaerobic species.[12,36,74,83,122]

In looking at the spectrum of described pathogens, a few patterns warrant discussion. Certain host factors seem to predispose toward particular pathogens. Intravenous drug abuse has long been recognized to carry an increased risk of infection with *Pseudomonas aeruginosa*.[26,28,57,69,88,98,119] This is particularly germane to a discussion of cervical osteomyelitis given the unusual predilection for cervical involvement of intravenous drug abusers. Genitourinary sources have been shown to account for nearly 50% of vertebral infections in some series, a large percentage of which are Gram-negative organisms.[57,58,89] In the absence of urinary tract instrumentation or manipulation, benign prostatic hypertrophy appears to be a significant risk factor for bacteremias and hematogenous seeding.[12,57] Liebergall et al[57] found this to be a contributing factor in 42% of their patients.

Direct bacteriologic confirmation of the diagnosis is variable, and is obtained in 57–100% of cases.[12,28,57,62,69,105] Needle biopsies are diagnostic in 70–80% of cases.[98,116] Operative tissue samples have a slightly higher yield – 86%.[116] In those instances where biopsy material fails to grow an organism, or is unavailable, the diagnosis may be supported by laboratory data, histopathology, imaging studies, other cultures (blood, urine, sputum, etc.), and the response to treatment. Blood cultures have been positive in 24–43% of cases.[57,89,116] The reasons for negative cultures may include prior administration of antibiotics, sampling error in needle biopsies, poor timing of blood cultures, delay in specimen processing, and poor culture techniques. In discussing the remarkably low incidence of anaerobic spinal infections, Raff and Melo[83] speculated that poor culture techniques probably lead to significant underestimation of prevalence. It may be reasonable to assume that a portion of the culture-negative cases of osteomyelitis may be caused by anaerobic organisms. Due consideration must be given to this in the cervical spine because of the large numbers of anaerobic organisms in the oropharynx.

Treatment

In cervical osteomyelitis, as elsewhere in the spine, the goals of treatment are to sterilize the infection, relieve

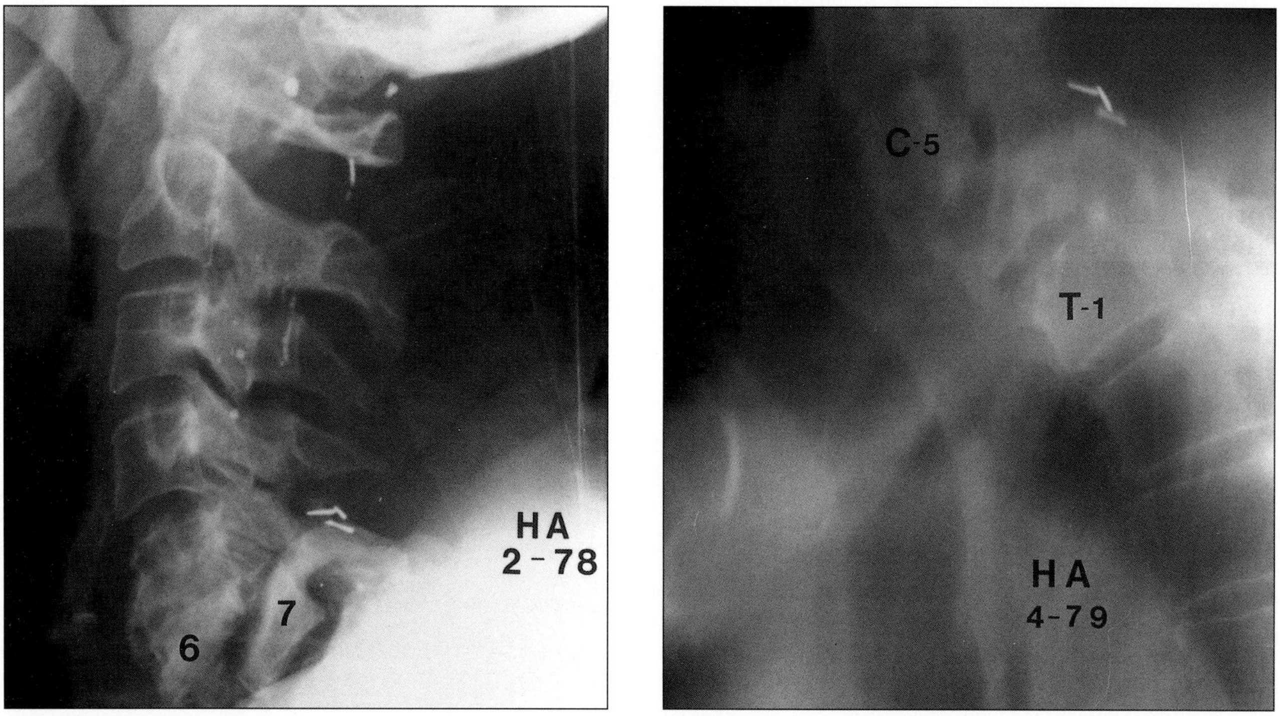

a b

Figure 16.3
Patient HA presented with progressive quadriplegia secondary to a cervical epidural abscess. The osseous involvement anteriorly was not appreciated. He was treated with laminectomies of C5–C7. Shortly afterwards he dislocated C6 on C7 (a), and his neurologic status deteriorated. Skeletal traction was used to reduce the dislocation, and indirectly to decompress his spinal cord until an anterior decompression and reconstruction was performed (b). He recovered normal neurologic function. (Reproduced from Bohlman[9] with permission)

neurologic compression, and maintain or restore spinal stability. Although some authors have reported satisfactory results with medical management of vertebral osteomyelitis, treatment in the cervical region is largely surgical. The cervical spine is highly mobile and readily accessible with low morbidity, whereas patients can ill afford the risk of catastrophic neurologic deficits that occur when medical treatment fails. Care should be used in the interpretation of the work of Liebergall et al[57] in which they claim equivalent results with medical and surgical management. In their series, surgery was reserved for the sickest and most severely involved patients. In the cervical spine, the physician should not wait to see if a significant deterioration will occur, but treatment should be instituted when the diagnosis is appreciated.

Surgical management should adhere to the principles of Hodgson and Stock.[45] Pathology is usually confined to the anterior column and ventral epidural space, and, accordingly, the surgical approach should be anterior. Radical excision of the involved tissues is essential. If epidural extension of the infection is known or suspected, then the posterior longitudinal ligament must be excised to ensure adequate débridement. A note of caution is in order for the cervical spine. The degree of bone destruction by the infection can be extensive, and extend to the foramen transversarium. Smith et al[96] have reported on intraoperative injury to the vertebral artery under such circumstances, with significant associated morbidity.

When vertebral fracture and collapse have contributed to kyphosis and spinal canal compromise, preoperative skeletal traction may restore normal alignment, indirectly decompressing the spinal cord. If not, resection of diseased tissue will allow gradual realignment to occur during surgery. However, it should be noted that the amount of traction applied should be significantly reduced under general anesthesia. Somatosensory evoked potentials should be monitored to warn of any ill effects of either the surgical procedure or the realignment.

The extent of the resection will vary from a single disc space with a few millimeters of adjacent bone to multiple complete corpectomies. As the mean number of vertebrae involved is two,[62] a two-level corpectomy is the most common procedure required; immediate reconstruction of the defect with autograft bone should be performed.[12,26,27,55,57,98,116] Iliac crest grafts may accommodate defects of two vertebrae or less, whereas fibular strut grafts are better suited to resections of two or more levels. Anterior cervical plates are probably contraindicated under these circumstances, as they may be a *locus minoris resistentiae* for bacteria. Care must be taken to key these grafts securely into position, as described in Chapter 9.

Postoperative bracing requirements will vary with the extent of the procedure performed, the quality of host bone, and the quality of graft fixation achieved. In general, cervicothoracic orthoses will suffice for resections involving less than two corpectomies. For more extensive débridement, a halo vest is recommended. For corpectomies involving three or more levels, or for patients with impaired healing potential, the author recommends a supplemental posterior arthrodesis (see Fig. 16.1). If technically possible, and the surgeon possesses adequate experience, the addition of posterior, lateral, mass plate fixation may obviate the need for the halo. Similar to the author's philosophy of surgical treatment of metastatic disease of the spine, there is a low threshold for complementing any anterior reconstruction procedure with a posterior arthrodesis.

Antibiotic therapy should be guided by culture and sensitivity data when available. Parenteral administration should be continued for not less than 4 weeks,[26,55,62,89] because shorter courses carry an increased risk of recurrence.[55] The decision to continue treatment with oral antibiotics must be made on an individual basis according to the virulence of the organism, the clinical response to treatment, the sedimentation rate, and host factors, such as nutritional status, immune competence, and compliance. Successful eradication of the infection will be reflected in complete healing of the strut graft and normalization of the sedimentation rate, usually within 3 months. Delayed graft healing is indicative of excessive motion, persistent infection, or both.

The results of aggressive anterior surgical management have been quite favorable. Spinal alignment and stability can be predictably restored. The probability of neurologic improvement is high, with a minimum associated risk of neurologic deterioration.[12,26,57,62,98] The same cannot be said of laminectomies performed in this clinical setting (Fig. 16.3).[9] As the anterior column is destroyed by the infection, the posterior elements provide what little inherent stability remains. Eismont et al[26] found prior laminectomy to predispose to neurologic decline in their series. Numerous others have reaffirmed this opinion.[9,46,47,49,69]

TUBERCULOUS INFECTIONS OF THE CERVICAL SPINE

Tuberculous infections of the cervical spine are quite rare. It has been estimated that only 4% of all spinal tuberculosis cases affect this region, with the subaxial cervical spine accounting for almost 80% of such instances. The bulk of information regarding Pott's disease in the neck comes from Hong Kong. After reviewing their experience with 1100 cases of Pott's disease treated between 1956 and 1983, Hsu and Leong,[46] and Fang et al[31] published reports on tuberculous involvement of the subaxial and cervicocranial regions, respectively. Among the 1100 cases treated, 40 patients had disease between C2 and C7. The mean number of vertebrae involved was 2.6, whereas C6 was the most commonly affected level. Bone destruction was characteristically anterior, and 11 patients presented with cervical hump or gibbus deformities. The average amount of kyphosis was 26° and neurologic deficits were present in 43% of patients. Paresis or paralysis usually developed within 1–2 months of the onset of symptoms, with pain being the most common primary complaint.

Classification

Hsu and Leong[46] classified these cases into two groups based on the clinical features and the age of presentation. The 'child' type tended to occur in patients less than 10 years of age. This subgroup tended to have more vertebral levels involved, which the authors presumed to be the result of the decreased immunity in this age group. Alternatively, the vascular supply to the child's intervertebral disc space may facilitate spread. The prevertebral fascia and anterior longitudinal ligament act to contain local abscess formation, but facilitate vertical extension to adjacent levels. As these abscesses increase in size within the retropharyngeal space, they may produce swallowing problems or airway obstruction. Asthma Millari is a life-threatening syndrome involving airway obstruction secondary to tracheal compression by a large paraspinal abscess. Fortunately, this subgroup had a significantly lower incidence of neurologic deficits compared to the 'adult' type. The overall rate of paresis or paralysis was only 17% in those under 10 years of age.

The 'adult' type was distinguished by its older age at presentation, more focal involvement, smaller abscesses, and higher incidence of neurologic deficit. Hsu and Leong[46] noted neurologic deficits in 81% of patients over 10 years of age at the time of presentation. The explanation for this phenomenon is not clear, but it may be a result of more confined disease. The tendency toward more focal involvement and less purulence is presumably a function of a more mature immune system. The normal involution of the intervertebral disc's vascular supply may also serve to restrict spread to adjacent levels. Local osseous and ligamentous anatomy is not likely to be an important influence, because many of these patients are still far from skeletal maturity.

Tuberculous Infection of the Upper Cervical Spine

Tuberculous involvement of the upper cervical spine is even less common. Fang et al[31] reported only six cases of C1–C2 involvement among 1100 (0.5%) patients with Pott's disease. In a larger series of 5393 cases of spinal tuberculosis, Wang[109] had only 15 cases (0.3%) involving the atlantoaxial level. These patients also present with non-specific symptoms, which commonly include neck pain and headaches. Most patients eventually develop focal and striking complaints such as torticollis, dysphagia, or asphyxia resulting from the effect of a retropharyngeal mass. Patients may also present with significant spinal cord dysfunction.[31,46,72,109] The differential diagnosis is similar to that of lower cervical involvement, but the differential diagnosis of torticollis must also be included. The history, physical examination, and radiographic studies should help to exclude the possibility of traumatic atlantoaxial rotatory subluxation, displaced odontoid fractures, Grisel's syndrome, or primary or metastatic tumors. When a retropharyngeal mass is observed or palpated, Neal et al[72] have suggested that extension across the midline favors the diagnosis of tuberculosis rather than neoplasms or pyogenic abscesses. The median raphe normally functions as an effective barrier to contralateral extension of the latter processes.

Deformity is quite likely in upper cervical Pott's disease. Among their six patients, Fang et al[31] reported five instances of torticollis and one fixed flexion deformity. Tuberculosis of the subaxial cervical spine does not share the marked propensity toward deformity seen in either the upper cervical or the thoracic spine. As this region is lordotic, two-thirds of axial loads are distributed through the posterior elements.[76] The more posterior weight-bearing line may exert a protective influence. However, the lack of kyphosis does not seem to protect the 'adult' group from a high incidence of neurologic complications. From their surgical and autopsy findings, Hsu and Leong attributed most spinal cord compression to abscess formation, not to gibbus deformities. The increased mobility of the cervical spine may also have an influence on the incidence of neurologic complications, particularly in comparison to the thoracic spine where the rib cage provides inherent stability.

Clinical History, Physical Findings, and Differential Diagnosis

The diagnosis of cervical tuberculosis is usually delayed,[46,47,72,108] which is to be expected, given its rarity and the non-specific initial symptoms. As pain is the presenting complaint in 90% of patients,[108] little heed may be given to the symptom in the absence of other more dramatic clinical features, especially in adults. However, spinal pain in children should be taken as clinical evidence of a tumor or infection until proven otherwise. The presence of adenopathy or masses should be sought during the initial physical examination, alerting the physician to the appropriate diagnosis. Unfortunately, such palpable findings are only present in about half the patients.

The differential diagnosis of cervical Pott's disease includes pyogenic and fungal osteomyelitis, pyogenic retropharyngeal abscesses, metastatic disease, primary benign or malignant bone tumors, recent trauma, and degenerative disease. The age of the patient may be of some help. In children, metastatic disease is very uncommon, whereas intervertebral discitis, hematogenous osteomyelitis, retropharyngeal abscesses, lymphoma, eosinophilic granulomata, and osteoblastomas are quite compatible with this age group. Among older patients, neck pain is a common and non-specific complaint frequently associated with spondylosis. Radiographic evidence of bone destruction should raise the possibility of lytic metastases, multiple myeloma or osteomyelitis. Palpable masses or prevertebral soft-tissue enlargement on plain radiographs should alert the physician to the possibility of local soft-tissue abscesses or primary head and neck tumors. An appropriately detailed patient history and selective diagnostic investigations should rapidly narrow the possibilities. However, as Walker[108] wrote in reference to the failure of early recognition of skeletal tuberculosis, 'to make a diagnosis of tuberculosis one must first consider it as a possibility. Tuberculosis has now joined syphilis as a great deceiver largely because its rarity so often excludes it from consideration in the differential diagnosis'. Walker's remark deserves added emphasis in a time when the prevalence of immunocompromised hosts and opportunist infections is increasing.

Treatment

Treatment of cervical tuberculosis is according to the principles established by Hodgson and Stock in 1956.[45] The spine must be stabilized to prevent further neurologic injury, while sources of spinal cord compression must be eliminated. Patients presenting with neurologic deficits warrant emergency evaluation. In the absence of pathologic fracture or instability, the presence of an epidural abscess must be sought. Currently, MRI provides the most rapid and anatomically relevant means of identifying epidural abscesses, and any involved vertebrae or disc spaces. For those patients with fractures and kyphosis, immediate skeletal traction is advised to protect the spinal cord, and to achieve some indirect decompression through improved alignment. The extent of the disease and source of spinal canal compromise should then be defined with appropriate studies. Myelography with post-myelography computed tomography, MRI, or both, will provide the necessary information for preoperative planning.

The treatment of cervical Pott's disease is surgical, followed by an adequate period of chemotherapy. As the disease affects the vertebral body, and rarely the posterior elements, the primary approach is anterior. Radical anterior decompression of all involved tissues, including the posterior longitudinal ligament, if necessary, is followed by reconstruction with iliac or fibular autograft. If more than a one-level corpectomy is necessary, supplemental stabilization may be necessary. Traditionally, halo support has been a useful adjunct. However, supplemental posterior fusions, particularly with the addition of lateral mass plating, may obviate the need for such a restrictive external support.

The role of posterior surgical procedures is strictly adjunctive. Posterior fusions alone have proved inadequate to maintain spinal alignment, or prevent late kyphosis and progressive neurologic deficit.[1,31,45–47] Supplemental posterior stabilization is particularly important in the upper cervical spine if the nature of the anterior disease has required transoral decompression. Acute bone grafting and reconstruction through such an approach carries too high a risk of infection, although not achieving suitable mechanical stability to promote union. Laminectomy for cervical tuberculosis is mentioned only to be condemned:[46,47,49] this procedure only creates further instability and neurologic complications.

DIRECT INOCULATION AS A SOURCE OF CERVICAL SPINE INFECTIONS

Infections of the cervical spine can occur as the result of local inoculation with organisms. The methods of introduction range from inadvertent contamination during a diagnostic or therapeutic procedure to penetrating trauma. Blunt trauma may even play an indirect role in some infections if the injury results in rupture of the cervical viscera. This section will deal with the broad spectrum of locally introduced infections of the cervical spine ranging from postoperative wound infections to those associated with penetrating and blunt visceral trauma.

Postoperative Wound Infections

The risk of infection is inherent to any invasive procedure. Once local barriers to bacterial invasion have been breached, a host of variables influences the risk of infection. It is beyond the scope of this chapter to discuss in detail those local and systemic factors which might influence the rate of wound infection; the reader is referred elsewhere for comprehensive reviews of these issues.[41,42,65] However, the literature does suggest some conclusions about cervical spine patients which are worthy of note. The incidence of infection must be discussed in the context of the type of procedure being performed as the figures will vary.

Currently, anterior approaches to the cervical spine are by far the most commonly performed procedures. The vast majority follow the surgical plane between the carotid sheath and the medial viscera. In unusual circumstances, pathoanatomy of the upper cervical region may necessitate a transoral approach in which the surgical incision occurs through a contaminated surface. Early experience with the transoral approach was fraught with complications. Fang and Ong[32] reported their experience with the transoral and transthyrohyoid exposures in 1962. Among their six transoral cases, one patient succumbed to infection. They urged further consideration of the technique with due regard to its inherent risks. Although two extrapharyngeal approaches to the upper cervical spine have been developed,[67,114,115] the transoral exposure still warrants consideration. Recent series have documented considerably less risk of infection. When it is performed for the purpose of decompression alone, the risk of infection is minimal, provided adequate prophylactic antibiotics are used.[2,37,97] Hadley et al[37] have reported their experience with 53 transoral procedures with only one infection and no deaths.

In the event that bone grafting will be required to reconstruct a defect, opinions vary regarding the advisability of transoral exposure. Whereas McAfee et al[67] warn against inserting bone grafts through this approach, Ashraf and Crockard[4] have reported three cases of successful transoral fusion without infection. One of the cases among the 53 reported by Hadley et al[37] was successfully grafted without becoming infected. Proponents of the procedure point out that oral surgeons frequently employ autogenous bone graft in their reconstructive procedures with little concern for infection. However, as Fang and Ong[32] reported, the consequences of infection for the transoral approach may be life threatening. Therefore, if technically possible, extrapharyngeal exposures should be considered the exposure of choice when bone grafting is anticipated. Transoral grafts cannot be recommended when alternatives exist, and are probably contraindicated if the dura is violated during the decompression.

The incidence of infections reported after anterior extrapharyngeal cervical spine procedures ranges from 0%

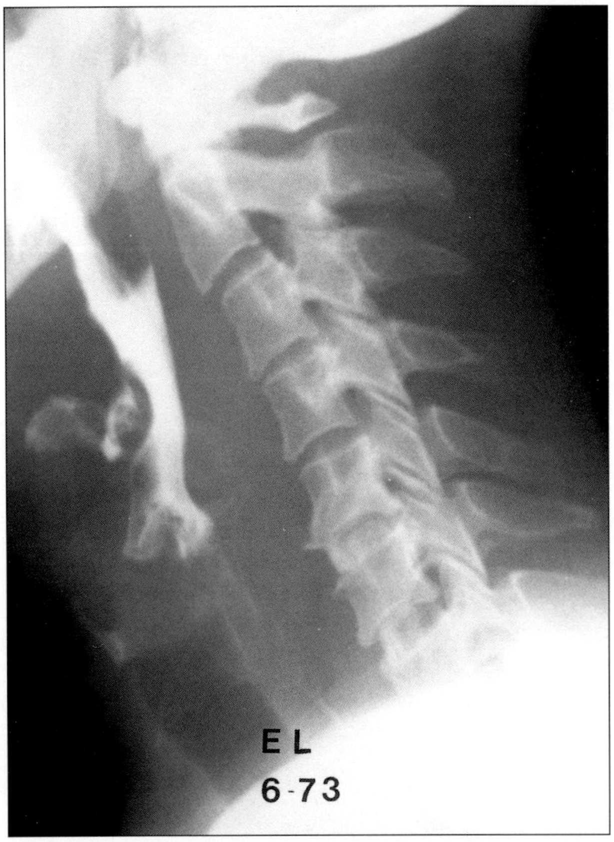

a

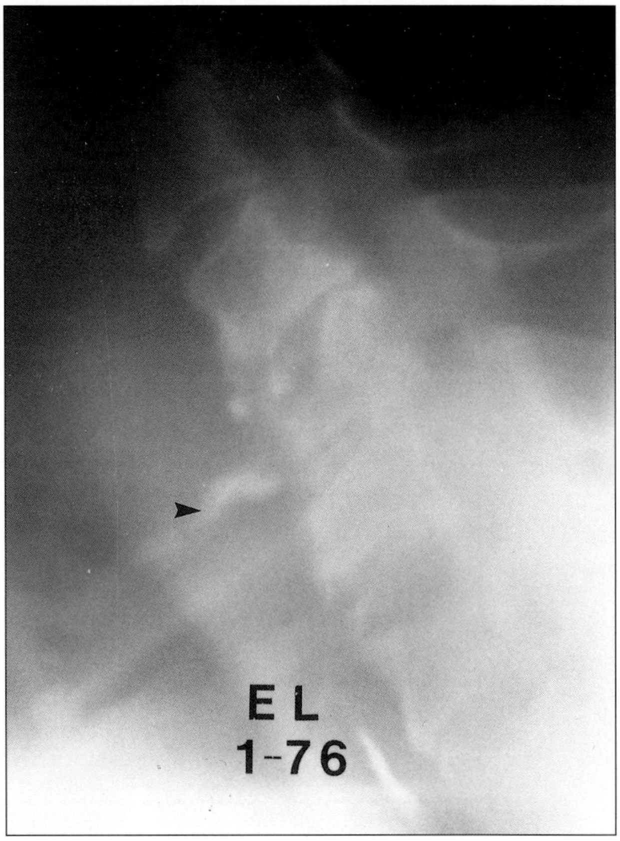

c

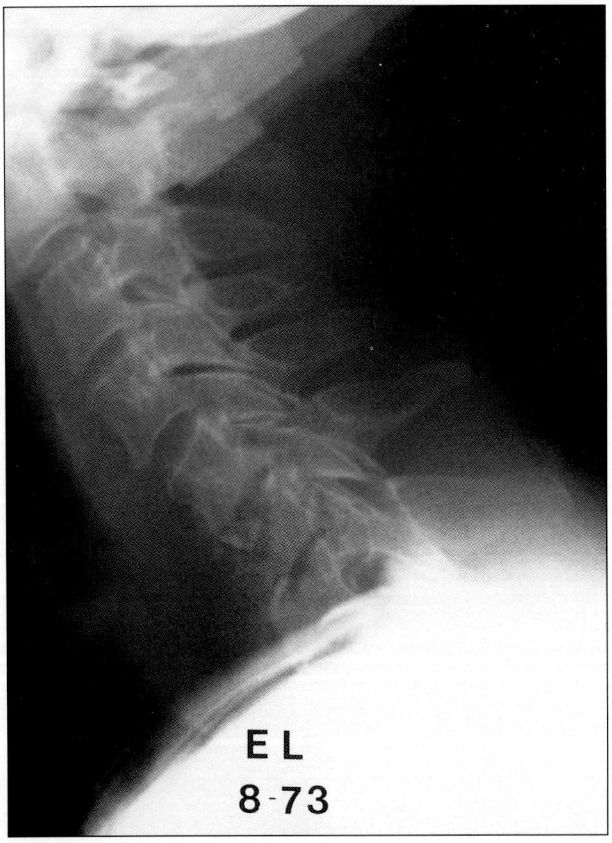

b

Figure 16.4
Patient EL underwent anterior cervical discectomies and fusion at C5–C6 and C6–C7. The postoperative course was complicated by a deep wound infection which was not appreciated for some time. An esophogram was performed for complaints of dysphagia (a). Note the marked prevertebral soft-tissue swelling. Two months later, radiographs demonstrated graft collapse, resorption, and osteolysis of the adjacent vertebral bodies with kyphosis (b). Treatment with parenteral antibiotics was unsuccessful. (c) Fistulogram performed for a chronic draining sinus 2½ years later. (Courtesy of H H Bohlman)

to 2%.[8,13,19,59,67,102] Whether the incidence varies with the type of procedure performed is unclear. Lumbar operations involving implants and/or bone grafts are associated with an increased risk of wound infection.[41,42,65] For anterior cervical cases performed without fusion, the incidence of infection varies from 0.6% to 2%.[8,29,40,61] Among the series of anterior procedures, including fusions, the frequency of infection is virtually identical, from 0% to 1.5% (Fig. 16.4).[13,19,59,61,67,102,107] Unfortunately, there are few series reported which allow direct comparison of the two techniques. Among their 253 patients, Lunsford et al[61] performed 148 anterior cervical discectomies without fusions and 137 with autograft fusions. The incidence of infection was half that among patients without fusions: 0.7% compared to 1.5%. However, the converse was found among the 1106 patients reviewed by Esperson et al[29] In a smaller series, Martins[63] compared 25 patients undergoing a Cloward-style anterior cervical discectomy and fusion to 26 patients undergoing discectomy alone. The one infection occurred in the discectomy group. No meaningful comparison of incidence could be made from such a small sample population.

Data about the rate of infection for posterior cervical laminectomies are available. The two largest series included 1.2% and 1.5% infection rates. Henderson et al[43] reported on their results for 846 patients: ten patients (1.2%) developed wound infections. The authors did not state whether any of these procedures incorporated posterior fusions, and, furthermore, they did not comment on the number of levels operated on or whether this might have influenced the incidence of infection.[43] Among his 205 patients, Raaf[82] observed three infections (1.5%). Fager[30] has reported an infection rate of 2.9% following posterior cervical procedures for spondylotic myelopathy in 35 patients. The small number of patients probably makes such an estimate inherently unreliable.

Posterior cervical fusion procedures, such as those in the lumbar spine, appear to engender a higher risk of infection. The reported incidence of wound infections varies from 0% to 15%.[15,48,87,91,110,112] Rheumatoid patients undergoing posterior cervical fusion are generally considered at increased risk for wound infections,[15,48,87] although Weiland and McAfee[110] did not observe any such difference. They reported no infections among 100 procedures, 27 of which were rheumatoid.

In spite of the higher and more rapid rates of union, and the lower incidence of graft collapse associated with autograft, various types of allograft are employed for anterior cervical fusions. Whether or not allograft carries an increased risk of wound infection is unclear in the cervical spine. Tomford et al[104] have suggested that this might be the case. However, the data from the literature are inconclusive. In their massive study, Esperson et al[29] analyzed their clinical results according to the type of graft used. They claimed no difference in the functional outcome of those treated with autograft, allograft, or xenograft (calf bone). However, they did note reoperation rates of 6%, 9%, and 22%, respectively. Unfortunately, they did not analyze their infection rates by graft type or specify the reason for reoperation. In another series of patients using only calf bone, Taheri and Gueramy[99] reported two infections among 200 patients.

Given the reproducible increase in observed infection rates among instrumented lumbar fusions,[41,42,65] similar results might be suspected in the anterior cervical spine. However, this does not seem to be the case. Among the series of instrumented anterior cervical fusions reported in recent years, the incidence of infection appears remarkably similar to uninstrumented rates: 0.0% to 3.6%.[13,59,101,102] The highest incidence was reported by Tippets and Apfelbaum[101] in 1988; they had one infection among their first 28 cases. However, at the Twentieth Annual Meeting of the Cervical Spine Research Society in 1992, they reported updated information on their first 220 patients. The infection rate had fallen to 0.45%.[102] The newer incidence figure was probably a reflection of both increased experience on the part of the surgeons and a larger sample size. Nevertheless, the reader is cautioned not to conclude that anterior cervical plating is benign with respect to infections. Longer follow-up and larger series are likely to provide more reliable incidence figures because delayed implant failure has been associated with esophageal rupture and infection.[73]

The incidence of infection among instrumented, posterior, cervical spine procedures ranges from 0% to 18%.[10,11,16,17,24,33,85,91,94,110,117,121] The highest rates, as noted above, have been reported for patients with rheumatoid arthritis[11,15,48,85,87,112,117] and Down's syndrome.[91] Among these patients, decreased host resistance undoubtedly plays an important role. If all such series are excluded, there is still a range of infection from 0% to 4.5%.[10,16,17,24,33,94,121] Overall, the incidence of infection is probably higher than with instrumented anterior fusions. This may be a reflection of the more extensive dissection and tissue trauma associated with the posterior procedures.

Methyl methacrylate has been shown to compromise local immune mechanisms and contribute to an increased risk of infection.[77,78] The data for the cervical spine seem to support these observations (Fig. 16.5). When looking at the rate of wound infection associated with methyl methacrylate, this complication may be seen in up to 18% of patients. Eismont and Bohlman,[25] and McAfee et al[66] have cautioned against the use of methyl methacrylate because of both mechanical inadequacy and increased rates of infection. If all the series of patients with rheumatoid arthritis are excluded, the incidence of wound infections with methyl methacrylate is still increased. Among 52 traumatic lesions stabilized with methyl methacrylate, Duff et al[24] had a 2% infection rate. Likewise Branch et al[10] reported infections in 3 of 99 patients similarly treated for traumatic instabilities.

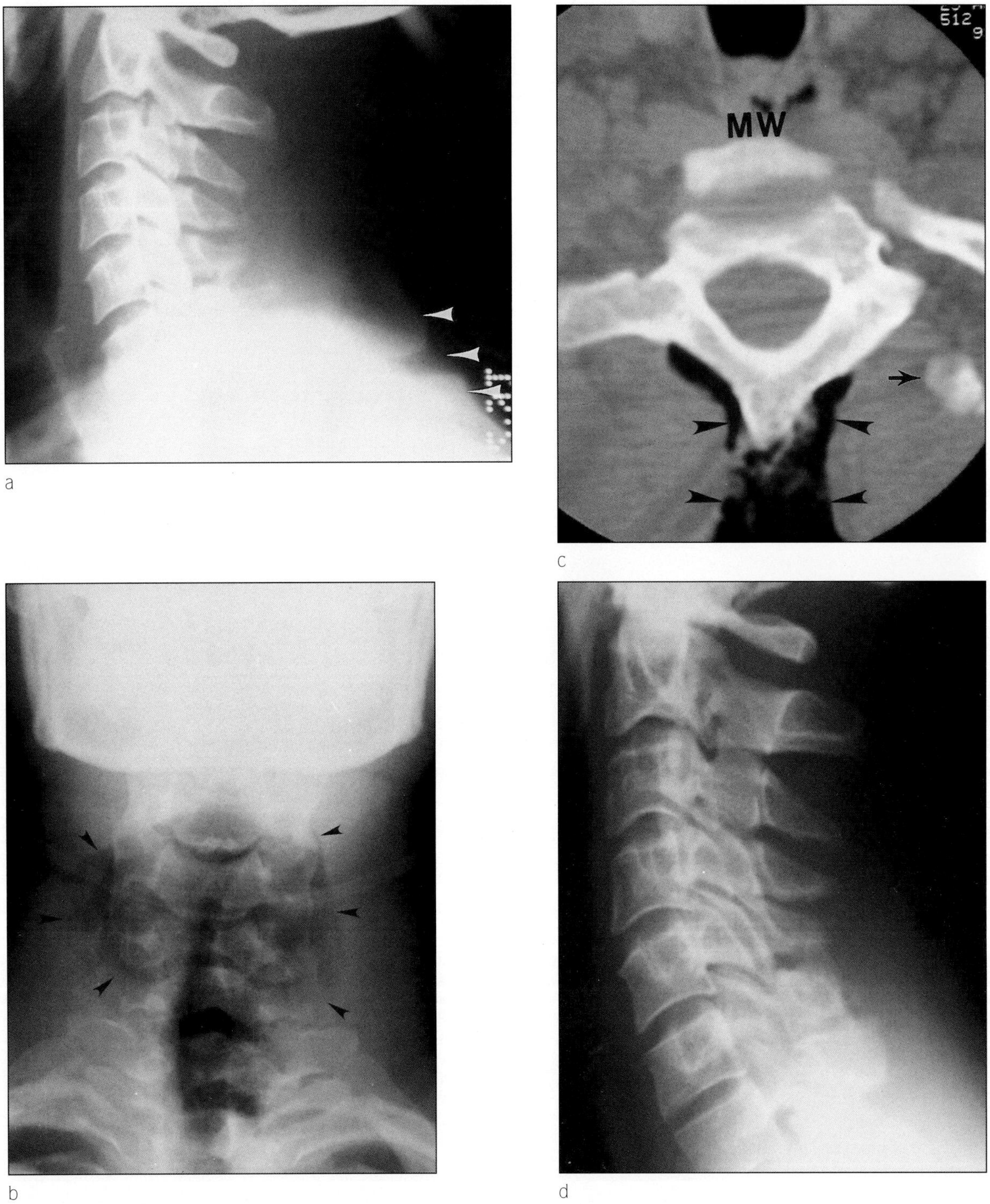

Figure 16.5
Patient MW sustained a flexion distraction injury at C6–C7. He was initially treated with posterior methyl methacrylate fixation without bone graft. A wound infection developed which was treated with débridement and parenteral antibiotics. He was referred for evaluation because of persistent drainage with an open wound. The (a) lateral and (b) posteroanterior radiographs taken at the time of referral indicate the extent of the wound dehiscence (arrowheads). (c) The computed tomogram illustrating the open wound margins better (arrowheads), as well as the retained methyl methacrylate (arrow) responsible for the persistent infection. Definitive treatment consisted of thorough débridement, parenteral antibiotics, and a delayed onlay grafting with primary closure over drains. A lateral radiograph one year after surgery shows a mature C6–C7 interspinous fusion

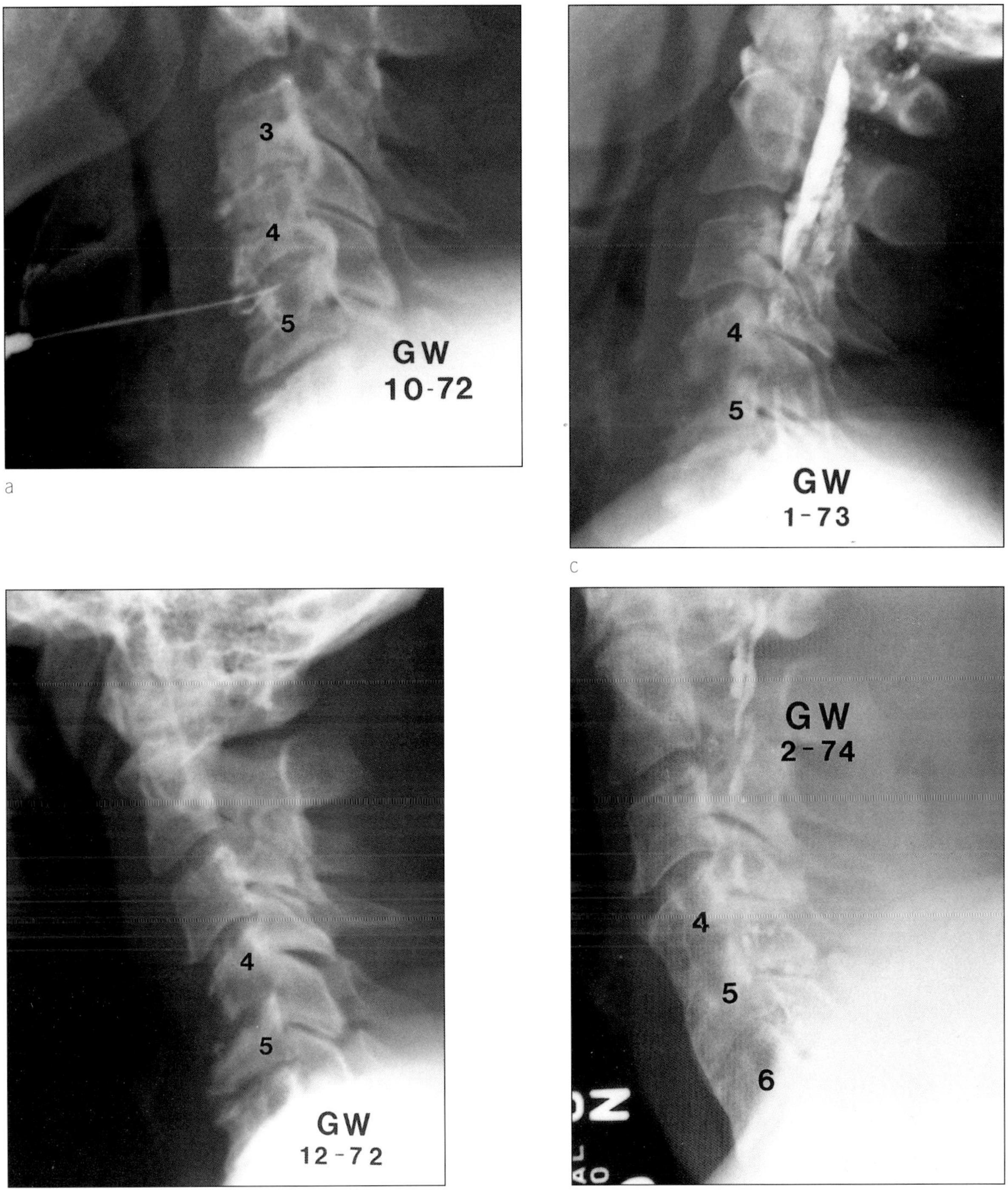

Figure 16.6
Patient GW was treated for neck pain with cervical discography (a), and simultaneous intradiscal injection of steroids. He subsequently developed *Staphylococcus aureus* osteomyelitis of C4, C5, and C6 (b) with an epidural abscess. Note the complete myelographic block (c). The patient remained quadriplegic until his demise, despite using autofusion from C4 to C6 while in a halo vest (d). (Reproduced from Bohlman[9] with permission)

Nosocomial Infections

Percutaneous diagnostic and therapeutic procedures may also result in nosocomial infections. Cervical discography (Fig. 16.6), epidural, prevertebral, and intradiscal steroid injections, and angiography have all been associated with infectious complications. The types of infection encountered cover the entire spectrum from intervertebral discitis and osteomyelitis to prevertebral and epidural abscesses, or any combination of the above. The incidence of infection associated with these procedures is not known. First, the use of these techniques is much less common in the cervical spine than in the lumbar region. Second, most cases have been reported in series discussing the type of infection, not the procedure responsible for its inception. Darden and Connor[21] recently reported on the complications associated with 31 cervical discograms. There were two significant complications (6.5%): one patient developed intervertebral discitis and the other acquired an epidural abscess which led to quadriplegia. The serious nature of such complications compels the responsible physician to evaluate the advisability of and need for these procedures critically. At the very least, due respect should be given to sterile technique, and appropriate antibiotic prophylaxis should be considered. Patients who subsequently complain of increasing neck pain or neurologic symptoms should be carefully evaluated with the above diagnoses in mind.

Penetrating Trauma

Penetrating trauma is another source of inoculation for cervical infections.[19,20] The contamination may be either direct or indirect; direct introduction of organisms may occur if they are present on the penetrating weapon, although this is more likely to be the case with stab or bite wounds. Gunshot wounds are less likely to introduce organisms directly; more often they will induce infection indirectly through trauma to the cervical viscera. Fractures or neurologic injuries inflicted by penetrating trauma rarely require surgical exploration or stabilization.[53] However, each victim of penetrating neck trauma must be carefully evaluated to exclude the possibility of significant visceral injuries. Astute clinical observation combined with the judicious use of arteriography, panendoscopy, and radiographic contrast studies should identify the majority of such patients. Surgical exploration is indicated in the event of positive diagnostic studies, expanding hematomas, tracheal deviation, airway compromise, or a widened mediastinum. Schaefer et al[90] have demonstrated the need for aggressive intervention in these circumstances to reduce the risk of soft-tissue and bone infections, and their associated morbidity.

Blunt Trauma

Infections resulting from injuries to the esophagus and hypopharynx may also be the result of blunt trauma. Although most spine surgeons are aware of the possibility of such injuries occurring during[73,95,106] or after surgery,[19,54,73,111,113,120] or with penetrating trauma, they have also been reported in association with cervical fractures and dislocations.[80] Pollock et al[80] reported four cases of infection caused by visceral trauma in acute cervical spinal cord injury patients. The diagnosis was delayed in all cases. In general, these patients will develop unexplained fever, swelling of the neck, dysphagia, odynophagia, and/or leukocytosis. If undiagnosed for a sufficient period of time, these infections can have serious consequences. One esophageal injury resulted in mediastinitis. Another prevertebral abscess led to airway compromise and probably contributed to a respiratory arrest. As with esophageal tears recognized at the time of surgery, immediate primary repair results in rapid healing with little morbidity.[73,106] Delays in diagnosis complicate management, result in prolonged hospitalization, and carry an increased mortality risk.[73,106]

EPIDURAL ABSCESS FORMATION IN THE CERVICAL SPINE

Infections of the epidural space are uncommon. The overall incidence has been reported to vary from 0.2 to 1.2 cases per 10 000 hospital admissions.[5,20,44] However, recent evidence suggests that the incidence may be increasing. Danner and Hartman[20] reported a significant increase in the frequency of epidural abscesses from 0.18 cases per 10 000 in the early 1970s to 2.8 cases per 10 000 admissions by 1982. Whether this is an isolated observation or a real change paralleling an increase in the population at risk is unclear. Blunt trauma,[14] vertebral fractures,[51] diabetes, malignancy, spinal surgery, discography,[20,86,89,111] epidural anesthesia,[75] remote infectious foci, alcohol abuse, and immunosuppression have been noted as predisposing factors.[36,39,44,50] The thoracic spine is most often involved, but cervical occurrences are noted in 6–18% of reported series.[5,20,35,39,44,56]

Clinical History, Physical Symptoms, and Laboratory Findings

The clinical presentation has been described as rather predictable, even monotonous, but is often hard to appreciate at an early stage. The initial complaint is uniformly axial pain. Fever or other symptoms of infection are present about half the time. The progression and time course of symptoms are astoundingly uniform from this point forward. Within 3 days, the patient will note root symptoms, followed within another day and a half by weakness.[20,38,44] Rapid deterioration to paralysis typically ensues within the next 24 hours. This evolution of symptoms has been so uniform that some authors have suggested that it establishes the diagnosis until proved otherwise (Fig. 16.7). In spite of this, Danner and Hartman[20] noted that only 20% of their patients were properly diagnosed at the time of admission. Others have observed higher rates of initial misdiagnosis.[5,44] This is particularly important because the prognosis is directly proportional to the speed of diagnosis and institution of treatment.

As with other spinal infections, laboratory findings are not usually helpful. Fever and leukocytosis are suggestive when present, but are absent in over half the cases. The erythrocyte sedimentation rate is almost universally elevated. Unfortunately, this finding is true for other spinal infections as well as some tumors. In addition, because remote infectious foci of hematogenous seeding are present in up to three-quarters of patients, the abnormal erythrocyte sedimentation rate may be attributed to the wrong process. Clinical suspicion and judicious use of imaging technology are the keys to a timely diagnosis. As with other infections, radionuclide scans may identify the process, but they are limited by inherent delays, lack of specificity, and sensitivity to previous antibiotic administration.

Radiographic Studies

Myelography combined with computed tomography is quite useful. Lateral C1–C2 puncture is recommended under most circumstances. The study will identify the upper level of the epidural mass, but may not define its lower extent or any skip lesions. A second puncture below any myelographic block will be required to appreciate the full extent of the abscess. Myelography has the added benefit of providing a sample of cerebrospinal fluid (CSF) for analysis and culture. Most often the findings will reflect a nonspecific pattern consistent with parameningeal inflammation, although 7–13% of patients will have concurrent meningitis.[5,20] The degree of local bone destruction from associated vertebral osteomyelitis is best appreciated on computed tomograms, and this information may be particularly helpful in preoperative planning.

The advent of MRI has provided a powerful tool in the diagnosis of these patients. If available, its speed and ability to identify inflammatory foci, as well as to define regional anatomy, probably render MRI the diagnostic imaging modality of choice. The findings of epidural abscesses are quite characteristic.[52] The epidural mass may be iso- or hypointense on T1-weighted images, whereas it will be hyperintense on T2-weighted images (Fig. 16.7). In those few reported instances where gadolinium has been administered, marked enhancement of the mass has been noted.[42,52] Gardner et al[35] have reported on the use of MRI in diagnosing cervical epidural abscesses, but offered one caution. The presence of an abscess was not appreciated in one case because of its extensive nature: it spanned 21 levels, so its upper and lower margins were not well seen. It is possible that gadolinium would have helped in such a circumstance. Magnetic resonance imaging may provide the additional benefit of identifying previously unsuspected intervertebral discitis or vertebral osteomyelitis. In such circumstances, this information could lead to modifications in the treatment plan.[35] The principal shortcomings of MRI are its tendency to overestimate bone involvement, and the lack of ability to identify meningitis when present. Supplemental computed tomograms are recommended to aid preoperative planning in the presence of osteomyelitis. Lateral cervical puncture should be done to obtain CSF if clinical suspicion of meningitis exists.

Differential Diagnosis

Epidural abscesses must be considered in the differential diagnosis of someone presenting with unexplained, rapidly increasing spinal pain, especially in the setting of fever, altered mental status, or sepsis. However, the other diagnoses to be considered may not be readily distinguishable from epidural abscesses. Among the other diagnostic possibilities are acute transverse myelitis, meningitis, osteomyelitis, discitis, subdural or intramedullary abscesses, epidural hematoma, intraspinal tumors, vascular lesions, and disc herniations.

Acute transverse myelitis is considerably more common than epidural abscesses, but may initially be indistinguishable. Factors favoring the diagnosis of acute transverse myelitis include a more rapid evolution of neurologic deficits, a lack of significant pain, myelographic block, or recent infections. Evidence of osteomyelitis on plain radiographs will probably exclude the presence of acute transverse myelitis.[3]

Microbiology of Epidural Abscesses

The bacteriology of epidural abscesses includes the same spectrum of organisms as vertebral osteomyelitis. Gram-positive cocci account for 78% of cases in Danner and Hartman's series;[20] they cultured *Staphylococcus aureus* in

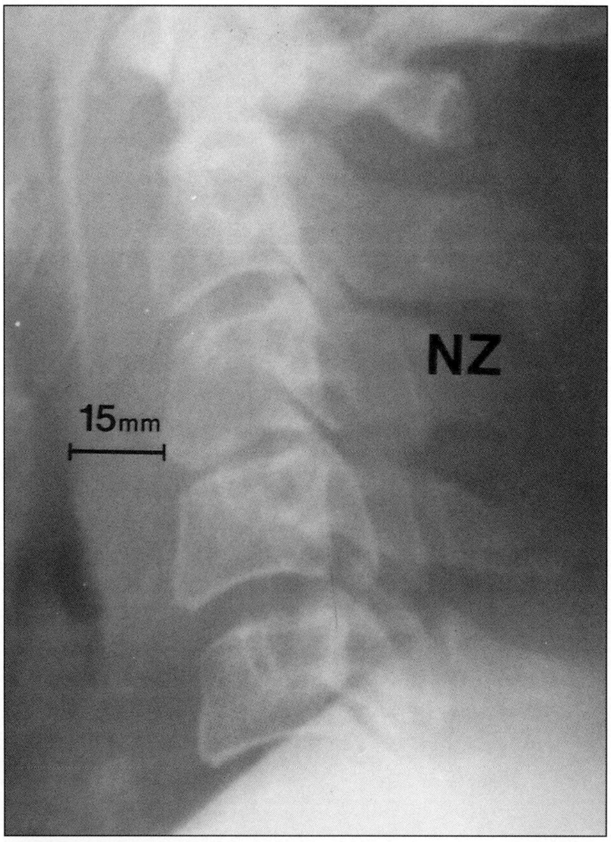

a

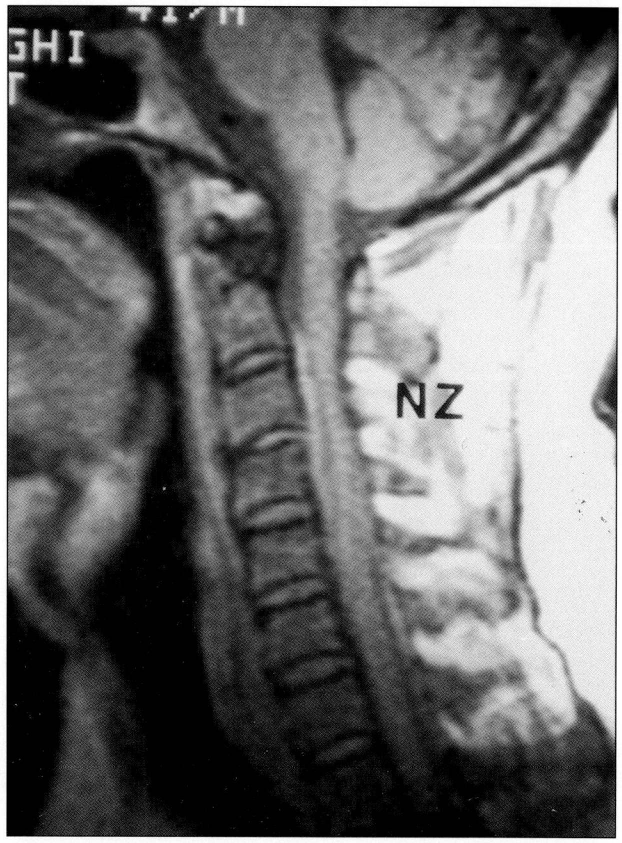

c

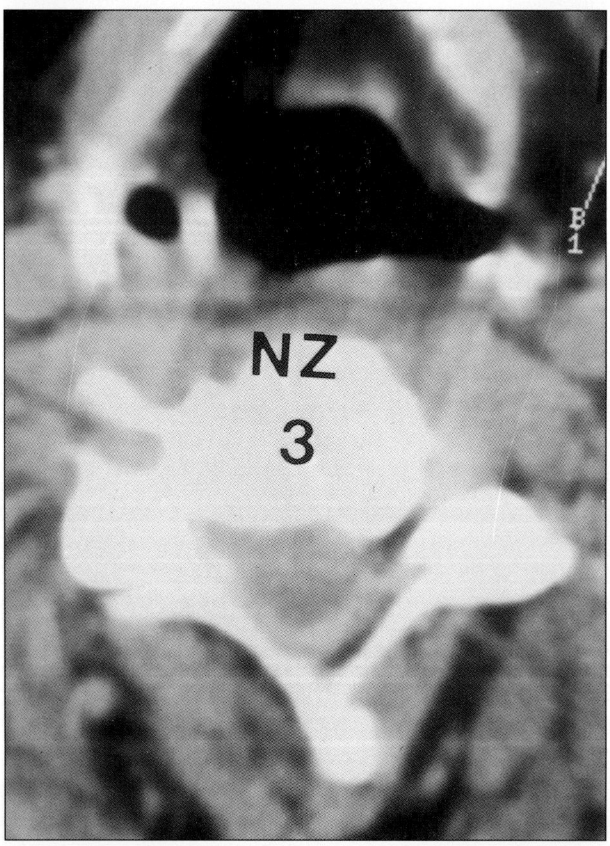

b

Figure 16.7
Patient NZ presented with 2 days of progressively severe neck pain, headaches, and upper extremity paresthesiae. He was febrile but neurologically intact. He had no known risk factors for spinal infection. The lateral radiograph at the time of admission (a) demonstrated decreased disc height at C3–C4 in association with abnormal prevertebral soft-tissue width. (b) Computed tomogram with intrathecal contrast revealing spinal cord compression by a ventral extradural soft-tissue mass. T1 and T2 (c, d, respectively) signal characteristics on the sagittal MR images were diagnostic of an epidural abscess associated with intervertebral discitis. (e) Transaxial MRI from the same level as the computed tomogram, included for comparison. Note how well MRI delineated the extent of the abscess and identified the discitis. The patient was treated by anterior decompression and fusion

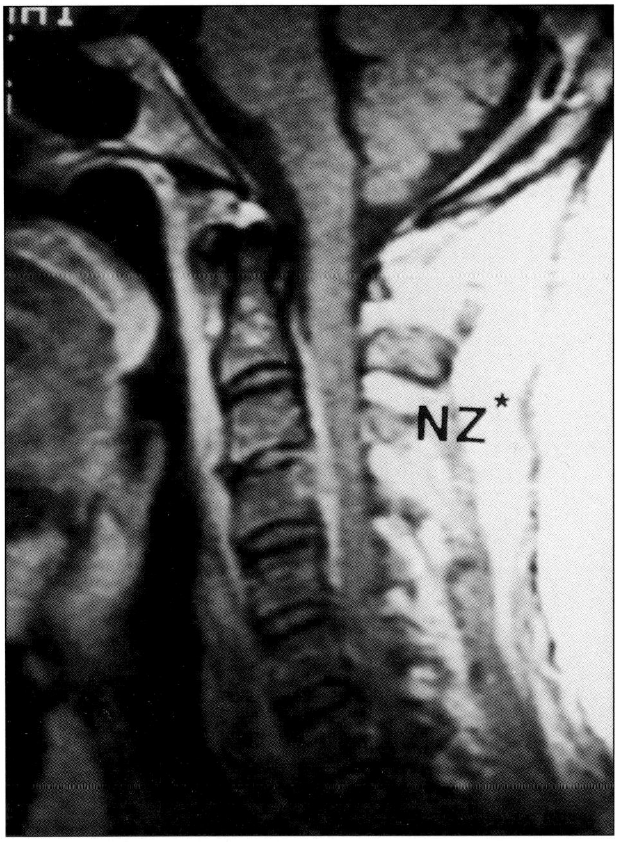

d

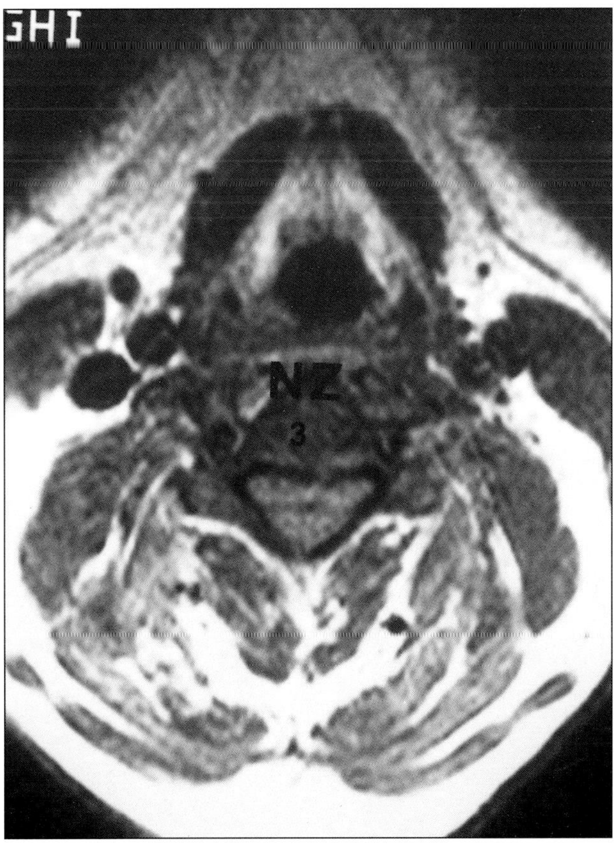

e

54% of cases. The remaining organisms were predominantly Gram-negative rods, but occasional anaerobes have been identified.[36] Diligent search will usually identify cutaneous, respiratory, or genitourinary sources of the infection, and a clue to the offending organism.[5,14,20,36,38,39,52,56] In the absence of such information, the initial choice of antibiotics should provide broad-spectrum coverage and good blood–brain barrier penetration. Modification of the drug regimen can then be based on definitive culture data. The duration of therapy must be individualized, but should not be less than 6 weeks in the presence of osteomyelitis. Shorter courses may be reasonable for isolated soft-tissue infections. Consultation with an infectious disease specialist is recommended.

The prognosis for patients with cervical epidural abscesses is generally worse than for those with abscesses in the thoracic or lumbar spine. They have a propensity to develop more severe neurologic deficits, and a correspondingly higher mortality rate.[26,35] Baker et al[5] reported an overall mortality of 18% for epidural abscesses in general. Gardner et al[35] found that 38% of their patients with cervical epidural abscesses died in spite of aggressive treatment. The worse prognosis for cervical abscesses may result from the same factor that has been offered to explain the lower incidence of cervical involvement: the cervical epidural space is much smaller than elsewhere in the spine.[39,56] Although this region may be somewhat resistant to hematogenous seeding, once infection is established there is little room to accommodate the abscess. Significant spinal cord compromise can be expected earlier in the disease.

Treatment

Treatment of cervical epidural abscesses is a surgical emergency. Regardless of the time course of evolution, decompression should be undertaken at once.[20] Any further neurologic progression compromises the patient's potential for recovery.[20,38] Hakin et al[38] demonstrated that neurologic recovery is inversely proportional to the severity of the paralysis and delay in treatment. Incomplete cord lesions, manifested by sensory sparing, indicated some probability of recovery, as did treatment undertaken within 24 hours of the onset of paralysis. Among their patients treated more than 36 hours after the onset of paralysis, none recovered useful function.[38]

Cervical epidural abscesses tend to occur anteriorly, whereas posterior locations are more common in the thoracic and lumbar spine.[20,39,50,52,75,118] The increased incidence of vertebral osteomyelitis or discitis associated with cervical epidural abscesses has been offered as an explanation for this observation.[39,52] Whatever the cause, the surgical decompression must address the location and extent of the spinal cord compression, as well as restoring spinal alignment and stability. Posterior cervical procedures are reserved for posterior abscesses in the absence of any anterior pathology, such as discitis or osteomyelitis. Most procedures will require an anterior approach for direct decompression of the epidural space, resection of involved disc and bone, and acute reconstruction of the spine (see Fig. 16.7). The abscess generally spans two to four levels, but may extend the entire length of the spinal canal.[20,35,38,39,44,52] The information available from the preoperative MRI scans and computed tomograms will help the surgeon formulate a rational operative plan.

Meningitis

Meningitis may be not only indistinguishable from cervical epidural abscesses, but coexistent in up to 13% of cases.[5,20] Cerebrospinal fluid analysis will be diagnostic of meningitis, whereas the CSF itself will show patterns consistent with parameningeal inflammation in the presence of epidural, subdural, or intramedullary abscesses.[5,20,23,60]

Subdural Abscess

Subdural abscesses are truly rare, and were probably clinically and radiographically indistinguishable from epidural abscesses until the advent of MRI.[34,60,103] Otherwise their clinical courses and treatment are similar.

Intramedullary Abscess

Intramedullary spinal abscesses are infrequent, but are usually far more delayed in their diagnosis. The clinical course is insidious, and delays in diagnosis may have increased paradoxically in the antibiotic era. The cervical spine is involved 24% of the time. The risk factors are similar to those for epidural abscesses with the notable addition of dermal sinuses and the relative youth of patients. They occur mainly in infants or teenagers. Intramedullary abscesses are probably best appreciated with pre- and post-gadolinium MRI. These represent surgical emergencies and require open drainage.[23,103]

Epidural hematomas are often spontaneous, but may also occur after trauma. The patients are less likely to have signs or symptoms of infection, but may experience progressive and profound neurologic deficits. Once diagnosed, they also require decompression if neurologic compromise exists.

GRISEL'S SYNDROME

Non-traumatic atlantoaxial subluxation resulting from ligamentous laxity, induced by peripharyngeal inflammatory processes, is known as Grisel's syndrome. The process was initially described in 1830,[7] but an explanation was not available until 1984. Parke et al identified reproducible lymphovenous anastomoses between the posterosuperior nasopharynx and the upper cervical epidural sinuses, by way of the periodontal venous plexus. Their retrograde venous injection studies demonstrated a network of venous tributaries which drained the peripharyngeal region, and then penetrated the prevertebral fascia and atlanto-occipital membrane to join the network of veins around the odontoid process. Parke et al felt that this could function as a pathway for the spread of inflammatory or neoplastic processes to the atlanto-occipital joint. This, in turn, could be responsible for the induced laxity or rupture of the atlantoaxial ligaments, and subsequent subluxation or dislocation.

Clinical, Laboratory, and Radiographic Findings

This infrequent syndrome affects young people. Most patients are less than 30 years old with peaks of incidence in children less than 10 years and young adults aged between 20 and 30. Patients present with increasing pain in the cervical spine which may become quite severe and generalized to the trapezial or shoulder region. Headaches are frequent and often distressing. Motion of the head and neck usually exacerbates pain. Supine rest with support of the head and neck may provide some relief, but torticollis may develop at varying intervals after the onset of symptoms, or not at all. A history of some prodromal viral respiratory or nasopharyngeal illness, or surgical procedure on the head and neck, is common. This should alert the physician to the possibility of either a local infection or Grisel's syndrome.

Patients frequently present supporting their head in their hands, declining to move their head. Changes in position, especially from supine to upright, may be quite distressing. In children, one should consider the possibility of an occult odontoid fracture.[92] Regional tenderness and spasm may be prominent. Torticollis and its associated physical findings may be apparent, such as the 'cock robin' position (a retropharyngeal prominence caused by the anterior arch of the subluxated atlas vertebra) or Sudek's sign. The last finding consists of a palpable C2 spinous process deviated from the midline in the direction toward which the head has rotated. Manual traction may alleviate some of the pain, whereas compression or passive rotation may exacerbate it. Neurologic deficits are only reported to occur in 15% of patients, but they may be catastrophic, given the potential level of cord injury.

Laboratory or imaging studies may be helpful, but the findings are often non-specific. The leukocyte count and differential are often normal, but the sedimentation rate is frequently elevated. In the absence of torticollis, static plain radiographs of the cervical spine are usually unremarkable, unless they reveal prevertebral soft-tissue abnormalities or locally destructive processes. Lateral flexion–extension radiographs may demonstrate occult ligamentous laxity, provided the patient is able to comply with the requested motion arch. If the plain radiographs look bizarre at first glance, examine the bony landmarks on the anteroposterior and lateral views to be sure all the elements are seen in proper profile. Careful scrutiny of the facial bones, mandibular angles, and posterior arch of the atlas will disclose that they are abnormally rotated relative to the lower cervical spine. Abnormal findings also may be apparent on the open-mouth odontoid view, such as laterally displaced subaxial spinous processes, or asymmetry in the size and alignment of the C1 lateral masses or atlantoaxial joint spaces. Radionuclide bone scans may be positive.[22] If the patient appears acutely ill, has abnormal mental status, or excessive neck pain and stiffness, then emergency MRI of the spinal column should be considered to rule out an epidural abscess, followed by a spinal tap to exclude meningitis.

Treatment

Treatment of Grisel's syndrome is directed to the underlying nasopharyngeal process, while controlling atlantoaxial stability and protecting the neural elements. Antibiotic therapy and, occasionally, surgical drainage may be needed to treat local infections. A period of restricted activity and cervical bracing will allow the local cervical symptoms to subside. If the patient presents with torticollis and fixed atlantoaxial subluxation of short duration, skeletal traction should be instituted to effect reduction. Arthrodesis is reserved for patients who present with symptomatic spinal cord compression or residual instability.

REFERENCES

1 Tuberculous paraplegia [editorial]. *BMJ* **1**: 1442–1443, 1979.
2 Alonso WA, Black P, Connor GH, Uematsu S. Transoral transpalatal approach for resection of clival chordoma. *Laryngoscope* **81**: 1626–1631, 1971.
3 Altrocchi PH. Acute spinal epidural abscess versus acute transverse myelopathy: A plea for neurosurgical caution. *Arch Neurol* **9**: 17–25, 1963.
4 Ashraf J, Crockard HA. Transoral fusion for high cervical fractures. *J Bone Joint Surg [Br]* **72**: 76–79, 1990.
5 Baker AS, Ojemann RG, Swartz MN, Richardson EP. Spinal epidural abscess. *N Engl J Med* **293**: 463–468, 1975.
6 Barron MM. Cervical spine injury masquerading as a medical emergency. *Am J Emerg Med* **7**: 54–56, 1989.
7 Bell C. *The Nervous System of the Human Body*. London: Longman, 1830.
8 Bertalanffy H, Eggert HR. Complications of anterior cervical discectomy without fusion in 450 consecutive patients. *Acta Neurochir* **99**: 41–50, 1989.
9 Bohlman HH. Complications of treatment of fractures and dislocations of the cervical spine. In Epps C (ed.) *Complications of Orthopaedic Surgery*, 897–918. Philadelphia: JB Lippincott, 1985.
10 Branch CL, Kelly DL, Davis CH, McWhorter JM. Fixation of fractures of the lower cervical spine using methylmethacrylate and wire: Technique and results in 99 patients. *Neurosurg* 1989; **25**: 503–513.
11 Bryan WJ, Inglis AE, Sculco TP, Ranawat CS. Methylmethacrylate stabilization for enhancement of posterior cervical arthrodesis in rheumatoid arthritis. *J Bone Joint Surg [Am]* **64**: 1045–1050, 1982.
12 Cahill DW, Love LC, Rechtine GR. Pyogenic osteomyelitis of the spine in the elderly. *J Neurosurg* **74**: 878–886, 1991.
13 Cahill DW, Rechtine GR. The use of the Morscher anterior cervical plate system to enhance fusion in the cervical spine: 40 consecutive cases (abstract). Presented at the Twentieth Annual Meeting of the Cervical Spine Research Society, Palm Desert, California, December 1992.
14 Chen JY, Chen WJ, Huang TJ, Shih CH. Spinal epidural abscess complicating cervical spine fracture with hypopharyngeal perforation: A case report. *Spine* **17**: 971–974, 1992.
15 Clark CR, Goetz DD, Menezes AH. Arthrodesis of the cervical spine in rheumatoid arthritis. *J Bone Joint Surg [Am]* **71**: 381–392, 1989.
16 Clark CR, Keggi KJ, Panjabi MM. Methylmethacrylate stabilization of the cervical spine. *J Bone Joint Surg [Am]* **66**: 40–46, 1984.
17 Cooper PR, Cohen A, Rosiello A, Koslow M. Posterior stabilization of cervical spine fractures and subluxations using plates and screws. *Neurosurgery* **23**: 300–306, 1988.
18 Craig JB. Cervical spine osteomyelitis with delayed onset tetraparesis after penetrating wounds of the neck. *S Afr Med J* **69**: 197–199, 1986.
19 Cuatico W. Anterior cervical discectomy without interbody fusion: An analysis of 81 cases. *Acta Neurochir* **57**: 269–274, 1981.
20 Danner RL, Hartman BJ. Update of spinal epidural abscess: 35 cases and review of the literature. *Rev Infect Dis* **9**: 265–274, 1987.
21 Darden BV, Connor PM. Cervical discography: Complications and clinical efficacy (abstract). Presented at the Twentieth Annual Meeting of the Cervical Spine Research Society, Palm Desert, CA, December 1992.
22 Digby JM, Kersley JB. Pyogenic non-tuberculous spinal infection: An analysis of thirty cases. *J Bone Joint Surg [Br]* **61**: 47–55, 1979.

23 DiTullio MV. Intramedullary spinal abscess: A case report with a review of 53 previously described cases. *Surg Neurol* **7**: 351–354, 1977.
24 Duff TA, Khan A, Corbett JE. Surgical stabilization of cervical spine fractures using methyl methacrylate. *J Neurosurg* **76**: 440–443, 1992.
25 Eismont FJ, Bohlman HH. Posterior methylmethacrylate fixation for cervical trauma. *Spine* **6**: 347–353, 1981
26 Eismont FJ, Bohlman HH, Soni PL, Goldberg VM, Freehafer AA. Pyogenic and fungal vertebral osteomyelitis with paralysis. *J Bone Joint Surg [Am]* **65**: 19–29, 1983.
27 Emery SE, Chan DPK, Woodward HR. Treatment of hematogenous pyogenic vertebral osteomyelitis with anterior debridement and primary bone grafting. *Spine* **14**: 284–291, 1989.
28 Endress C, Guyot DR, Fata J, Salcicciol G. Cervical osteomyelitis due to IV heroin use: Radiologic findings in 14 patients. *Am J Roentgenol* **155**: 333–335, 1990.
29 Esperson JO, Buhl M, Eriksen EF et al Treatment of cervical disc disease using Cloward's technique: I. General results, effect of different operative methods, and complications in 1,106 patients. *Acta Neurochir* **70**: 97–114, 1984.
30 Fager CA. Results of adequate posterior decompression in the relief of spondylotic cervical myelopathy. *J Neurosurg* **38**: 684–692, 1973.
31 Fang D, Leong JCY, Fang HSY. Tuberculosis of the upper cervical spine. *J Bone Joint Surg [Br]* **65**: 47–50, 1983.
32 Fang SY, Ong GB. Direct anterior approach to the upper cervical spine. *J Bone Joint Surg [Am]* **44**: 1588–1604, 1962.
33 Fehlings MG, Cooper PR, Errico T, DiBartolo T. Posterior plates in the management of cervical instability: Long term results in a consecutive series (abstract). Presented at the Twentieth Annual Meeting of the Cervical Spine Research Society, Palm Desert, California, December 1992.
34 Fraser RAR, Ratzan K, Wolpert SM, Weinstein L. Spinal subdural empyema. *Arch Neurol* **28**: 235–238, 1973.
35 Gardner R, Eismont FJ, Cammisa F. Cervical epidural abscesses (abstract). Presented at the Sixteenth Annual Meeting of the Cervical Spine Research Society, Key Biscayne, Florida, December 1988.
36 Guerrero IC, Slap GB, MacGregor RR, Lawner P, Ruggeri S, Gennarelli T. Anaerobic spinal epidural abscess: Case report. *J Neurosurg* **48**: 465–469, 1978.
37 Hadley MN, Spetzler RF, Sonntag VKH. The transoral approach to the superior cervical spine: A review of 53 cases of extradural cervicomedullary compression. *J Neurosurg* **71**: 16–23, 1989.
38 Hakin RN, Burt AA, Cook JB. Acute spinal epidural abscess. *Paraplegia* **17**: 330–336, 1980.
39 Hancock DO. A study of 49 patients with acute spinal extradural abscess. *Paraplegia* **10**: 285–288, 1973.
40 Hankinson HL, Wilson CB. Use of the operating microscope in anterior cervical discectomy without fusion. *J Neurosurg* **43**: 452–456, 1975.
41 Heller JG. Postoperative infections of the spine. In Rothman RH, Simeone FA (eds) *The Spine*, 3rd ed, 817–837. Philadelphia: WB Saunders, 1992.
42 Heller JG, Garfin SR. Postoperative infection of the spine. *Semin Spine Surg* **2**: 268–282, 1990.
43 Henderson CM, Hennessy RG, Shuey HM, Shackelford EG. Posterior–lateral foraminotomy as an exclusive operative technique for cervical radiculopathy: A review of 846 consecutively operated cases. *Neurosurgery* **13**: 504–512, 1983.
44 Heusner AP. Nontuberculous spinal epidural infections. *N Engl J Med* **239**: 845–854, 1948.
45 Hodgson AR, Stock FE. Anterior spinal fusion: A preliminary communication on the radical treatment of Pott's disease in adults. *Br J Surg* **44**: 266–75, 1956.
46 Hsu LCS, Leong JCY. Tuberculosis of the lower cervical spine (C2 to C7): A report on 40 cases. *J Bone Joint Surg [Br]* **66**: 1–5, 1984.
47 Hsu LCS, Yau ACMC. Infections: Tuberculosis. In Sherk HH, Dunn EJ, Eismont FJ et al (eds), *The Cervical Spine*, 2nd ed, 544–551. Cervical Spine Research Society. Philadelphia: JB Lippincott, 1989.
48 Itoh TI, Tsuji H, Katoh Y, Yonezawa T, Kitagawa H. Occipitocervical fusion reinforced by Luque's segmental spinal instrumentation for rheumatoid arthritis. *Spine* **13**: 1234–1238, 1988.
49 Kemp HBS, Jackson JW, Shaw NC. Laminectomy in paraplegia due to infective spondylosis. *Br J Surg* **61**: 66–72, 1974.
50 Keon-Cohen BT. Epidural abscess simulating disc hernia. *J Bone Joint Surg [Br]* **50**: 128–130, 1968.
51 Korovessis P, Sidiropoulos P, Piperos G, Karagiannis A. Spinal epidural abacess complicated closed vertebral fracture. *Spine* **18**: 671–674, 1993.
52 Kricun R, Shoemaker EI, Chovanes GI, Stephens HW. Epidural abscess of the cervical spine: MR findings in five cases. *Am J Roentgenol* **158**: 1145–1149, 1992.
53 Kupcha PC, An HS, Cotler JM. Gunshot wounds to the cervical spine. *Spine* **15**: 1058–1063, 1990.
54 Kuriloff DB, Blaugrund S, Ryan J, O'Leary P. Delayed neck infection following anterior spine surgery. *Laryngoscope* **97**: 1094–1098, 1987.
55 La Rocca SH, Eismont FJ. Infections: Other infectious diseases. In Sherk HH, Dunn EJ, Eismont FJ et al (eds) *The Cervical Spine*, 2nd ed, 552–563. Cervical Spine Research Society. Philadelphia: JB Lippincott, 1989.
56 Lasker BR, Harter DH. Cervical epidural abscess. *Neurology* **37**: 1747–1753, 1987.
57 Liebergall M, Chaimsky G, Lowe J, Robin GC, Floman Y. Pyogenic vertebral osteomyelitis with paralysis: Prognosis and treatment. *Clin Orthop* **269**: 142–150, 1991.
58 Lowe J, Kaplan L, Liebergall M, Floman Y. Serratia osteomyelitis causing neurological deterioration after spine fracture: A report of two cases. *J Bone Joint Surg [Br]* **71**: 256–258, 1989.
59 Lowery GL, Reuter MW, Sutterlin CE. Anterior cervical interbody arthrodesis with plate stabilization for degenerative disc disease (abstract). Presented at the Twentieth Annual Meeting of the Cervical Spine Research Society, Palm Desert, California, December 1992.
60 Lownie SP, Ferguson GG. Spinal subdural empyema complicating cervical discography. *Spine* **14**: 1415–1417, 1989.
61 Lunsford LD, Bissonette DJ, Jannetta PJ, Sheptak PE, Zorub DS. Anterior surgery for cervical disc disease. Part 1: Treatment of lateral cervical disc herniation in 253 cases. *J Neurosurg* **53**: 1–11, 1980.
62 Malawski SK, Lukawski S. Pyogenic infection of the spine. *Clin Orthop* **272**: 58–66, 1991.
63 Martins AN. Anterior cervical discectomy with and without interbody bone graft. *J Neurosurg* **44**: 290–295, 1976.

64 Maruyama H, Gejyo F, Arakawa M. Clinical studies of destructive spondyloarthropathy in long-term hemodialysis patients. *Nephron* **61**: 37–44, 1992.

65 Massie JB, Heller JG, Abitbol JJ, McPherson D, Garfin SR. Postoperative posterior spinal wound infections. *Clin Orthop* **284**: 99–108, 1992.

66 McAfee PC, Bohlman HH, Ducker T. Failure of stabilization of the spine with methylmethacrylate: A retrospective analysis of twenty four cases. *J Bone Joint Surg [Am]* **68**: 1145–1157, 1986.

67 McAfee PC, Bohlman HH, Riley LH, Robinson RA, Southwick WO, Nachlas NE. The anterior retropharyngeal approach to the upper part of the cervical spine. *J Bone Joint Surg [Am]* **69**: 1371–1383, 1987.

68 McGrath H, McCormick C, Carey ME. Pyogenic cervical osteomyelitis presenting as a massive prevertebral abscess in a patient with rheumatoid arthritis. *Am J Med* **84**: 363–365, 1988.

69 Messer HD, Litvinoff J. Pyogenic cervical osteomyelitis: Chondro-osteomyelitis of the cervical spine frequently associated with parenteral drug use. *Arch Neurol* **33**: 571–576, 1976;

70 Modic MT, Feiglin DH, Piraino DW, et al. Vertebral osteomyelitis: Assessment using MR. *Radiology* **157**: 157–166, 1985.

71 Murakami DM, Bassett LW, Seeger LL. Advances in imaging of rheumatoid arthritis. *Clin Orthop* **265**: 83–95, 1991.

72 Neal SL, Kearns MJ, Seelig JM, Harris JP. Manifestations of Pott's disease in the head and neck. *Laryngoscope* **96**: 494–497, 1986.

73 Newhouse KE, Lindsey RW, Clark CR, Lieponis J, Murphy MJ. Esophageal perforation following anterior cervical spine surgery. *Spine* **14**: 1051–1053, 1989.

74 Noble RC, Overman SB. *Propionibacterium acnes* osteomyelitis: Case report and review of the literature. *J Clin Microbiol* **25**: 251–254, 1987.

75 North JB, Brophy BP. Epidural abscess: A hazard of spinal epidural anaesthesia. *Aust NZ J Surg* **49**: 484–485, 1979.

76 Pal GP, Sherk HH. The vertical stability of the cervical spine. *Spine* **13**: 447–449, 1988.

77 Petty W. The effect of methylmethacrylate on chemotaxis of polymorphonuclear leukocytes. *J Bone Joint Surg [Am]* **60**: 492–498, 1978.

78 Petty W. The effect of methylmethacrylate on bacterial phagocytosis and killing by human polymorphonuclear leukocytes. *J Bone Joint Surg [Am]* **60**: 752–757, 1978.

79 Pinckney LE, Currarino G, Highgenboten CL. Osteomyelitis of the cervcial spine following dental extraction. *Radiology* **135**: 335–337, 1980.

80 Pollock RA, Purvis JM, Apple DF, Murray HH. Esophageal and hypopharyngeal perforation injuries in patients with cervical spine trauma. *Ann Otol* **90**: 323–327, 1981.

81 Post MJD, Sze G, Quencer RM, Eismont FJ, Green BA, Gahbauer H. Gadolinium-enhanced MR in spinal infection. *J Comput Assist Tomogr* **14**: 721–729, 1990.

82 Raaf JE. Surgical treatment of patients with cervical disk lesions. *J Trauma* **9**: 327–338, 1969.

83 Raff MJ, Melo JC. Anaerobic osteomyelitis. *Medicine* **57**: 83–103, 1978.

84 Rafto SE, Dalinka MK, Schiebler ML, Burk DL, Kricun ME. Spondyloarthropathy of the cervical spine in long-term hemodialysis. *Radiology* **166**: 201–204, 1988.

85 Rao S. Neurological and clinical outcome of surgical stabilization for cervical rheumatoid arthritis (abstract). Presented at the Twentieth Annual Meeting of the Cervical Spine Research Society, Palm Desert, California, December 1992.

86 Redekop GJ, Del Maestro RF. Diagnosis and management of spinal epidural abscess. *Can J Neurol Sci* **19**: 180–187, 1992.

87 Santavirta S, Slatis P, Kankaapaa U, Sandelin J, Laasonen E. Treatment of the cervical spine in rheumatoid arthritis. *J Bone Joint Surg [Am]* **70**: 658–667, 1988.

88 Sapico FL, Montgomerie JZ. Vertebral osteomyelitis in intravenous drug abusers: Report of three cases and review of the literature. *Rev Infect Dis* **2**: 196–206, 1980.

89 Sapico FL, Montgomerie JZ. Vertebral osteomyelitis. *Infect Dis Clin North Am* **4**: 539–550, 1990.

90 Schaefer SD, Bucholz RW, Jones RE, Carder HM. The management of transpharyngeal gunshot wounds to the cervical spine. *Surg Gynecol Obstet* **152**: 27–29, 1981.

91 Segal LS, Drummond DS, Zanotti RM, Ecker ML, Mubarak SJ. Complications of posterior arthrodesis of the cervical spine in patients who have Down syndrome. *J Bone Joint Surg [Am]* **73**: 1547–1554, 1991.

92 Seimon LP. Fracture of the odontoid process in young children. *J Bone Joint Surg [Am]* **59**: 943–948, 1977.

93 Smith DF, Smith FW, Douglas JG. Tuberculous polyradiculopathy: The value of magnetic resonance imaging of the neck. *Tubercle* **70**: 213–216, 1989.

94 Smith MD, Anderson P. Occipital-cervical arthrodesis using contoured reconstruction plates: An early report on a versatile technique for internal fixation (abstract). Presented at the Twentieth Annual Meeting of the Cervical Spine Research Society, Palm Desert, California, December 1992.

95 Smith MD, Bolesta MJ. Esophageal perforation after anterior cervical plate fixation: A report of two cases. *J Spinal Dis* **5**: 357–362, 1992.

96 Smith MD, Emery SE, Dudley A, Murray KJ, Leventhal M. Iatrogenic vertebral artery injuries during anterior cervical spine procedures: A report of ten patients (abstract). Presented at the Nineteenth Annual Meeting of the Cervical Spine Research Society, Philadelphia, Pennsylvania, December 1991.

97 Spetzler RF, Selman WR, Nash CL, Brown RH. Transoral microsurgical odontoid resection and spinal cord monitoring. *Spine* **4**: 506–510, 1979.

98 Stone JL, Cybulski GR, Rodriguez J, Gryfinski ME, Kant R. Anterior cervical debridement and strut-grafting for osteomyelitis of the cervical spine. *J Neurosurg* **70**: 879–883, 1989.

99 Taheri ZE, Gueramy M. Experience with calf bone in cervical interbody spinal fusion. *J Neurosurg* **36**: 67–71, 1972.

100 Tami TA, Burkus JK, Strom CG. Cervical osteomyelitis: An unusual complication of tonsillectomy. *Arch Otolaryngol Head Neck Surg* **113**: 992–994, 1987.

101 Tippets RH, Apfelbaum RI. Anterior cervical fusion with the Caspar instrumentation system. *Neurosurgery* **22**: 1008–1013, 1988.

102 Tippets RH, Apfelbaum RI. Technical and clinical complications with Caspar plating (abstract). Presented at the Twentieth Annual Meeting of the Cervical Spine Research Society, Palm Desert, California, December 1992.

103 Tom BM, Power TC. Diagnosis of spinal column infections. *Spine* **2**: 395–406, 1988.

104 Tomford WW, Starkweather RJ, Goldman MH. A study of the clinical incidence of infection in the use of banked allograft bone. *J Bone Joint Surg [Am]* **63**: 244–248, 1981.

105 Transfeldt E, Macnab I, Kostuik JP, Morley TP. The spectrum and natural history of pyogenic vertebral osteomyelitis (abstract). *J Bone Joint Surg [Br]* **66**: 299, 1984.

106 van Berge Henegouwen DP, Roukema JA, de Nile JC, van der Werken C. Esophageal perforation during surgery on the cervical spine. *Neurosurgery* **29**: 766–768, 1991.

107 Verbiest H, Paz Y Geuse HD. Anterolateral surgery for cervical spondylosis in cases of myelopathy or nerve root compression. *J Neurosurg* **25**: 611–622, 1966.

108 Walker GF. Failure of early recognition of skeletal tuberculosis. *BMJ* **1**: 682–683, 1968.

109 Wang, LX. Peroral focal debridement for treatment of tuberculosis of the atlas and axis. *Chin J Orthop* **1**: 207–209, 1981.

110 Weiland DJ, McAfee PC. Posterior cervical fusion with triple-wire strut graft technique: 100 consecutive patients. *J Spinal Dis* **4**: 15–21, 1991.

111 Welsh LW, Welsh JJ, Chinnici JC. Dysphagia due to cervical spine surgery. *Ann Otol Rhinol Laryngol* **96**: 112–115, 1987.

112 Wertheim SB, Bohlman HH. Occipitocervical fusion: Indications, technique, and long-term results in thirteen patients. *J Bone Joint Surg [Am]* **69**: 833–836, 1987.

113 Whitehill R, Sima EC, Young DC, Cantrell RW. Late esophageal perforation from an autogenous bone graft. *J Bone Joint Surg [Am]* **67**: 644–645, 1985.

114 Whitesides TE Jr. Lateral retropharyngeal approach to the upper cervical spine. In Sherk HH, Dunn EJ, Eismont FJ et al (eds), *The Cervical Spine*, 2nd ed, 796–80. Cervical Spine Research Society. Philadelphia: JB Lippincott4, 1989.

115 Whitesides TE Jr, McDonald AP. Lateral retropharyngeal approach to the upper cervical spine. *Orthop Clin North Am* **9**: 1115–1127, 1978.

116 Wilber RG, Frantz NA. Cervical spine infections. In Camins MB, O'Leary PF (eds), *Disorders of the Cervical Spine*. Baltimore: Williams & Wilkins, 465–471, 1992.

117 Wilde GP, Hopkins JS. The use of acrylic bone cement for cervical fusion in patients with rheumatoid arthritis. *J R Soc Med* **81**: 523–525, 1988.

118 Williams JW, Powell T. Epidural abscess of the cervical spine: Case report and literature review. *Br J Radiol* **63**: 576–578, 1990.

119 Yang EC, Neuwirth MG. *Pseudomonas aeruginosa* as a causative agent of cervical osteomyelitis: Case report and review of the literature. *Clin Orthop* **231**: 229–233, 1988.

120 Yee GKH, Terry AF. Esophageal penetration by an anterior cervical fixation device: A case report. *Spine* **18**: 522–527, 1993.

121 Zeidman SM, Ducker TB. Posterolateral local bone fusion to prevent post-laminectomy kyphosis: Review of 30 cases (abstract). Presented at the Twentieth Annual Meeting of the Cervical Spine Research Society, Palm Desert, California, December 1992.

122 Zigler JE, Bohlman HH, Robinson RA, Riley LH, Dodge LD. Pyogenic osteomyelitis of the occiput, the atlas, and the axis. *J Bone Joint Surg [Am]* **69**: 1069–1073, 1987.

17 Rheumatoid arthritis of the cervical spine: surgical decision-making

Scott D. Boden and Henry H. Bohlman

INTRODUCTION

The anatomic abnormalities in the cervical spine involved with rheumatoid arthritis are thought to be a consequence of the destruction of synovial joints, ligaments, and bone. Inflammatory synovitis can result in erosion of both bone and ligament; this then results in pain, instability, bony subluxations, and ultimately spinal cord compression. Compression of the cervical spinal cord and/or brain stem may result from either direct compression by synovial pannus or indirect compression caused by cervical subluxations. Although much is known about the natural history, pathophysiology, pharmacologic management, and surgical stabilization of patients with rheumatoid disease in the cervical spine, the clinically relevant question of when to undertake surgical intervention remains somewhat unclear.

Surgical stabilization or arthrodesis has traditionally been reserved for patients with severe progressive neurologic deficit or intractable pain.[10] The early experience with many of these patients demonstrated a high surgical morbidity as well as variable neurologic recovery once significant paralysis had occurred. To further complicate the surgical decision, although many patients have radiographic evidence of cervical spine involvement, not all go on to have progression of their cervical disease and development of paralysis. Thus, the difficult question remains how to detect patients clinically before they develop irreversible neurologic deficit and then to proceed with surgical stabilization in this select group. Although the answer to this question is still not completely known, we can shed some light on it by examining what is known about predictors of paralysis as well as predictors of the potential for neurologic recovery following surgery in patients with rheumatoid disease in their cervical spine. After such an analysis is undertaken, a rational scheme can then be devised to monitor patients safely and cost effectively, to decide when secondary neurodiagnostic imaging studies should be performed, and to offer recommendations for the timing of surgical stabilization. As the techniques of surgical stabilization are covered elsewhere, this chapter will focus primarily on a strategy for evaluation and management of these patients.

PREDICTORS OF PARALYSIS

Natural History

Analysis of what is known about the natural history of cervical disease in patients with rheumatoid arthritis shows great variation depending upon the particular series reviewed. Neck pain is reported in 40–88% cervical subluxations have been observed in 43–86%. It is significant to note that neurologic deficit is reported in only 7–34%.[17] Thus, a significant number of patients with pain and radiographic instability do not develop neurologic deficit. In addition, an alarming statistic is the estimation that some 10% of these patients may die from medullary compression unrecognized before death.[16] The most common type of cervical subluxation in rheumatoid patients is atlantoaxial subluxation, and this represents 65%. Among these patients the vast majority of the subluxation is anterior, although there are approximately 20% who may have lateral subluxations and less than 10% with posterior subluxation. Approximately 20% of rheumatoid subluxations involve basilar invagination (cranial settling) alone or in combination with atlantoaxial subluxation. Some 15% of rheumatoid arthritic patients may also have subaxial subluxation which frequently occurs at many levels.

Clinical Manifestions

Clinical manifestations of cervical rheumatoid arthritis include pain, neurologic deficit, and potentially death. Pain is typically in the neck, and frequently at the craniocervical junction. Occipital headache is not uncommon and may be accompanied by stiffness and crepitus. Neurologic symptoms are multiple and can be vague, ranging from paresthesiae in the hands to Lhermitte's phenomenon with an electric shock sensation traveling through the body. Vertebrobasilar insufficiency, especially with basilar invagination, may cause tinnitus, vertigo, loss of equilibrium, visual disturbance, diplopia, and dysphagia. Subtle changes in physical examination in patients with rheumatoid arthritis may be masked because of severe peripheral rheumatoid disease, which can result in weakness from articular involvement, tenosynovitis, and tendon rupture. Thus, the clinician must be astute in detecting subtle changes resulting from cervical neurologic compression which may be masked until it is too late.

Many studies have attempted to examine the natural history of patients with rheumatoid arthritis for progression of disease in the cervical spine.[15] In patients with neck symptoms, radiographic progression has been observed in 35–80% of patients; neurologic progression has been estimated to occur in 15–36%. In addition, in one study it has been estimated that the 5-year mortality rate for such patients may be as high as 17%. Several potential risk factors for progression of cervical disease have been identified, including male sex, severe peripheral disease, and use of corticosteroids. It is difficult to say whether the use of corticosteroids is truly an independent risk factor, or whether it merely shows a high association in patients with severe peripheral disease.

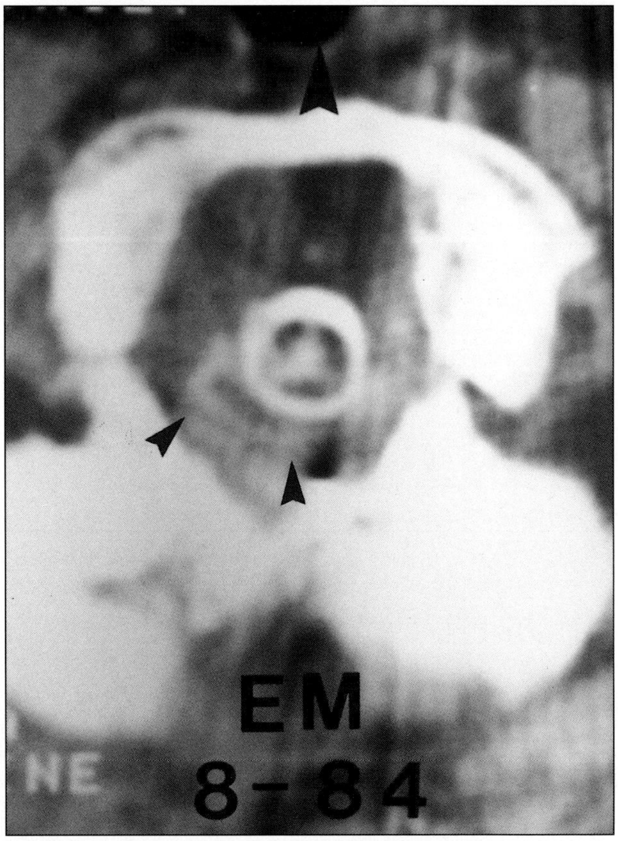

Figure 17.1
Computed tomogram–myelogram in a rheumatoid patient with anterior C1–C2 subluxation. Ventral compression of the spinal cord (arrows) by the dens is noted as well as an increased anterior atlantodental interval

RADIOGRAPHIC PREDICTORS OF PARALYSIS

Computed Tomography

Prediction of the onset of paralysis in any given patient is therefore difficult on the basis of what is known about the natural history and the relationship of clinical symptoms to neurologic progression. Many have investigated the use of diagnostic imaging studies to predict and correlate with paralysis in patients with rheumatoid disease. Computed tomography, particularly when used after a myelogram with intrathecal contrast, can be particularly useful for demonstrating spinal cord compression in patients with upper cervical rheumatoid disease (Fig. 17.1). It has been shown to have a much higher correlation with neurologic status and development of paralysis than the measurement of the traditional anterior atlantodental interval from lateral cervical radiographs.[2] In one study of 19 patients identified with a widened anterior atlantodental interval, computed tomography demonstrated spinal cord compression in 11 and the absence of any neurologic compression in 8.[20] In other studies, multiplanar computed tomography demonstrated unsuspected areas of compromise in 9 of 14 patients with rheumatoid arthritis, frequently resulting in altered surgical plans.[13]

Polytomography

Tomograms are particularly useful for the quantification of the amount of basilar invagination that is present in the cervical spine; they should be obtained if there is any suggestion of this deformity on plain radiographs.

Protrusion of the tip of the dens above the opening of the foramen magnum defines basilar invagination; another definition is protrusion >4.5 mm above McGregor's line (drawn from the top of the hard palate to the base of the occiput). Several other lines and measurements can be made to quantify the extent of settling; however, the most important point is simply to recognize any degree of basilar invagination when present and to determine if it is a fixed or a mobile deformity.

Magnetic Resonance Imaging

Magnetic resonance imaging (MRI) has afforded an increased ability to visualize spinal cord compression, frequently present in rheumatoid arthritis, not only from bone, but also from the soft-tissue pannus. Dvorak et al[9] showed that two-thirds of rheumatoid arthritic patients with atlantoaxial subluxation had a pannus >3 mm in diameter. The implication of this finding is that the space available for the spinal cord can frequently be considerably less than the bony canal diameter available on plain radiographs. It was also observed in this study that the space available for the cord was decreased with flexion. Measurements of the spinal cord diameter in neutral position and in flexion were made and correlated with clinical findings; the recommendation from this series was that surgery should be recommended if the spinal cord diameter was <6 mm in flexion.

Another investigation by Kawaida et al[14] showed that there was spinal cord compression in all rheumatoid arthritic patients when the space available for the cord was ≤13 mm. In contrast, spinal cord compression was only variably present in patients who had an anterior atlantodental interval ≥8 mm. They only observed a moderate correlation between the anterior atlantodental interval and the space available for the cord. The explanation for this phenomenon lies in the variability of the soft-tissue pannus behind the dens, as well as the variability in the width of the dens and the anterior and posterior interval in different patients. The pannus has been observed to decrease in size after solid fusion is achieved.[24] Another important finding available on MRI is the cervicomedullary angle which is normally 135–175°. Rheumatoid patients with a cervicomedullary angle of <135° showed a high correlation with the presence of clinical myelopathy and paralysis.[4]

Plain Radiography

Although MRI is the superior imaging modality for distinguishing cord compression from subluxation or synovial pannus, it is expensive and somewhat time-consuming, and therefore not practical to use on a routine basis to screen all rheumatoid arthritic patients. Thus, it is important to review plain radiographs and see what can and cannot be learned from these studies. An increasing number of studies which look at the measurements made from plain lateral cervical radiographs have shown that the anterior atlantodental interval is unreliable in the discrimination of rheumatoid arthritic patients with or without neurologic deficit. One example is a study by Collins et al[6] which showed that 61% of rheumatoid patients undergoing total joint replacement surgery had radiographic evidence of atlantoaxial instability, and yet only 50% of these patients had any signs or symptoms of their cervical disease.[6] Several studies have attempted to use the anterior atlantodental interval as a potential surgical criterion for recommending surgery in patients with rheumatoid arthritis that affects the cervical spine (Fig. 17.2). Although the normal atlantodental interval is 3 mm, a value of >5 mm at sublux-

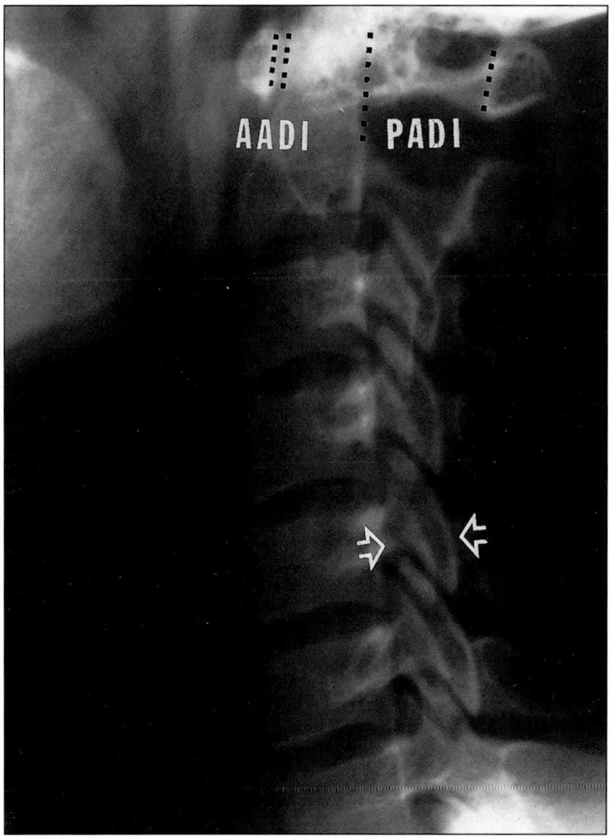

Figure 17.2
Cervical subluxations in rheumatoid arthritis may occur at the craniocervical junction, atlantoaxial joint, or in the subaxial cervical spine. Measurements made on lateral cervical radiographs may include the anterior and posterior atlantodental intervals (AADI + PADI) and the subaxial canal diameter

ation is considered to represent atlantoaxial instability.[11] Studies looking at rheumatoid patients have recommended surgery for an atlantodental interval >8 mm, >9 mm, or >10 mm, depending on the series.[5,18,21] Others have suggested that it is not the absolute amount of subluxation, but the degree of mobility, that is most important.[12] In addition, there is a general impression that neurologic progression is inevitable once any degree of cord compromise is present. However, no correlation has been found between vertebral subluxation on plain radiographs and cord compression on MRI.[3]

Traditionally, the anterior atlantodental interval as measured from lateral cervical radiographs has been used clinically to follow patients with rheumatoid arthritis affecting the cervical spine. Unfortunately, the ability of this measurement to identify patients with paralysis before its onset is somewhat unreliable. This can be more clearly documented by examining the sensitivity, specificity, accuracy, and positive and negative predictive values; the last values are calculated for the anterior atlantodental interval in the prediction of paralysis, depending on where the cut-off value for the interval is set. For example, if the critical anterior atlantodental interval is set at ≥8 mm the sensitivity, or ability to detect those with paralysis, is 59%; however, the specificity, or the ability to remain normal in the absence of clinical disease, is only 58%. Although increasing the cut-off of the anterior atlantodental interval to ≥10 mm raises the specificity of the test to 90%, it decreases the sensitivity and ability to detect those with paralysis to 35%. More importantly, the negative predictive value, which represents the percentage of patients below that interval who would not have paralysis, is only 56%.

The posterior atlantodental interval is measured from the posterior wall of the dens to the anterior aspect of the C1 lamina. This measurement was extensively evaluated and compared with the traditional anterior interval in a recent long-term series.[1] The use of the posterior atlantodental interval with a cut-off of ≤14 mm yields a sensitivity of 97%, far superior to that of the anterior interval (Table 17.1). The specificity using the posterior interval is only 52%, comparable to the anterior interval. More importantly, the negative predictive value using the posterior atlantodental interval rises to 94%. The significance of this latter phenomenon is that with a posterior atlantodental interval of ≥14 mm, there is a 94% chance that the patient will not have paralysis. In fact, the negative predictive value is probably the most important value to examine for a diagnostic test to be used as a screening tool in the indication of those patients requiring further study or even of those who can undergo surgery. The primary goal of such a screening test is first to avoid missing patients with disease or paralysis, and second to minimize the number of false positives.

For similar reasons, in patients with subaxial subluxations, the remaining posterior canal diameter is more useful than measurement of the percentage of anterior vertebral slippage. As with the anterior atlantodental interval, these measurements from plain lateral radiographs are *not* equal to the space available for the cord; this is the result of the unknown thickness of the synovial pannus not seen on plain radiographs. Thus, although a posterior atlantodental interval ≥14 mm is generally safe, a patient with a value of 13 mm could have from 12 mm to 8 or 9 mm available for the cord, depending on the thickness of pannus.[1]

Table 17.1 Reliability of anterior and posterior atlantodental intervals in predicting paralysis in patients with rheumatoid arthritis

Test		*Sensitivity (%)*	*Specificity (%)*	*Accuracy (%)*	*PPV*	*NPV*
AADI	≥ 8 mm	59	58	58	61	56
	≥ 9 mm	41	77	58	67	55
	≥ 10 mm	35	90	62	80	56
	≥ 11 mm	18	97	55	86	52
PADI	≤ 12 mm	76	90	83	90	78
	≤ 13 mm	91	71	82	78	88
	≤ 14 mm	97	52	75	69	94

These numbers were calculated from a series of 73 patients.[1]
AADI, anterior atlantodental interval; PADI, posterior atlantodental interval; PPV, positive predictive value; NPV, negative predictive value.

PREDICTORS OF NEUROLOGIC RECOVERY

Studies on predictors of the potential for neurologic recovery following surgery in rheumatoid arthritic patients are far fewer than those on the natural history of the condition. There are several factors which do not seem to be strongly correlated with recovery after surgery: age, sex, duration of paralysis before surgery, preoperative anterior atlantodental interval (in patients with atlantoaxial subluxation), and the percentage preoperative slippage of the vertebral body (in patients with subaxial subluxation).

Several factors have also shown such a correlation. The classification of Ranawat et al[19] is a rough gauge for the presence and severity of neurologic deficit (Table 17.2), which seems to have a correlation with recovery after surgery in that patients with more severe deficits tend to show less recovery and a higher morbidity. Another prognostic indication for recovery is the location of rheumatoid pathology within the cervical spine – patients with any significant degree of basilar invagination appear to have a poorer prognosis. Pseudoarthrosis after an attempted fusion also shows a correlation with poor recovery.

More recently, data are available which suggest that the *preoperative* posterior atlantodental interval (in patients with atlantoaxial subluxation) and the *postoperative* subaxial canal diameter (in patients with subaxial subluxation) may be predictors of the potential for neurologic return following surgery.[1] Those with posterior atlantodental intervals of <10 mm before surgery have a poor prognosis; in contrast, patients who have posterior intervals of ≥14 mm tend to experience significant motor recovery after appropriate surgery, and those with a residual postoperative subaxial canal diameter of <14 mm tend to show less recovery.

Table 17.2 Classification of Ranawat et al of neurologic deficit[19]

Class	*Signs*
I	Pain, no neurologic deficit
I	Subjective weakness, hyperreflexia, dysesthesiae
III	Objective weakness, long-tract signs
III A	Ambulatory
III B	Non-ambulatory

From Ranawak et al.[19]

SCHEME FOR SERIAL EVALUATION AND TIMING OF SURGICAL INTERVENTION

With an understanding of both the predictors of paralysis and the predictors of the potential for recovery following surgical stabilization, we can then begin to put together a rational scheme for the serial evaluation of patients who undergo non-operative management, as well as key check points at which surgery should be considered. The goals of management of these patients are threefold: first, to avoid the development of an irreversible neurologic deficit; second, to avoid the onset of sudden death caused by unrecognized spinal cord compression; and third, to avoid unnecessary surgery. Ideally, these three goals should be accomplished with a scheme that is cost-effective and easy to follow. The basis for such a management scheme must include three important concepts:

1. There is a common belief that earlier surgery yields a better outcome; this stems from the seemingly increased morbidity in patients with more severe neurologic deficits who undergo operation.[24]
2. Some 10% of all rheumatoid arthritic patients may experience sudden death from unrecognized cord compression, and this must be prevented.
3. As 50% of rheumatoid patients with radiographic evidence of instability (measured by the anterior atlantodental interval) remain asymptomatic,[17] it is also important that surgery is avoided in these patients.

With these concepts in mind, we can now focus on a rational scheme for serial patient evaluation and indications for surgery in patients with rheumatoid arthritis of the cervical spine.

Patients with intractable pain and/or a clear-cut neurologic deficit are generally candidates for surgical management. However, rheumatoid patients with some degree of pain or no pain and radiographic evidence of instability make up a more controversial group for surgery. Discussion will focus on this group. The most cost-effective way of screening patients for rheumatoid involvement in the cervical spine is plain radiographs followed by tomography if there is any suggestion of basilar invagination. On the basis of these two studies, patients can be separated into those with atlantoaxial subluxation, basilar invagination, subaxial subluxation, or some combination of the three.

ATLANTOAXIAL SUBLUXATION

In patients with atlantoaxial subluxation and no neurologic deficit, it is generally safe to continue just with observation of these patients, provided the posterior atlantodental interval is ≥14 mm on plain radiographs. If, however, the posterior atlantodental interval is ≤14 mm, an MRI would be advisable to evaluate the true space available for the cord, taking into account for the amount of space occupied by the synovial pannus. If MRI demonstrates a cervicomedullary angle of <135°, cord diameter in flexion of <6 mm, or space available for the cord of <13 mm, a posterior atlantoaxial fusion would be recommended.

A halo ring is applied just before surgery to maintain traction during the operation and to facilitate vest application after surgery. If traction is not required, the patient can be fitted before surgery with a posteriorly opened halo ring and the vest. A midline incision from the occiput to C4 is made. The tips of the spinous processes are exposed and subperiosteal dissection carried out along the laminae of C2 and the posterior arch of C1. All soft tissues are then carefully removed from the bony surfaces. The arch of C1 should not be exposed >1.5 cm from the midline in adults and >1 cm in children to avoid injury to the vertebral arteries. Great care must be taken not to fracture the posterior ring of C1 while dissecting the ligamentum flavum.

Fielding advocates the use of a modified Gallie H graft from the iliac crest, contouring it to fit over the posterior arches of C1 and C2.[11] A doubled, U-shaped, 18- or 20-gauge wire is passed under the arch of C1 in an inferosuperior direction. A bone block is taken from the posterior iliac crest and shaped to fit between C1 and C2, and the wires. The loop of the wire goes over the bone block and the spinous process of C2, and the ends are tightened around the graft between C1 and C2. The deep cancellous surfaces of the graft must be contoured to fit over the curved posterior surface of C1 and C2 so that the graft is in firm contact with the underlying vertebrae, immobilizing the involved segment. Additional cancellous bone chips are placed lateral to the main graft as far as possible over the laminae.

In the Brooks-type fusion, doubled, twisted, 24-gauge wires are passed under the arch of C1 and then under the lamina of C2. Rectangular, iliac crest, bone grafts are harvested and beveled to fit the interval between the arch of C1 and each lamina of the axis. The wires are then tightened, securing the graft in proper position.

Some authors suggest preoperative halo traction followed by posterior fusion reinforced with metal mesh, wire, and polymethylmethacrylate to enhance stability in the osteoporotic patients.[5,15] Adequate external immobilization should be carried out for approximately 12 weeks with a halo vest or cast.

Basilar Invagination

In patients with atlantoaxial subluxation and any significant degree of basilar invagination, but no neurologic deficit, an MRI scan in flexion is still advisable to evaluate specifically the amount of spinal cord compression that is present (Fig. 17.3). As a result of the high morbidity of surgery in patients with progressive basilar invagination, and the poor potential for recovery, evaluation and treatment should take a more aggressive approach. If there is any evidence of cord compression, cervical traction is appropriate and, if reduction is achieved, then occipitocervical fusion should be performed. If cord compression is not relieved with traction, then either a C1 laminectomy or an anterior resection of the odontoid should be performed in addition to the occipitocervical fusion.[8] Patients who have isolated and fixed basilar invagination with no symptoms and no evidence of significant cord compression may continue with just observation.

In the transoral approach, the patient is supine with the head placed in a hyperextended position. Although routine tracheotomy is advocated by many, endotracheal anesthesia may be used as well. The soft palate is turned back on itself and held in position with a stay suture. A 5-cm midline incision is then made in the posterior pharyngeal wall with its center 1 cm inferior to the palpable anterior tubercle of the atlas. The incision is carried down to bone. The posterior pharyngeal wall is then dissected subperiosteally as far lateral as the lateral masses of the atlas and axis, exposing the anterior arch of C1 and the body of C2. The anterior arch of C1 is then removed with a rongeur, exposing the odontoid process. The odontoid is removed, preferably with a high-speed drill; excision of a superiorly migrated and posteriorly angulated odontoid process may be difficult. Careful dissection is required, freeing the odontoid of all soft tissue. If lateral C1–C2 fusion is done, articular cartilage from the C1–C2 articulation is removed and filled with wedge iliac crest graft. A single layer closure is recommended by most authors to allow for drainage, and oral intake is deferred for 6–7 days.

Figure 17.3
This rheumatoid patient with cervical pain experienced progression of cervical spine involvement from (a) 1985 to (b) 1988 with atlantoaxial subluxation, basilar invagination, and subaxial subluxation at C3–C4. (c) Gadolinium-enhanced MRI demonstrates the erosion of the odontoid from posterior pannus which enhances and indents the brain stem (arrows). (d) The patient had a successful posterior fusion from the occiput to C2, and experienced spontaneous fusion at C3–C4. (Reproduced with permission from *Rheumatology*, ed. J Klippel, P Dieppe. Gower, London, 1994)

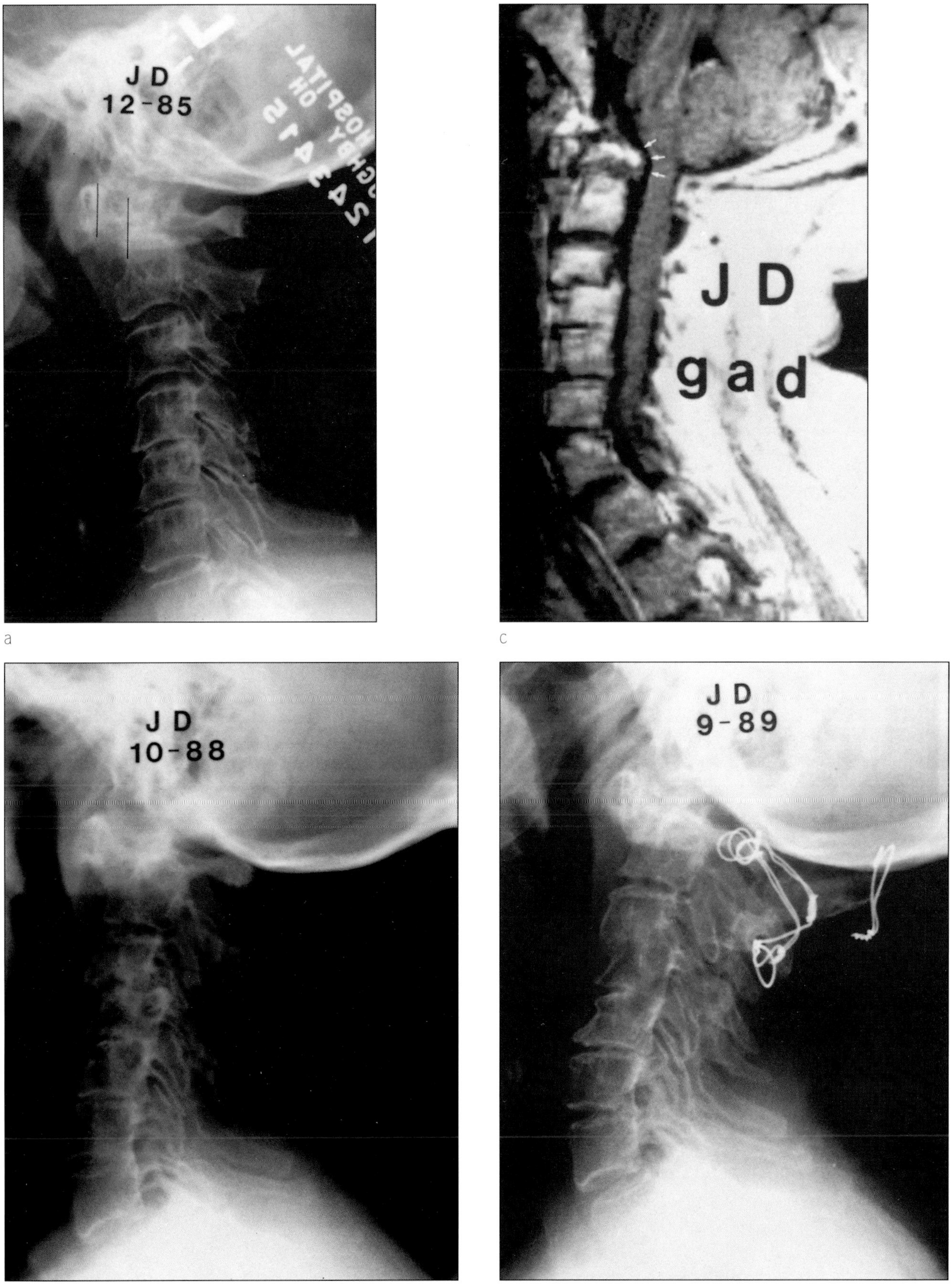

a c b d

In patients with progressive basilar invagination, occipitocervical fusion is indicated. Several techniques have been described, although the authors prefer the method described by Wertheim and Bohlman.[22] A midline posterior approach is made, with exposure from the external occipital protuberance to the fourth cervical vertebra. Sharp, subperiosteal dissection is completed exposing the occiput and the cervical laminae. The external occipital protuberance is thick and represents the ideal location for passage of wires without having to go through both tables of the skull. A high-speed diamond burr is used to create a trough on both sides of the protuberance at a level 2 cm above the foramen magnum. A towel clip is then used to create a hole in the ridge, and an 18-gauge wire passed through the hole and twisted over the ridge. A second wire loop is passed around the arch of C1 and a third is passed through and around the base of the spinous process of C2. The posterior iliac crest is then exposed and a large, thick, slightly curved graft of corticocancellous bone of appropriate width and length is obtained. The graft is divided and three drill holes placed in each graft. The occiput is decorticated and the grafts anchored in place by the wires. Additional cancellous bone is then packed between the two grafts. Finally, halo-vest immobilization is required for 12 weeks.

Subaxial Subluxation

Patients with subaxial subluxation and no neurologic deficit should be followed with plain cervical radiographs (Fig. 17.4). If the subaxial canal diameter is >14 mm in the area of interest, it is generally safe to continue observation. If, however, the posterior subaxial canal diameter is <14 mm, an MRI should be obtained to evaluate the true space available for the cord. If the space available for the cord is <13 mm or a significant degree of mobility is present at that segment, surgical arthrodesis is recommended. In most cases, a posterior cervical fusion is the procedure of choice. However, if significant deficit is present, and the subluxation is not readily reduced, an anterior decompression and fusion instead of or in addition to the posterior stabilization may be advisable.

Combined Subluxations

Patients with combinations of upper cervical and lower cervical subluxations must have these dealt with together; frequently an occipitocervical fusion will need to be carried down into the subaxial cervical spine to avoid deterioration below an upper fusion. Although some have suggested that there is accelerated progression of subaxial disease following atlantoaxial fusion, this is difficult to confirm from the data available.

Certainly some may consider a prophylactic arthrodesis to be overly aggressive when based on radiographic instability in patients who are not yet experiencing clinical symptoms or neurologic deficit. However, it is also clear that many patients present with an initial deficit so severe that it is potentially irreversible. When patients have not yet developed severe myelopathy, outcome after surgical arthrodesis is good. In addition, surgical morbidity and anesthetic complications are less common when surgery is performed earlier in the course of surgical disease. Monitoring a patient's disease progression by following the anterior atlantodental interval on plain lateral radiographs is an unreliable method at best. Plain radiographs are still useful if the posterior atlantodental interval and subaxial canal diameters are followed instead. These radiographs can and should be used as the screening tool; they can be followed up with MRI scans only when indicated, this decision being based on the criteria already outlined. With the increase in work on somatosensory and motor evoked potentials, such electrophysiologic diagnostic studies may also prove useful in predicting the potential for neurologic recovery following surgery. Once significant demyelination has occurred, it cannot be reversed.

Clinical Outcomes and Surgical Complications

The clinical success rate for cervical fusions in rheumatoid patients ranges from 60% to 90%. This variance is partly explained by variable disease severity at the time of surgery and partly by the precise definition of clinical success in a patient with a progressive systemic disease. The most common complications of cervical spine surgery in rheumatoid arthritis include death (5–10%), infection, wound dehiscence, wire breakage and loss of reduction, non-union (5–20%), and late subaxial subluxation below a fused segment.[7] Thus, anatomically involved levels should be incorporated into a fusion even if distal to the site of the primary pathology. In addition, previously asymptomatic levels can develop subluxation below rigid segments, so continued clinical monitoring is imperative. Not all non-unions are symptomatic and management must be on an individual basis.

SUMMARY

The primary goal in management of patients with rheumatoid arthritis of the cervical spine is to prevent the onset of irreversible neurologic deficit. Patients should be

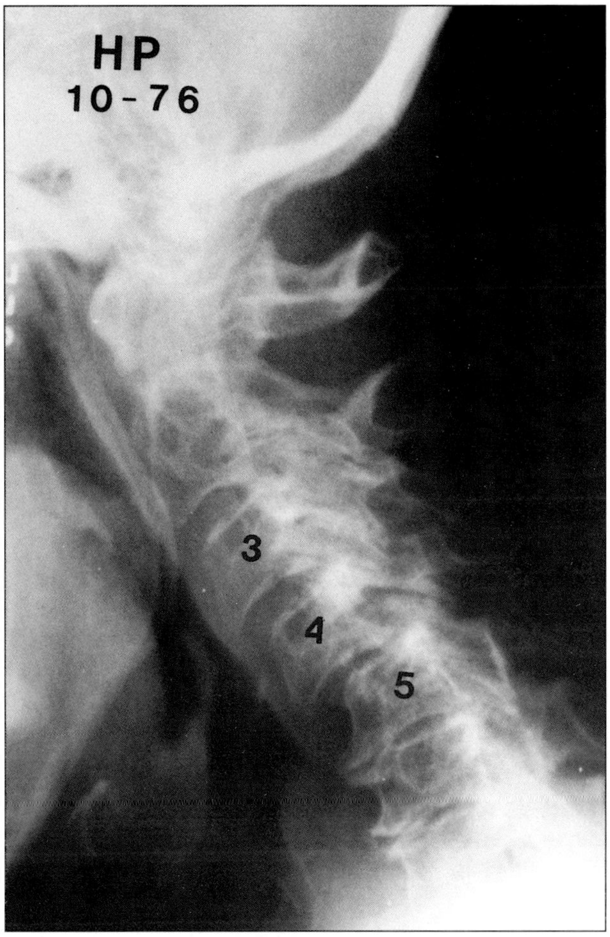

a

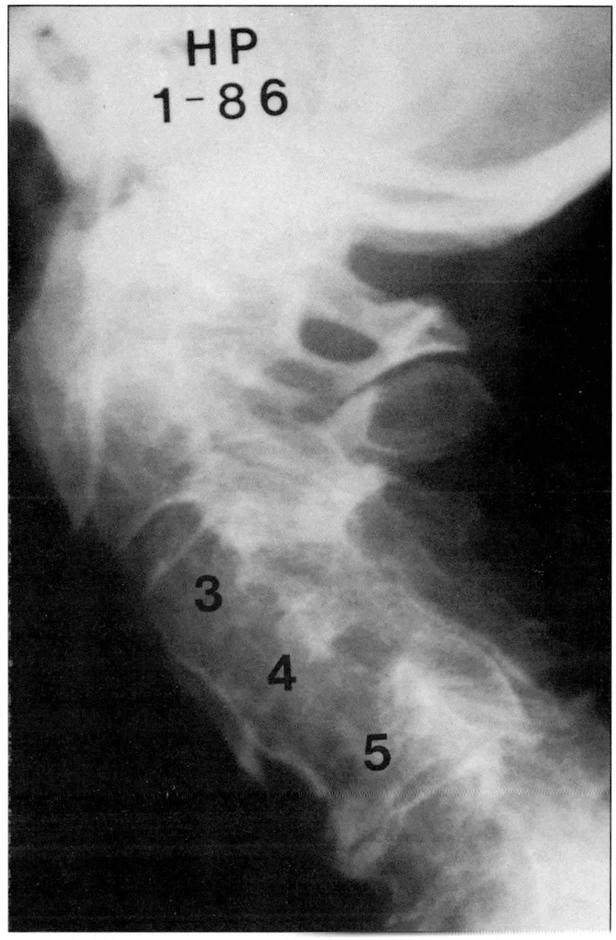

c

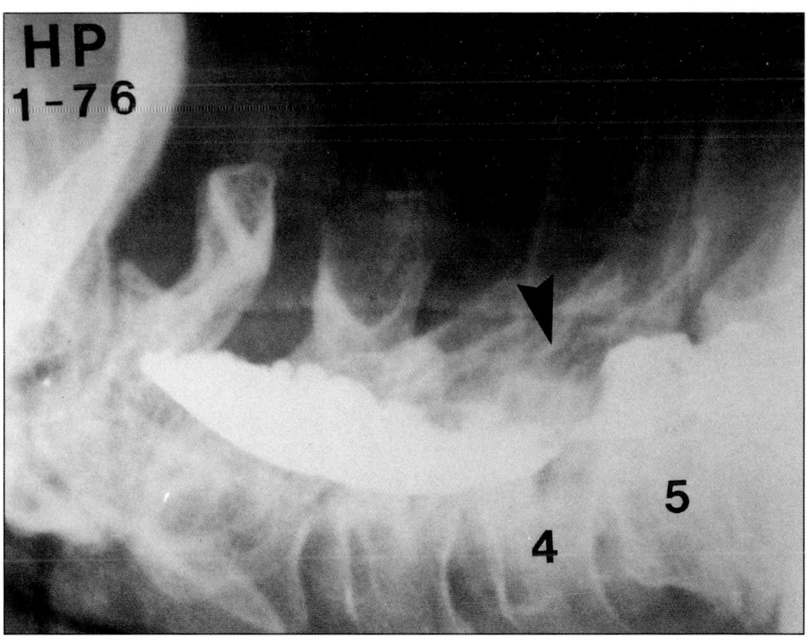

b

Figure 17.4
This 71-year-old woman with rheumatoid arthritis had neck pain and mild myelopathy for one year. (a) Plain radiographs demonstrated subaxial subluxation at C3–C4 and C4–C5. (b) The myelogram reveals anterior cord compression at C4–C5. (c) The patient underwent an anterior decompression and C3–C5 fusion and continued to have good pain relief and full motor recovery at 10-year follow-up

followed and evaluated by careful physical examination to avoid the masking of subtle changes of myelopathy by severe peripheral joint disease. Use of the posterior atlantodental interval and subaxial canal diameters measured on plain lateral cervical radiographs is a reliable screening tool to identify high-risk patients who require further evaluation with MRI or computed tomogram–myelogram. The primary technical objective of surgery is stabilization of diseased spinal segments and relief of spinal cord compression via reduction of subluxation or decompression. Complications are not uncommon, but tend to occur less frequently in patients who have surgical intervention before the onset of severe myelopathy. Pain relief is generally good when a solid arthrodesis is achieved, and neurologic recovery is most favorable when severe cord compression is not present before surgery.

REFERENCES

1 Boden SD, Dodge LD, Bohlman HH, Rechtine GR. Rheumatoid arthritis of the cervical spine: A long-term analysis with predictors of paralysis and recovery. *J Bone Joint Surg [Am]* **75**: 000–000, 1993.
2 Braunstein EM, Weissman BN, Seltzer SE, Sosman JL, Wang AM, Zamani A. Computed tomography and conventional radiographs of the craniocervical region in rheumatoid arthritis: A comparison. *Arthr Rheum* **27**: 26–31, 1984.
3 Breedveld FC, Algra PR, Vielvoye CJ, Cats A. Magnetic resonance imaging in the evaluation of patients with rheumatoid arthritis and subluxations of the cervical spine. *Arthr Rheum* **30**: 624–629, 1987.
4 Bundschuh C, Modic MT, Kearney F, Morris R, Deaf C. Rheumatoid arthritis of the cervical spine. *Am J Roentgenol* **151**: 181–187, 1988.
5 Clark CR, Goetz DD, Menezes AH. Arthrodesis of the cervical spine in rheumatoid arthritis. *J Bone Joint Surg [Am]* **71**: 381–392, 1989.
6 Collins DN, Barnes CL, FitzRandolph RL. Cervical spine instability in rheumatoid patients having total hip or knee arthroplasty. *Clin Orthop* **272**: 127–135, 1991.
7 Conaty JP, Mongan ES. Cervical fusion in rheumatoid arthritis. *J Bone Joint Surg [Am]* **63**: 1218–1227, 1981.
8 Crockard HA, Calder I, Ransford AO. One-stage transoral decompression and posterior fixation in rheumatoid atlanto-axial subluxation. *J Bone Joint Surg [Br]* **72**: 682–685, 1990.
9 Dvorak J, Grob D, Baumgartner H, Gschwend N, Grauer W, Larsson S. Functional evaluation of the spinal cord by magnetic resonance imaging in patients with rheumatoid arthritis and instability of upper cervical spine. *Spine* **14**: 1057–1064, 1989.
10 Ferlic D, Clayton ML, Leidholt JD, Gamble WE. Surgical treatment of the symptomatic unstable cervical spine in rheumatoid arthritis. *J Bone Joint Surg [Am]* **57**: 349–354, 1975.
11 Fielding JW, Hawkins RJ, Ratzan SA. Spine fusion for atlanto-axial instability. *J Bone Joint Surg [Am]* **58**: 400–407, 1976.
12 Heywood AWB, Learmonth ID, Thomas M. Cervical spine instability in rheumatoid arthritis. *J Bone Joint Surg [Br]* **70**: 702–707, 1993.
13 Kaufman RL, Glenn WV Jr. Rheumatoid cervical myelopathy: Evaluation by computerized tomography with multiplanar reconstruction. *J Rheum* **10**: 42–54, 1983.
14 Kawaida, H, Sakou T, Morizono Y, Yoshikuni N. Magnetic resonance imaging of upper cervical disorders in rheumatoid arthritis. *Spine* **14**: 1144–1148, 1989.
15 Lipson SJ. Rheumatoid arthritis in the cervical spine. *Clin Orthop* **239**: 121–127, 1989.
16 Mikulowski P, Wollheim FA, Rotmil P, Olsen I. Sudden death in rheumatoid arthritis with atlanto-axial dislocation. *Acta Med Scand* **198**: 445–451, 1975.
17 Pellicci PM, Ranawat CS, Tsairis P, Bryan WJ. A prospective study of the progression of rheumatoid arthritis of the cervical spine. *J Bone Joint Surg [Am]* **63**: 342–350, 1981.
18 Rana NA. Natural history of atlanto-axial subluxation in rheumatoid arthritis. *Spine* **14**: 1054–1056, 1989.
19 Ranawat CS, O'Leary P, Pellicci P, Tsairis P, Marchisello P, Dorr L. Cervical fusion in rheumatoid arthritis. *J Bone Joint Surg [Am]* **61**: 1003–1010, 1979.
20 Raskin RJ, Schnapf DJ, Wolf CR, Killian PJ, Lawless OJ. Computerized tomography in evaluation of atlantoaxial subluxation in rheumatoid arthritis. *J Rheum* **10**: 33–41, 1983.
21 Weissman BNW, Aliabadi P, Weinfeld MS, Thomas WH, Sosman JL. Prognostic features of atlantoaxial subluxation in rheumatoid arthritis patients. *Radiology* **144**: 745–751, 1982.
22. Wertheim, SB, Bohlman HH. Occipitocervical fusion. Indications, technique and long term results in thirteen patients. *J Bone Joint Surg [Am]* **69**: 833, 1987.
23 Zoma A, Sturrock RD, Fisher WD, Freeman PA, Hamblen DL. Surgical stabilisation of the rheumatoid cervical spine: A review of indications and results. *J Bone Joint Surg [Am]* **69**: 8–12, 1987.
24 Zygmunt S, Saveland H, Brattstrom H, Ljunggren B, Larsson EM, Wollheim F. Reduction of rheumatoid periodontoid pannus following posterior occipito-cervical fusion visualized by magnetic resonance imaging. *Br J Neurosurg* **2**: 315–320, 1988.

18 Cervical kyphosis

Thomas A. Zdeblick

The normal cervical spine has a gentle sloping, lordotic curve from C1 to C7. Loss of lordosis or straightening of the cervical spine is often seen after acute injury secondary to paraspinal muscle spasm.[9] However, reversal of the lordotic curve into a cervical kyphosis is much less common and can be due to degenerative, inflammatory, traumatic, or neoplastic conditions in the child and adult. Regardless of the cause, cervical kyphosis poses significant treatment problems. The cervical spinal cord is normally tethered in its position within the cervical spine by both the laterally directed nerve roots and the dentate ligaments.[3] With reversal of the normal lordotic curvature, the cervical spinal cord becomes draped over the posterior elements of the vertebral bodies,[21,52] potentially increasing the tension within the spinal cord itself.[10] This increased tension may lead to direct neuronal damage but, more importantly, can lead to ischemia. Increased tension within the cord stretches the longitudinally directed vessels, narrowing their lumen and diminishing the blood flow.[10]

In addition, because of the weight of the head and the relatively poor mechanical advantage of the posterior cervical paraspinal muscles, cervical kyphosis tends to be progressive.[40,42,50] In particular, when kyphosis is associated with myelopathy, surgical treatment is often indicated as a result of the poor natural history of these combined findings.[5,6,21,49,52]

Childhood cervical kyphosis may occur in association with scoliosis. This is most common with congenital deformities including the Klippel–Feil syndrome, congenital block or wedge vertebrae, and sharply angulated upper thoracic curves.[22,45] Childhood cervical kyphosis may also occur secondary to spinal cord tumor and/or laminectomy performed for tumor resection.[1,4,14,27,28,34,6,48,51] In the adult, cervical kyphosis may occur as a result of ankylosing spondylitis, where development of a fixed kyphosis may lead to significant functional disability. Kyphosis may also occur following cervical trauma, either due to collapse of the vertebral body with compression or burst fracture, or due to unrecognized posterior ligamentous injury.[7,8,21,33,46] Degenerative cervical kyphosis may result from sequential vertebral subluxation and disc space collapse as seen in spondylosis, rheumatoid arthritis, or as a result of posterior laminectomy and partial facetectomy.[11,14,15,25,26,28,31,32,34,41,42] Each of these etiologic factors will be discussed and treatment options offered.

CHILDHOOD DEFORMITY

Cervical kyphosis associated with idiopathic scoliosis is extremely rare. High thoracic curves may generate a compensatory curve in the lower cervical spine; however, this portion of the curve rarely requires treatment. Congenital scoliosis may involve the cervical spine. Congenital cervical–thoracic scoliosis is unusual, but has the potential to be severely disfiguring. These curves often include sharp, angular deformities which may also be associated with significant torticollis, shoulder decompensation, scapular elevation, and late instability.[22,37] These are best treated with an in situ posterior arthrodesis. Correction and/or instrumentation are often unnecessary. Postoperative immobilization using a CTLSO or halo cast is recommended. Posterior spinal instrumentation for the correction of cervical scoliosis is not recommended. Sublaminar hooks placed in the cervical spine are often ill-fitting and may lead to neurologic injury. Should extension of a thoracic instrumentation be required into the cervical spine, posterior spinous process wiring using Wisconsin buttons is a safer alternative.

Although post-laminectomy kyphosis may occur in any age group, it is most frequently found in children and young adults.[42,50,51] Cattell and Clark described cervical kyphosis occurring soon after multiple laminectomies were

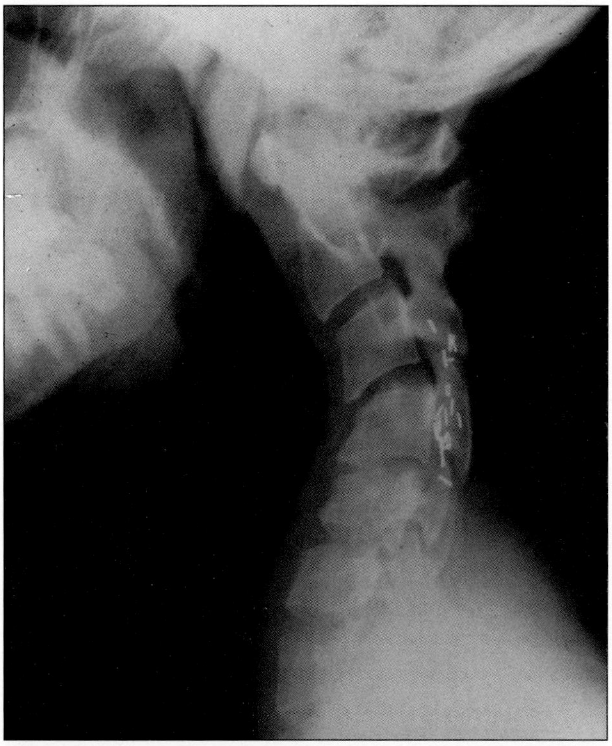

a

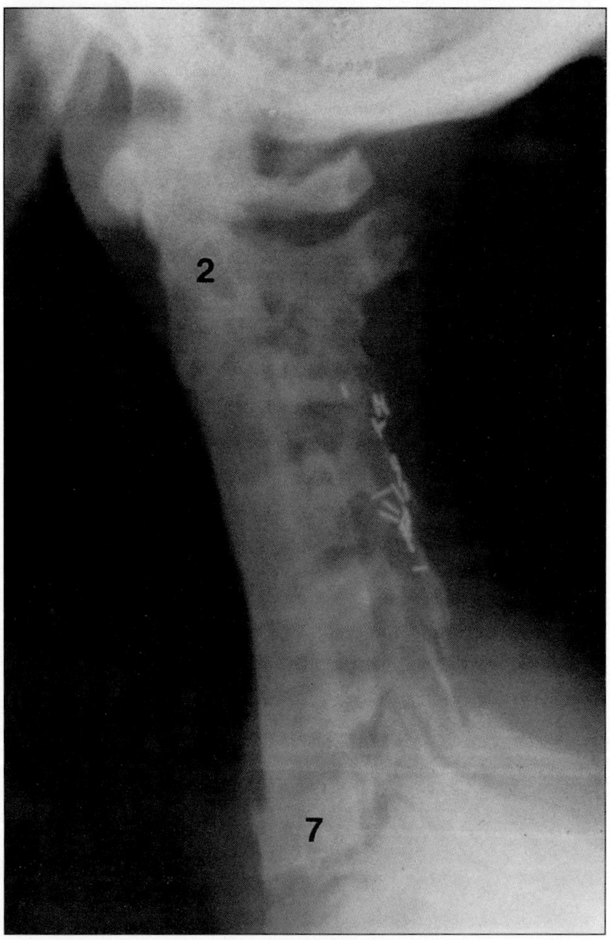

b

performed for tumor excision.[14] This report brought the potential problem to the attention of the present author, but did not delineate its incidence, treatment, or prevention. Tachdjian and Matson[48] studied 24 patients who underwent cervical laminectomy for spinal cord tumor excision. No patient in this series developed post-laminectomy kyphosis.[48] However, Bell and co-workers[4] reviewed 89 multi-level cervical laminectomies in children for a variety of problems.[4] These patients were followed for an average of 5.5 years with 53% developing a significant deformity. The kyphotic deformity in this group varied from 5° to 120° with the peak incidence occurring at the age of 10 years.

Children are at greater risk of kyphotic deformity following laminectomy because of several factors. First, the vertebral body is more subject to biologic plasticity than the adult vertebra. Secondly, children have greater ligamentous laxity, which when compromised by laminectomy, posterior ligamentous resection, and possibly partial facet capsule resection, may lead to subluxation. Finally, there is less development of the cervical paraspinal musculature and a greater weight of the head in relationship to the body, which may lead to an increasing cervical kyphosis.[31,32,34,40,50]

The immature patient undergoing cervical laminectomy is at risk of postoperative cervical instability (Fig. 18.1). Should facet resection be required at the time of tumor excision, then stabilization should be performed at the same operative setting.[11,36] Facet wiring, posterior cervical plating, or simply in situ onlay bone grafting with subsequent halo immobilization represent treatment alternatives. In the author's view lateral mass plating is the procedure

Figure 18.1

(a) This young man had progressive quadriparesis and pain in the neck due to an arteriovenous malformation at the third cervical level. This was treated with laminectomy from the third to the sixth cervical vertebrae, myelotomy, excision of the tumor, and drainage of a syrinx. After the operation, the patient remained quadriparetic (grade 3 motor strength). Four years later, a progressive kyphosis developed, as did quadriplegia. The kyphosis measured 43°. (b) A multi-level decompression was performed through an anterior approach. To do this, subtotal corpectomies were carried out from the third to the sixth cervical vertebra level. Traction was applied to reduce the kyphosis, and a fibular strut graft was inserted to provide stability. After 34 months, there was a solid fusion with minimal residual kyphosis. Motor strength had returned to grade 3. (Reproduced with permission of the authors) of choice should sufficient facet remain for purchase of a screw.[17] If there is insufficient bone stock posteriorly after decompression, then a multi-level anterior fusion via strut grafting would be preferable.[2,21,49] Cervical laminectomy performed in children without facet resection can safely be observed. These patients should be seen at regular intervals and sequential radiographs taken. Should a kyphotic deformity develop, surgical fusion is then recommended. This is most easily performed via an anterior approach, particularly in young children, and the best procedure is by creation of an anterior trough spanning multiple disc spaces, reduction of the deformity, and insertion of an autogenous fibular strut graft.[21,49]

Severe cervical kyphosis with progressive neurologic involvement may occur when posterior laminectomy is combined with radiation for tumor (Fig. 18.2). This can lead to development of a sharp, angular kyphosis due to growth arrest and possibly necrosis of the vertebral body secondary to radiation, and loss of posterior tensile supporting structures secondary to laminectomy.[48] Once the deformity is recognized, these patients should be treated with preoperative traction for reduction followed by multiple anterior releases and strut grafting. If kyphosis develops secondary to radiation-induced vertebral body collapse without laminectomy, the posterior elements remain intact, producing a fixed deformity. With such a deformity, the initial operative intervention could potentially include multiple posterior cervical osteotomies, followed by anterior releases, traction, reduction, and possibly anterior strut fusion.

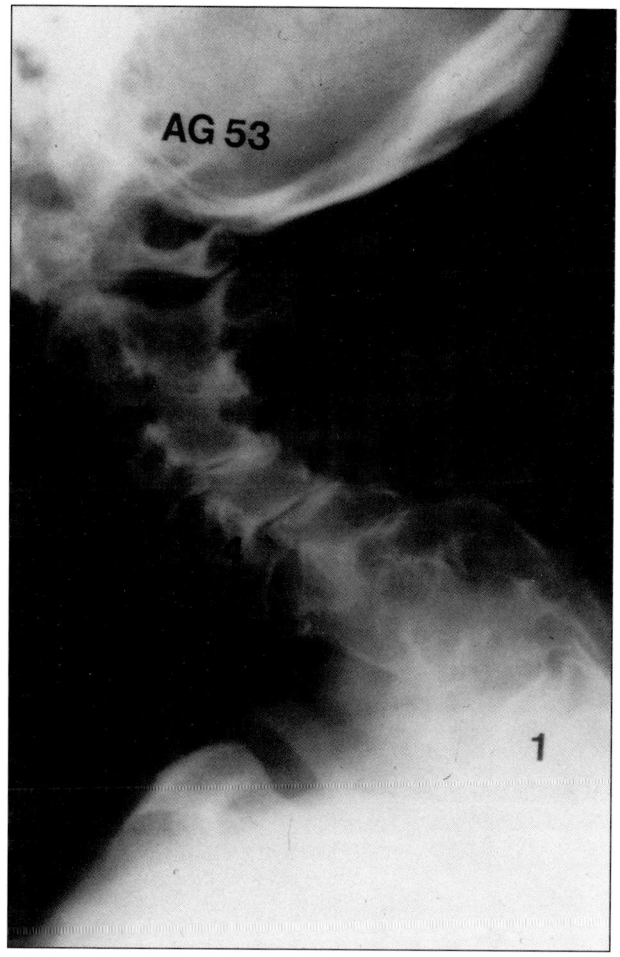

a

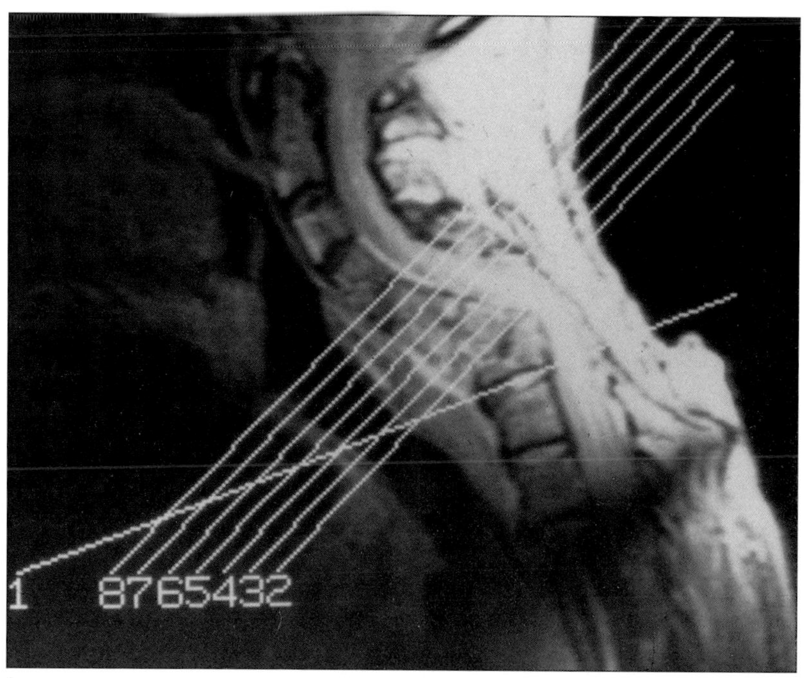

b

Figure 18.2
Cervical spine metastatic tumors causing unremitting pain and/or neurologic deficit are best treated with anterior excision, stabilization, and adjunctive radiotherapy. Laminectomy is rarely indicated for vertebral body lesions with angular deformity. If treated with laminectomy, severe angular kyphosis may result

Finally, post-infectious kyphosis may be seen in the cervical spines of children. Tuberculosis remains an etiologic agent in many countries, with tuberculous abscess formation with kyphosis leading to cord compression and neurologic symptoms in approximately 40% of cases. Recommended treatment includes multi-drug chemotherapy, anterior excision of the diseased bone, and anterior strut grafting.

For reduction of severe cervical-thoracic kyphoscoliosis, anterior releases may be required. Micheli and Hood[30] have described a combined anterior exposure of the cervical–thoracic spine, including an anterolateral cervical incision and a transpleural transthoracic incision. This allowed exposure from C3 to T9, with mobilization of the great vessels and anterior releases being performed. This then allowed for a subsequent safe posterior reduction and stabilization.

ANKYLOSING SPONDYLITIS

Kyphosis of the spine may be an unfortunate and debilitating consequence of ankylosing spondylitis. Kyphosis most commonly occurs in the thoracolumbar spine and the mid-thoracic spine, although cervical kyphosis may also occur, and can be the result of several factors. There is an element of primary muscle disease in ankylosing spondylitis which weakens the posterior paraspinal muscle support.[20,43] Facet inflammation may become painful and patients may tend to stand in a more flexed posture. Once ankylosis occurs, the weight of the head and upper body and gravity may tend to pull the patient further into kyphosis. With time, a severe 'chin-on-chest' type of deformity may result from a combination of thoracic and cervical kyphosis. Fixed deformity in this position leads to severe disability, with inability to see the horizon, and difficulties with swallowing, chewing, and speech.

In ankylosing spondylitis deformities of this nature are best treated by prevention. Once the diagnosis of ankylosing spondylitis is made, a physical therapy program should be instituted to maintain the erect posture. Such a program, combined with occasional use of a lightweight brace and anti-inflammatory medication, may be successful in preventing kyphosis. However, once deformity occurs and is fixed, treatment becomes much more difficult. For deformities of the thoracolumbar spine, multi-level osteotomies using posterior spinal segmental fixation represent the procedure of choice. For deformity in the mid-thoracic spine, anterior release followed by posterior osteotomy and instrumentation may correct the deformity. In the cervical spine, Simmons has popularized a C7-based extension osteotomy of the cervical spine. The details of this procedure are discussed in Chapter 9.

Cervical kyphosis may also occur in patients with ankylosing spondylitis after trauma. Fractures in an ankylosed spine can be extremely difficult to diagnose,[7,8] and any significant fall or motor vehicle accident must be evaluated carefully in patients with ankylosed spines. Should a fracture be detected, treatment is directed towards placing the spine in its pre-morbid position and allowing healing. This may be done either with external immobilization (i.e. halo cast) or with internal fixation. Unrecognized injury may accelerate the process of kyphosis.

'Chin-on-chest' deformity may also result without ankylosis. Patients with thoracic kyphosis from a number of causes may eventually develop a dynamic hyperflexion deformity of the cervical spine, primarily due to muscle weakness of the posterior paraspinal musculature.[20,43] In these patients, who can be passively corrected to the neutral position, an in situ fusion in the neutral position is indicated, performed through multi-level spinous process wiring and onlay grafts, or with contoured posterior lateral mass plates. It may be necessary in some cases to extend fixation into the thoracic spine for which custom-made implants may be required.

Post-laminectomy Kyphosis

Decompression of the cervical spinal cord and cervical nerve roots can be accomplished through an anterior or posterior approach. Posteriorly, laminectomy is required for decompression of the cord, and foraminotomy for decompression of the nerve roots.[18,19] A portion of the cervical facet (zygo-apophyseal) joint must be resected to expose and decompress the nerve root. A laminectomy and a foraminotomy effectively decompress the cord and roots, but may render the spine unstable, leading to progressive kyphosis and worsening of the patient's neurologic status.

The incidence of post-laminectomy kyphosis is not known. Certainly, in the child or skeletally immature adult, kyphosis is much more prevalent after laminectomy. In the adult, Mikawa et al[31] noted a 14% incidence of kyphosis after cervical laminectomy in the treatment of spondylosis. They found that the degree of facet resection correlates with the eventual development of this spinal deformity.

Several biomechanical studies have been performed in an attempt to shed light on this phenomenon.[23,24,34,35,37,38,47,53] Biomechanical research on the spine is most useful when it can provide clinically relevant information. Spinal instability can be defined as excessive segmental motion under physiological loading conditions.[53] Goel et al[24] tested intact cervical spines before and after laminectomy at the C5 and C6 cervical levels.[24] They found that flexion–extension motion increased by 10% after laminectomy alone. They did not

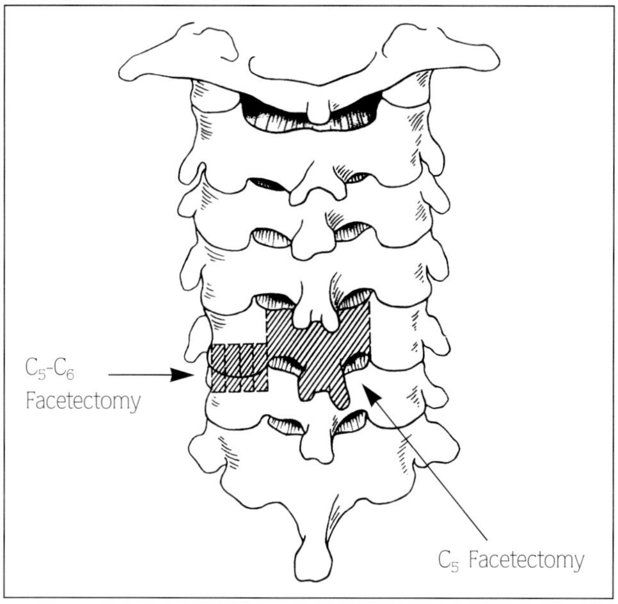

a

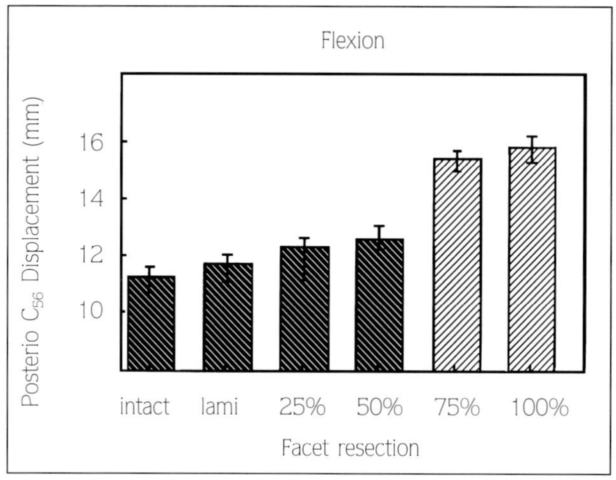

b

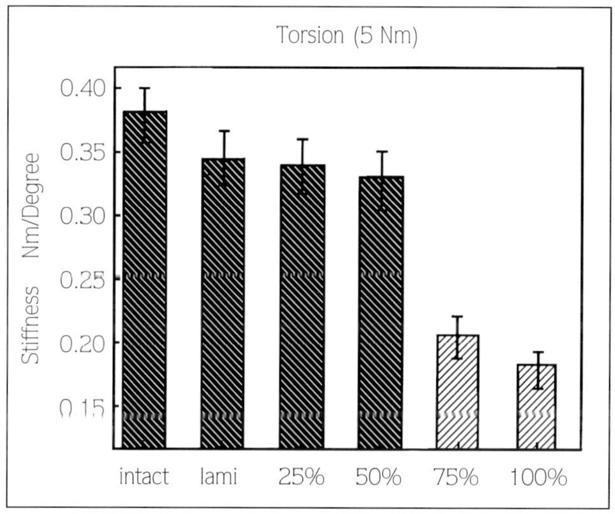

c

Figure 18.3
Biomechanically, instability is defined as segmental hypermobility under physiologic loading. The cervical spines of human cadavers were tested to determine what amount of facet resection would lead to instability. Progressive, staged facetectomy was performed. In (b) flexion or (c) torsion of 5 Nm, hypermobility resulted if more than 50% of the facet was resected

feel that this was unstable. Facet wiring effectively restored spinal stiffness to four times that of the intact spine.

Raynor et al[37,38] have investigated the effect of facet joint resection on spinal stability. They tested single vertebral motion segments in shear loading, with all specimens tested to failure. Failure occurred with fracture of the facet in all four specimens treated with 70% facetectomy. In five specimens treated with only 50% facet joint resection, failure occurred at the interface of the specimen and the potting jig. The authors concluded that resection of more than 50% of the facet resulted in instability.

Cusick et al[16] have also tested a single vertebral motion segment of the cervical spine. They performed a complete facetectomy and then tested the spines in flexion and compression loading. Unilateral facetectomy diminished the strength of the spine by 31% and bilateral facetectomy by 53%. They concluded that complete facetectomy will lead to spinal instability. Zdeblick et al[53] tested the cervical spines of 12 human cadavers after sequential laminectomy and facetectomy at the C5–C6 level (Fig. 18.3). Loads of axial compression, flexion and extension moments, and torsion were used in the tests and each test was repeated after laminectomy and facetectomy of 25%, 50%, 75%, and 100%. They found that, in flexion, the flexion displacement increased significantly with facetectomy of 75% or 100%. Similarly, in torsion, torsional stiffness decreased significantly with facetectomy of 75% or 100%. They concluded that laminectomy and facet resection up to 50% did not lead to acute hypermobility of the cervical spine. However, segmental hypermobility occurred if foraminotomy involved resection of more than 50% of the facet. Based on these findings, spine stabilization is recommended if more than 50% facetectomy is required for decompression.

Numerous factors come into play in the attempt to determine whether, in fact, a post-laminectomy kyphosis may develop. Mikawa et al[31] followed 64 adult patients who had undergone multi-level cervical laminectomy, including those with cervical spondylosis, ossification of the posterior longitudinal ligament (OPLL), and spinal cord tumors. Thirty-six percent of their patients showed postoperative changes in spinal stability, including 14% who developed kyphosis. They found that cervical mobility was reduced in general after laminectomy. Although kyphosis developed in 14% of patients, no patient required further operation for instability or severe deformity. They concluded that cervical laminectomy had little effect on long-term stability of the spine.

Saito et al[40] performed a finite element analysis to simulate post-laminectomy cervical spine deformities. Their simulation revealed the primary cause for development of post-laminectomy kyphosis to be the resection of the spinous processes and posterior ligaments, including ligamentum flavum, supraspinous, and intraspinous ligaments. They felt that, with the removal of these structures, the tensile stresses that were preoperatively distributed through the posterior ligaments were then transferred to the facets in the post-laminectomy state. This led to an imbalance of stresses, which, when combined with the gravitational pull to the head, would determine whether deformity would develop. They felt that kyphosis was more common in children because of the relatively larger size of the head and its more anteriorly located center of gravity.

Post-laminectomy cervical kyphosis, when it occurs, can be quite difficult to treat. The treatment of post-laminectomy kyphosis is guided to some degree by neurologic involvement. If cervical myelopathy is present in addition to the kyphotic deformity, posterior management alone may not be sufficient. Draping of the spinal cord over the kyphotic segment may lead to anterior spinal cord impingement and long tract dysfunction. When any evidence of myelopathy exists, treatment needs to be directed to both correction of the deformity and anterior decompression of the spinal cord. Anterior discectomy alone is often not sufficient to remove the midline osteophytes that are present. Multiple level corpectomy is often required for cord decompression. Kyphosis correction can then be obtained through manipulation and traction, followed by anterior strut grafting.[52]

Fielding and Tolli[21] felt that the best surgical treatment for cervical kyphosis was via the anterior approach. They felt that preoperative correction in halo or traction was important, followed by multi-level anterior corpectomies and strut grafting. For one- or two-level corpectomies, an autogenous iliac crest strut is used, whereas autogenous fibular strut graft is used for three or more levels. These grafts are wedged into place by carefully undercutting the vertebral end-plates at either end of the decompression, applying traction, and keying the graft into these end-plate depressions. Fielding recommended postoperative halo immobilization.

Newer anterior fixation techniques may obviate the need for postoperative halo. The use of the anterior cervical plate does provide adequate anterior stabilization, as well as fixation into the strut graft.[12,13] Two different plating techniques are currently used. The non-locking plate (Caspar plate from Aesculap, Inc.) enforces the need to penetrate the posterior cortex of the vertebral body for adequate purchase. The titanium locking plate (Synthes, Inc.) does not require penetration of the posterior cortex. This plate has a screw inset which expands the head of the screw, thus holding it more rigidly to the plate. Both these techniques are demanding, and require meticulous attention to detail in order to obtain adequate anterior fixation.

It is the experience of the present author that the reduction of the kyphosis achieved through use of traction and anterior corpectomy is sufficient. True osteotomies of the cervical spine for post-laminectomy deformity are rarely indicated. When performing reduction, care must be taken to use intraoperative radiography or fluoroscopy to document the amount of reduction. Use of intraoperative spinal cord monitoring is strongly encouraged.

Whitecloud and LaRocca have confirmed these results in their series of 26 anterior arthrodeses using fibular strut grafts.[49] They reported a high rate of success, although three grafts extruded in the postoperative period. The use of a halo vest and/or an anterior cervical plate may prevent these postoperative graft dislocations.

Post-laminectomy kyphosis may be difficult to treat by use of an isolated posterior approach. With no evidence of spinal cord pathology, the deformity may be reducible through preoperative and intraoperative traction and manipulation; an in situ fusion may then be performed. Simple onlay grafting of the remaining facet joints, followed by postoperative halo immobilization, is the least complicated procedure which can successfully lead to posterior fusion. However, due to the lack of immediate stability, Callahan et al[11] introduced a form of segmental fixation for these procedures. They used stainless steel wires placed through each of the remaining facets and wired to onlay rib strut grafts. For this procedure to succeed, a sufficient portion of the facet joint must remain for wire placement and purchase. Furthermore, the stability of the construct can be limited by the quality of the patient's cervical bone and rib graft which can be poor, especially in the elderly patient.

The introduction of lateral mass screw and plate constructs has significantly increased the ability of the spinal surgeon to obtain stability following cervical laminectomy.[17] If a patient's deformity is passively correctable with preoperative manipulation and/or traction, then positioning in the operating room followed by in-situ plating and fusion is indicated. If adequate correction cannot be obtained with traction alone, anterior releases may first be required. The present author prefers to perform these cases on a turning frame, such as a Stryker frame, where first a standard anterior approach is performed with releases through the appropriate disc spaces.[39] Care must be taken to take these releases back to the posterior longitudinal ligament, so that cancellous bone graft can then be placed within the disc spaces. The patient is turned on the turning frame and the posterior cervical approach performed. Gentle manipulation may be required for correction, together with spinal cord monitoring. In situ plating with contoured lateral mass plates will then maintain the correction that is achieved. Care should be taken to maintain the patient's neck in traction throughout the operative process.

POST-TRAUMATIC DEFORMITY

Cervical kyphosis can also result following trauma, and may be due to unrecognized tearing of the infraspinous and supraspinous posterior ligament complexes, unrecognized facet subluxation, or progressive collapse due to vertebral body fracture (Fig. 18.4).[7,8,46] Additionally, kyphotic deformities which develop after injury to the cervical spine and spinal cord may result from a laminectomy performed for decompressive purposes. Morgan et al[33] found that 68% of patients who had been treated with laminectomy for a cervical injury required a secondary arthrodesis. Laminectomy is rarely required for traumatic burst fractures, compression fractures, or disc herniations. Cervical laminectomy may be required for laminar or facet fractures with impaction.

Kyphotic deformities which develop after cervical trauma are most commonly due to disruption of the posterior ligaments. Stauffer and Kelly[46] described the development of kyphosis and collapse in patients who underwent an anterior Cloward arthrodesis for treatment of traumatic

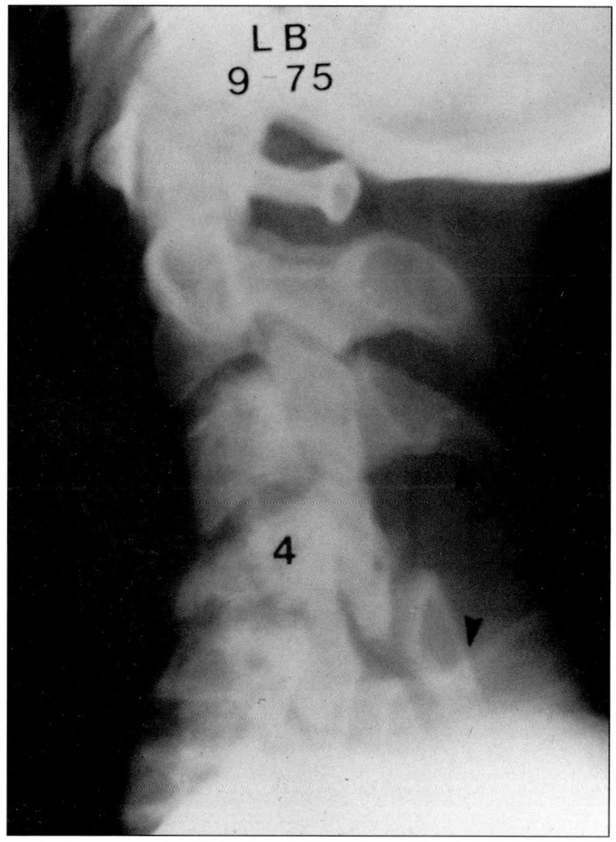

a

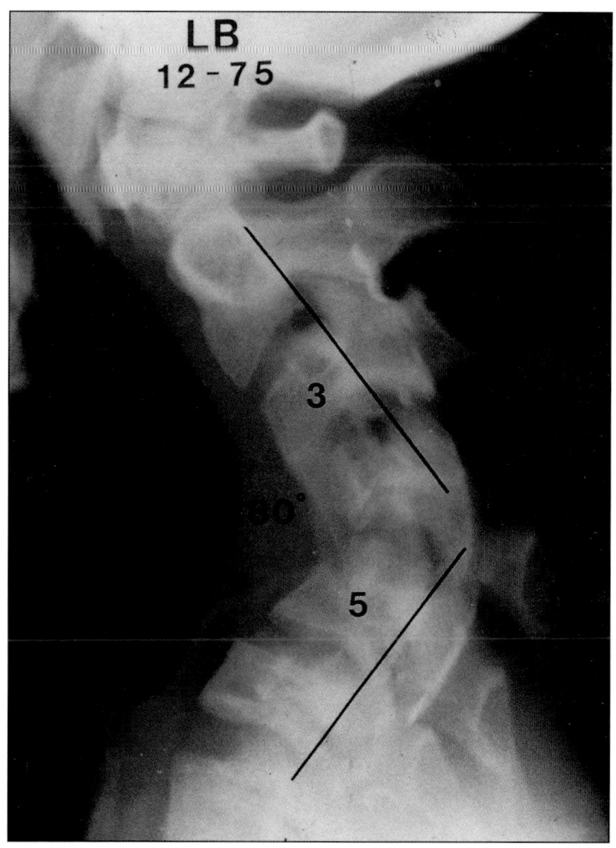

b

Figure 18.4
Axial load injuries with flexion may cause a burst fracture as well as posterior ligamentous injury. Spreading of the spinous processes indicates posterior instability, and treatment should include either anterior and posterior fusion or instrumentation to obtain rigidity. This patient had an unrecognized posterior instability which was allowed to heal with significant kyphosis

injury.[46] In all 16 of these patients they found widening of one or more of the interspinous spaces on preoperative lateral radiographs. Once disrupted, the posterior ligamentous complex does not heal and posterior arthrodesis is required to prevent angular deformity. If posterior ligamentous tearing is recognized before the operation, then ensuing deformity can often be prevented. If a burst fracture is associated with posterior ligamentous disruption, surgical treatment often includes corpectomy for decompression followed by anterior strut grafting. The postoperative employment of a halo vest may prevent late kyphotic deformity. However, because of the marked instability of this injury, it is preferable to supplement the strut graft with an anterior cervical plate in the reduced position, or perform a simultaneous circumferential arthrodesis by completing a posterior fusion at the same sitting. McAfee and Bohlman[29] reported 24 patients who they had treated with simultaneous anterior and posterior stabilization. They felt that this approach was well tolerated by the patient and led to excellent results. Certainly, the key to the prevention of cervical kyphosis after trauma is preoperative recognition of the type and extent of injury.

Once cervical kyphosis develops after an unrecognized posterior ligamentous injury, reduction and stabilization become more difficult. If the anterior fusion has healed in the kyphotic position, anterior release through the fusion mass followed by manipulation and posterior plating is the procedure of choice. Prior to fusion healing, manipulation and placement in a halo may correct the kyphotic deformity.

Degenerative Causes

Kyphosis associated with cervical spondylosis is the result of progressive subluxation of the intervertebral joints secondary to degeneration of the discs and facet joints. In a patient with cervical spondylosis and kyphosis, laminectomy will not improve the neurologic situation. For laminectomy to improve spinal cord function, there must be a neutral or lordotic position of the cervical spine.[3] This then allows migration of the spinal cord posteriorly away from the offending osteophytes. With a kyphotic segment of the spine, laminectomy performed for stenosis and/or radiculopathy may worsen the deformity. Patients with a kyphotic segment and symptoms of radiculopathy may often be treated with anterior cervical discectomies and fusion at the appropriate levels.[39] However, if myelopathy is present, a single or multi-level corpectomy is generally required for full decompression of the spinal canal. Zdeblick and Bohlman[52] reported on 14 patients with combined myelopathy and kyphosis treated with corpectomy and strut grafting. Eight of these patients were primarily cervical spondylosis cases. The results in these patients were excellent with resolution of preoperative myelopathy and radicular symptoms, obtaining solid fusion of the strut graft by 4 months. It is important when performing multiple discectomies or multiple corpectomies to treat all levels involved in the kyphotic segment. Leaving an unfused degenerated segment within the kyphosis will lead to further instability and late progression of symptoms. Careful review of radiographic studies, whether it be myelography, computed tomography, or magnetic resonance imaging, is required to assess all the levels contributing to neural compression. When performing multiple anterior corpectomies for kyphosis, the posterior osteophytes must be removed if myelopathy is present. If deformity is the primary reason for surgery, a thin shell of posterior cortex may be left intact before manipulation and strut grafting.

Surgical technique

A technique for anterior multi-level corpectomy and strut graft fusion is shown in Fig. 18.5. First, spinal cord monitoring leads are applied to the scalp, neck, and extremities. After induction of general anesthesia, 6.75 kg (15 lb) of skeletal traction is applied through a halo ring or skull tongs. The patient is then carefully positioned in the supine position on a Mayfield horseshoe headrest. An intraoperative lateral radiograph is taken before the surgical preparations to document the position of the cervical spine. An anterior Smith–Robinson approach[44] can then be carried out through a horizontal right- or left-sided skin incision depending on the surgeon's preference. A three- or four-level corpectomy can be performed through a horizontal incision, although most feel that an oblique incision, paralleling the medial border of the sternocleidomastoid, is preferable. When using a horizontal incision, it must be placed at the midpoint of the decompression and must be long enough to allow mobilization of tissues, both superiorly and inferiorly. Under these circumstances, a vertical skin incision is not necessary. After the longus colli muscle is identified and elevated over the entire length of the decompression, anterior discectomies are performed at the appropriate levels. It is important to visualize the uncovertebral joints on the right and left sides during the completion of the discectomies. This allows orientation to the midline during the corpectomy phase. The central two-thirds of the frontal plane of each vertebral body is then removed using rongeurs and a power burr, creating a trough that extends the full length of the kyphosis. As the posterior aspect of each vertebral body is approached, the high-speed burr is used to thin the posterior cortex. Once it is appropriately thinned, small angled curettes are introduced to free the osteophytes. An angled 3.0 curette is

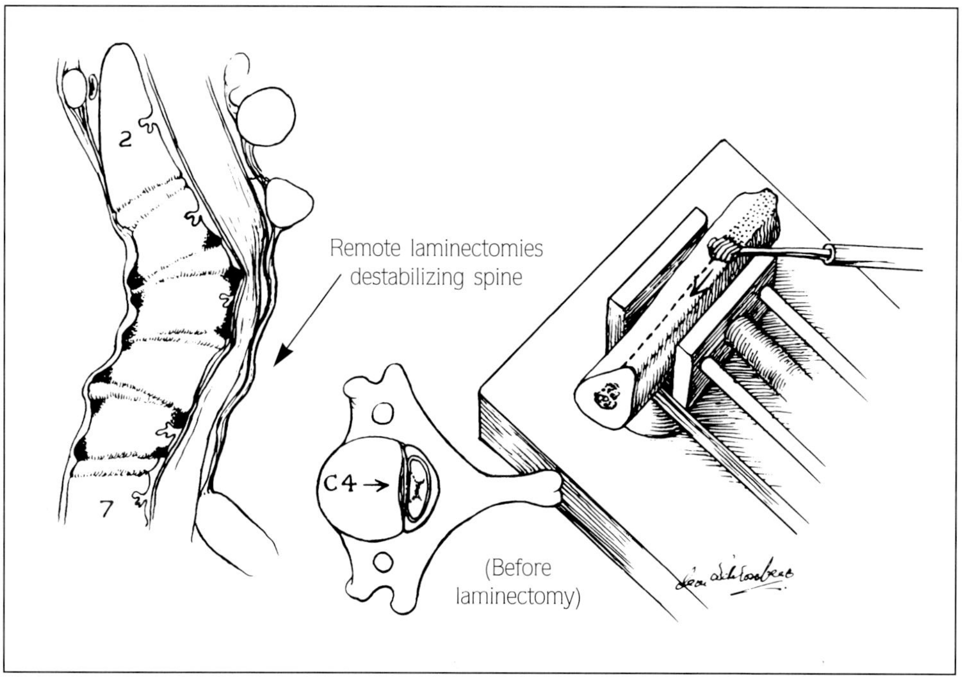

a

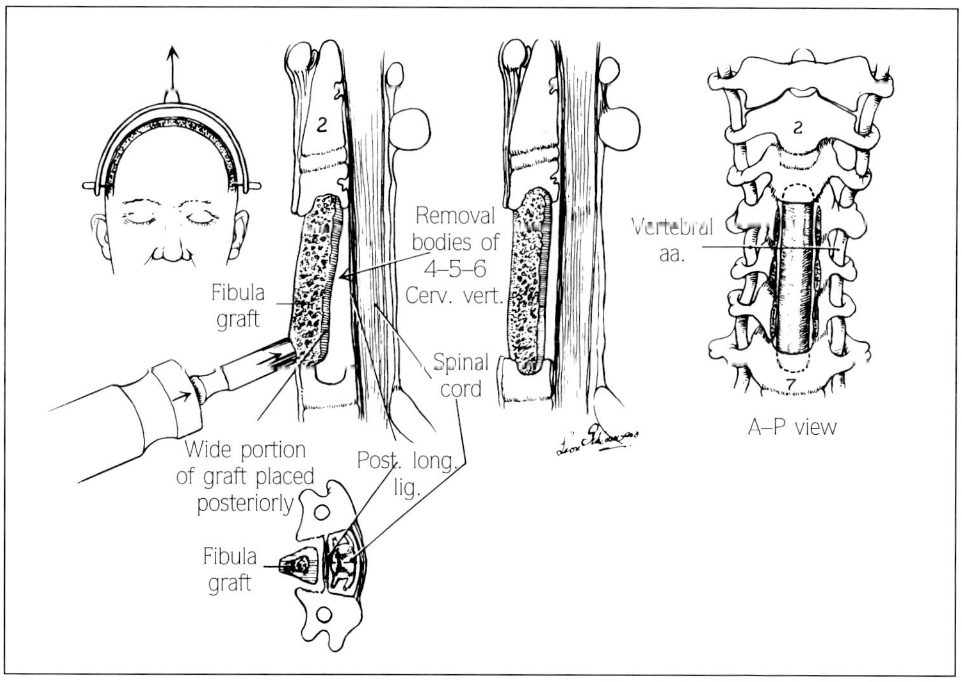

b

Figure 18.5
(a) Drawing showing marked compression of the spinal cord from posterior osteophytes, despite a laminectomy. After the fibular strut is harvested, it is shaped using a burr. A small vise facilitates preparation of the bone graft. (b) The steps of the procedure that are performed after anterior corpectomy and decompression. Skeletal traction is increased to reduce the kyphosis. Extension of the neck may also be needed. Seating holes are made in the end-plates of the superior and inferior intact vertebral bodies with a burr. The ends of the graft are then rounded, and the graft is impacted into place. When traction is released, the graft is locked into place. (Reproduced with permission of the *Journal of Bone and Joint Surgery*)

especially useful in peeling this thin shell of posterior cortical bone away from the posterior longitudinal ligament. These fragments are pulled anteriorly and removed, completing the decompression. Magnifying loupes and a headlamp are required for adequate visualization, although some surgeons prefer an operating microscope. If the posterior longitudinal ligament is calcified or absent, the dura will be exposed. However, should the soft posterior longitudinal ligament remain, it is left intact. Once the decompression has been completed, seating holes are burred into the middle of the vertebral end-plates at either end of the trough. The skeletal traction is increased to 13.5 or 18 kg (30 or 40 lb) by the anesthesiologist. This traction aids in the reduction of the kyphosis and facilitates graft placement. If adequate correction is not obtained during this maneuver, the surgeon breaks scrub and gently extends the neck over a rolled sheet. Radiographs are then taken to document the reduction. Thereafter, no effort is made to obtain further reduction.

The length of the graft to be inserted is determined by measuring from the superior to the inferior seating hole using a malleable probe or calliper. The type of graft is determined on the basis of the segments to be resected. An iliac crest graft is used for a one- or two-level corpectomy, whereas an autogenous fibular strut graft is used for a longer arthrodesis. The ends of the graft are contoured with the burr so that they will fit snugly into the previously made seating holes. The graft is held with a vise during preparation.

Finally, the graft is impacted into position and the traction is reduced to 2.25 kg (5 lb), thereby locking the graft securely in place. Additional radiographs are taken to confirm the reduction and the correct position of the graft.

If anterior and posterior simultaneous arthrodesis is to be performed, the patient is then turned on the turning frame. After radiographic confirmation, the posterior arthrodesis is carried out in situ. The author's group prefers to maintain postoperative traction for 24–48 hours in the intensive care unit. If the respiratory status is stable at that time, the team then proceeds with the placement of a cervical orthosis and/or halo vest. The external support is worn for 8–12 weeks or until the graft appears on radiograph to be incorporated.

In summary, there are multiple causes for cervical kyphosis. The most effective treatment for all causes is prevention. Careful observation and evaluation for potential instability developing in children treated with laminectomies are required. Recognition of posterior ligamentous injuries in traumatic injuries will help prevent the late kyphotic instabilities. Cervical spondylosis, if kyphosis is present, is best treated via the anterior approach. Cervical laminectomy alone should not lead to late instability. Should facetectomy be required for nerve root decompression, it should be limited to less than 50% of the facet. Should kyphosis occur despite these precautions, the appropriate surgical management should be pursued as outlined in this chapter.

REFERENCES

1 Aronson DD, Kahn RJ, Canady A. Cervical spine instability following suboccipital decompression and cervical laminectomy for Arnold–Chiari syndrome (abstract). Presented at the Fifty-Sixth Annual Meeting of the American Academy of Orthopedic Surgeons, Las Vegas, Nevada, February 1989.

2 Bailey RW, Badgley CE. Stabilization of the cervical spine by anterior fusion. *J Bone Joint Surg [Am]* **42**: 565–594, 1960.

3 Batzdorf U, Batzdorf A. Analysis of cervical spine curvature in patients with cervical spondylosis. *Neurosurgery* **22**: 827–836, 1988.

4 Bell DF, Walker J., O'Connor G. Spinal deformity following multiple level cervical laminectomy in children (abstract). Presented at the Fifty-sixth Annual Meeting of the American Academy of Orthopedic Surgeons, Las Vegas, Nevada, February 1989.

5 Bernard TN, Whitecloud TS. Cervical spondylotic myelopathy and myeloradiculopathy: Anterior decompression and stabilization with autogenous fibula strut graft. *Clin Orthop* **221**: 149–160, 1987.

6 Bohlmann HH. Cervical spondylosis with moderate to severe myelopathy. A report of seventeen cases treated by Robinson anterior cervical discectomy and fusion. *Spine* **2**: 151–162, 1977.

7 Bohlman HH. Complications of treatment of fractures and dislocations of the cervical spine. In Epps CN Jr (ed) *Complications in Orthopaedic Surgery*, 611–641. Philadelphia: JB Lippincott 1978.

8 Bohlmann HH. Surgical management of cervical spine fractures and dislocations. The American Academy of Orthopedic Surgeons, *Instructional Course Lectures*, St Louis, CV Mosby, **34**: 163–187, 1985.

9 Braakman M, Braakman R. Hyperflexion sprain of the cervical spine. Follow-up of forty-five cases. *Acta Orthop Scand* **58**: 388–393, 1987.

10 Breig A. Adverse mechanical tension in the central nervous system. An analysis of cause and effect. In *Relief by Functional Neurosurgery*. New York: John Wiley 1978.

11 Callahan RA, Johnson RM, Margolis RN, Keggi KJ, Albright JA, Southwick WO. Cervical facet fusion for control of instability after laminectomy. *J Bone Joint Surg [Am]* **59**: 991–1002, 1977.

12 Capen DA, Garland DE, Waters RL. Surgical stabilization of the cervical spine. A comparative analysis of anterior and posterior spine fusions. *Clin Orthop* **196**: 229–237, 1985.

13 Caspar W. Anterior stabilization with the trapezoidal osteosynthetic plate technique in cervical spine injuries. In Kehr P, Weidner A (eds) *Cervical Spine I*, 198–204. Wien, New York: Springer-Verlag, 1987.

14 Cattell HS, Clark GL. Cervical kyphosis and instability after multiple laminectomies in children. *J Bone Joint Surg [Am]* **49**: 713–720, 1967.

15 Crandall PH, Gregorius FK. Long-term follow-up of surgical treatment of cervical spondylotic myelopathy. *Spine* **2**: 139–146, 1977.

16 Cusick JF, Yoganandan N, Pintar F, Myklebust J, Hussain H. Biomechanics of cervical spine facetectomy and fixation techniques. *Spine* **13**: 808–812, 1988.

17 Ebraheim NA, An HS, Jackson WT, Brown JA. Internal fixation of the unstable cervical spine using posterior Roy–Camille plate: Preliminary report. *J Orthop Trauma* **3**: 23–28, 1989.

18 Epstein JA. The surgical management of cervical spinal stenosis, spondylosis, and myeloradiculopathy by means of the posterior approach. *Spine* **13**: 864–869, 1988.

19 Fager CA. Results of adequate posterior decompression in the relief of spondylotic cervical myelopathy. *J Neurosurg* **38**: 684–692, 1973.

20 Fielding JW quoted in Simmons EH, Bradley DD. Neuro-myopathic flexion deformities of the cervical spine. *Spine* **13**: 760, 1988.

21 Fielding JW, Tolli TC. Surgical management of postlaminectomy kyphosis. *Semin Spine Surg* **1**: 271–275, 1989.

22 Francis WR Jr, Noble DP. Treatment of cervical kyphosis in children. *Spine* **13**: 883–887, 1988.

23 Gill K, Paschal S, Corin J, Ashman R, Bucholz RW. Posterior plating of the cervical spine: A biomechanical comparison of different posterior fusion techniques. *Spine* **13**: 813–816, 1988.

24 Goel VK, Clark CR, Harris KG, Kim YE, Schulte KR. Evaluation of effectiveness of a facet wiring technique: An in-vitro biomechanical investigation. *Ann Biomed Eng* **17**: 115–126, 1989.

25 Jenkins DHR. Extensive cervical laminectomy: Long-term results. *Br J Surg* **60**: 852–854, 1973.

26 Kamioka Y, Yamamoto H, Tani T, Ishida K, Sawamoto T. Posterior instability of cervical CPLL and cervical radiculomyelopathy. *Spine* **14**: 1177–1183, 1989.

27 Katsumi Y, Honma T, Nakamura T. Analysis of cervical instability resulting from laminectomies for removal of spinal cord tumor. *Spine* **14**: 1172–1176, 1989.

28 Lonstein JE. Post-laminectomy kyphosis. *Clin Orthop* **128**: 93–100, 1977.

29 McAfee PC, Bohlman HH. One-stage anterior cervical decompression and posterior stabilization with circumferential arthrodesis. A study of twenty-four patients who had a traumatic or neoplastic lesion. *J Bone Joint Surg [Am]* **71**: 78–88, 1989.

30 Micheli LJ, Hood RW. Anterior exposure of the cervicothoracic spine using a combined cervical and thoracic approach. *J Bone Joint Surg [Am]* **65**: 992–997, 1983.

31 Mikawa Y, Shikata J, Yamamuro T. Spinal deformity and instability after multilevel cervical laminectomy. *Spine* **12**: 6–11, 1987.

32 Miyazaki K, Tada K, Matsuda Y, Okuno M, Yasuda T, Murakami H. Posterior extensive simultaneous multisegment decompression with posterolateral fusion for cervical instability and kyphotic and/or S-shaped deformities. *Spine* **14**: 1160–1170, 1989.

33 Morgan TH, Wharton GW, Austin GN. The results of laminectomy in patients with incomplete spinal cord injuries. *J Bone Joint Surg [Am]* **52**: 822, 1970.

34 Munechika Y. Influence of laminectomy on the stability of the spine: An experimental study with special reference to the extent of laminectomy and the resection of the intervertebral joint. *Nippon Seikeigeka Gakkai Zasshi* **47**: 111–125, 1973.

35 Nolan JP Jr, Sherk HH. Biomechanical evaluation of the extensor musculature of the cervical spine. *Spine* **13**: 9–11, 1988.

36 Raimondi AJ, Gutierrez FA, DiRocco C. Laminotomy and total reconstruction of the posterior spinal arch for spinal canal surgery in childhood. *J Neurosurg* **45**: 555–560, 1976.

37 Raynor RB, Moskovich R, Zidel P, Pugh J. Alterations in primary and coupled neck motions after facetectomy. *Neurosurgery* **21**: 681–687, 1987.

38 Raynor RB, Pugh J, Shapiro I. Cervical facetectomy and its effect on spine strength. *J Neurosurg* **63**: 278–282, 1985.

39 Robinson RA, Southwick WO. Surgical approaches to the cervical spine. The American Academy of Orthopedic Surgeons, *Instructional Course Lectures*, St Louis, CV Mosby, **17**: 299–330, 1961.

40 Saito T, Yamamuro T, Shikata J, Oka M, Tsutsumi S. Analysis and prevention of spinal column deformity following cervical laminectomy. I. Pathogenetic analysis of postlaminectomy deformities. *Spine* **16**: 494–502, 1991.

41 Scoville WB. Cervical spondylosis treated by bilateral facetectomy and laminectomy. *J Neurosurg* **18**: 423–428, 1961.

42 Sim FH, Svien HJ, Bickel WH, Janes JM. Swan-neck deformity following extensive cervical laminectomy. A review of twenty-one cases. *J Bone Joint Surg [Am]* **59**: 564–580, 1974.

43 Simmons EH, Bradley DD. Neuro-myopathic flexion deformities of the cervical spine. *Spine* **13**: 756–762, 1988.

44 Smith GW, Robinson RA. The treatment of certain cervical spine disorders by anterior removal of intervertebral disc and interbody fusion. *J Bone Joint Surg [Am]* **40**: 607–624, 1958.

45 Smith MD. Fusion for congenital cervicothoracic scoliosis: An analysis of twenty patients with long-term follow-up. Presented at the Scoliosis Research Society Annual Meeting, Minneapolis, Minnesota, 1991.

46 Stauffer ES, Kelly EG. Fracture dislocations of the cervical spine. Instability and recurrent deformity following treatment by interbody fusion. *J Bone Joint Surg [Am]* **59**: 45–48, 1977.

47 Sutterlin CE III, McAfee PC, Warden KE, Rey RM Jr, Farey ID. A biomechanical evaluation of cervical spinal stabilization methods in a bovine model: Static and cyclical loading. *Spine* **13**: 795–802, 1988.

48 Tachdjian MO, Matson DD. Orthopedic aspects of intra-spinal tumors in children. *J Bone Joint Surg [Am]* **47**: 223–248, 1965.

49 Whitecloud TS III, LaRocca H. Fibular strut graft in reconstructive surgery of the cervical spine. *Spine* **1**: 33–43, 1976.

50 Yasouka S, Peterson HA, Laws ER, MacCarty CS. Pathogenesis and prophylaxis of postlaminectomy deformity of the spine after multiple level laminectomy: Difference between children and adults. *Neurosurgery* **9**: 145–152, 1981.

51 Yasouka S, Peterson HA, MacCarty CS. Incidence of spinal column deformity after multilevel laminectomy in children and adults. *J Neurosurg* **57**: 441–445, 1982.

52 Zdeblick TA, Bohlman HH. Cervical kyphosis and myelopathy. Treatment by anterior corpectomy and strut-grafting. *J Bone Joint Surg [Am]* **71**: 170–182, 1989.

53 Zdeblick TA, Zou D, Warden KE, McCabe R, Kunz D, Vanderby R. Cervical stability after foraminotomy: A biomechanical in-vitro analysis. *J Bone Joint Surg [Am]* **74**: 22–27, 1992.

19 Spinal instrumentation of the cervical spine

Howard S. An and
J. Michael Simpson

There are numerous techniques available for stabilization of the cervical spine. Wiring techniques are still commonly used for posterior stabilization, but other forms of posterior stabilization have been recently reported. Spinal implants can also be used anteriorly, although indications for their use are more limited. There are advantages and disadvantages of each method, and the surgeon must choose an appropriate method based on the mechanism of injury, the pathoanatomy of the lesion, and familiarity with the various techniques. Various posterior wiring methods and more rigid stabilization techniques of anterior and posterior cervical fixation are discussed and the indications, techniques, and potential complications of these techniques presented.

POSTERIOR CERVICAL SPINE

Upper Cervical Spine

The indications for posterior atlantoaxial stabilization include traumatic atlantoaxial instability with rupture of the transverse ligament-type II odontoid fractures with high risk of non-union, as in older patients with a significant displacement, and late atlantoaxial instability caused by Jefferson's fracture of the C1 ring or odontoid non-union. Atlantoaxial instabilities may also be caused by non-traumatic disorders such as rheumatoid arthritis,[40] congenital anomalies, and metabolic problems. Anterior atlantoaxial subluxation is assessed radiographically by measuring the atlantodental interval from the midposterior margin of the anterior ring of C1 to the anterior surface of the dens. An atlantodental interval >3 mm in the adult or >4 mm in the child on flexion–extension views is accepted as being unstable or potentially unstable. In non-traumatic disorders, an atlantoaxial interval >3 mm is not necessarily an indication for surgery. For example, in rheumatoid arthritis, indications for surgery include significant progressive neurological deterioration, intractable pain, or severe instability (>9 mm). Many patients with an atlantoaxial interval >3 mm as a result of non-traumatic disorders do well because the disease process may be protracted and non-progressive.

Posterior atlantoaxial arthrodesis may be performed using either the Gallie or the Brooks technique.[11,27,31] The former technique is safer because the spinous process of C2 is used in place of a sublaminar wire, although the latter provides additional rotational stability when compared to the Gallie technique. The author recommends the Gallie technique for most flexion injuries, but the Brooks technique is preferred for all extension injuries, and in cases where more rigid fixation is required. Autogenous iliac crest graft material is preferable, but allograft material can be supplemented if the pelvic bone is insufficient or osteoporotic. The fusion should extend to the occiput when the arch of C1 is deficient or when the patient exhibits superior migration of the odontoid, as in rheumatoid arthritis. The author recommends halo-vest external support in the postoperative period for a period of approximately 3–4 months.

Posterior Atlantoaxial Arthrodesis

A halo ring is applied just before surgery to maintain traction during surgery and to facilitate vest application after surgery. Preoperative halo traction may be helpful in cases where significant deformity is present. If traction is not required, the patient can be fitted with a posterior opened halo ring and vest before surgery. A midline incision from the occiput to the third cervical vertebra is made. The tips of the spinous processes are exposed and

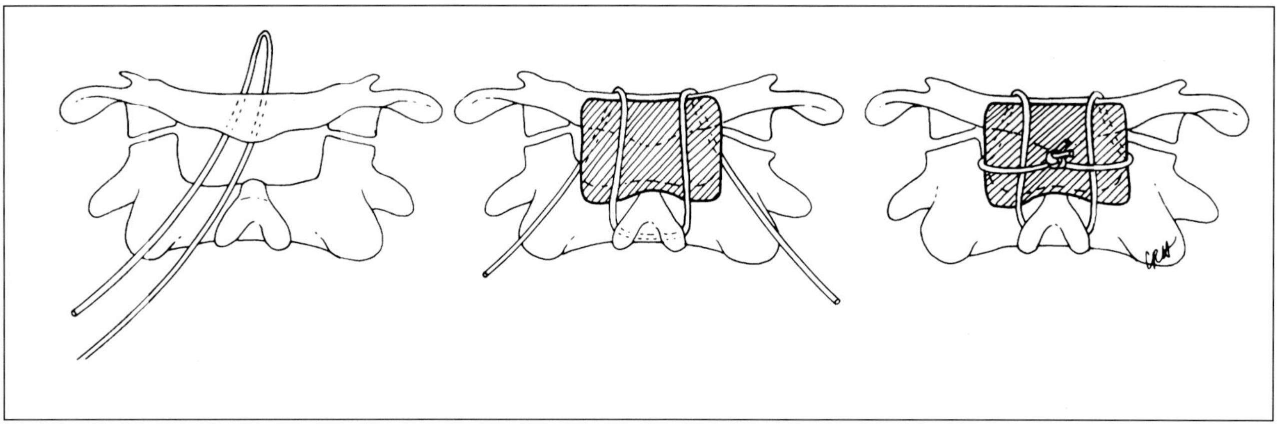

Figure 19.1
A modified Gallie H graft from the iliac crest over the posterior arches of C1 and C2. Left: a doubled, U-shaped, 18- or 20-gauge wire is passed under the arch of C1 from inferior to superior. Middle: a bone block is taken from the posterior iliac crest and shaped to fit between C1 and C2, and the wires. Right: the loop of the wire goes over the bone block and the spinous process of C2, and the ends of the wire are tightened around the graft between C1 and C2

subperiosteal dissection carried out along the lamina of C2 and the posterior arch of C1. All soft tissues are carefully removed from the bony surfaces. The arch of C1 should not be exposed >1.5 cm from the midline in adults and >1 cm in children to avoid injury to the vertebral arteries. Great care must be taken not to fracture the posterior ring of C1 while dissecting the ligamentum flavum. Muscular insertions on the spinous process of C2 should be preserved as much as possible to prevent instability at C2–C3.

There are several modified Gallie types of wiring. The author prefers a technique by Simmons,[65] who uses a modified Gallie H graft from the iliac crest, contouring it to fit over the posterior arches of C1 and C2. A doubled, U-shaped 18- or 20-gauge wire is passed under the arch of C1 in a caudal-to-cranial direction. A bone block is taken from the posterior iliac crest and shaped to fit between C1 and C2 (Fig. 19.1). The loop of the wire goes over the bone block and the spinous process of C2, with the ends of the wire tightened around the graft between C1 and C2. The deep cancellous surfaces of the graft must be contoured to fit over the curved posterior surface of C1 and C2 so that the graft is in firm contact with the underlying vertebrae, immobilizing the involved segment. Additional cancellous bone chips are placed in defects to promote fusion.

In the Brooks-type fusion, doubled, twisted, 24-gauge wires are passed under the arch of C1, and then under the lamina of C2 (Fig. 19.2). Rectangular iliac crest bone grafts (1.25 × 3.5 cm) are harvested, and beveled to fit in the interval between the arch of C1 and each lamina of the axis. The wires are then tightened, securing the graft in proper position.

There have been other reports on C1–C2 fixation techniques. Aprin and Harf[5] recommend internal fixation of C1–C2 by passing two 18-gauge, stainless steel wires beneath the posterior arch of the atlas and around a threaded Steinman pin, which is drilled through the base of the spinous process of the axis.[5] They reported excellent results in eight patients treated with this technique. Meyer's technique is a variation of the Brooks technique, in that sublaminar wires are placed under C1 and C2, followed by fixing the bone grafts with the wires that threaded through holes in the grafts instead of wiring over the grafts[48] (Fig. 19.3). Fielding et al[26] have also described other Gallie technique modifications for atlantoaxial stabilization. The triple-wire technique is another good method of stabilizing the upper cervical spine.[79]

Although wiring and bone graft fixation methods give satisfactory stabilization in most cases, other forms of internal C1–C2 fixation have been reported in the literature in recent years. One method of posterior atlantoaxial arthrodesis uses an interlaminar clamp.[20,36,49,69] These clamps may be used in selected cases where sublaminar wires would be difficult or dangerous to pass (Fig. 19.4). Potential problems with interlaminar clamp fixation are implant slippage, difficulty with bone grafting, and pseudoarthrosis. Another method of atlantoaxial stabilization is Magerl's

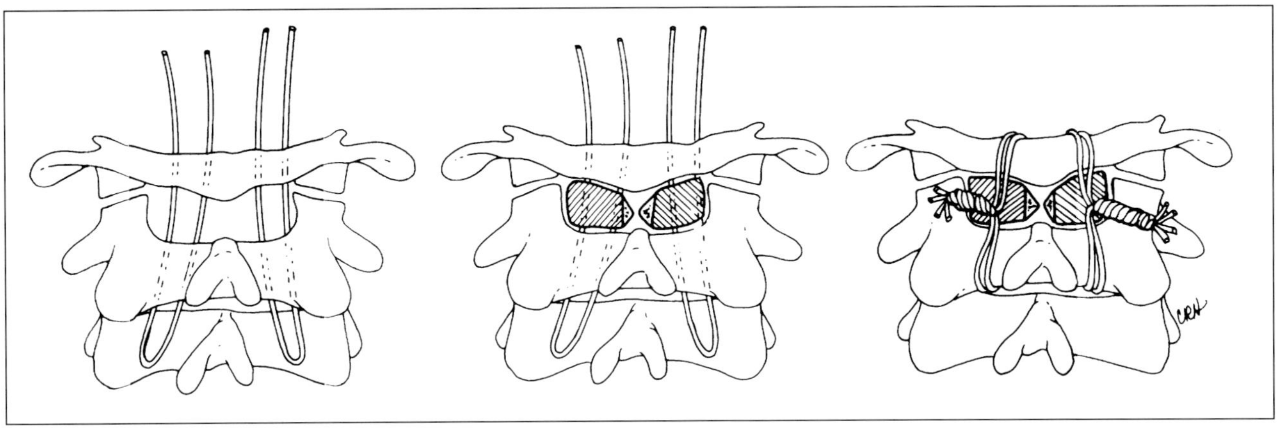

a

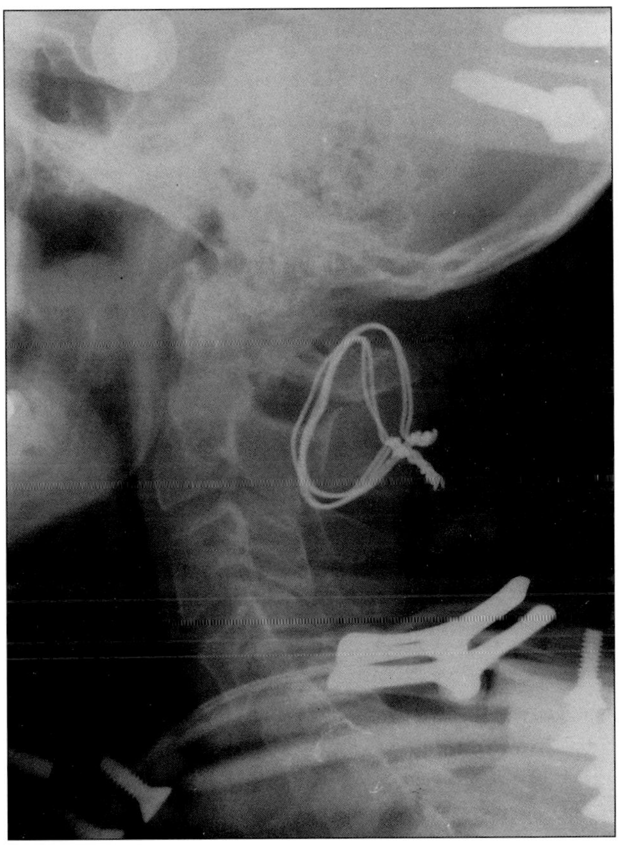

b

Figure 19.2

(a) The Brooks-type fusion. Left: doubled twisted 24-gauge wires are passed under the arch of C1 and then under the lamina of C2. Middle: rectangular iliac crest bone grafts (1.25 cm × 3.5 cm) are harvested and beveled to fit in the interval between the arch of C1 and each lamina of the axis. Right: the wires are then tightened securing the graft. (b) Lateral radiograph of a patient who underwent a Brooks wiring and fusion

transarticular screw fixation.[45,70] This procedure provides rigid fixation, but requires thorough knowledge of surgical anatomy and meticulous technique. A midline approach is used to expose the region from the occiput to C3. Subperiosteal dissection is completed over the lateral and cranial aspect of C2 to expose the C1–C2 facet joints bilaterally. Magerl recommends the use of K wires to retract the soft tissues containing the greater occipital nerve and its accompanying venous plexus. The screws are inserted by entering C2 at the inferior aspect and exiting at the posterior aspect of the upper articular process. The screws are placed through the facet joints into the lateral masses of C1 (Fig. 19.5). In a recent biomechanical study, this Magerl technique was found to be significantly stiffer in rotation than the Gallie wiring technique.[50] Magerl recommends Gallie wiring and fusion in addition to transarticular screws in patients with an intact C1 ring.[44,45,70] Recently, a technique of atlantoaxial stabilization using pediatric Cotrel–Dubousset rods and hooks has been reported as well.[68]

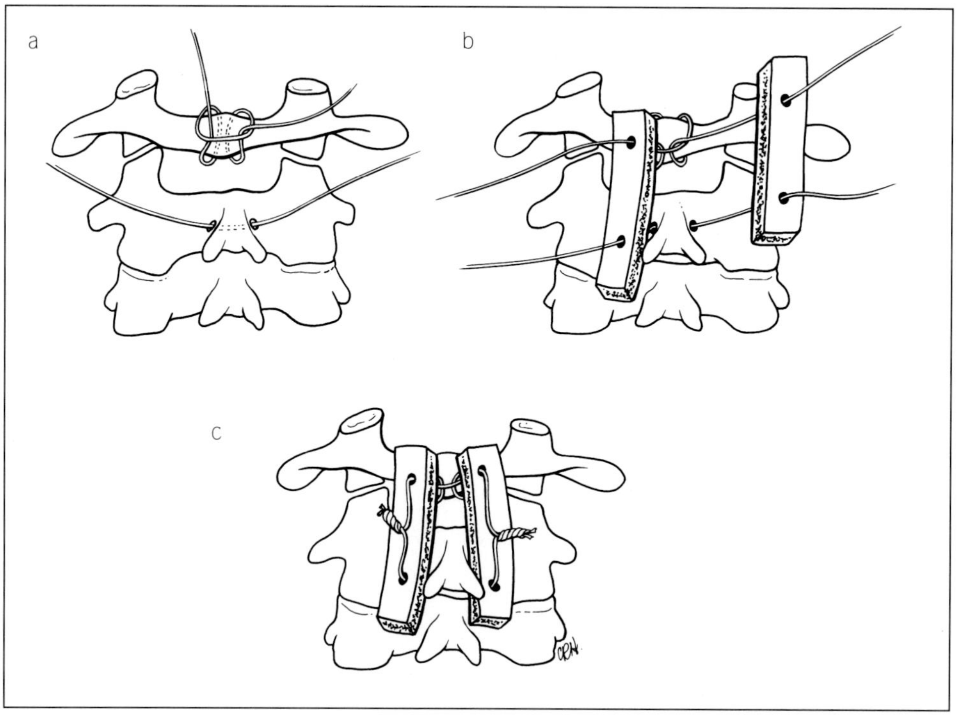

Figure 19.3
Meyer's technique of C1–C2 fusion: (a) a sublaminar wire is placed under C1 and spinous process wire is passed through the base of C2; (b) wires are threaded through holes in the grafts; (c) wires are tightened over the grafts

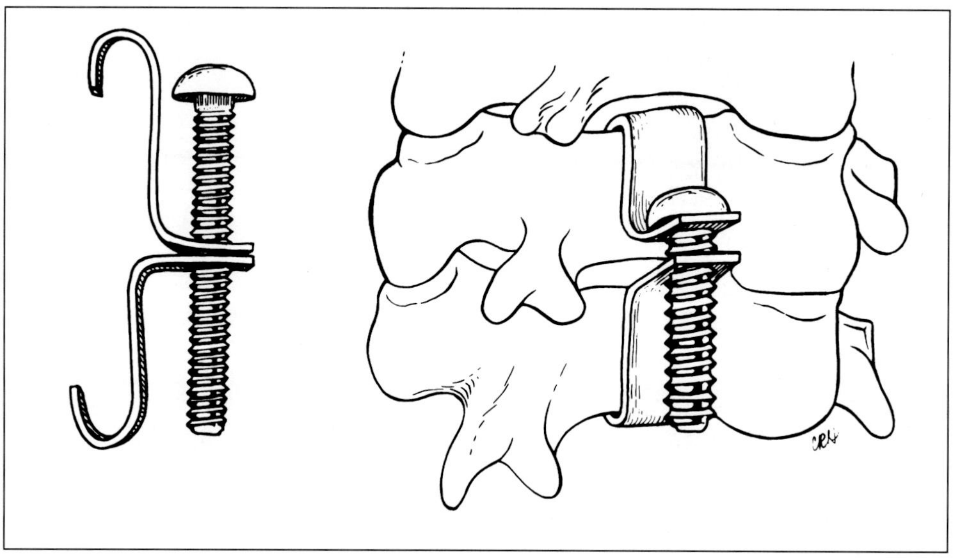

Figure 19.4
Halifax clamp for C1–C2 stabilization

Posterior Occipitocervical Fusion

Several techniques have been described. The authors prefer the method described by Wertheim and Bohlman (Fig. 19.6).[72] A midline posterior approach is made, exposing from the external occipital protuberance to the fourth cervical vertebra. Sharp, subperiosteal dissection is completed exposing the occiput and the cervical laminae. The external occipital protuberance is thick and represents the ideal location for passage of wires without having to go through both tables of the skull. A high-speed diamond burr is used to create a trough on both sides of the protuberance at a level 2 cm above the foramen magnum. A towel clip is then used to create a hole in the ridge, and an 18-gauge wire passed through the hole, and twisted over the ridge. A second wire loop is passed around the

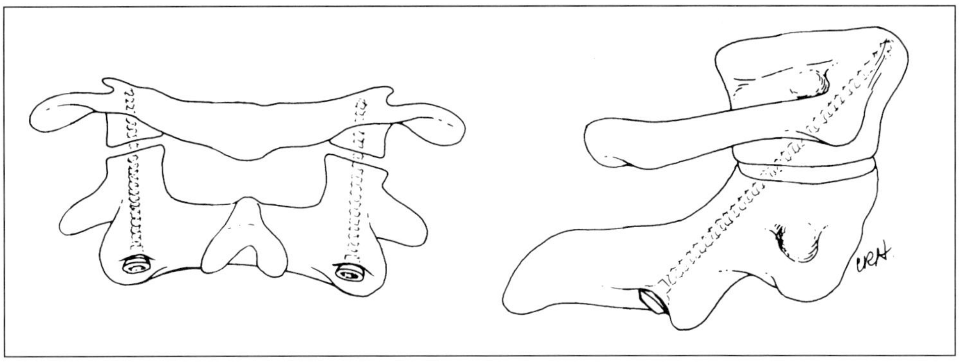

a

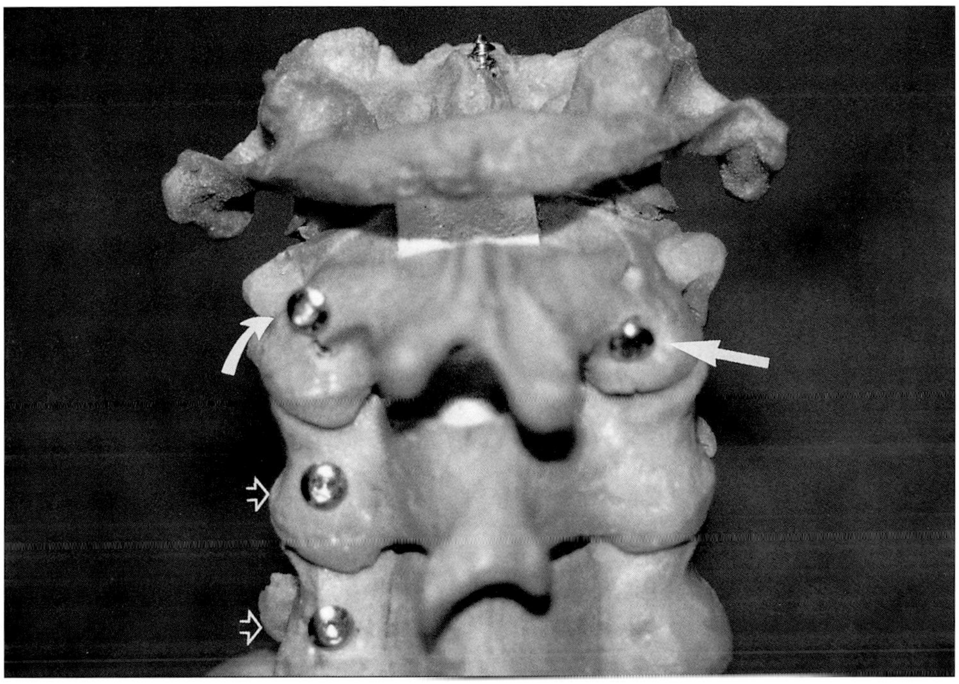

b

Figure 19.5
Magerl's technique of C1–C2 screw fixation. (a) Left: the screws are inserted by entering C2 at the inferior aspect and exiting at the posterior aspect of upper articular process. Right: the screws are placed through the facet joints into the lateral masses of C1. (b) A photograph of a cervical spine, saw bone model demonstrating C1–C2 screw (straight arrow), pedicle screw of C2 (curved arrow), and lateral mass screws (open arrows)

arch of C1, and a third is passed through and around the base of the spinous process of C2. The posterior iliac crest is then exposed, and a large, thick, slightly curved graft of corticocancellous bone of appropriate width and length is obtained. The graft is then divided, and three drill holes placed in each graft. The occiput is decorticated, and the grafts are anchored in place by the wires. Additional cancellous bone is then packed between the two grafts. Finally, halo-cast immobilization is required for 12 weeks.

There have been other occipitocervical fusion techniques described in the literature.[30,35,48,57] Some authors use the occipital bone just above the atlanto-occipital space, penetrating the opposite cortex for the passage of wires. Great care should be taken not to injure the dura or venous structures. Although isolated successful cases have been reported,[52] occipitocervical arthrodesis with onlay grafts and no internal fixation is not generally recommended. Without internal fixation, the patient may require prolonged bedrest, and a higher rate of pseudoarthrosis is expected. However, this technique may be adequate in young children if patients are immobilized after surgery by halo fixation.[42]

Occipitocervical fusion can also be achieved by using Luque segmental instrumentation[10,37,55] (Fig. 19.7). These techniques provide a stronger fixation, but potential complications associated with sublaminar wiring prohibit routine use. Recently, screw fixation into the occiput has

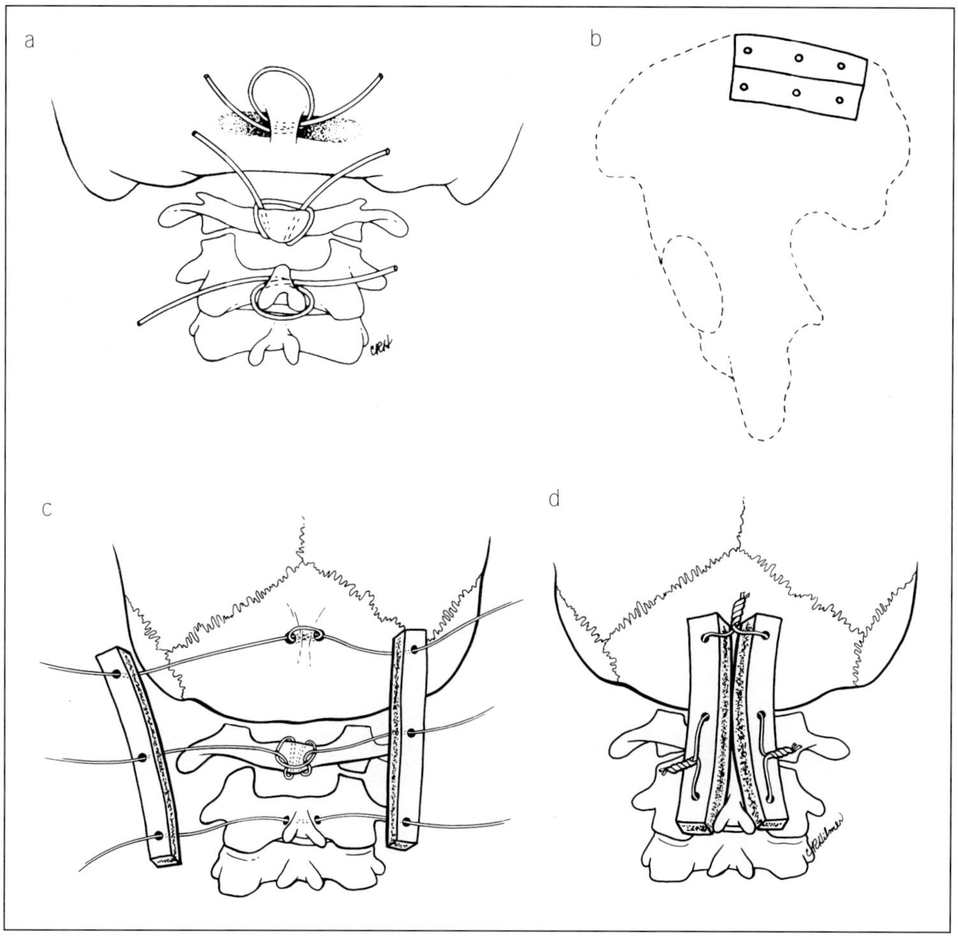

Figure 19.6
Wertheim and Bohlman's method of occipitocervical fusion. (a) A wire is looped around the external occipital protuberance at a level 2 cm above the foramen magnum. A towel clip is then used to create a hole in the ridge, and an 18-gauge wire passed through the hole and twisted over the ridge. A second wire loop is passed around the arch of C1 and a third is passed through and around the base of the spinous process of C2. (b) The outer iliac crest is used for bone grafts. (c) Drill holes are made in the bone grafts and wires are passed through the holes. (d) The wires are tightened

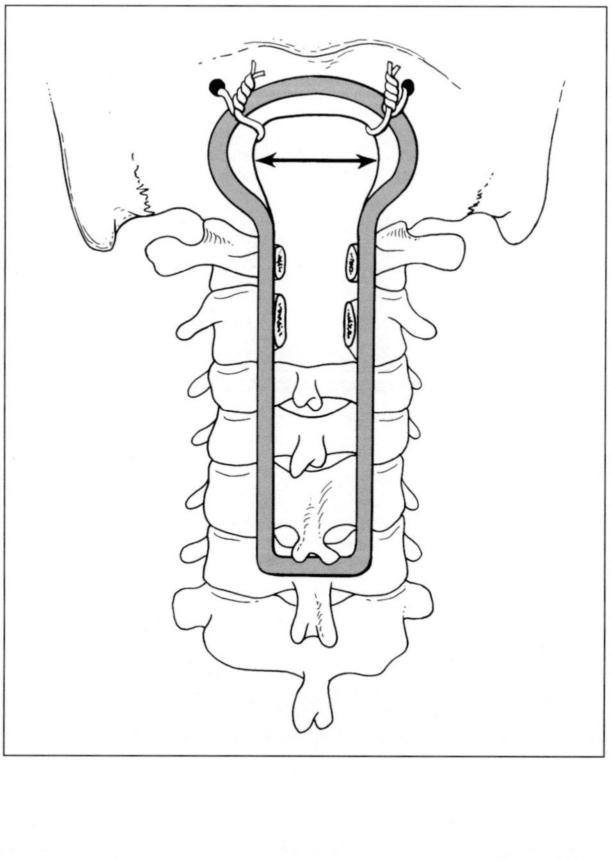

Figure 19.7
A diagram of a Luque ring or Hartshell Ransford rectangle for upper cervical fixation. Sublaminar wires are usually used to stabilize the ring but spinous process wires may be used

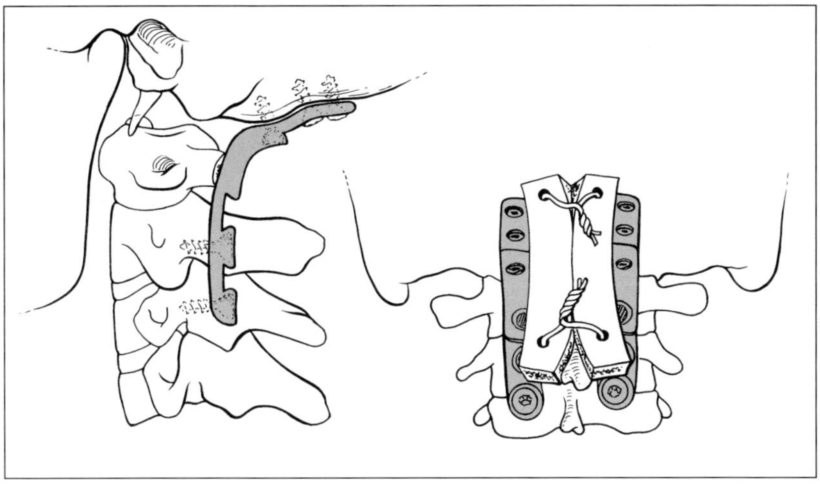

a

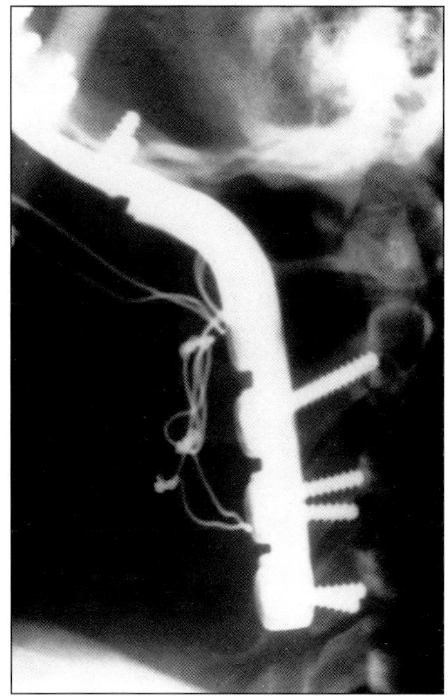

b

Figure 19.8
Roy-Camille technique of occipitocervical fixation. (a) Diagram of the contoured occipitocervical plate and screw fixation. (b) Lateral radiograph of a patient who underwent occiput–C4 fixation using the Roy-Camille plate

been described.[10,25,32–34,60,61,68] This technique may be advantageous in patients who undergo decompressive laminectomy or who require multi-level fixation from the occiput to the lower cervical spine. Roy-Camille et al[60,61] have devised an occipitocervical plate that is contoured to fit the occipitocervical junction (Fig. 19.8). AO reconstruction plates may also be contoured and fit over the occipitocervical junction (Fig. 19.9). Fidler presented three patients with metastatic cervical spine disease who underwent plate–screw fixation to the occiput, and sublaminar wire fixation of the upper cervical spine.[25] This plate is screwed to the midline of the occiput, where the bone is thicker. A modified Cotrel–Dubousset system is also available for use in the occipitocervical spine. This system uses screws in the occipital bone, and hooks in the upper cervical spine.[41] No clinical series have been reported at this time.

Methylmethacrylate can also be used as adjunct fixation for occipitocervical stabilization. Recently, Stambough and associates described a technique of occipitocervical stabilization with bone cement in the osteoporotic spine. Posterior fusion, reinforced with metal mesh or polymethyl methacrylate in patients with severe osteoporosis or malignancy, has been reported in the literature, but it should be regarded as temporary adjunctive fixation.[9,12,16,17,46,54]

Complications associated with posterior fusion of the upper cervical spine may be serious. Care is required during passage of the wires or application of the screws to

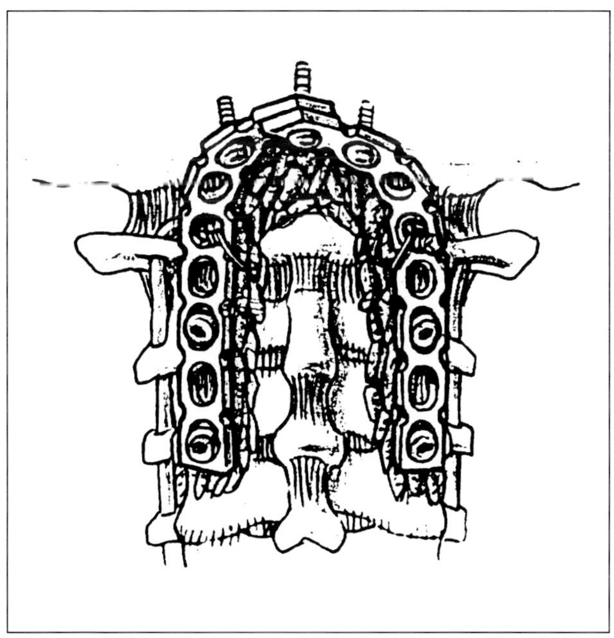

Figure 19.9
Posterior plating of the occipitocervical spine using AO reconstruction plates overlapping in the midline. (From Aebi M. Surgical treatment of cervical spine fractures by AO spine techniques. In Bridwell KH, Dewald RL, eds, *The Textbook of Spinal Surgery*, 1083. Philadelphia: JB Lippincott)

prevent injury to the brain or spinal cord. Somatosensory evoked potential monitoring is recommended in high-risk procedures. Dissection on the ring of the atlas must be done in a gentle manner, because direct pressure may result in fracture or slippage of an instrument. Laterally only 1.5 cm should be dissected because the vertebral artery is at risk. Also dissection of the foramen magnum should be avoided because the inferior edge is needed to prevent uncontrollable venous bleeding. Halo-vest immobilization after surgery is recommended to prevent failure of the surgical construct and to lessen the likelihood of pseudo-arthrosis.

Lower Cervical Spine

Posterior fusion of the lower cervical spine may be indicated in patients with traumatic instabilities, extensive laminectomies for neural decompression, or destruction of bony elements by neoplasm. The goals of the treatment include stabilization, maintenance of alignment, fusion, and early rehabilitation. There are many methods of posterior stabilization of the cervical spine; each has advantages and disadvantages, and the surgeon should choose the appropriate procedure depending on the particular circumstances of the individual case.

Wiring Procedures

Since Rogers initially described a method of cervical wiring and fusion,[58] other techniques have been described in the literature.[8,13,15,24,48,53,58,63,71] Wiring techniques are quite effective in preventing flexion, but less effective in preventing extension or rotation. The authors favor an interspinous process, a triple-wire technique which compresses the bone grafts to the underlying laminae (Fig. 19.10). This triple-wire technique has been shown to be safe and effective, and biomechanically superior to many other constructs.[8,47]

The patient should be in cranial tong traction on the Stryker frame to maintain alignment. After preparation and draping of the patient, the skin and subcutaneous tissue are dissected down to the midline fascia. At this time, a lateral radiograph is taken to be certain of the level. Subperiosteal dissection is then completed to expose the spinous processes, lamina, and necessary facet joints. Caution is necessary to avoid dissection beyond fusion sites and to prevent creeping fusion extension. A 3-mm burr is used to drill a hole at the base of the spinous process on both sides. The drill hole site should be at the proximal aspect of the cephalad spinous process and at the distal aspect of the caudad spinous process. A towel clip is gently passed through the holes to create a tunnel for wires. A single 18- or 20-gauge wire is then passed through both spinous processes (for a single-level fusion) and tightened. If more than one level is to be fused, figure-of-eight wiring is used to incorporate the middle spinous process in the wiring construct. If the middle spinous process or lamina is fractured, wiring should be avoided at this level. The second and third wires are passed through the cephalad and caudad holes in the base of the processes, respectively. Decortication of the lamina and facets is done carefully using a power burr. Corticocancellous bone grafts of appropriate length are next taken from the outer table of the iliac crest. Two drill holes are placed in each graft for passage of wires. The grafts are then slid over the wires, and contact made between the graft and laminae. The posterior cortical edge of the graft should be placed just under the bulbous spinous process to enhance the stability of the construct and maximize graft–lamina contact. The wires on each side of the spine are then simultaneously tightened. Additional cancellous chips are placed on the exposed lamina or facets. The patient is usually kept in a cervicothoracic orthosis or halo vest for 6 weeks, depending on the stability of the construct and the compliance of the patient.

Sublaminar fixation is generally not recommended in the lower cervical spine as this technique is associated with a greater risk of neurologic injury (Fig. 19.11a). An alternative fixation is the 'Dewar procedure', in which Kirschner wires are inserted through the bases of the spinous processes and secured with wire in a loop fashion[21,59,64] (Fig. 19.11b). Another method involves Wisconsin button and wires with a Luque ring (Fig. 19.12). This technique provides a good fixation without sublaminar wires

Facet fracture or subluxation can be managed with an oblique wiring technique or wire loop by passing the wire through the lateral mass.[13,24,74] In post-laminectomy conditions requiring stabilization, interfacet wiring and fusion can be performed.[14] In the oblique wiring technique, the facet wire is passed by placing a small Penfield dissector into the facet joint, followed by making a 2-mm drill hole into the facet in a superoinferior direction. Wire (20 or 22 gauge) is passed through this hole and looped around the inferior spinous process for one-level fusion as required in most unilateral facet dislocations (Fig. 19.13). Facet wires may be extended to adjacent facets for multi-level facet stabilization as in post-laminectomy instability (Fig. 19.14). The facet wires may be tied to bone grafts for fusion and also can be tied to metallic rods for additional stability[28,51] (Figs 19.15 and 19.16).

Complications associated with posterior interspinous wiring in the cervical spine are relatively infrequent. One must avoid unnecessary exposure of the cervical levels beyond fusion areas to prevent creeping fusions to adjacent vertebrae. Inadvertent penetration into the ligamentum flavum and the spinal canal can occur if care is not taken during subperiosteal dissection. Dural penetration can also occur during drilling or passage of wires if the

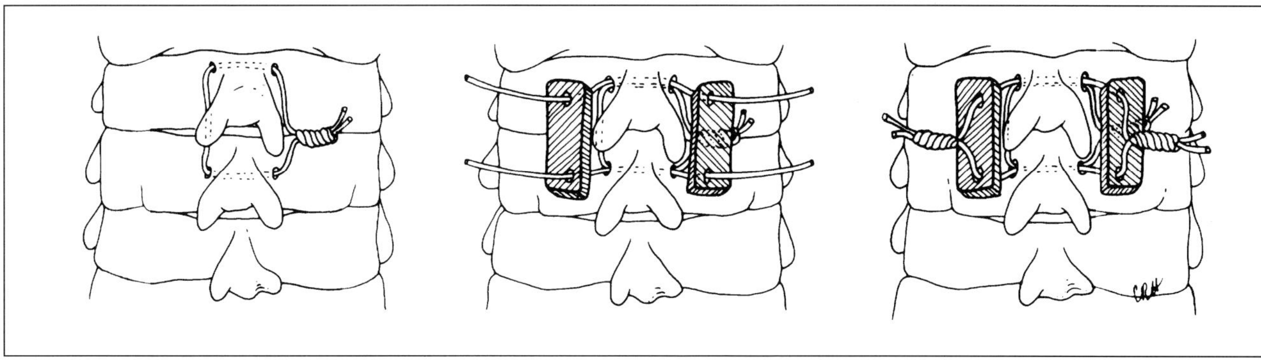

Figure 19.10
A triple-wire technique with interspinous process wires. Left: a wire passed from the cephalad part of the superior spinous process to the inferior part of the caudad spinous process. Middle: the second and third wires are passed through the cephalad and caudad holes in the base of the processes, respectively. After decortication of the lamina and facets, corticocancellous bone grafts from the outer table of the iliac crest are placed. Right: wires are tightened over the grafts and additional cancellous chips are laid down on the exposed lamina or facets

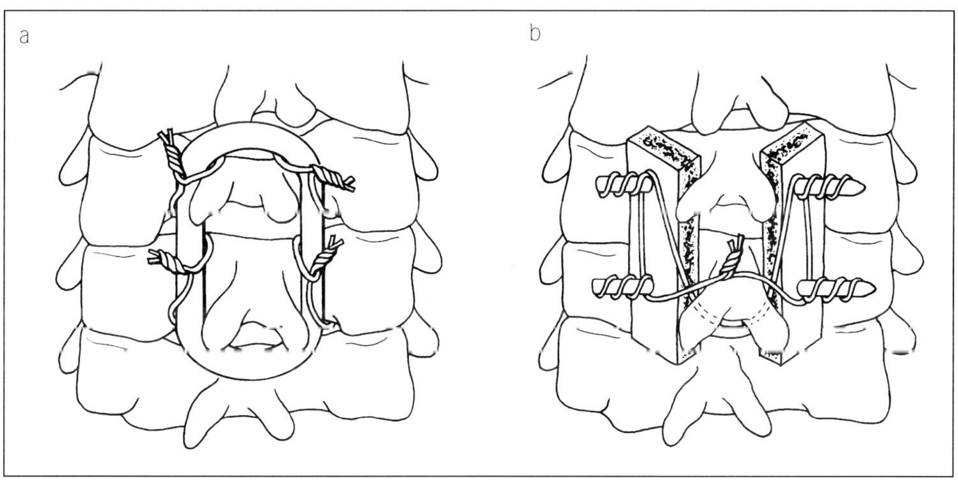

Figure 19.11
(a) A sublaminar fixation with a Luque ring; (b) the Dewar procedure in which Kirschner wires are inserted through the bases of the spinous processes and secured with a figure-of-eight wire

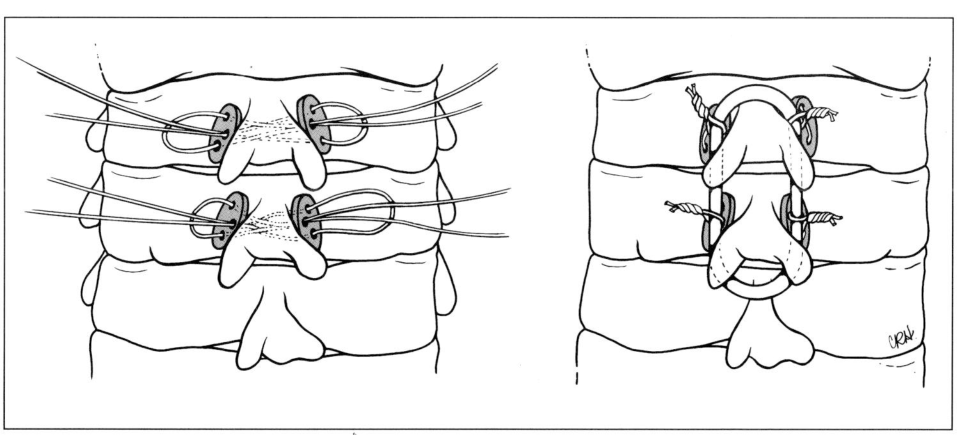

Figure 19.12
Cervical spine fixation using Wisconsin buttons and spinous process wires

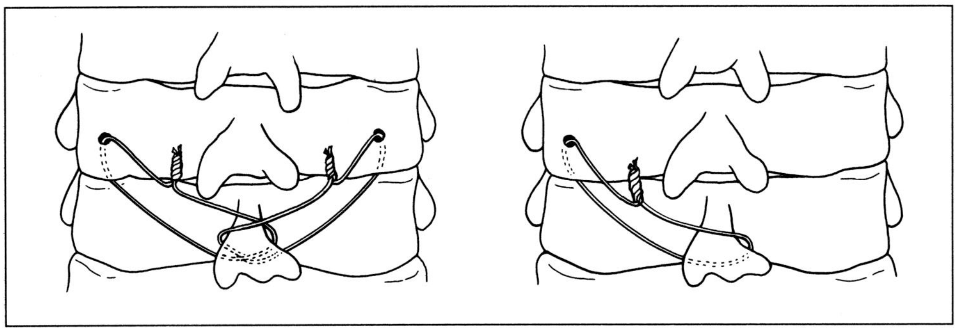

Figure 19.13
(a) Bilateral oblique wiring technique; (b) unilateral oblique wiring technique

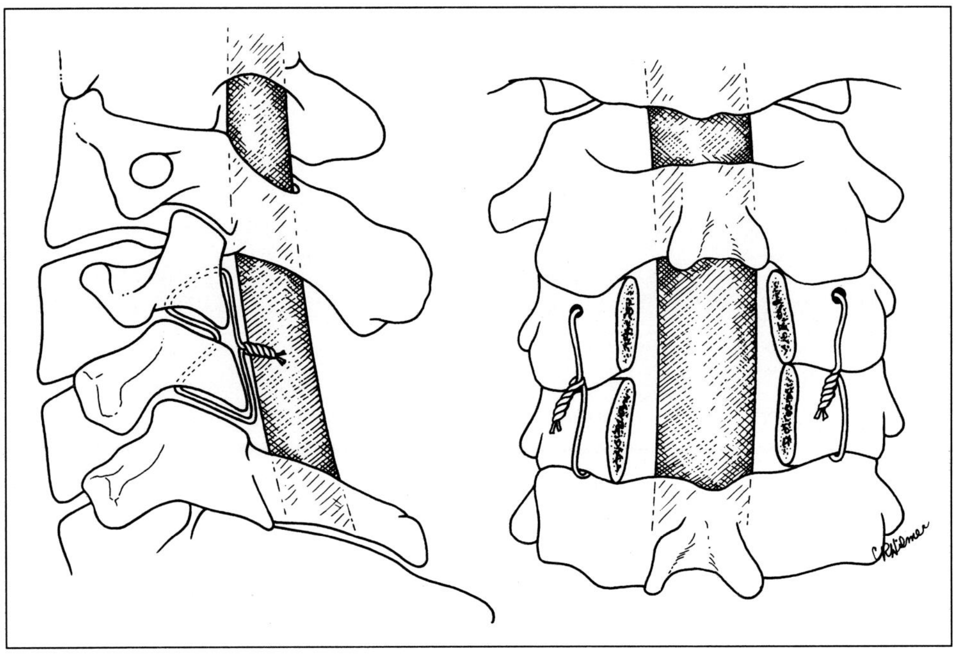

Figure 19.14
Interfacet wiring after laminectomy: wires are passed through the facet joint and holes in the lateral mass

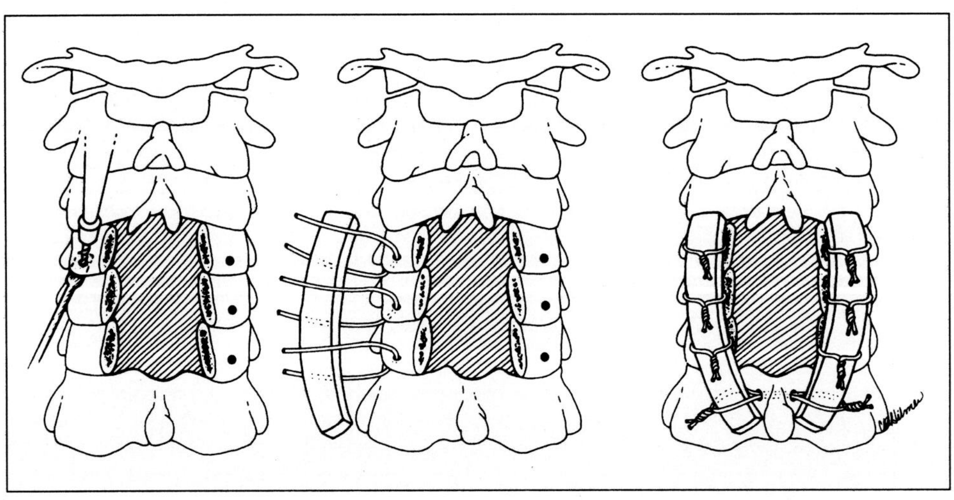

Figure 19.15
Multi-level fixation after laminectomy. Left: the facet wire is passed after making drill holes into the facet from superior to inferior. Middle: wires are looped around the bone grafts. Right: wires are tightened over the grafts

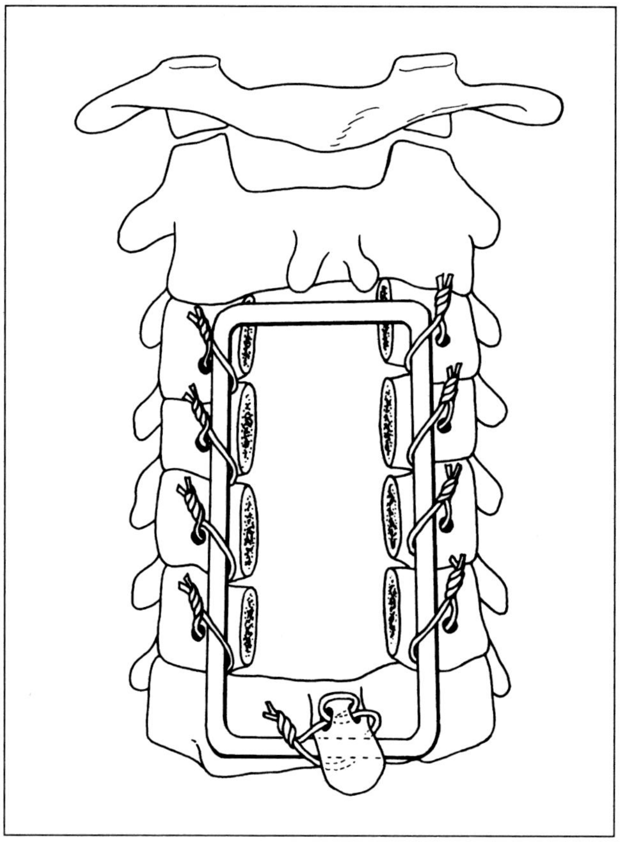

Figure 19.16
Luque ring fixation with facet wires after laminectomy

holes are placed too close to the dura. The most common complication associated with the wiring procedure in the cervical spine is loss of fixation and subsequent recurrence of deformity. This complication is often related to the surgeon's technique, and type of postoperative external support. If a relatively rigid construct is accomplished, such as with the triple-wire and bone block procedure, the patient can be managed simply with a cervicothoracic orthosis in the postoperative period. However, if the surgical construct is not quite stable, or if the patient's compliance is questionable, a halo-vest orthosis should be used for postoperative external stabilization.

Rigid Internal Fixation

Although most patients with instability of the cervical spine can be treated with wiring methods, there are situations in which more rigid internal fixation is indicated. Most apparent are instances in which the spinous processes are absent or deficient, as in post-laminectomy cases and fractures of the spinous processes. Also, stable fixation of many levels is another advantage of other techniques that use instrumentation such as rods or plates. More rigid fixation is of greater benefit either in patients with multi-level injuries or in those who have extensive neoplasticity at many levels. Rigid fixation also allows for earlier mobilization of the patient with minimal postoperative external support, which may be paramount in the treatment of multiple trauma victims.

There are numerous types of instrumentation of the cervical spine which provide greater stability. Harrington or Luque rods with wires have been used in the cervical spine.[28,51] Pediatric Cotrel–Dubousset hooks can be used in the adult cervical spine for hook–rod fixation. The Halifax interlaminar clamp has been mentioned before under the upper cervical spine. This device uses the lamina, and provides good stability against flexion, but not against extension or rotation.[20,36,49,69,73]

Posterior stabilization of the cervical spine using screws and plates has been pioneered by Roy-Camille in Paris[60,61] (Figs 19.17 and 19.18). Louis uses a similar type of plate–screw fixation onto the lateral masses.[32–34,43] Magerl devised a plate–screw system for the cervical spine, in which the inferior portion of the plate is a hook configuration[32–34,38,44,45] (Fig. 19.19). Recently, Anderson and associates[4] presented 30 patients with unstable cervical spines, who underwent a posterior arthrodesis with AO reconstruction plates. All had solid fusions with no neurologic or vascular complications, and three patients had screw loosening without clinical sequelae. Biomechanical strengths of these plates have been shown to be superior to posterior wiring, especially in extension and torsion.[19] Clinical reports to date are also quite encouraging.[4,19,22,23,39,63] These reports showed good correction of deformity and maintenance of alignment until fusion. Although the authors have not experienced any significant complications, potential problems associated with posterior plating with screws include injury of the vertebral artery or cervical nerve roots. Thorough familiarity with the articular pillar anatomy and surgical technique is important in the prevention of these complications.

A cadaveric study was done to find out potential dangers of posterior plate–screw osteosynthesis of the cervical spine.[2,3] The vertebral artery and spinal cord were virtually free of danger with known techniques. The nerve root exits at the anterolateral portion of the superior facet. Medial angulation and excessive angulation of the screw are more likely to impinge on the nerve root. The ideal exit point of the drill was determined to be the juncture

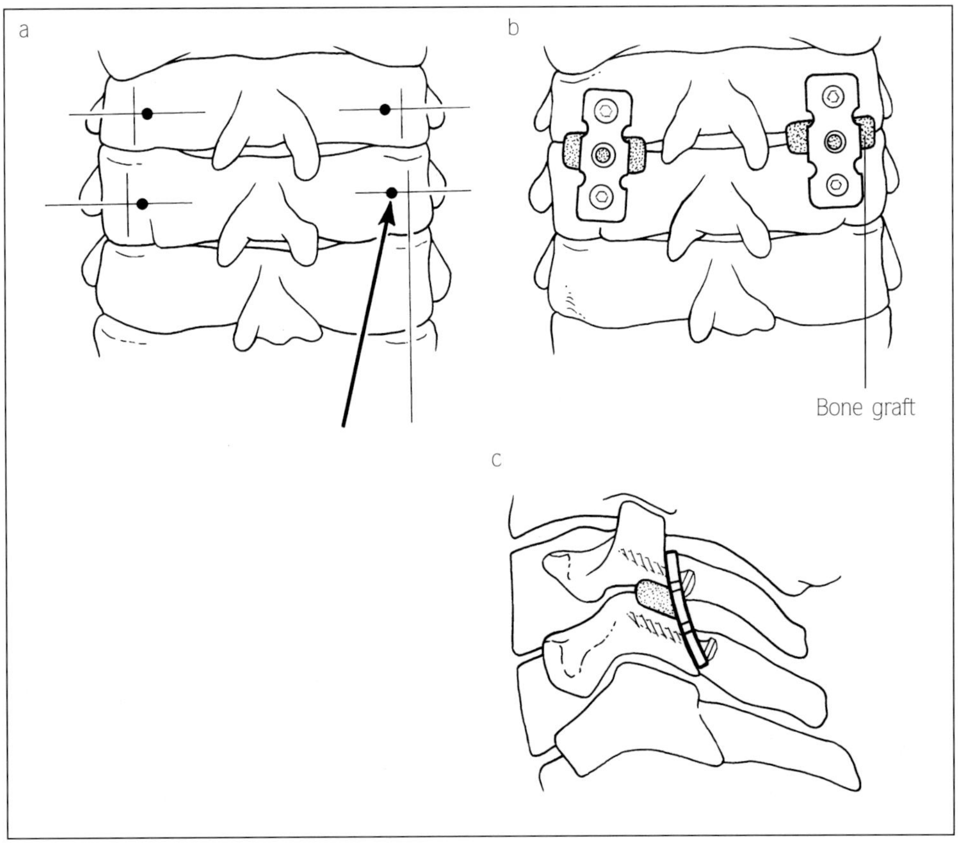

Figure 19.17
Posterior plate–screw fixation of the cervical spine. (a) the ideal drilling technique for safety of the nerve root. The starting point is 1 mm medial to the center of the lateral mass and the drill is directed 25–30° laterally and 15° cranially. (b) Plate–screw fixation on the lateral masses of the cervical spine with bone grafts between the facet joints. (c) The plates should be slightly contoured to cervical lordosis

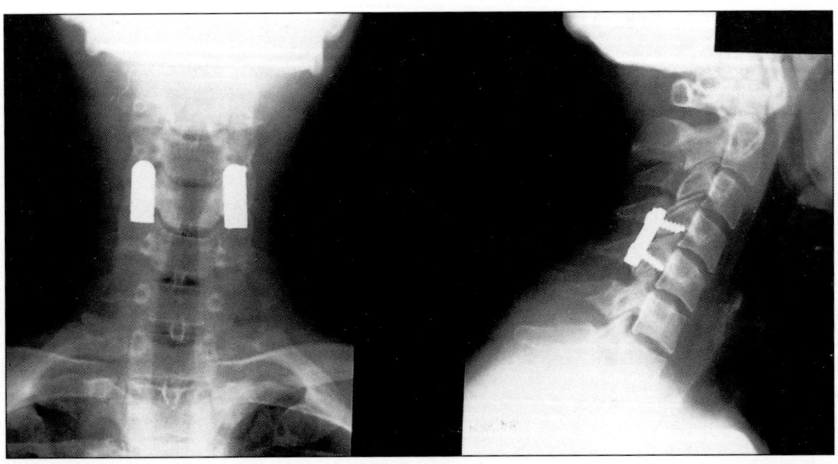
a

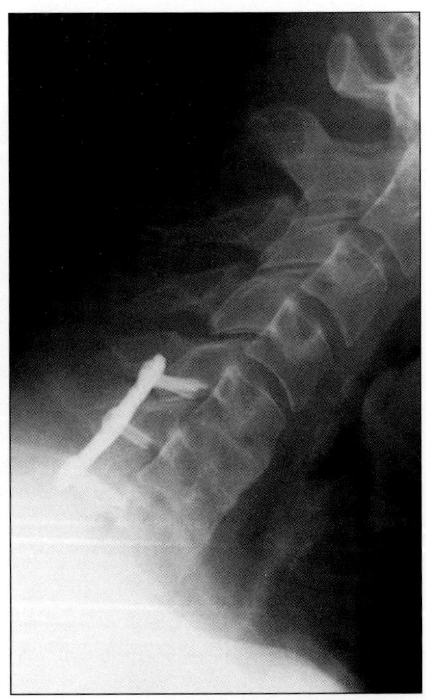
b

Figure 19.18
(a) Anteroposterior and lateral radiographs of a patient who underwent posterior Roy-Camille plating for C4–C5 instability. (b) Another patient who was symptomatic from C6–C7 pseudoarthrosis underwent posterior foraminotomy and titanium plate fixation from C5 to C7

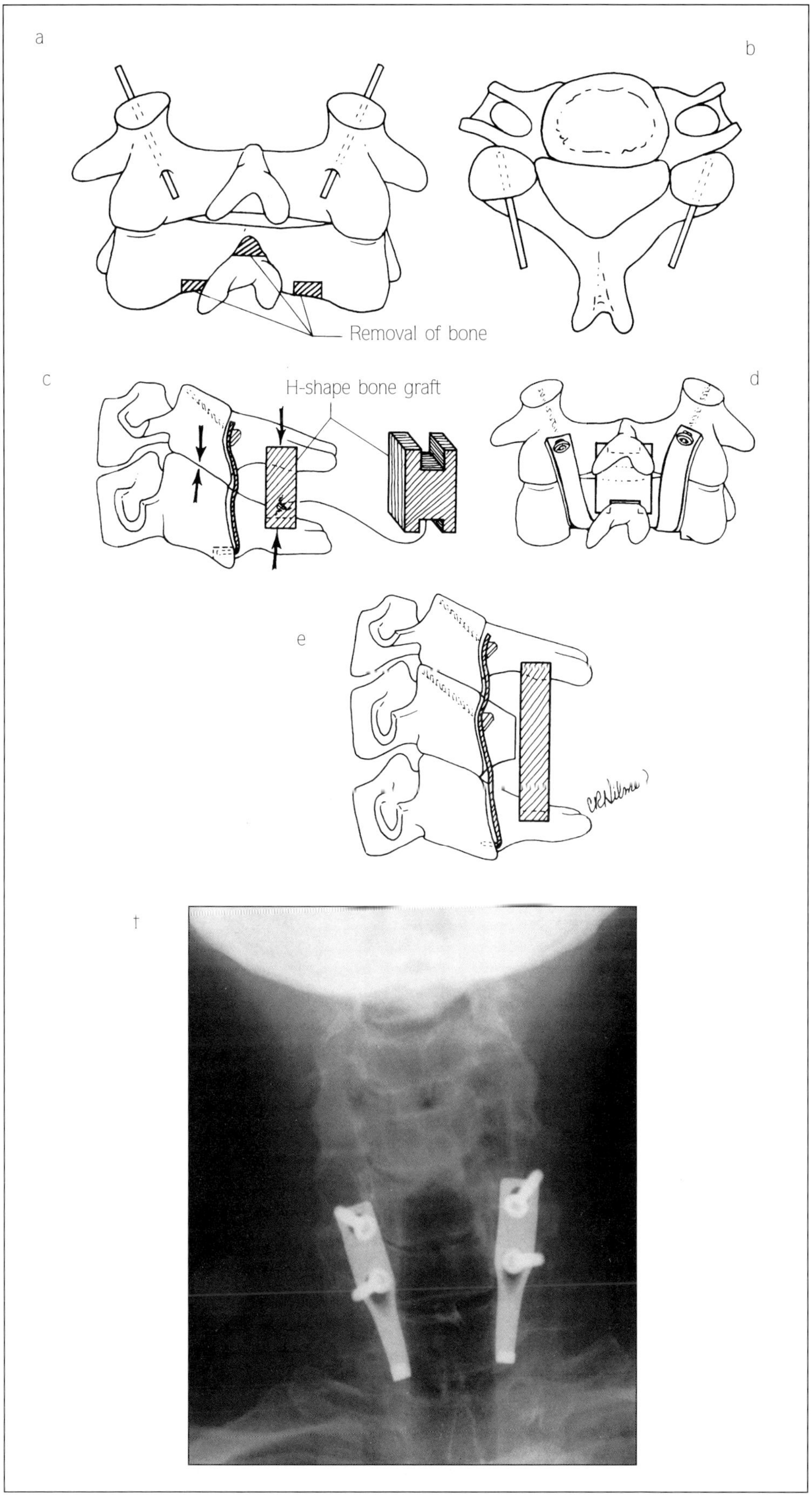

Figure 19.19
Magerl's hook–plate fixation of the cervical spine. (a) Superior angulation is 45° to parallel the facet joint. Bone from the inferior lamina is removed as shown. (b) Lateral angulation of the screw at 25°. (c) H-shaped bone graft between spinous processes. (d) Hook–plate is placed and secured with screws. (e) This technique avoids lateral mass screw inferiorly which may be advantageous at C7, where the lateral mass is thin. (f) Anteroposterior radiograph of patient who underwent C5–C7 hook–plate fixation

between the transverse process and the facet. The safest screw direction is determined to be 30° lateral and 15° cephalad, starting 1 mm medial to the center of the lateral mass for the C3–C6 vertebrae. The lateral mass is quite thin at the transitional C7 level. Attempts to place a lateral mass screw at this level are dangerous to the underlying nerve root and may disrupt the facet joint. Hook–plate designs are preferred at the C7 region. This cadaveric study allowed for measurement of the interfacet distances from the center of the lateral mass to the next lateral mass from C3 to C7. Results show that interfacet distances vary widely among different individuals, ranging from 9 mm to 16 mm with an average of 13 mm. A new plate design with oblong holes is necessary for better accommodation of the differences of interfacet distances among different patients and different levels.

Posterior plate–screw fixation of the cervical spine must be done with thorough knowledge of lateral mass anatomy. Bilateral exposure to the limits of the lateral masses is made. The center of the articular pillar is located, and the cortex pierced with an awl or small burr 1 mm medial to the center. As mentioned before, there are many techniques of drilling depending on various authors. Based on anatomic dissection to avoid potential injury to the nerve root, the pillar is drilled at 30° laterally and 15° cephalad for C3–C6, using a 2.5-mm drill bit. At C2, drilling should be directed about 10–15° medially and 35° superiorly to avoid injury to the vertebral artery. The opposite cortex is penetrated, using a drill with a stop guide. The drill hole is tapped with a 3.5-mm tap. A contoured posterior cervical plate and 3.5 mm diameter cortical screws of appropriate length are placed and secured. In addition to Roy-Camille plates, other plates, such as AO reconstruction plates, titanium plates, and Harm's posterior cervical plates, are becoming available. A titanium device has the advantage of magnetic resonance imaging capability after implantation. The posterior elements adjacent to the plates are decorticated, and bone grafts are added. Complications associated with rigid posterior fixations of the cervical spine can be numerous. Devices such as a Harrington or pediatric Cotrel–Dubousset hook should be used cautiously, because hooks may impinge on the underlying dura, particularly if used bilaterally at the same level. Laminar hooks should be avoided in the injured level, where the spinal cord has already been compromised by edema or mechanical compression. Screw–plate fixation on the lateral mass may be complicated by injuries to the spinal cord, vertebral artery, or the nerve roots. Meticulous exposure of the lateral mass, and strict adherence to surgical technique will prevent these complications. Implant loosening may occur if postoperative external support is ignored or pseudoarthrosis results. If rigid fixation has been achieved, halo-vest external immobilization is generally unnecessary except in non-compliant patients.

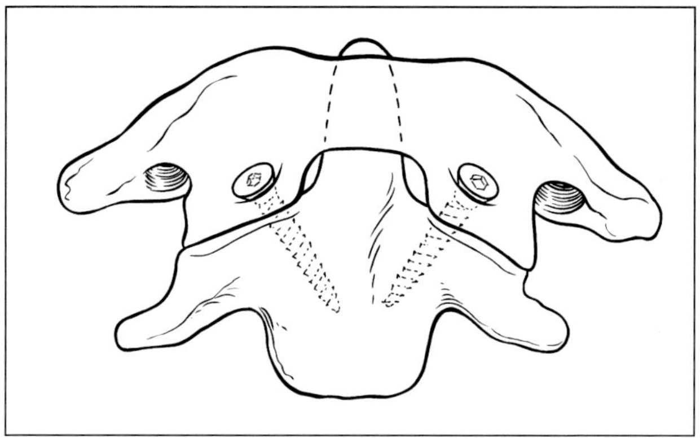

Figure 19.20
Anterior C1–C2 screw stabilization

Summary

Posterior fixation of the cervical spine may be done by either a simple and reliable triple-wire method or other rigid fixation methods, depending on the pathoanatomic process of the lesion. One must be thoroughly familiar with the surgical anatomy, surgical techniques, and potential complications before using a particular method of stabilization of the cervical spine.

ANTERIOR CERVICAL SPINE

Anterior C1–C2 Screw Stabilization

Anterior C1–C2 screw stabilization can be attempted for C1–C2 instability and fractures. Although the authors generally advise a posterior approach for such conditions, it remains a useful technique for patients with previously failed posterior procedures, and for patients with an absent posterior element.

The transoral surgical approach is not advised for any procedure involving insertion of hardware. High rates of infection are assured, which may be life-threatening. Bilateral lateral retropharyngeal approaches are required, as described in Chapter 2. Dissection along the transverse process of the atlas leads to the lateral mass and atlantoaxial joint. Capsular tissues about the joint are removed for visualization of landmarks required for screw placement.

Drilling is completed in a posteroinferior direction, and averages 10° posteriorly and 25° inferiorly for a distance of 20–25 mm (Fig. 19.20). The articular surfaces of the atlantoaxial articulations are cleared of cartilage, and cancellous bone packed into the interface before insertion of the screw. An AO malleolar lag screw, usually 26 mm in length, is then inserted but not secured, until the opposite side of the patient is exposed and prepared in a similar fashion. Once screws have been placed bilaterally, they are tightened, and the articulation stabilized.

This approach offers no significant functional advantage over posterior C1–C2 fusion techniques, and hence its usefulness is limited. The authors have only limited experience with this technique, but feel that the required bilateral exposures are time-consuming, cumbersome, and technically demanding, when compared to posterior arthrodesis techniques.

Complications with this technique mostly include those inherent to the surgical approach; those specific to the technique itself have not been well described.

Anterior Screw Stabilization of the Odontoid

Anterior screw stabilization of the odontoid is a procedure advocated by many for acute fracture and non-union of the dens. Odontoid fractures are relatively common, and account for 10–14% of all cervical spine fractures.[1] The traditional approach to treatment of odontoid fractures has been conservative. These authors still prefer conservative management through halo immobilization, because a large percentage of these fractures heal uneventfully. However, for widely displaced type II fractures, early surgical stabilization may be contemplated to enhance both the potential for fracture healing and the patient's functional recovery.

Traditionally, surgery for fracture of the odontoid process has been posteriorly directed. In most cases, these patients are immobilized in a halo-vest device before surgery, and a posterior C1–C2 arthrodesis performed using either a Brooks or Gallie technique. However, this surgical approach eliminates rotation about the C1–C2 articulation, which is the rationale for direct anterior fixation of such fractures, because this preserves rotation while providing rigid internal fixation with no requirement for restrictive bracing; it also avoids the additional complications associated with bone-grafting techniques. Advocates of this approach feel that patient morbidity is lessened, and that operative blood loss is minimal.

The surgical approach to the cervical spine is a standard anteromedial one. A right-sided transverse incision is made just above the level of the cricoid cartilage, and extends 6–8 cm laterally. The platysma muscle is split in a longitudinal fashion at the medial border of the sternocleidomastoid muscle. The contents of the carotid sheath are identified, and the retropharyngeal space then accessed just medial to the palpable carotid pulse. Blunt finger dissection is continued to the prevertebral fascia and anterior longitudinal ligament, and the anterior tubercle of the atlas is palpably identified. The prevertebral fascia and anterior longitudinal ligament are split in the midline over the body of the axis, and extended in a cranial fashion, exposing the odontoid process and fracture site.

In the operating room, before actual surgery is started, time must be taken to obtain sufficient radiographic imaging in both anteroposterior and lateral planes (Fig. 19.21). Reduction of the fracture may be completed by closed means through application of skeletal traction, although this

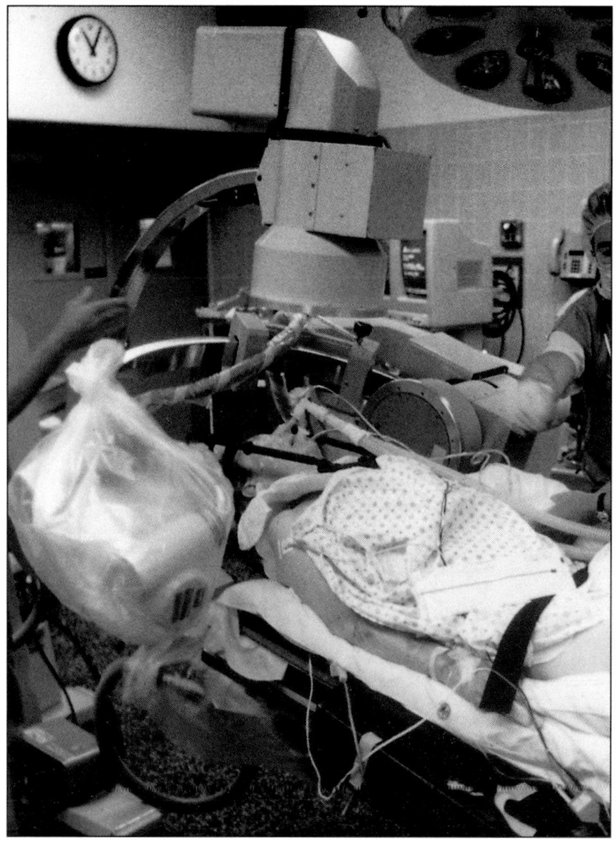

Figure 19.21
Photograph of patient positioning and simultaneous anteroposterior and lateral fluoroscopy for anterior screw fixation of the odontoid

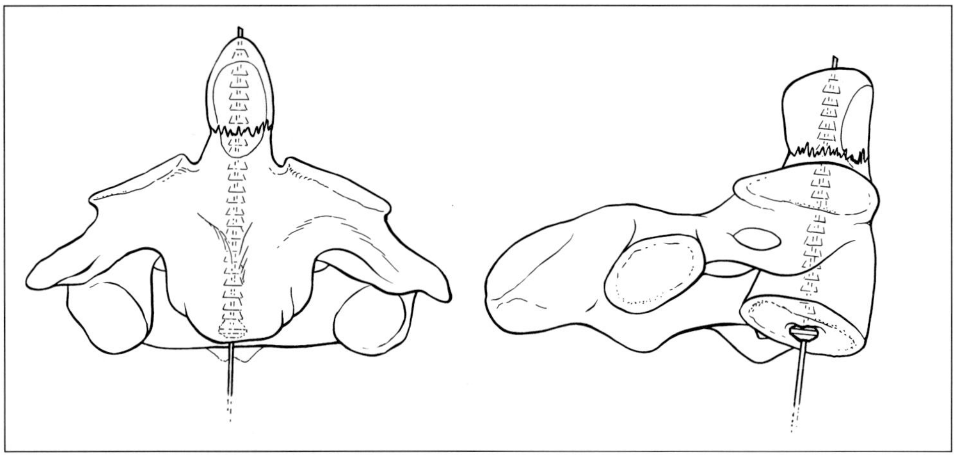

Figure 19.22
Anterior screw fixation for type II fractures of the odontoid: a 2.0-mm Kirschner wire is placed under image intensification through the body of C2 into the odontoid process. Once secured in this position, the hole is tapped, and a 3.5-mm cannulated cortical screw placed using a lag technique

should not be attempted vigorously. For displaced fractures, unreduced by skeletal traction, the odontoid process may require mobilization and realignment before fixation. Once reduction of the odontoid process is complete, the anteroinferior border of the C2 body is used as the starting point for drilling. The authors prefer using 2.0-mm Kirschner wires, which are placed by image intensification through the body of C2 into the odontoid process. One or two wires are placed across the fracture site (Fig. 19.22). Once secured in this position, the wire is then removed, the hole tapped, and a 3.5-mm cortical screw placed using a lag technique. The average length of the screw usually approximates 40 mm. General advice from the authors is to place the tip of the screw through the apical cortex of the odontoid, which seems to enhance fixation greatly. After surgery, the authors still prefer adjunct halo-vest immobilization, although others feel safe with less restrictive devices.

Böhler[7] had the largest series of odontoid fractures treated in this manner. Based on the results of treatment in patients with non-union and acute fracture, he no longer advocates anterior screw fixation for the treatment of non-union. The indications for this technically demanding procedure seem to be displaced odontoid fractures which cannot be reduced adequately through skeletal traction or use of a halo device. In addition, patients with fractures of the odontoid associated with a concomitant C1 ring fracture are also reasonable candidates for this operative technique.

Anterior Instrumentation of the Lower Cervical Spine

Over the last 20 years, several devices have been developed and implemented for osteosynthesis of the anterior cervical spine; the most common indication for such surgery is still a degenerative condition. This approach was first noted in the literature by Bailey and Badgley,[6] Smith and Robinson,[66] and Cloward.[18] The particular techniques that they have described have been widely accepted and successful for degenerative conditions with reliance on the bone graft for stability of the affected motion segment. However, these techniques, when applied to the acutely unstable cervical spine, do not offer sufficient stability and, as isolated procedures, have been plagued with complications. As such, additional methods and techniques for augmentation of cervical immobilization have been employed, including concomitant posterior arthrodesis, prolonged immobilization in a halo-vest device or other external cervical orthosis, and prolonged bedrest with cranial tong traction. These alternatives do not, however, allow for early patient mobilization and rehabilitation, which it is now realized is an important factor in the treatment and survival of the spinal cord-injured patient. Anterior decompressive procedures, followed by stabilized reconstructive techniques, potentially offer sufficient stability through a single surgical approach and minimize patient morbidity.

Although anterior cervical plating is not routinely used by the authors in cervical spine surgery, indications may include reconstruction of the spine after vertebral body excision or cases of fracture, spondylosis, tumor, or infection. Additional indications may include anterior ligamentous disruption secondary to hyperextension injuries with resulting instability and, less commonly, stabilization of interbody fusions after excision of the intervertebral disc.

In this chapter, rather than dwelling on the particular advantages or disadvantages of this technique for varying conditions, the technique of anterior cervical plating is reviewed in detail with the commonly employed and commercially available systems. The specific indications for implementation of anterior plate fixation are reviewed in appropriate chapters elsewhere in this book.

Surgical Technique

As for other planned surgeries of the spine, proper preoperative planning, including considerations for intubation, positioning, and stabilization during the operative period, is imperative. For most fractures and dislocations, degenerative disorders, tumors, and infections, skeletal traction is applied via cranial tongs to secure the patient's head and control the cervical spine. Most acutely injured patients are brought to the operating room in traction and on a Stryker frame, which facilitates patient care. This frame may also be used as the operative table, allowing atraumatic transport and turning of the patient.

The surgical approach for most conditions include a standard anteromedial Smith–Robinson technique. A transverse incision generally suffices, although a longitudinal incision along the anterior border of the sternocleidomastoid may be required in some cases. After the skin is incised, the platysma muscle is split in line with its fibers. Alternatively, it may be incised in a transverse fashion. The carotid artery is palpated, and contents of the carotid sheath retracted laterally. Blunt finger dissection is then carried down to the prevertebral fascia and anterior longitudinal ligament. Once the proper level is identified, the longus colli muscles are elevated in a subperiosteal fashion, starting in the midline of the cervical spine. Self-retaining retractor blades are then placed under the longus colli muscle to protect the vital structures. Once the retractor is placed, the temporal artery pulse is palpated by the anesthesiologist to ensure safety of the carotid artery. The decompression is then performed, depending on the identified preoperative pathology. Fusion may simply involve an interbody arthrodesis rather than a vertebral body reconstruction with fibular strut or tricortical iliac crest graft. Again, the specific techniques for these procedures are addressed in the appropriate chapters.

Once the graft is inserted, some decision has to be made concerning the need for supplemental anterior fixation. For three-column injuries to the cervical spine, anterior plating is a requirement when attempting to avoid either a concomitant posterior arthrodesis or complications associated with anterior grafting not involving fixation. For reconstructive procedures where sufficient stability is not obtained with graft implantation, and in many tumor conditions where methylmethacrylate spacers are used, adjunct stabilization with fixation devices is also useful.

The process of instrumentation is first started by selection of an appropriately sized cervical plate, which must extend from the midportion of the superior uninvolved vertebra to the midportion of the adjacent inferior uninvolved vertebra. The plate is then contoured to the anterolateral surfaces of the cervical spine, maximizing contact to the plate. When osteophytes are present on the vertebral bodies, their removal with a high-speed burr or rongeur is required to maximize bony contact to the plate, and thus enhance stability of the construct.

At this point, there are several alternatives. The authors often prefer to stabilize the plate to the graft using a centrally located unicortical screw. Depending on the type of graft used, either a cortical or cancellous screw is inserted for this purpose. Once the plate is stabilized in this manner, screws may be implanted at either the proximal or distal poles of the plate. With the Caspar system, these holes may be drilled manually or with an air-driven, adjustable, drill guide. It is important when using an air-powered drill to measure the anteroposterior depth of the adjacent intact vertebrae, which most frequently approximates 16–20 mm. With the plate stabilized, the hole is drilled through a drill guide allowing no more than 16–18 mm of penetration. The drilling should parallel the end-plates of the vertebral body, and be directed slightly toward the midline. Some prefer the use of a K wire, which may give the surgeon a better feel for the posterior cortical wall. The drill bit or K wire is then removed, and the drill hole palpated with a depth gauge. If the posterior cortex has not been successfully penetrated, the drill guide is readjusted to allow for an additional 2 mm of drilling. This sequence is repeated as necessary until the posterior wall is perforated. Once the hole is completed, it is then tapped with a 3.5-mm cortical tap through both the anterior and posterior vertebral walls. A 3.5-mm cortical screw is then inserted, and only lightly tightened until the remaining screws are placed.

This sequence of events is repeated for each of the three remaining holes. Bicortical approaches are advocated at each involved vertebra to obtain maximal purchase and prevent complications. Once all the screws are placed, an intraoperative radiograph is taken to verify the position and length of the screws, and then they are firmly tightened (Fig. 19.23). If, for any reason, there is a less than adequate purchase into the vertebral body, the screws should be removed and redirected. If this procedure also fails to obtain adequate bony purchase, a small amount of methyl

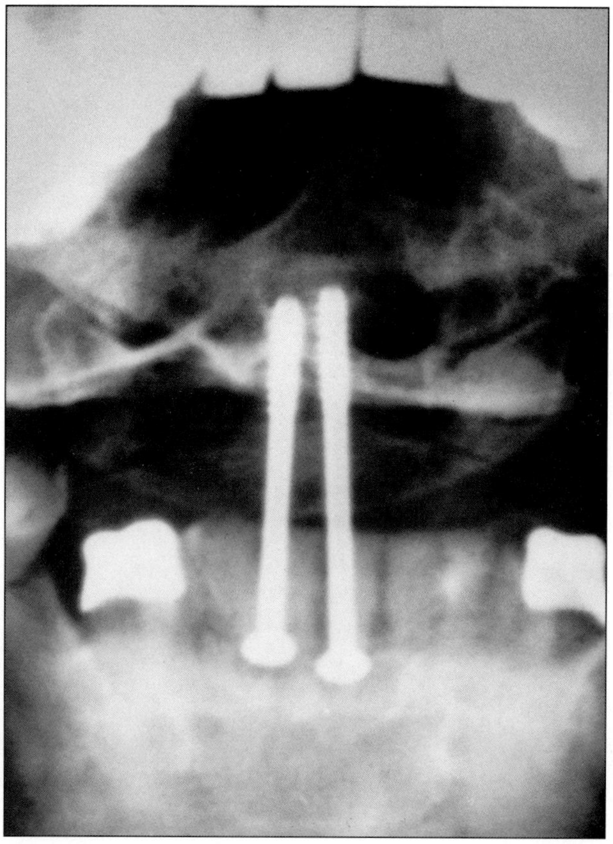

a

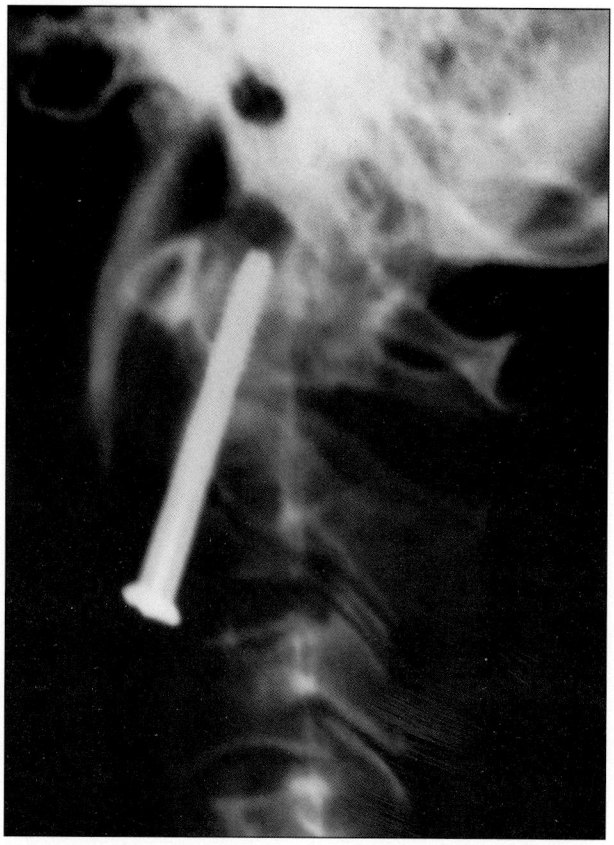

b

Figure 19.23
Anteroposterior (a) and lateral (b) radiographs of a patient who underwent screw fixation for type II odontoid fracture

methacrylate may be used to enhance screw fixation adjunctively.

Once the procedure is completed, drains are placed, and the wound closed in a routine fashion. After surgery, consideration must be given to the patient's respiratory status. With prolonged operative procedures, there is a risk of edematous changes which may, in fact, lead to respiratory compromise. Therefore, for procedures exceeding 6–8 hours, it is often wise to keep these patients intubated for a period of 24–48 hours. Before the patient is awakened from the anesthetic, adjunct external stabilization of the neck is required with the appropriate cervical orthosis. For most patients, operative time is considerably less than 6 hours. These patients can be extubated directly after surgery, and mobilized the day following surgery with an external orthosis.

The Caspar and AO–Orozco plate systems are composed of stainless steel (Fig. 19.24). These plates come in various sizes. The AO–Orozco plate is available in sizes from 5 to 20 holes, and ranges in length from 23 to 133 mm. Screw hole placement is also variable, and ranges from 16 to 21 mm in each of the various lengths. These plates can be cut and contoured easily to the surfaces of the anterior cervical spine. This system uses 3.5-mm screws, as described earlier, and allows variable placement of the screws through the holes of the plate up to 45°.

The authors often prefer using the AO–Morscher pure titanium cervical plate (Fig. 19.25). This plate is available in five- and eight-hole configurations with length varying from 24 to 63 mm. Hole spacing is also variable from 16 to 55 mm. At one end of the plate, screw direction is set at a 12° angle to facilitate insertion of the screw where the anatomy does not allow right-angle application. There are several screws available for application with this plate. A standard 3.5-mm titanium screw is available for conventional bicortical purchase, as described earlier. However,

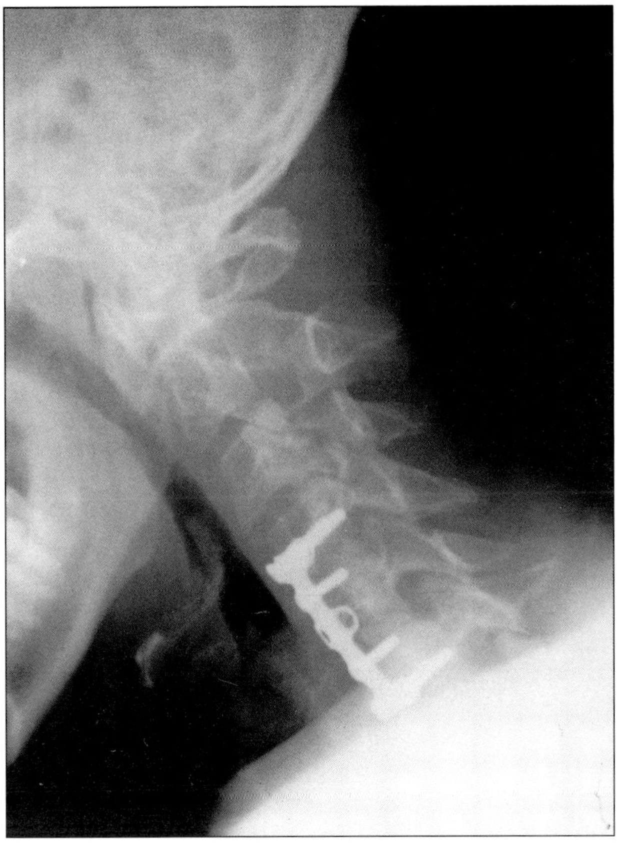

Figure 19.24
Lateral radiograph of a patient who underwent anterior vertebrectomy and fusion and stabilization with AO–Orozco plate

the most commonly used screw with this plate is the 14-mm expansion head screw, which comes in a 4-mm diameter. This expansion head screw comes in perforated and non-perforated forms. The proximal portion of the screw is hollowed out and has an expansile shoulder. Once the 4-mm diameter expansion head screw is placed through the plate and into the vertebral body, it is then locked to the plate with use of the smaller expansion screw. The expansion screw fits into the hollowed-out cylindrical portion of the expansion head screw and, with tightening, widens the shoulder of the expansion head screw, locking it to the cervical plate. The benefits of this screw are primarily related to the fact that bicortical purchase is not required. The stability of this configuration is, however, dependent on the screw purchase to the bone, and its stability may be inferior to the plate–screw system with bicortical purchase.

Complications

Any of the complications inherent to the anterior cervical approach still apply with attempts at anterior cervical instrumentation. Meticulous technique during surgical exposure, without undue pressure on the vital structures of this region, will allow easy access to the spine. Self-retaining retractors with blunt tip blades placed under the longus colli muscle, coupled with additional retraction with similar self-retaining blades in a superoinferior fashion, will facilitate this portion of the operative procedure.

Potential complications directly referable to anterior instrumentation are many. Certainly the most feared complication is that of iatrogenic neurologic injury, which would be most often encountered with use of excessively long screws; these penetrate the posterior cortex and directly injure the dura and underlying neurologic structures. Such injury may also occur during the drilling process. It is important to use a drill guide that prevents inadvertent posterior penetration. An alternative to using a power drill is to use a hand-held drill bit. This may provide the surgeon with additional tactile and proprioceptive feedback which can prevent such penetration.

Dural penetration may also be of concern. Leaks of cerebrospinal fluid under these circumstances may not even be noticed by the operating surgeon. Clinically, however, these have not been shown to represent a significant problem. Repair of visualized dural tears may be attempted, although this represents a technically difficult procedure and may not be possible. Under these circumstances, a small piece of Gelfoam or fascia can be laid across the region; this generally suffices. Undue penetration of the posterior wall can be eliminated with use of the AO–Morscher titanium cervical plate system which, as indicated earlier, uses an expansion head screw.

An additional and relatively common complication of anterior cervical plating is misplacement of the screw into the supra-adjacent or infra-adjacent disc space. This is a complication that should be recognized during surgery. Radiographs should be obtained once the screws are placed for confirmation of position. With penetration into a disc space, there is relative assurance that eventual loosening of the screw can occur, because of movement across that particular motion segment. These screws should be removed and redirected when possible. Such screw misplacement often occurs as a result of improper plate sizing. It is critical that the chosen plate extend only from the midportion of the vertebral bodies above and below the decompressed segment. If the operating surgeon is uncertain of the superior and inferior borders of the respective vertebral bodies, the plate may be appropriately placed on the anterior surface of the cervical spine, and a radiograph taken to verify the position and length of the plate before screw insertion. This may prevent improper plate sizing and penetration of the screw into the disc space.

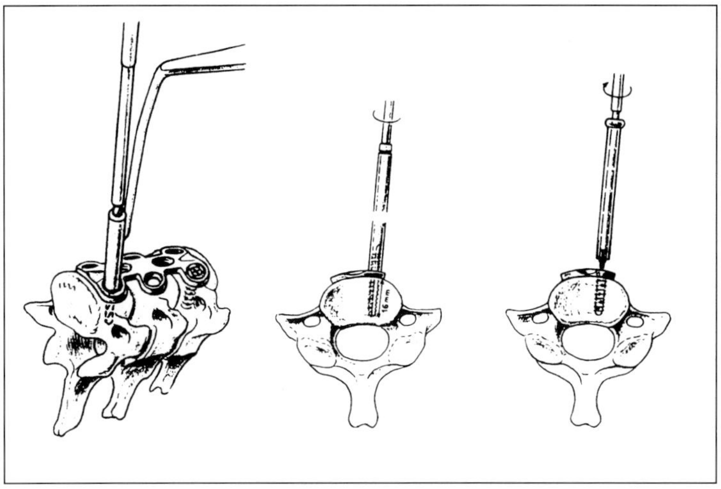

a

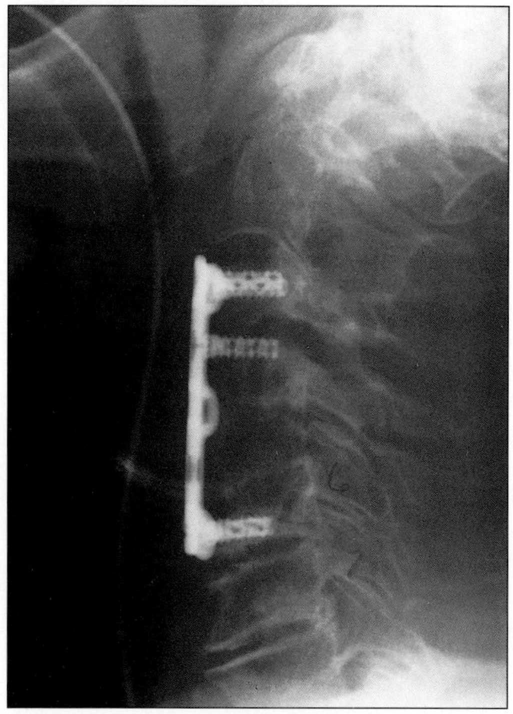

b

Figure 19.25
(a) AO–Morscher titanium cervical plating. Left: appropriate sized plate is centered over the vertebral body. Center: drilling and tapping is done down to 16 mm. Right: screw is inserted followed by expansion screw. (b) Lateral radiograph of a patient with AO–Morscher titanium plate–screw stabilization

Potentially, the most severe complication associated with anterior instrumentation of the cervical spine is that of hardware loosening and subsequent injury to surrounding vital structures and organs. Hardware loosening may be the result of osteoporosis with insufficient bony purchase, technical difficulties where multiple attempts at insertion lead to inadequate purchase, and finally, improper postoperative immobilization of the patient. Use of anterior cervical plate fixation is strongly discouraged in the osteoporotic patient, because the authors feel that the potential risks outweigh the benefits under these circumstances. Technical mishaps may be minimized by following the appropriate surgical steps and experience. The choice of a postoperative orthosis is dependent on the overall stability of the construct. Of course, the patient must be compliant with the orthosis. Use of anterior plate fixation should not be used in the uncooperative patient. Although reports of screw loosening were of obvious concern, more recent reports indicate such plating techniques to be safe when used in the proper patient. In a series of 92 patients reported by Meyer and colleagues, only 2% of these cases had complications as a direct result of screw implantation. In those cases where screw loosening was recognized, it was thought to be secondary to incorrect screw placement or improper plate positioning at the time of surgery. Again, it must be remembered that strict adherence to the demanding technique of screw insertion is imperative for avoidance of such complication. In this study,[56] all screws were placed with posterior cortical purchase. The posterior cortex was also penetrated with the drill bit. However, no neurologic complications or dural leaks were encountered in the series.

Summary

Anterior cervical plating is being popularized as a method of cervical spine fixation. With experience and proper patient selection, use of such instrumentation may preempt the need for additional posterior surgical techniques and, as such, avoid potential complication with the posterior surgical approach, and decrease operative time. The authors do not believe that any such anterior cervical plating system abolishes the need for posterior stabilization procedures, but it does add to the armamentarium available to spinal surgeons.

REFERENCES

1. Althoff B. Fracture of the odontoid process. An experimental and clinical study. *Acta Orthop Scand Suppl* **177**: 1–95, 1979.
2. An HS, Gordin R, Renner K. Anatomic consideration for plate-screw fixation of the cervical spine. *Spine* 16(105): 548–551, 1991.
3. An HS, Vaccaro A, Cotler JM. Spinal disorders at the cervicothoracic junction. Presented at the Cervical Spine Research Society Annual Meeting, San Antonio, Texas, November 1990.
4. Anderson PA, Henley MB, Grady MS, Montesano PX, Winn HR. Posterior cervical arthrodesis with AO reconstruction plates and bone graft. *Spine* **16**(Suppl): S72–S79, 1991.
5. Aprin H, Harf R. Stabilization of atlantoaxial instability. *Orthopaedics* **11**: 1687–1693, 1988.
6. Bailey RW, Badgley CE. Stabilization of the cervical spine by anterior fusion. *J Bone Joint Surg [Am]* **42:** 565–594, 1960.
7. Böhler J. Anterior stabilization of acute fractures and nonunions of the dens. *J Bone Joint Surg [Am]* **64**: 18, 1982.
8. Bohlman HH. Acute fractures and dislocations of the cervical spine: an analysis of 300 hospitalized patients and review of the literature. *J Bone Joint Surg [Am]* **61:** 1119–1142, 1979.
9. Brattstrom H, Granholm L. Atlanto-axial fusion in rheumatoid arthritis: a new method of fixation with wire and bone cement. *Acta Orthop Scand* **47**: 619–628, 1976.
10. Bridwell K. Treatment of markedly displaced Hangman's fracture with a Luque rectangle and a posterior fusion in a 71-year-old man. *Spine* **11**: 49–52, 1986.
11. Brooks AL, Jenkins EB. Atlanto-axial arthrodesis by the wedge compression method. *J Bone Joint Surg [Am]* **60**: 279–284, 1978.
12. Bryan WJ, Inglis AE, Sculco TP, Ranawat CS. Methyl methacrylate stabilization for enhancement of posterior cervical arthrodesis in rheumatoid arthritis. *J Bone Joint Surg [Am]* **64:** 1045–1050, 1982.
13. Cahill DW, Bellegarrigue R, Ducker TB. Bilateral facet to spinous process fusion: a new technique for posterior spinal fusion after trauma. *Neurosurgery* **13**: 1–4, 1983.
14. Callahan RA, Johnson RM, Margolis RN, Keggi KJ, Albright JA, Southwick WO. Cervical facet fusion for control of instability following laminectomy. *J Bone Joint Surg [Am]* **59:** 991–1002, 1977.
15. Capen D, Zigler J, Garland D. Surgical stabilization in cervical spine trauma. *Contempt Orthop* **14**: 25–32, 1987.
16. Clark CR, Goetz DD, Menezes AH. Arthrodesis of the cervical spine in rheumatoid arthritis. *J Bone Joint Surg [Am]* **71**: 381–392, 1990.
17. Clark CR, Keggi KJ, Panjabi MM. Methyl methacrylate stabilization of the cervical spine. *J Bone Joint Surg [Am]* **66**: 40–46, 1984.
18. Cloward RB. Treatment of acute fractures and fracture-dislocations of the cervical spine by vertebral-body fusion: a report of eleven cases. *J Neurosurg* **18**: 201–209, 1961.
19. Cooper PR. Posterior stabilization of the cervical spine using Roy-Camille plates: a North American experience. *Trans Orthop* **12**: 43, 1988.
20. Cybulski GR, Stone JL, Crowell RM, Rifai MH, Gandhi Y, Glick R: use of Halifax interlaminar clamps for posterior C1–C2 arthrodesis. *Neurosurgery* **22**: 429–431, 1988.
21. Davey JR, Rorabeck CH, Bailey SI, Bourne RB, Dewar FP. A technique of posterior fusion for instability of the cervical spine. *Spine* **10**: 722–728, 1985.
22. Dominella G, Berlanda P, Bassi G. Posterior approach osteosynthesis of the lower cervical spine by the R. Roy-Camille technique. *Ital J Orthop Trauma* **8**: 235–244, 1982.
23. Ebraheim NA, An HS, Jackson WT, Brown JA. Internal fixation of the unstable cervical spine using posterior Roy-Camille plates: preliminary report. *J Orthop Trauma* **3**: 23–28, 1989.
24. Edwards CC, Matz SO, Levine AM. The oblique wiring techniques for rotational injuries of the cervical spine. *Trans Orthop* **9**: 142, 1985.
25. Fidler MW. Pathological fractures of the cervical spine. *J Bone Joint Surg [Br]* **67**: 352–357, 1985.
26. Fielding JW, Hawkins RJ, Ratzan SA. Spine fusion for atlanto-axial instability. *J Bone Joint Surg [Am]* **58**: 400–407, 1976.
27. Gallie WE. Fractures and dislocations of the cervical spine. *Am J Surg* **46**: 495–499, 1939.
28. Garfin SR, Moore MR, Marshall LF. A modified technique for cervical facet fusions. *Clin Orthop* **230**: 149–153, 1988.
29. Glynn MK, Sheehan JM. Fusion of the cervical spine for instability. *Clin Orthop* **179**: 97–101, 1983.
30. Grantham SA, Dick HM, Thompson RC, Stinchfield FC. Occipitocervical arthrodesis. *Clin Orthop* **65**: 118–129, 1969.
31. Griswold DM, Albright JA, Schiffman E, Johnson R, Southwick WO. Atlanto-axial fusion for instability. *J Bone Joint Surg [Am]* **60**: 285–292, 1978.
32. Grob D, Dvorak J, Panjabi M, Froehlich M, Hayek J. Posterior occipitocervical fusion. A preliminary report of a new technique. *Spine* **16** (Suppl): S17–S24, 1991.
33. Grob D.Magerl F. Surgical stabilization of C1 and C2 fractures. *Orthopaedics* **16**: 46–54, 1987.
34. Grob D, Magerl F. Dorsal spondylosis of the cervical spine using a hooked plate. *Orthopaedics* **16**: 55–61, 1987.
35. Hamblen DL. Occipito cervical fusion. *J Bone Joint Surg [Br]* **49**: 33–45, 1967.
36. Holness RO, Huestis W, Howes WJ, Langille RA. Posterior stabilization with an interlaminar clamp in cervical injuries: technical note and review of the long term experience with the method. *Neurosurgery* **14**: 318–322, 1984.
37. Itoh T, Tsuji H, Katoh Y, Ynenzawa T, Kitagawa H. Occipito-cervical fusion reinforced by Luque's segmental spinal instrumentation for rheumatoid diseases. *Spine* **13**: 1234–1238, 1988.
38. Jeanneret B, Magerl F, Halterward E, Ward JC. Posterior stabilization of the cervical spine with hook plates. *Spine* **16** (Suppl): S56–S63, 1991.
39. Karlstrom G, Olerud S. Internal fixation of fractures and dislocations in the cervical spine. *Orthopaedics* **10**: 1549–1558, 1987.
40. Larsson S, Toolanen G. Posterior fusion for atlanto-axial subluxation in rheumatoid arthritis. *Spine* **11**: 525–530, 1986.
41. Lesoin F, Autricque A, Jomin M. Use of C-D instrumentation for cranio-cervical junction osteosynthesis. Proceedings of the Sixth International Congress on Cotrel-Dubousset Instrumentation, Montpellier, France, Sauramps Medical, 1989: 249.
42. Letts M, Slutsky D. Occipitocervical arthrodesis in children. *J Bone Joint Surg [Am]* **72**: 1166–70, 1990.

43. Louis RP. *Surgery of the Spine*, 49–83. Berlin: Springer-Verlag, 1983.
44. Magerl F, Grob D, Seeman PS. Stable dorsal fusion of the cervical spine (C2–T1) using hook plates. In Kehr P, Weidner A (eds), *Cervical Spine*, 217–221. Vienna, New York: Springer-Verlag, 1987.
45. Magerl F, Seeman PS. Stable posterior fusion of the atlas and axis by transarticular screw fixation. In Kehr P, Weidner A (eds), *Cervical Spine*, 322–327. Vienna, New York: Springer-Verlag, 1987.
46. McAfee PC. Bohlman HH, Ducker T, Eismont FJ. Failure of stabilization of the spine with methyl methacrylate: a retrospective analysis of twenty-four cases. *J Bone Joint Surg [Am]* **68**: 1145–1157, 1986.
47. McAfee PC, Bohlman HH, Wilson WL. The triple wire fixation technique for stabilization of acute cervical fracture-dislocations: a biomechanical analysis. *Trans Orthop* **9**: 142, 1985.
48. Meyer PR Jr. Surgical stabilization of the cervical spine. In Meyer PR (ed.), *Surgery of Spine Trauma*, 11–49. New York: Churchill Livingstone, 1989.
49. Mitsui H. A new operation for atlanto-axial arthrodesis. *J Bone Joint Surg [Br]* **66**: 422–425, 1984.
50. Montesano PX, Juach EC, Anderson PA, Benson DR, Hanson RB. Biomechanics of cervical spine internal fixation. *Spine* **16** (Suppl.): S10–S16, 1991.
51. Murphy MJ, Daniaux H, Southwick WO. Posterior cervical fusion with rigid internal fixation. *Orthop Clin North Am* **17**: 55–65, 1986.
52. Newman P, Sweetnam R. Occipito-cervical fusion. *J Bone Joint Surg [Br]* **51**: 423–431, 1969.
53. Oro JJ, Watts C. Sublaminar and epilaminar wire fusion: a new technique for posterior subluxation injuries of lower cervical spine. *Trans Orthop* **9**: 142, 1985.
54. Ranawat CS, O'Leary P, Pellici P, Tsairis P, Marchisello P, Dorr L. Cervical spine fusion in rheumatoid arthritis. *J Bone Joint Surg [Am]* **61**: 1003–1010, 1979.
55. Ransford AO, Crockard HA, Pozo JL, Nelson IW. Craniocervical instability treated by contoured loop fixation. *J Bone Joint Surg [Br]* **68**: 173–177, 1986.
56. Ripa DR, Dowall MG, Meyer PR, Rusin JJ. Series of 92 traumatic cervical spine injuries stabilized with anterior ASIF plate fusion technique. *Spine* **16** (Suppl.): S46–S55, 1991.
57. Robinson RA, Southwick WO. Surgical approaches to the cervical spine. In: American Academy of Orthopaedic Surgeons, *Instructional Course Lectures*, Vol XVII, 299–330. St Louis: CV Mosby, 1960.
58. Rogers WA. Fractures and dislocations of the cervical spine: an end-result study. *J Bone Joint Surg* **39**: 341–376, 1957.
59. Rorabeck CH, Rock MG, Hawkins RJ, Bourne RB. Unilateral facet dislocation of the cervical spine. An analysis of the results of treatment in 26 patients. *Spine* **12**: 23–27, 1987.
60. Roy-Camille R, Mazel C, Saillant G. Treatment of cervical spine injuries by a posterior osteosynthesis with plates and screws. In: Kehr P, Weidner A (eds), *Cervical Spine*, p. 163. Vienna, New York: Springer-Verlag, 1987.
61. Roy-Camille R, Saillant G, Mazel C. Internal fixation of the unstable cervical spine by a posterior osteosynthesis with plates and screws. In: Sherk HH, Dunn EJ, Eismont FJ, *et al.*, (eds), *The Cervical Spine*, 2nd ed, 390–403, The Cervical Spine Research Society. Philadelphia: JB Lippincott, 1989.
62. Savini R, Parisini P, Cevellati S. The surgical treatment of late instability of flexion-rotation injuries in the lower cervical spine. *Spine* **12**: 178–182, 1987.
63. Schlicke LH, Schulak DJ. Wiring of the cervical spinous process. *Clin Orthop* **154**: 319–320, 1981.
64. Segal D, Whitelaw GP, Gumbs V, Pick RY. Tension band fixation of acute cervical spine fractures. *Clin Orthop* **159**: 211–222, 1981.
65. Simmons EH. Surgery of the spine in rheumatoid arthritis and ankylosing spondylitis. In: Evarts CM (ed.) *Surgery of the Musculoskeletal System*, Vol. 2, 4:85–151. New York: Churchill Livingstone, 1983.
66. Smith GW, Robinson RA. Treatment of certain cervical spine disorders by anterior removal of the intervertebral disc and interbody fusion. *J Bone Joint Surg [Am]* **40**: 607–23, 1958.
67. Stambough JL, Balderston RA, Grey S. Technique for occipito-cervical fusion in osteopenic patients. *J Spinal Dis* **3**: 404–407, 1990.
68. Steib JP, Kehr P, Mitteau M. C1–C2 instrumentation with C-D pediatric material. Proceedings of the Sixth International Congress on Cotrel-Dubousset Instrumentation. Montpellier, France, Sauramps Medical, 245, 1989.
69. Tucker HH. Technical report: method of fixation of subluxed or dislocated cervical spine below C1–2. *Can J Neurol Sci* **2**: 381–382, 1975.
70. Weidner A. Internal fixation with metal plates and screws. In: Sherk HH, Dunn EJ, Eismont FJ, *et al.* (eds), *The Cervical Spine*, 2nd ed, 404–421, The Cervical Spine Research Society. Philadelphia: JB Lippincott, 1989.
71. Weiland DJ, McAfee PC. Posterior cervical fusion with triple-wire strut graft technique: one hundred consecutive patients. *J Spinal Dis* **4**: 15–21, 1991.
72. Wertheim SB, Bohlman HH. Occipitocervical fusion. *J Bone Joint Surg [Am]* **69**: 833–836, 1987.
73. White AA, Panjabi MM. *Clinical Biomechanics of the Spine*, 2nd Ed. Philadelphia: JB Lippincott, 1990.
74. Wilber RG, Peters JG, Likaver MJ. Surgical techniques in cervical spine surgery. In: Errico TJ, Bauer RD, Waugh T (eds), *Spinal Trauma*, 2nd ed, 145–158. Philadelphia: JB Lippincott, 1991.

20 Complications of cervical spine surgery

Thomas G. Andreshak and Howard S. An

Cervical spine surgery can be gratifying and beneficial for the patient when the appropriate procedure is selected and performed with skill. Complications can destroy the best of results and lead to patient morbidity and mortality. Careful patient selection, preoperative planning, surgical expertise and experience, and proper identification of the underlying pathology will help to avert complication in cervical spine surgery. Each of the different procedures and surgical approaches, used to treat the various disease processes, have inherent risks and potential for complication that are unique to the particular technique. There are also complications common to all forms and techniques in cervical spine surgery. Cervical spine surgery can be performed anteriorly or posteriorly and, on occasion, may require a combined anterior and posterior approach, for conditions including disc disease, trauma, tumors, and inflammatory disorders. Specific complications inherent in the treatment of each condition will be discussed, in addition to a list of general complications which may occur in any cervical spine surgery.

Knowledge of the underlying disease process and various treatment options will help the surgeon to identify which patient may benefit from surgical intervention. Potential for complications may occur at any stage of the treatment process and include: selection of the wrong patient, operating on the wrong level, and use of the wrong surgical approach for a given lesion. Vascular injury, neural injury, dural tears, infection, instability, non-union, recurrence, injury to the trachea or esophagus, graft failure, donor site morbidity, and errors in positioning are all complications that can occur but are minimized with appropriate planning and meticulous surgical technique.

The patient with cervical disc disease usually has one of five clinical syndromes:

1. Discogenic axial pain with or without referred patterns of pain.
2. Radicular patterns of pain from acute soft lateral herniated disc.
3. Radicular pain from chronic disc degeneration.
4. Acute myelopathic symptoms from central disc herniation.
5. Cervical spondylotic myelopathy from multi-level cervical disc degeneration.[52,171]

The syndromes of myelopathy and radiculopathy require thorough preoperative evaluation, with the selected surgical approach dependent on the pathoanatomy of the disease. Each of the available procedures has its own pitfalls and complications.

Cervical trauma is best treated by early recognition of the pathology and pattern of injury with the specifics of surgical treatment dependent on the stability of the spinal segment and presence or absence of neurologic compromise. The potential for late segmental instability as a result of the injury or treatment may complicate patient care and should be recognized.

COMPLICATIONS OF ANTERIOR CERVICAL SPINE SURGERY

Anterior cervical spine surgery is performed for cervical disc disease, cervical trauma, and decompression of anterior pathology. Perhaps the most critical element in the decision to use an anterior approach is proper identification of the underlying pathology. An anterior approach has potential for more complication than a posterior approach as a result of the various organs and great vessels that are encountered during the exposure of the cervical spine. These include the carotid artery, vertebral artery, internal jugular vein, thyroid arteries, trachea, esophagus, sympathetic nerves, laryngeal nerves, thoracic duct, and possibly the dura and spinal cord. Fortunately, most of these injuries are rare, and all can be avoided with meticulous, careful surgical technique.

Vascular Injury

Although low in incidence, the magnitude of any injury to the vertebral or carotid artery can be catastrophic and result in significant associated morbidity or mortality. Injuries to the carotid artery or jugular vein are exceedingly rare, although the actual incidence is not well known. The injuries are generally the result of over-zealous retraction or an accidental, iatrogenic laceration. The importance of knowing the anatomy and approach cannot be overemphasized. Exposure of the anterior cervical spine medial to the sternocleidomastoid and carotid sheath places the internal jugular vein and common carotid artery at risk. The carotid may be lacerated during the approach, occluded during retraction or produce emboli of plaque resulting in stroke.[53,190] Tew and Mayfield[191] reported no vascular injuries in their review of more than 500 cases of anterior spine surgery. Hohf[95] reported 16 cases of injury of the carotid artery and detailed four cases of injury to the carotid artery including three lacerations and one division. Phillips[142] reported no cases of vascular injury to the carotid artery using the Cloward retractor but felt that the carotid sheath was at 'some risk'. It is important to check for the temporal arterial pulse after placement of the retractor. Absence of the pulse signifies compression of the carotid artery which may be productive of ischemia, stroke,[190] or aphasia.[97] A laceration of the carotid artery should be repaired directly and promptly.

The vertebral artery can be lacerated or inadvertently injured with dissection lateral to the uncinate process. This artery enters the foramen transversarium most commonly at C6 (89.1%), and C5 (6%).[5] Aggressive dissection should not be performed too far laterally as the vertebral artery is at risk. Inadvertent penetration with a curette or power burr may cause significant injury.[177] Packing of the bleeding site may control hemorrhage, but it is preferable actually to expose the site and directly repair the vessel in the foramen.[190] The costotransverse lamellae may require exposure, after mobilization of the longus colli, to allow for visualization of the vertebral artery.[199] Ligation of the vertebral artery has a low risk of neurologic deficit,[166] but a case of Wallenberg's syndrome has been reported following thrombosis secondary to a vertebral spreader.[97] Rizzoli (personal communication)[149] reported a case of vertebral artery laceration from a pituitary rongeur used too far laterally. Bleeding was controlled in this case by packing without further complication or sequelae. Vertebral artery injury has also been described during transoral approaches for treatment of upper cervical spine injuries.[64]

Each patient has some unique anatomical feature which adds to the risk of vascular injury. During the anterior approach, the superior thyroid artery is most commonly seen above C4 and the inferior thyroid artery is seen below C6. However, this is variable. These vessels are at risk for injury and may require ligation. Avoiding ligation of these vessels is generally advised, however, as the superior laryngeal nerve, a branch of the inferior ganglion of the vagus nerve, accompanies the superior thyroid artery to innervate the cricothyroid muscle. Unrecognized injury to these vessels may lead to a large hematoma. Injury to the external jugular vein during the approach may also result in hemorrhage and postoperative hematoma, if neglected. Hematoma formation is relatively common with one series reporting an incidence of 9%.[170] Hematoma may complicate wound healing, but is rarely responsible for obstruction of the airway or spinal cord compression.[159] Epidural hematoma may cause spinal cord compression or even death.[113] Elevation of the head of the bed in the immediate postoperative period will control some of the venous bleeding that may be present. The use of meticulous hemostasis and routine placement of a drain is advised to avoid these complications.

Esophageal Injury

Esophageal injury during anterior cervical procedures is uncommon. The severity of injury may range from simple edema and dysphagia to frank perforation. Dysphagia after anterior cervical surgery is relatively common, but is fortunately a temporary condition, in most cases. The various etiologies of dysphagia include postoperative edema, hemorrhage, denervation, graft extrusion, or infection.[121,203] It may also be related to aspiration resulting from laryngeal nerve dysfunction. Edema is felt to be the result of retraction against the rigid endotracheal tube and esophagus, and usually results in mild symptoms of dysphagia. Persistent dysphagia should always be evaluated with a barium swallow or endoscopy. Esophageal perforation is a rare but serious complication of anterior cervical spine surgery.[10,39,45,62,72,211] It occurs in about 1 of 500 procedures.[190] Such esophageal injuries generally result from excessive retraction, use of sharp-tipped retractors or, rarely, inadvertent perforation or tear by use of surgical instruments. Esophageal perforation is usually not recognized during surgery. In the postoperative period, however, the patient may develop an abscess, tracheo-esophageal fistula, or fulminating mediastinitis.[39,71,94,136] Osteomyelitis or an esophagocutaneous fistula may also develop if not recognized and treated early. A survey of the Cervical Spine Research Society[80] compiled 22 cases. Six were recognized at the time of surgery, six after surgery and ten during the recovery phase from 10 weeks to several months after surgery. One-quarter of these cases involved the use of hardware with esophageal injury occurring some time after the operation. All patients were hospitalized for a prolonged course and one patient died of related complications.

In surgery for traumatic injuries of the cervical spine, Kewalramani and Riggins[102] reported one case of esophageal

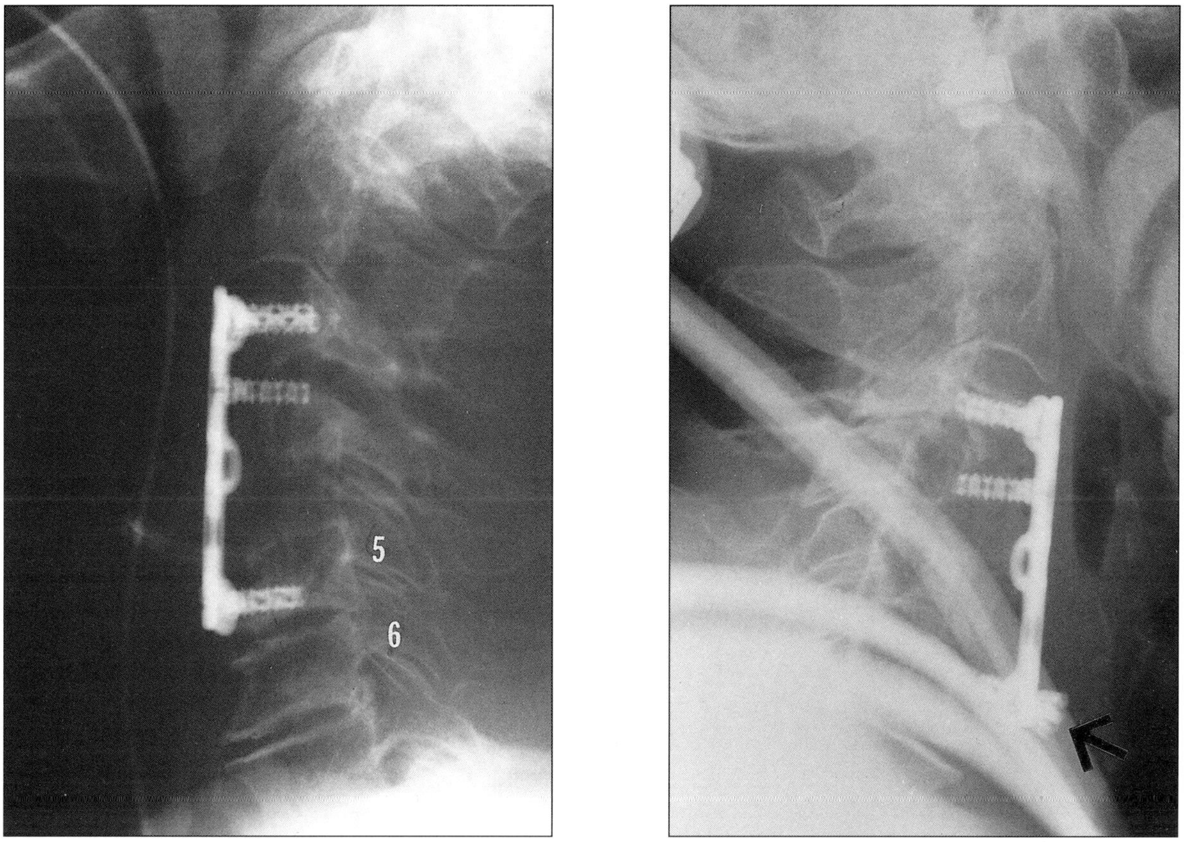

Figure 20.1
(a) Postoperative lateral radiograph demonstrating an iliac crest strut graft with an anterior cervical plate after corpectomy for cervical spondylotic myelopathy. (b) Lateral radiograph 3 days after surgery demonstrates that the plate has displaced with loosening and cutting out of the inferior screws (arrow). The patient developed an esophageal tear and subsequent infection and the plate was removed

perforation in 41 patients. Bohlman and Eismont,[20] in a series of 75 anterior cervical corpectomies, also noted a single case. Newhouse et al[136] reported that 25% of patients who developed esophageal dysfunction after surgery for acute injuries had anterior hardware inserted for the purpose of stabilization, with many of these patients developing perforation. Materials used in the treatment and stabilization of grafts and fractures, including wires, plates and screws, and methylmethacrylate have been known to result in esophageal perforation (Fig. 20.1).[15] The use of screws and plates for anterior stabilization of cervical spine injuries has become widespread. However, these constructs are biomechanically weak in flexion and the screws may become loose and subsequently perforate the esophagus.[43] The perforation need not occur immediately in the postoperative period as wires used for securing anterior grafts have been known to erode into the esophagus after bone remodeling.[15] The esophagus is a pulsatile structure which, over time, may erode over a more rigid, fixed structure.

A traction diverticulum of the hypopharynx has been reported[77,152] with others emphasizing the early recognition and treatment of such injuries in an expedient fashion.[152,197] The presence of crepitus in the neck or mediastinal air on chest radiographs is suggestive of the diagnosis. Definitive testing should then be completed by esophagography followed by computed tomography.[136] Drainage and parenteral antibiotics are the recommended course of treatment.[136] Early consultation with a head and neck surgeon is recommended for consideration of surgical débridement and repair.

Tracheal and Laryngeal Injury, and Respiratory Complications

The anterior approach to the cervical spine places the trachea and larynx at risk for direct and indirect injury. Significant, penetrating injury to the larynx is a rare injury. When such an injury occurs, however, direct repair is indicated. Hoarseness is a common complaint in the initial postoperative period, and generally results from edema secondary to retraction against the rigid endotracheal tube. This mild edema will usually resolve in a few days. Persistent hoarseness may be the result of injury of the superior laryngeal nerve which may also result in aspiration as a result of laryngeal sensory loss. The superior laryngeal nerve is a branch of the inferior ganglion of the vagus nerve and travels along with the superior thyroid artery to innervate the cricothyroid muscle. This may result in hoarseness, but more commonly produces easy fatiguing of the voice. The inferior laryngeal nerve is a recurrent nerve which is protected in the tracheoesophageal groove on the patient's left side, but is vulnerable to injury on the right. It usually follows the inferior thyroid artery.[158] Recurrent laryngeal nerve palsy may be the culprit in patients with persistent hoarseness. The reported incidence of injury is generally felt to be 1%,[190] with one report showing an incidence of 11%. Henneman[89] found in his review that 11% of patients complained of postoperative voice changes, with three patients demonstrating permanent vocal cord paralysis. The true incidence of vocal cord paralysis is difficult to assess but is felt by Bulger et al[28] to approximate 2%. In more than 36 000 cases reviewed in a 1982 study, recurrent laryngeal nerve injury was the most frequent neurologic complication.[71] Most of the injuries are felt to be due to stretch injury rather than division of the nerve.

Severe laryngeal edema may occur in the postoperative period and lead to airway obstruction. Close perioperative monitoring of pulmonary function, the judicious use of drains, and aggressive postoperative pulmonary therapy should minimize any respiratory complication. Airway compromise should be suspected in any patient with dysphagia, stridor, or inability to clear oral secretions. Evidence of tracheal deviation or hematoma should be evaluated and emergency action taken as needed. Aronson[6] described a case that required emergency tracheotomy. A review of seven cases of upper airway obstruction was reported by Emery et al.[60] in which two patients died of complications related to obstruction. All seven patients had undergone multi-level anterior corpectomy and fusion for moderate-to-severe myelopathy. Additional risk factors included a history of heavy smoking and asthma. To avoid emergent re-intubation, Emery et al recommended maintenance of tracheal intubation for 24–48 hours after the operation, followed by direct laryngoscopic evaluation for edema or by deflating the cuff of the endotracheal tube and assessing airflow around the cuff.

Airway compromise following traumatic cervical spine injuries may be due to hematoma or swelling. Kuhn and Graziano[108] reported on 21 patients with airway compromise that were a result of retropharyngeal hematomas. Although airway compromise has not been reported below the C6 level, the risk for subsequent morbidity is such that it should be anticipated in all patients regardless of age, severity of trauma, or lack of symptoms. Risk factors for the development of pulmonary complications in cervical spine injury include a history of chronic obstructive pulmonary disease, age above 60 years, depression, and complete spinal cord lesions in the upper cervical spine.[12,18]

Neurologic Injury

Neurologic injury is probably the most feared complication to both patient and surgeon. Neurologic complications may arise during patient positioning, the surgical approach, or from direct injury to the spinal cord or nerve roots during decompression or stabilization efforts. Those patients with an unstable cervical spine, secondary to traumatic or inflammatory conditions, and those with compressive myelopathy, are at risk for neurologic injury during positioning and intubation. For many unstable injuries, preoperative immobilization in a halo device is the best choice, as long as it does not interfere with the planned operative procedure. Avoidance of cervical hyperextension in the myelopathic patient is imperative. Conscious fiberoptic intubation is generally advised in any patient susceptible to neurologic injury with passive manipulation of the head and neck.

Neurologic injury during anterior cervical surgical approaches probably represents the most common iatrogenically induced injury in cervical spine surgery. The surgeon must be totally familiar with the anatomy of this region and care must be taken to protect the superior laryngeal nerve, the recurrent laryngeal nerve, the hypoglossal nerve, and the sympathetic chain. These structures may be injured directly by division or more commonly through excessive retraction. The recurrent laryngeal nerve was found to be the most common neurologic injury in a review of over 36 000 cases.[71]

Horner's syndrome is a complication of the anterior approach to the cervical spine which may be overlooked initially. The cervical sympathetic chain lies on the anterior surface of the longus colli muscle and posterior to the carotid sheath. Injury may result from dissection carried too far lateral from the midline, use of electrocautery on the longus colli muscle, or overzealous retraction.[39,151] Subperiosteal dissection, which is started in the midline, and then extended laterally under the longus colli, is important to prevent direct damage to these nerves. The curved ends of the retractor blades should be placed into the developed pockets underlying the longus colli muscles. This holds the retractor down against the vertebral bodies and prevents them from popping out and injuring surrounding structures. Horner's syndrome is usually temporary but may be permanent in some cases.[97] Saunders reported a 2% incidence in his series,[161] with the incidence of permanent Horner's syndrome felt to be less than 1%.[71] Ophthalmologic consultation may be needed for treatment of ptosis.

Although injury to the recurrent laryngeal nerve has been reported to be the single most common neurologic injury, the one that is feared the most is that of permanent injury to the spinal cord or spinal nerves. Injury to these structures may be due to a retained disc fragment, graft dislodgement, neck hypertension during intubation, epidural hematoma, or percussive injury during graft impaction.[70,186,196] Flynn, reporting on the collective experience of 36 657 cases, noted 311 neurologic injuries;[71] of these 100 were found to have a permanent myelopathy or radiculomyelopathy. He reported that 53 of 70 postoperative myelopathic complications were immediate in onset. However, actual intraoperative trauma was recorded in only 38 cases. The incidence of myelopathic complication in other reports is low, ranging from 0% to 2.1% (Table 20.1). Unfortunate plunging of an instrument into the spinal cord has been reported by one author.[39] Spinal cord damage during anterior cervical surgery has been reported by others in the literature.[14,62,74,121,122,208]

Removal of the posterior longitudinal ligament is controversial, but believed to be necessary in some cases to remove perforating disc fragments or large osteophytes. This should be performed with the aid of the operating microscope to minimize the potential for injury to the dura or spinal cord. Violation of the posterior longitudinal ligament in anterior cervical surgery has been associated with an increase in direct spinal cord injuries.[14,15,17,21,141,150] When removing osteophytes, a burr is used first to thin the offending spurs. Frequent irrigation is useful to diminish the local thermal effects and improve visualization. Once adequately thinned, small curettes can be used to 'pluck' the remaining portion of the osteophyte in a posterior-to-anterior direction, facilitating removal and protecting the underlying dura and spinal cord from injury. Utmost care should be taken when removing osteophytes and disc material in the lateral corner near the uncovertebral joint to avoid nerve root injury. As stated earlier, vigorous attempts to remove osteophytes should be avoided.[14,106] By following these simple steps in spur removal, neurologic injury can be avoided.

Krause and Stauffer[106] reported on ten surgically induced spinal cord injuries; 50% of these were directly attributed to use of surgical instruments or bone graft insertion. There was one transverse myelitis thought to be secondary to use of electrocautery on the posterior longitudinal ligament. The etiology was unclear in the remaining patients; however, vascular compromise to the anterior arterial system was thought to be pathogenic.[106] The anterior spinal artery is essentially independent with no collateral circulation. An important radicular artery to the cervical cord enters at the C5–C6 or C6–C7 foramen and is second only in size to the artery of Adamkiewicz. Loss of this radicular artery or a significant decrease in blood flow through this vessel may cause ischemic changes in the cervical cord.[106]

Table 20.1 Incidence of myelopathic complications for anterior cervical spine surgery

Author	*No.*	*(%)*	*Reference*
DePalma	1 of 281	(0.35)	50
Flynn		(0.1)	71
Lesoin	4 of 800	(0.5)	114
Simmons	0 of 154	(0)	173
Yonenobu	2 of 95	(1.8)	216
Yonenobu	8 of 384	(2.1)	217

Spinal cord compression may also result from epidural hematoma formation or from a misplaced or dislodged bone graft. To prevent epidural hematoma formation, routine postoperative use of drains is recommended. Removal of the posterior longitudinal ligament is often associated with bleeding. Meticulous hemostasis with irrigating bipolar electrocautery, set at a lower setting, is recommended. With any evidence of early or late spinal cord compression secondary to bone graft protrusion or hematoma, expeditious re-exploration is required.[159]

Thoracic Duct Injury

Anterolateral approaches to the lower cervical spine on the left side and approaches to the cervicothoracic junction carry the added risk of injury to the thoracic duct. The thoracic duct ascends lateral to the esophagus in the chest and lies on the prevertebral fascia. It then courses over the subclavian artery at the level of T1, anterior to the scalenus anterior, and enters the subclavian vein. A chylomediastinum or chylous effusion may develop if injured and unrecognized. When injured, it is recommended that the thoracic duct be ligated twice on each stump.[117] In a series of 75 anterior cervical decompressions, Bohlman and Eismont[20] reported one case of thoracic duct injury which was successfully treated with bedrest.

Anterior Graft Complications

Complications associated with anterior bone grafting and fusion are common and may include graft extrusion, collapse, resorption, or non-union. A multitude of anterior cervical grafting techniques have been described, including those of Cloward, Smith–Robinson, Simmons, and Bailey–Badgely. All of these techniques can be used safely and effectively in routine surgery for cervical disc disease. Strut grafting techniques using fibula or iliac crest are used in cases requiring vertebrectomy for myelopathy, tumor, and infection.

The most commonly used graft is some modification of the Smith–Robinson interbody graft. The Smith–Robinson interbody fusion has been found to be biomechanically superior when compared to other described techniques, and is the one favored by the present authors. The graft ideally should be 8–9 mm in height, or 2 mm greater in height than the preoperative degenerated disc space, to obtain maximal compressive strength while maximally enlarging the neural foramina.[2,29] Overdistraction of the disc space by using a graft too large may result in narrowing of the adjacent neural foramina. Too small a graft may not relieve nerve compression and may lead to graft resorption. When preparing the end-plates for graft insertion, care should be taken to maintain the integrity of the subchondral plate, while allowing for sufficient vascular flow to the graft. Excessive removal or trimming of the subchondral plate may lead to interspace collapse and kyphosis. To avoid resorption, the graft should be at least 5 mm in height.[16] The incidence of graft collapse appears to be slightly higher for allograft than autograft. If graft collapse results in significant kyphosis, especially in patients who have undergone multiple vertebrectomies and strut grafting, revision surgery is required (Fig. 20.2).

Graft extrusion usually occurs anteriorly away from the spinal cord, and can be associated with tracheal obstruction, esophageal dysphagia, development of kyphosis, and neurologic symptoms. Esophageal perforation is a rare, but potential, risk of extrusion. Postoperative myelopathy may occur in cases with posteriorly displaced grafts.[41,106] The incidence of graft extrusion is variable, but reported from 1% to 13% (Table 20.2).[81] It has been noted that the incidence of quadriplegia secondary to graft extrusion is more common with use of the dowel technique.[106] Adherence to meticulous surgical technique is the key to prevention of these graft complications. Anterior graft extrusion can be avoided if the graft is countersunk 2 mm behind the anterior cortical margin of the vertebral body (Fig. 20.3). Posteriorly, when the end-plate is burred, a lip should be left to avoid retrodisplacement of the graft into the canal. If posterior graft displacement is associated with neurologic compromise, immediate surgical intervention is required. Routine use of an intraoperative lateral radiograph, and posterior palpation of the graft with a nerve

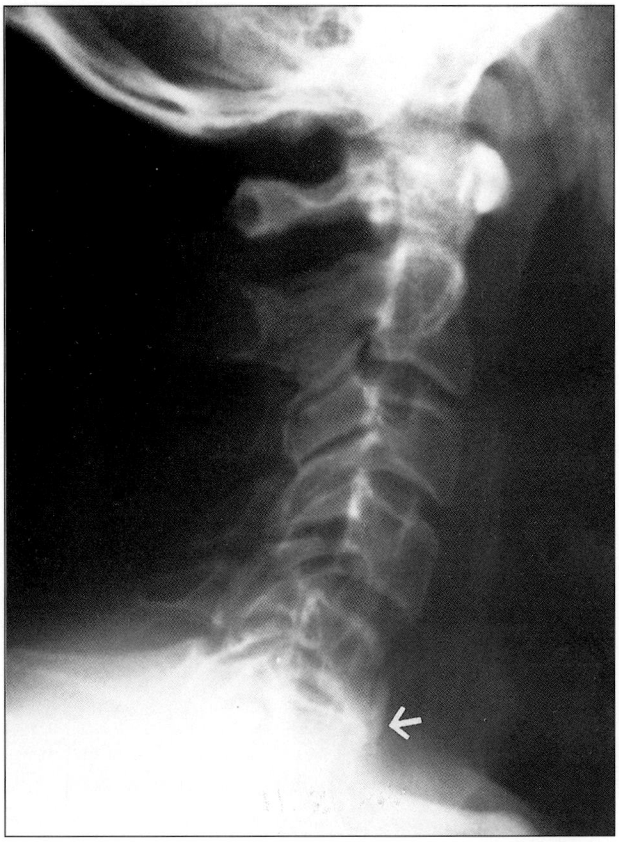

Figure 20.2
Anterior cervical fusion with subsequent collapse of allograft at C5–C6 level (arrow)

Table 20.2 Incidence of graft extrusion after anterior cervical fusion

Author	*Percentage*	*Reference*
DePalma	3	50
Gore	4.1	79
Lunsford	4.4	122
Simmons		173
Cloward	5.8	
Keystone	1.5	
Tew	2	191

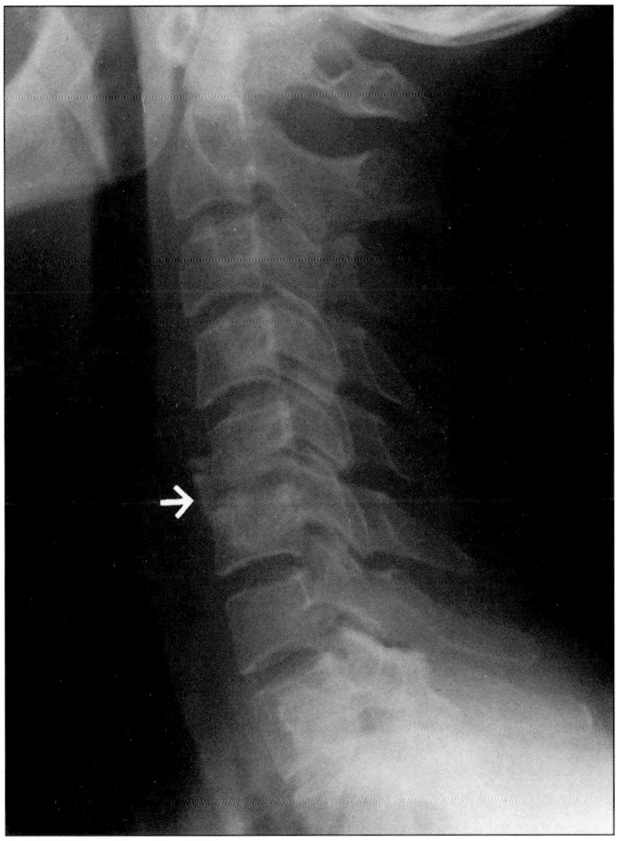

Figure 20.3
Anterior cervical fusion at C5–C6 with extrusion of allograft and subsequent fusion. Note the diminished disc height (arrow)

hook to ensure the presence of available space between the graft and dura, are advised to avoid this complication. Anterior extrusion of cervical grafts may be observed only as long as the patient is asymptomatic.

Anterior graft extrusion is a common complication in the postoperative period when an unrecognized posterior column injury is present.[11,40,67,143,182] Bell and Bailey[11] noted four graft displacements after performing anterior cervical fusions in patients with facet dislocations. Van Petegham and Schweigel[198] reported migration of anterior grafts in 6 of 12 patients with facet dislocation posterior ligament injury. In Bohlman's review[12] of 300 patients, 22 patients underwent anterior grafting after sustaining a flexion injury. Two grafts displaced in the two patients with posterior ligamentous injury. Stauffer and Kelly[182] reported a significant incidence of graft complication or late kyphotic deformities in those patients with unrecognized posterior ligamentous instability. Other studies have recommended and demonstrated the benefits of initial posterior stabilization before anterior reconstruction.[40,144]

Table 20.3 Pseudoarthrosis rate after anterior cervical fusion

Author	*Percentage*	*Reference*
Aronson	4	6
Connolly	21	45
DePalma	12	50
Gore	3	79
Riley	18	149
Robinson	12	152
Simmons		173
Cloward	18	
Keystone	0	
Stuck		185
Cloward	5	
White	26	208
Williams	10	214

Another complication of anterior cervical fusion is non-union (Figs 20.4 and 20.5). The incidence of pseudoarthrosis after anterior cervical fusion has been reported from 0% to 26% (Table 20.3). Failure of fusion is reported to be greater using the dowel technique,[172,198] whereas use of the trapezoidal graft described by Simmons in one series had no cases of non-union.[172,190] The use of a T-shaped graft has also demonstrated a low incidence of non-union in anterior cervical fusions.[20] Multi-level fusions have been associated with a higher rate of non-union compared with a single level fusion (Fig. 20.6).[116,148,207]

Fibula and iliac crest strut grafts can be used in multi-level vertebrectomy cases for myelopathy.[209] The potential for complication is greater for these grafts when compared to other described interbody fusions. Whitecloud and LaRocca[209] reported three cases of displaced fibular strut grafts in 19 patients. However, Roger[153] reported no cases of graft extrusion in his series. Many patients are asymptomatic despite radiographic evidence of non-union, and therefore require no treatment.[91,170] To prevent such complications, these grafts must be securely keyed into position. An adequate period of immobilization is required for healing, usually 6 months. With inadequate anterior

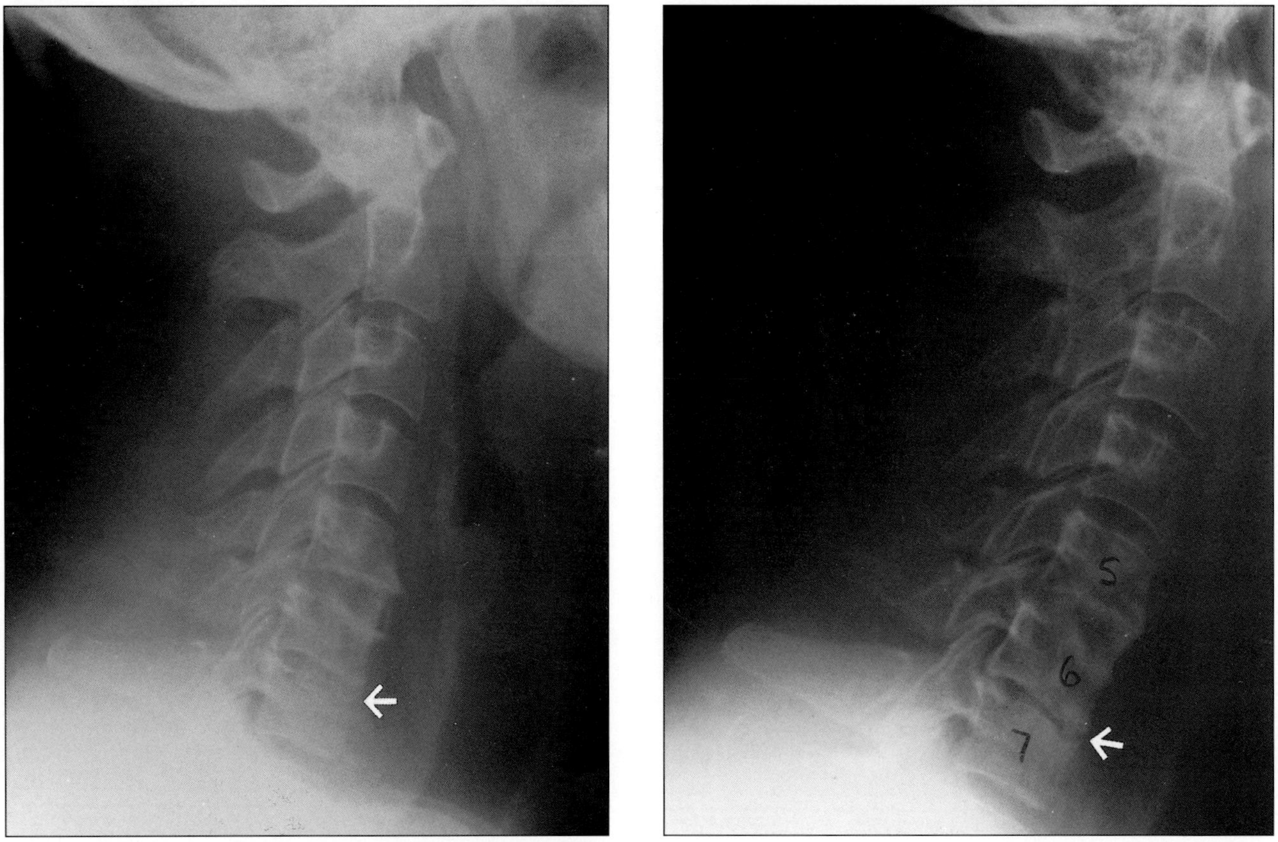

a b

Figure 20.4
(a) Lateral radiograph demonstrating an anterior cervical fusion with autogenous iliac crest graft at C5–C6, C6–C7. (b) Lateral radiograph demonstrating complete healing at C5–C6 and the development of a symptomatic pseudoarthrosis at C6–C7 with graft collapse (arrow)

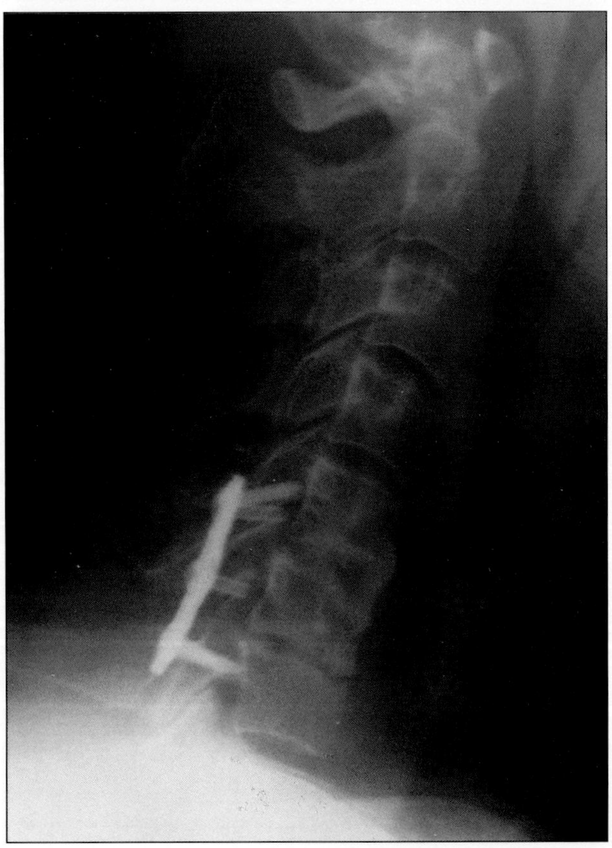

Figure 20.5
Treatment of symptomatic pseudoarthrosis by posterior fusion with plate and screw fixation

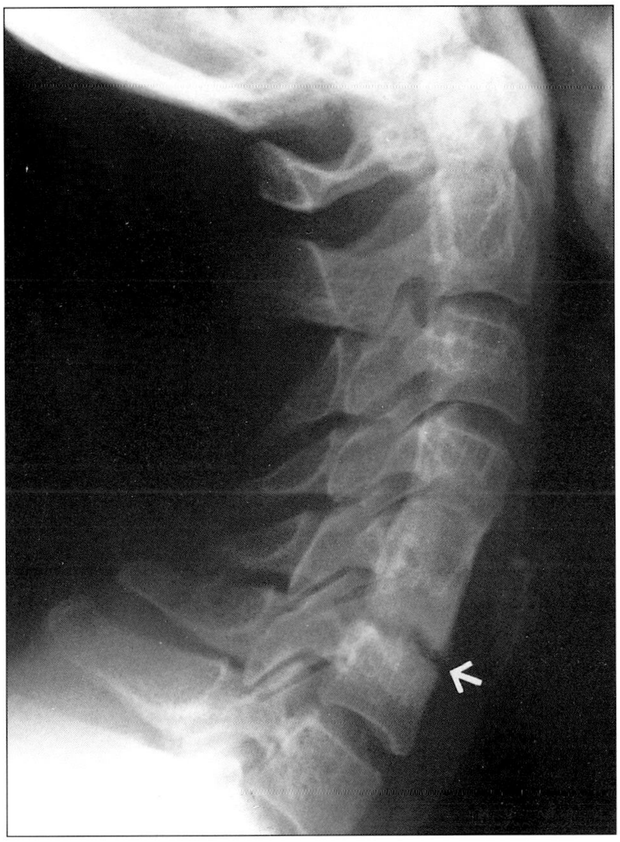

Figure 20.6
Pseudoarthrosis of C5–C6 after two-level anterior cervical fusion (arrow)

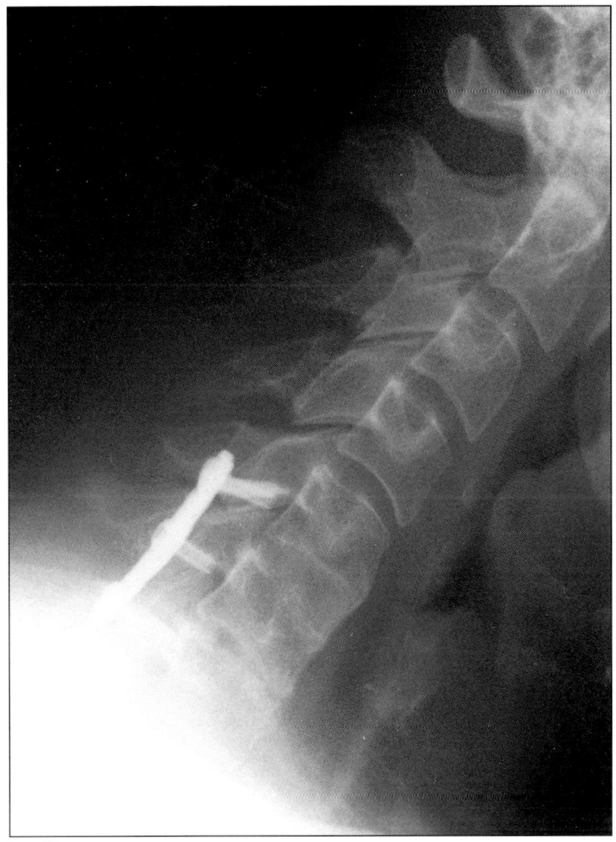

Figure 20.7
Treatment of a pseudoarthrosis at C6–C7 by posterior fusion with lateral mass screws and pelvic reconstruction plate

fixation, concomitant posterior stabilization should be contemplated. Fortunately, most pseudoarthroses are asymptomatic. However, for patients who experience pain refractory to conservative measures, a posterior fusion is preferredqover anterior revision surgery, due to post-operative scarring and the potential for injury to the esophagus and neurovascular structures of the neck (Fig. 20.7).

COMPLICATIONS OF POSTERIOR CERVICAL SPINE SURGERY

The posterior approach to the cervical spine is commonly used in treatment of cervical spine trauma, decompression of the spinal cord or nerve roots, excision of tumors, and most commonly in stabilization procedures of the cervical spine. The posterior approach is a safe and utilitarian approach which allows for an extensile exposure of the posterior cervical elements from the occipitocervical region to the cervicothoracic junction. The multitude of vital anatomic structures encountered in the anterior approach is not a factor; however, there are unique complications which may be encountered posteriorly and lead to significant morbidity and mortality.

Vascular Injury

Posterior cervical procedures have the inherent risk of injury to the vertebral artery at any point in its course from the foramen transversarium to the foramen magnum. The vertebral artery is most susceptible during upper cervical spine approaches for atlantoaxial and occipitocervical instability. Potential for injury to the vertebral arteries is greatest as they cross the C1–C2 articulation and then traverse the posterior ring of the atlas. Posterior dissection on C1 should stop 1.5 cm lateral to the posterior tubercle of C1 in adults, and 1.0 cm in children to minimize injury to the vertebral artery. Avoidance of vigorous dissection lateral to the dorsal ramus of C2, between the C1–C2 foramen, will also help avert injury to the vertebral artery as it exits the bony canal and courses towards the ring of C1. Reports of vertebral artery injury are rare from the posterior approach. Those reported have mostly been due to overzealous retraction or inadvertent placement of dissecting tools.[149,179] Electrocautery was the causative source in three cases reported by Rizzoli.[149] Stambough and Simeone[179] noted two cases which resulted from vigorous subperiosteal dissection for exposure of C1. No neurologic sequelae developed in either case in which the bleeding was simply controlled by packing.[179] Prolonged or excessive retraction of the vertebral artery may lead to occipital cortex ischemia when collateral circulation is compromised.[97] The neurologic sequelae of such ischemia generally include a bilateral homonymous hemianopia or cortical blindness. Injury may also result in a vertebral artery insufficiency syndrome if the collateral circulation is compromised. The vertebral artery may be ligated if needed with a low risk of deficit.[166]

The vertebral artery is at risk in the lower cervical spine, especially during insertion of lateral mass screws. Attention to detail, particularly in directing the drill bit and screw laterally, will tend to avoid this complication.

Injury to the central retinal artery of the eye secondary to pressure from a poorly positioned headrest in the prone position may result in thrombosis and subsequent blindness.[97] This may be averted by using a pinholder headrest, thereby alleviating the need to rest the face on any surface.

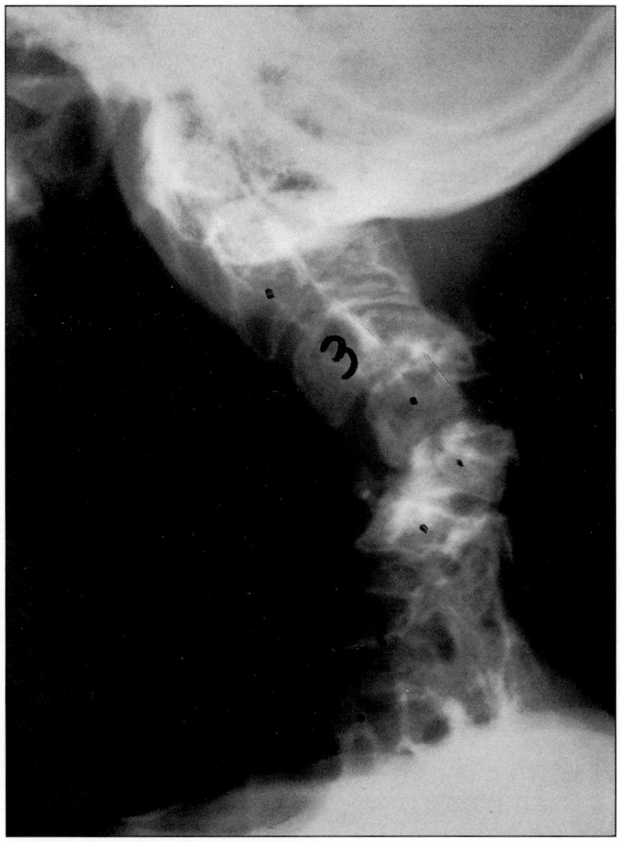

Figure 20.8
Lateral radiograph of a severe kyphotic deformity after laminectomy of the cervical spine without stabilization. Note the subluxation of C3 on C4 in addition to the angular deformity

Neurologic Injury

Posterior cervical spine surgery resulting in a spinal cord injury has rarely been reported in patients undergoing foraminotomy for cervical radiculopathy. However, such complications can and will occur in those patients undergoing complete laminectomy for myelopathy. The Cervical Spine Research Society polled its members, and reported in 1989[80] that the overall incidence of neurologic complication is higher (2.18%) in posterior surgery than reported in anterior procedures (0.64%). It is the authors' belief that somatosensory evoked potentials should be used in all myelopathy cases to minimize any injury that may result from decompression. Root injury during foraminotomy is usually the result of excessive nerve root manipulation. Such an injury may be severely disabling, particularly if it involves the C5 or C8 nerve root, but, fortunately, most of these deficits recover. Laminotomy and partial facetectomy without excision of the disc material may decrease the incidence of neural injury secondary to manipulation. Henderson et al[90] reported that foraminotomy alone gave good results and noted a postoperative sensory deficit in 5.7% and a motor deficit in 0.4% of patients. Sensory involvement is usually not of significance.

Laminectomy, in the treatment of cervical spine trauma, has been shown to result in loss of neural function, and is generally contraindicated as a decompressive procedure under these circumstances.[32] Of 300 cervical spine injuries reviewed by Bohlman,[12] 55 patients were treated with laminectomy. Of these, 22% had an increase in permanent neural loss as detected after surgery. Those treated nonoperatively or who underwent isolated stabilization procedures without decompression, sustained no additional permanent neurologic loss. Patients with incomplete neurologic injuries were noted to have significant deterioration following laminectomy (Fig. 20.8). It must be understood that posterior decompression for an anteriorly compressive lesion does not relieve cord compression,[12,17,128,134] and may allow for increased instability and translation of the involved segments. Such a result is neurologically counterproductive.[8,13,30,134,168,169,183] Laminectomy carries with it a significant risk for subsequent injury to the neural elements, estimated to be as high as 30%.[12,15,17,19,134] Quadriplegic patients have been reported to have a higher mortality rate after undergoing laminectomy.[12]

Respiratory Complications

Intraoperative injury to the upper cervical cord may lead to pulmonary complications including sleep-induced respiratory failure (Ondine's curse), which results from injury to the reticulospinal tracts.[12,57,68,69,105] Passage of sublaminar wires at the C1 level is commonly performed and rarely associated with neurologic compromise. However, at C2, the amount of free space available for the spinal cord is diminished.[12,15] The spinal cord may be contused from wire passage at this level, and lead to respiratory arrest.[69] Use of a strict and meticulous technique will prevent inadvertent injury. Cord retraction should never be attempted.

Posterior Graft Complications

Pseudoarthrosis of the cervical spine is multifactorial and can be related to the approach, surgical technique, age, use of allograft, and method of fixation and immobilization. Non-unions of the upper cervical spine have been well documented in surgically and non-surgically treated cases involving the occipitocervical, atlantoaxial, and odontoid regions.[12,19,72,88,93,125,130,133,137,154,162,163] Fielding et al.[68] reporting on 57 upper cervical fusions, including 46 Gallie-type atlantoaxial and 11 occipitocervical fusions, noted one non-union of a Gallie fusion and two occipitocervical non-unions. Edmunds and colleagues[56] reported 18 non-unions in 44 atlantoaxial fusions and 3 non-unions in 20 occipitocervical fusions. The use of wire fixation in performing such fusions added to stability of the surgical construct and improved fusion rate.[56] Other authors have reported success with occipitocervical fusions and clinical results.[44,87,118,204] Thompson and Mayer[193] reported a 90% fusion rate in 10 patients undergoing posterior C1–C2 fusions. Griswold et al,[82] reporting on C1–C2 fusions, noted four non-unions in 10 Gallie-type fusions and one non union in 30 Brooks-type fusions. The Brooks-type fusion, which uses sublaminar wires at both C1 and C2, has been shown to be superior in stability, especially rotation, when compared to the Gallie technique. Brooks and Jenkins[24] reported one pseudoarthrosis in 12 patients. White and associates[206] have demonstrated that lateral placement of these sublaminar wires helps to limit rotation, flexion, and extension.

Non-union of upper cervical fusions in children is less common. Koop[104] reviewed upper cervical fusions in children and noted one non-union in nine patients immobilized in just a halo vest orthosis. This patient was fused with allograft material. Stabler et al[178] reported on seven children with posterior cervical fusions with allograft and wire who developed non-union. Use of autogenous iliac crest bone graft is obviously advised.

Non-union of posterior fusions performed in the lower cervical spine is rare, and almost non-existent in children. Spontaneous fusion with extension of the fusion mass cephalad or caudad to the desired level is commonly seen. It is therefore prudent to expose only the involved levels to avoid unnecessary fused segments. The present authors prefer the triple-wire technique of posterior spine stabilization described by Bohlman.[12] In his review of 72 patients, there were no non-unions. Cadaveric studies confirm the rigidity of the construct with similar properties to posterior plating techniques.[43]

Cervical Instability as a Complication of Posterior Surgical Procedures

Deformities of the cervical spine can develop early or late in the treatment of posterior cervical diseases or injury and are usually the result of error in judgment regarding the treatment plan. Post-laminectomy cervical kyphosis is seen in a high percentage of children and adolescents,[33,86,119,120,184] but is uncommon in the adult.[63,99] It is more commonly seen in adults as a complication of partial facetectomy and in those patients with preoperative evidence of instability. Post-laminectomy instability is usually recognized as a progressive kyphotic deformity but may also present as a translational or extension type of deformity (Fig. 20.9). Johnson reported that spinal stability is compromised by 20% after cervical laminectomy. This increases to 60% with disruption of the facet joints.[100] Alteration of the load-bearing capabilities of the anterior or posterior structures is felt by White and colleagues[205] to lead to instability. Herkowitz[91] reported on 3 of 12 patients who underwent cervical laminectomy and bilateral partial facetectomy and developed kyphotic deformities within 2 years. It is generally felt that preoperative evidence of instability must be present for the adult to develop postoperative cervical kyphosis (Figs 20.10 and 20.11). This has been supported by the work of Mikawa in a series of 64 patients who underwent multiple level cervical laminectomies.[132]

Degenerative changes and development of instability above or below fusion masses are also of concern, and may lead to development of late neurologic symptoms of the juxtafused segments.[213,215] Altered biomechanics from the fused segments place additional stress on the adjacent motion segments and may accelerate degenerative change.[23,31,50,98]

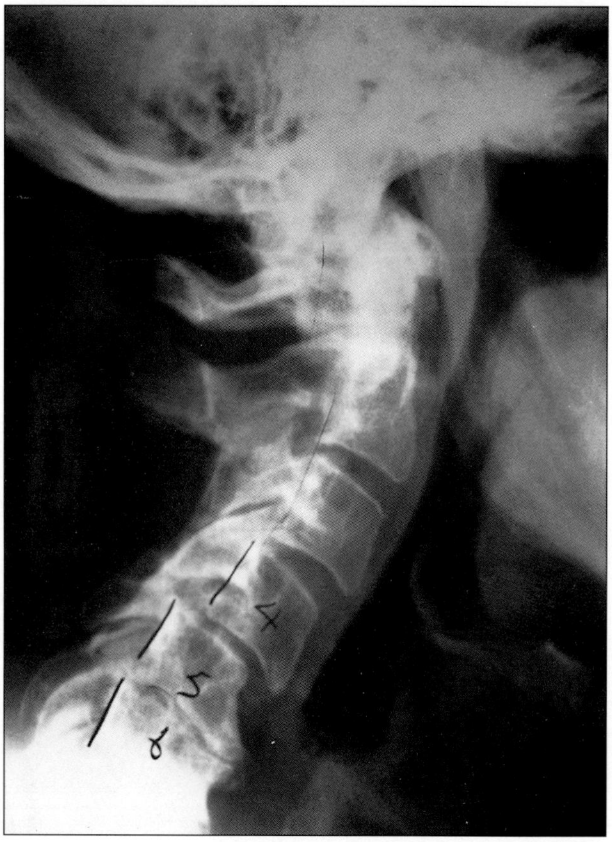

Figure 20.9
Post-laminectomy instability of the cervical spine with anterior vertebral subluxation of C4 over C5 and minimal angular deformity

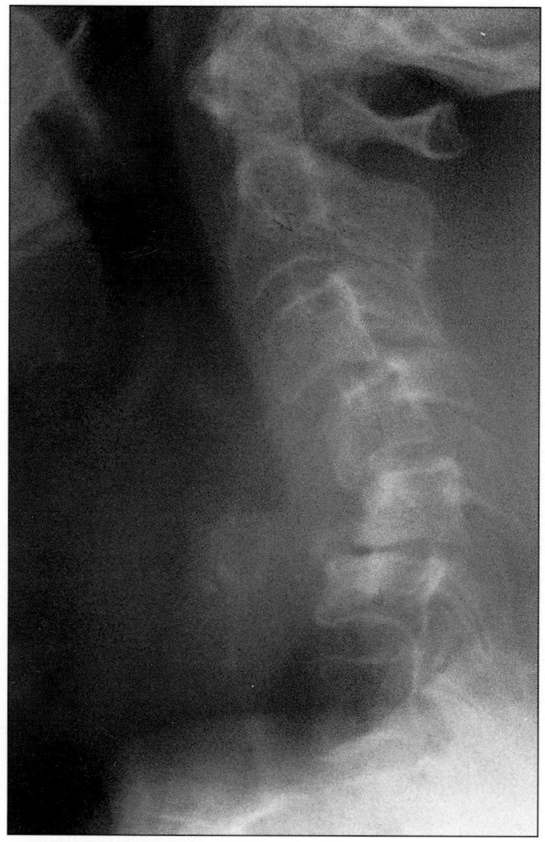

Figure 20.10
Radiograph of a progressive post-laminectomy instability and kyphotic deformity of C3–C6

Other potential errors which may lead to development of cervical deformity or instability include: failure to recognize the mechanism of injury in traumatic lesions, thereby failing to recognize the extent of ligamentous or bony injury; failure to employ proper surgical techniques needed for sufficient stability; improper or insufficient external immobilization until bony healing is adequate; and improper or inappropriate use of cervical instrumentation (Figs 20.12–20.14). The posterior cervical approach can result in increased permanent neurologic loss to the patient or development of late kyphosis, if posterior column injury is not recognized in cervical trauma.[12,15,30,114,135,169] Burst fractures of the cervical spine treated with isolated posterior fusion may also result in kyphosis. To prevent such deformity, surgical reconstruction of the anterior column is recommended. As noted earlier, decompressive laminectomy for traumatic cervical spinal cord injury may result in kyphosis and potentiate further neurologic injury.[8,15,30,35,165,183,189] Late development of neurologic symptoms with associated deformity may require extensive reconstructive procedures.[12,30] The development of cervical kyphosis in children has been well documented after laminectomy.[33,34,119,120] Its development can be quite rapid and severe resulting in complete neurologic injuries.[27,168] The potential for growth and plasticity of the pediatric spine may play a role in its progression.[35]

GENERAL COMPLICATIONS OF CERVICAL SPINE SURGERY

The preparation for cervical spine surgery is demanding and varies according to the pathomechanics and pathoanatomy of the surgical lesion. Errors may occur at any stage of the decision-making process, including selection of

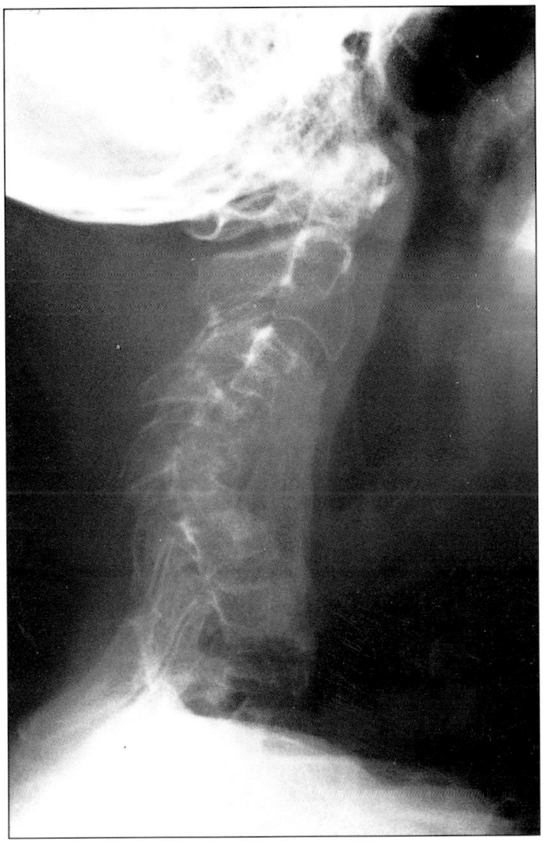

Figure 20.11
Lateral radiograph demonstrating solid fusion after anterior strut grafting and fusion from C3 to C7 for post-laminectomy instability and kyphosis

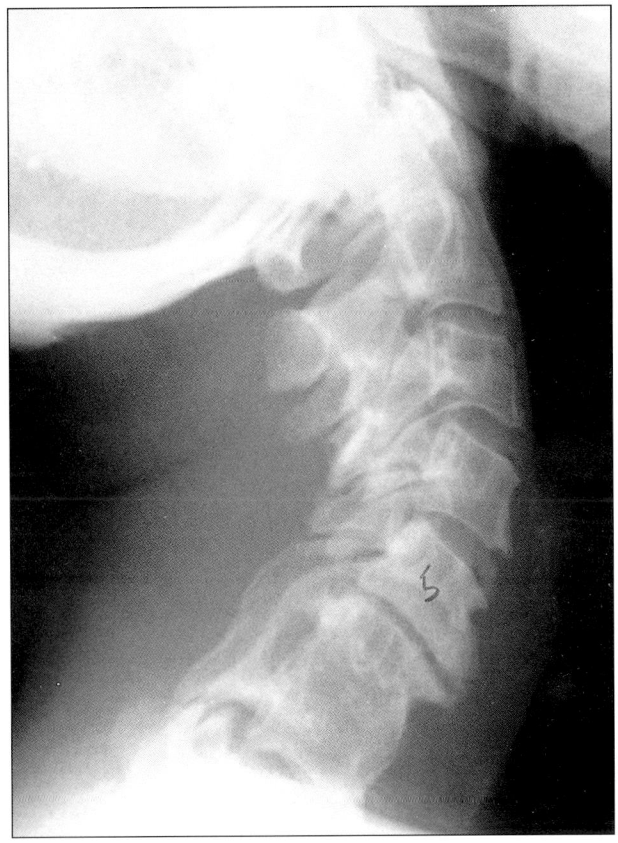

Figure 20.12
Lateral radiograph demonstrating post laminectomy instability with extension deformity and retrolisthesis of C3 on C4

surgical candidates, surgical approach and technique, and patient positioning. Various aspects of cervical spine surgery and the related complications will be discussed.

Complications of Positioning

Problems related to positioning are not unique to cervical spine surgery. Faulty positioning may ruin a technically perfect operation. Care should be taken to ensure that all peripheral nerves and the brachial plexus are protected during either prone or supine positioning. The brachial plexus is usually injured when the arm is extended over 90° in an anesthetized patient.[192] Parks[140] reported on 28 postoperative plexus injuries, with 14 each occurring in the supine and prone positions. The deficits may be mixed motor and sensory. Unfortunately, the motor loss tends to be much greater. The upper trunk of the brachial plexus tends to be more commonly involved. The ulnar nerve is the most common peripheral nerve that may be injured secondary to improper positioning. The nerve should be padded and protected to avoid direct pressure on the cubital tunnel.

Positioning of the head during cervical procedures requires careful attention to avoid spinal cord injury, especially in cases of myelopathy and instability. Extreme positions of the head should be avoided. Direct compression of the cervical cord by a spondylotic bar may occur with excessive flexion, extension, or rotation in patients with myelopathy. Intubation should be gentle and completed under fiberoptic guidance in patients with severe myelopathy. Somatosensory evoked potentials (SSEPs) should be monitored during the process of intubation as well as during the operative procedure. Care must be taken when moving the patient to avoid extreme positioning of the head. During the operative procedure, the head

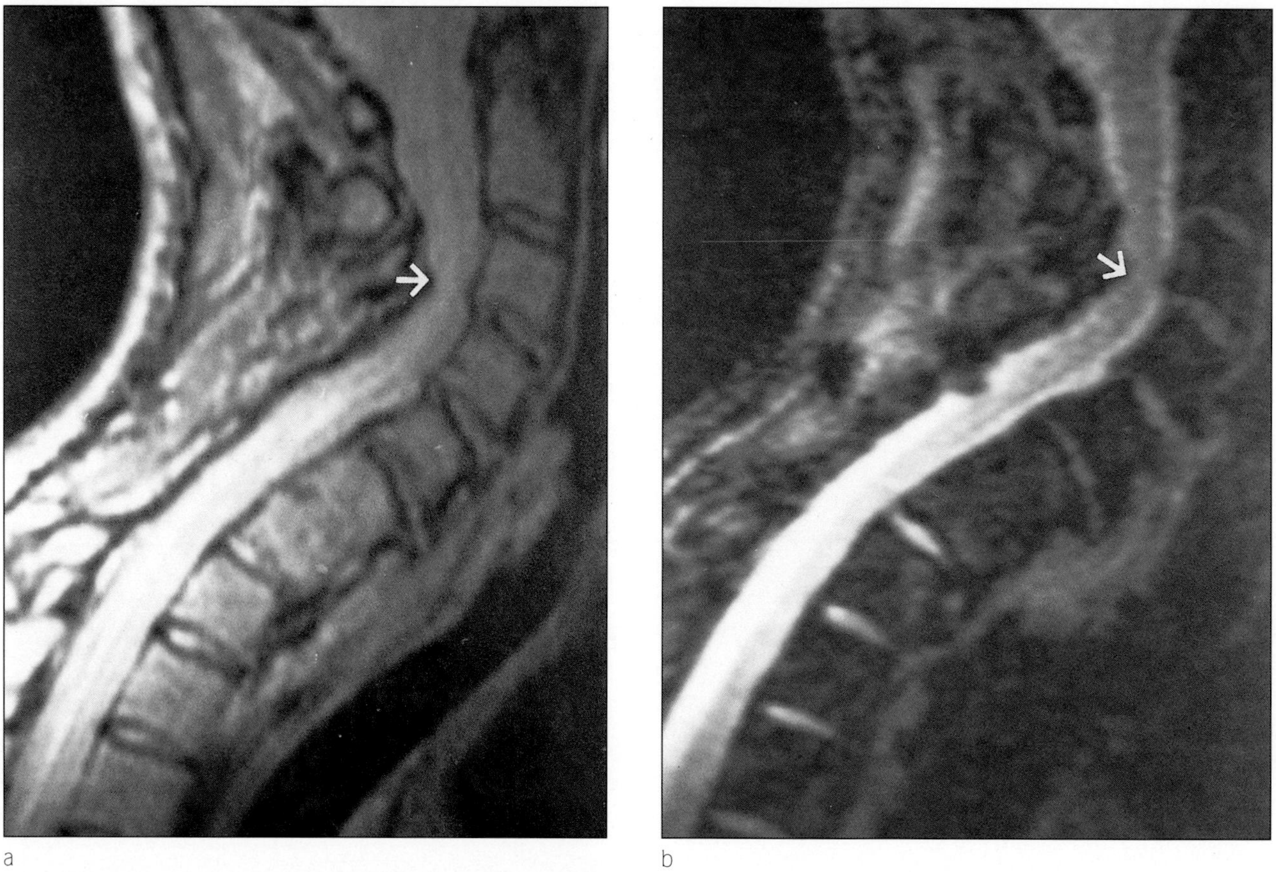

Figure 20.13
Magnetic resonance images of a symptomatic patient with post-laminectomy instability and an extension deformity. (a, b) T1- and T2-weighted images (respectively) showing compromise of the spinal cord at C3–C4 and C4–C5 (arrow)

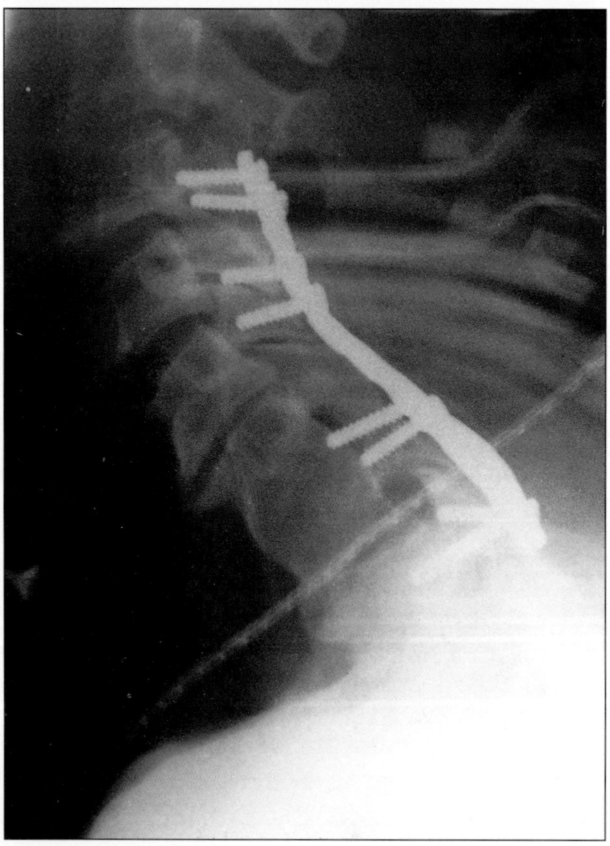

Figure 20.14
Stabilization and fusion of posterior cervical spine with plate and screws after decompression of cord impingement resulting from a post-laminectomy extension deformity

should be secured to a headrest or held firmly in a pinholder headrest. Generally, three to four fingerbreadths of space should be maintained between the chin and the sternum. The loss and reappearance of SSEPs during positioning has been recorded.[212]

Complications may arise from use of head-fixation devices. The horseshoe headrest is not commonly used in operative procedures performed in the prone position. It relys on taping of the head for stability, and has resulted in necrosis of forehead skin and blindness secondary to prolonged pressure on the eye.[97] Blindness, from retinal artery thrombosis, may occur as a result of circumferential pressure on the eye. These complications are generally averted by using the pinholder headrest. Use of this device eliminates all pressure points, while securely holding the head and neck in the desired position. However, its use has also been associated with complications, including infection or osteomyelitis, scalp lacerations, pressure necrosis of surrounding skin, and skull fracture or perforation.[7] Care should be taken to prepare the skin with appropriate antiseptics. Careful pin placement will prevent skin necrosis and lacerations. Avoiding unnecessary tightening of the clamp and its use in thin or soft skulls will prevent fracture or perforation of the inner table. The possibility of an existing skull fracture should be eliminated in cases of trauma to avoid subsequent dural penetration, brain abscess formation, or epidural hematomas.

The sitting position is used by many surgeons during posterior spine surgery as it greatly reduces venous bleeding. It is, however, associated with an increased risk of air embolism, which potentially is one of the most serious complications in cervical spine surgery. The degree of risk correlates directly with the gravitational gradient.[1,180,217] The higher the incision is placed above the level of the heart, the greater the risk of air embolism. Most air emboli are not clinically significant, but with sensitive monitoring techniques, have been reported to have an incidence of 25% in the sitting position.[1]

Complications of Anesthesia

In patients with known myelopathy, an unstable cervical spine, or an incomplete spinal cord injury, it is of paramount importance to use caution during intubation to avoid subsequent catastrophic neurologic injury. An awake nasotracheal or fiberoptic intubation is helpful in avoiding excessive manipulation of the spine. The controversy regarding oral versus nasal, and awake versus anesthetized, intubation was reviewed in a recent report by Suderman et al.[185] In this study, no significant progression or onset of neurologic symptoms was demonstrated with the various techniques.

Cervical trauma patients with spinal cord injury have a labile cardiovascular system in addition to instability of the cervical spine. Disruption of the sympathetic nervous system has been shown to increase the cardiovascular lability.[195] Reported cases of cardiopulmonary arrest after induction with succinylcholine have been found to result from a marked increase in serum potassium in spinal cord-injured patients.[9,84] The paralyzed muscles release high levels of potassium in response to succinylcholine.

The induction and surgical monitoring should be accompanied by SSEP monitoring in all cases of concern. Episodes of hypotension can produce cord anoxia which results from poor autoregulation of blood flow in patients with significant myelopathy.[97]

Dural Injury

Factors that may predispose a patient to dural injury include a history of previous surgery, inexperience of the operating surgeon, or failure to adhere to the basic principles of spinal surgery. Dural leaks are usually caused by the high-speed burr or other instrument during disc or bone removal. Dural leaks or tears after anterior spinal surgery are uncommon as most surgery preserves the posterior longitudinal ligament. If, however, removal of the posterior ligament is required to remove sequestered disc fragments or osteophytes, an operating microscope should be used to avoid injury to the dura. Dural repairs in the anterior cervical spine can be very difficult, if not impossible, to perform. If possible, a leak is best repaired using a small running suture on an atraumatic needle or using the suture technique described by Guity and Young.[85] If the leak cannot be repaired primarily, the use of a Surgicel patch covered with muscle or Gelfoam may often work, or a fascial graft usually suffices.[190] Other options may include use of a lyophilized dural graft combined with fibrin glue. There is a risk of HIV transmission with use of pooled fibrinogen. Use of the patient's own blood is optimal.[54,167] A case of Jakob–Creutzfeldt disease has been reported following use of a cadaveric dura mater graft.[214] Risk of dural injury is significantly greater during a complete laminectomy than with a unilateral foraminotomy. Pseudomeningocele has been reported after cervical laminectomy.[97] An identified dural tear should be closed in a meticulous manner and the incision closed watertight. A reverse Trendelenburg position decreases the hydrostatic pressure, and may facilitate surgical repair. Drains are usually not placed under these circumstances. Care must be taken to not compromise the intraluminal diameter of the dura during repair.[59] If the site of leak is seen but not suturable, fibrin glue may be effective.[164] Leaks in the cervical spine which cannot be repaired or patched may be effectively treated with bedrest, prophylactic antibiotics, and lumbar subarachnoid catheter drainage for a period of 72–96 hours to allow the wound to heal.[103] Re-exploration of the wound is necessary in recalcitrant cases who fail lumbar drainage. If a question arises as to the possibility of a leak or the formation of a pseudomeningocele, water-soluble contrast media with computed tomography or fluoroscopy may be used to localize it.[124]

Complications of Methylmethacrylate

Indications for use of methylmethacrylate in the treatment of cervical spine disorders are limited, and, to avoid complications, must be strictly adhered to.[129] Complications include, but are not limited to, failure of fixation, neurologic injury, infection, and dislodgement. The use of methylmethacrylate in the treatment of acute trauma should be condemned. McAfee et al[129] reported on the use of methylmethacrylate in 24 patients; 15 of these had sustained acute cervical injuries, 12 of whom developed loss of fixation. All of these failures involved posterior stabilization attempts. Eight of nine patients treated for spinal neoplasm also exhibited loss of fixation, with failure occurring at the bone–cement interface. Caution is needed when applying the principles of tumor stabilization to fracture–dislocations of the cervical spine. Loosening of these surgical constructs and dislodgement of cement struts occurs most often in regions of high mobility.[37,139] Failure at the bone–cement interface may eventually lead to fatiguing and breakage of wiring with subsequent loss of fracture reduction.[58,127] Perforation of the esophagus has been reported after loosening of a methylmethacrylate construct originally secured with two pins.[188] The risk of late infection and sepsis, usually from hematogenous spread, is greater with methylmethacrylate constructs in both tumor and fracture stabilization procedures.[58,139] Dunn, in reporting the results of a multicenter study, recommended the use of methylmethacrylate only in patients with metastatic disease or an unresectable primary tumor with a limited lifespan who could withstand surgery, and who may have severe pain or neurologic deficits which could be helped.[55] McAfee et al., in their review of 24 patients, felt that methylmethacrylate should only be used as a salvage technique in patients with a life expectancy of less than 1 year. They recommended further that use of methylmethacrylate be supplemented with autogenous bone grafts.[126,127] In brief, methylmethacrylate should be used for augmentation rather than for primary stabilization of these lesions.

Complications Associated with the Halo Orthosis

The halo orthosis is a frequently used device for immobilization of the unstable cervical spine. It is the only cervical orthosis to control rotation effectively, and its use can greatly facilitate early mobilization and rehabilitation of the patient. However, complications may occur during application of the device or during the period of immobilization. Pin-site loosening or infection is the most common complication, and can be prevented by proper application and daily pin care. Tight pins will remain sterile and will not become infected. The incidence of pin loosening has been reported to be 20% or more.[76] Infected pins should be removed and a new pin placed adjacent to the old site. The pins should be tightened to 6 inch pounds initially and then re-torqued to 6 inch pounds at 24–48 hours post-insertion. Continual tightening of the pins may lead to penetration of the skull with the potential for development of a brain abscess or meningitis. The pins should be placed laterally at the corner of the eyebrow, away from the supraorbital or supratrochlear nerves, to avoid injury. Discomfort and pin loosening will be common if the pins are placed in the temporal fossa.

The most serious problem with use of a halo orthosis is loss of reduction or position of the spine after reduction.[210] It must be understood that a change in position of the spine will occur with a change in position of the patient. Therefore, a very unstable spine may not be properly immobilized with a halo orthosis and require surgical stabilization. The vest must be correctly fitted to avoid shifting and change in spinal alignment. Constant vigilance should be used to prevent skin breakdown or pressure sores, particularly in quadriplegic patients.

Complications of Internal Fixation Devices

There are a multitude of internal fixation devices available for stabilization of the cervical spine. Anterior and posterior systems have been developed and may be beneficial in obtaining stability and promoting fusion, and yet, inappropriate or inadequate application of these devices may result in catastrophic consequences. The abundance of such instrumentation systems can lead to emphasis being mistakenly placed on mastering the technique of implant insertion, and to forgetting the primary goal of surgery, a solid bony fusion. All surgical implants will ultimately fail unless solid arthrodesis is obtained. Basic principles in spinal surgery must be strictly applied.

The use of wires in posterior fusion of the cervical spine can be associated with complications. The passage of sublaminar wires under C1 or C2 should be precise and controlled to avoid neurologic injury. Sublaminar wires should rarely, if ever, be passed under the lower cervical laminae. Spinous process wires are routinely used in the lower cervical spine and can be used safely. Care should be taken to pass the wires through a hole developed at the spinolaminar line, dorsal to the spinal cord, to avert neurologic injury or dural tear. Over-aggressive tightening of the spinous process wires should be avoided to prevent foraminal narrowing and subsequent nerve root compression at the involved segment. The technique of facet wiring provides biomechanically sound fixation, but it has the theoretical problem of accelerated degeneration of the adjacent unfused facets with the placement of wires. This is not a well-recognized problem in the literature, and clinically may be insignificant.

Transarticular screw fixation of the atlantoaxial joint is generally reserved for fixation of the C1–C2 articulation when there is a dens fracture with a concomitant posterior arch fracture of the atlas. This technique may also be used for an isolated odontoid fracture or odontoid non-union. Grob et al[83] reported on a cumulative series of 161 patients who had undergone posterior cervical fusion by transarticular screw fixation. There were only 10 complications directly related to screw insertion with no injuries reported to the vertebral artery or the medulla oblongata. Fractures of the dens can be treated with anterior or posterior fusion techniques. Clark and White[38] reported on a collection of patients with fractures of the dens and noted an increase in neurologic complications in those treated with an anterior procedure compared to posterior arthrodesis. Of 96 patients undergoing posterior cervical fusion, only one postoperative Brown–Séquard deficit was observed. Of eight patients undergoing anterior screw fixation for an odontoid fracture, there were two screw migrations with one resulting in ocular palsy, one patient with postoperative quadriparesis, and one patient with neurologic symptoms from a non-union requiring revision surgery.

The use of an interlaminar clamp to stabilize a motion segment in the cervical spine has been reported to give good results while avoiding the potential complications associated with passage of sublaminar wires in the upper or lower cervical spine. Holness and others[96] reported on the long-term results in 51 patients treated with the interlaminar Halifax clamp. Only two patients had loosening and slippage of the clamps requiring reoperation; this occurred early in the postoperative treatment period. There were no late displacements, no infections, and no neurologic deteriorations. Successful fusion was obtained without bone grafting in this series, but is not recommended by this author. Caution must be exercised when using the clamp for C1–C2 arthrodesis, as it is limited in its ability to control rotation and lateral bending. A risk of neurologic injury may result if the clamp is overtightened and the motion segment hyperextended.

Plate and screw fixation of the cervical spine can be used anteriorly and posteriorly in conditions of trauma, degenerative disease, and tumor surgery. The reason for using such devices is to obtain immediate rigid fixation while biologic fusion occurs. At no time should hardware be used alone in place of bony fusion. Posterior and anterior plating use different techniques and require meticulous surgical skills and attention to detail. A definite contraindication to plate screw fixation is severe osteoporosis. Potential complications include vertebral artery injury, neurologic injury, non-union, failure of fixation, and progressive kyphosis of the injured motion segment.

Posterior cervical plating requires a thorough knowledge of lateral mass anatomy, knowledge of neurovascular relationships to the lateral mass, and drill orientation. These techniques were pioneered by Roy-Camille in Paris.[155] Several techniques have been described for screw insertion to minimize potential for injury to the vertebral artery and nerve root, while avoiding facet impingement. An anatomic dissection was done to determine the safest direction of screw placement and the safest entry point of the drill bit.[3] The center of the articular pillar is identified, and the cortex penetrated with a small burr at a point 1 mm medial to the center or the 'hill'. Using a 2.5 mm drill bit, the pillar is drilled in a direction of 25–30° laterally and 15° cephalad for C3–C6. When drilling at C2, the drill should be angled 10–15° medially and 35° superiorly to avoid injuring the vertebral artery, which is exiting the foramen on its course to the C1 arch. The opposite cortex should be drilled, except at C2, and a drill stop used to avoid plunging. The seventh cervical vertebrae has a very thin lateral mass, and this presents a technical problem. Placement of a lateral mass screw at this level places the nerve root and facet joint at risk for injury. A hook-plate construct, as described by Magerl,[123] is preferred at the C7 region, as it provides good fixation without the need for an additional screw (see Fig. 20.15). Roy-Camille and colleagues[156] reported only four neurologic injuries in 238 cases of posterior cervical plating for lower cervical injuries.

There are various devices now available for anterior cervical fixation. Potential complications include vascular injury, loosening, esophageal erosion, and neurologic injury secondary to posterior cortex penetration.[201] Meyer et al[131] reported on their large series of 92 patients undergoing anterior cervical fusion with anterior plate stabilization. They noted four patients with screw loosening with only one requiring reoperation for dysphagia. There were no neurologic injuries directly related to bicortical fixation. Caspar[33] reported on 50 patients who underwent anterior cervical plating with a trapezoidal plate and noted four loosenings. Other authors have noted good clinical success and fusion rates with the use of the trapezoidal osteosynthetic plate.[4,146] Recommendations to minimize loosening of fixation include avoidance of screw placement across unfused disc spaces, thereby avoiding micromotion. Placement of the screws at least 2 mm from the adjacent end-plate will allow adequate screw purchase while minimizing potential for cutout or displacement into the disc space. External immobilization is recommended to facilitate early consolidation and fusion.

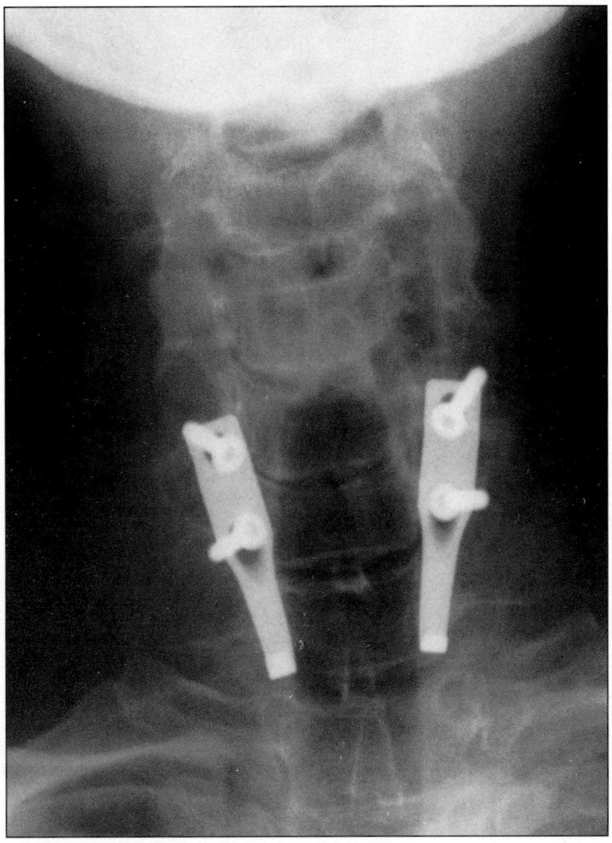

Figure 20.15
Posterior cervical fusion after laminectomy with a hook-plate system which avoids the placing of lateral mass or pedicle screws in the transitional lateral mass of C7

Complications of Autogenous Bone Grafting

The role of autogenous bone grafting in cervical spine surgery is very important, as it facilitates the fusion process and subsequently decreases rehabilitation time. This is particularly important after cervical spine injuries. The harvesting of autologous bone is not without complication, however, as it can be a source of chronic pain or disability for the patient.[46,49,50,73,110,138,147,170,172,181,208] Altered sensation over the donor site appears to be the most common complaint, and may be in the form of anesthesia, hyperesthesiae, dysesthesiae or chronic pain.[42,187,218] DePalma et al,[49] reporting on complications after anterior iliac crest harvest for anterior cervical fusions, noted a 9% incidence of hematoma and some degree of chronic pain in 36%. Dawson et a[48]. noted a 12% incidence of significant donor site pain, whereas Frymoyer et al[73] found 37% of patients to complain of donor site pain 10 or more years after their operations. The difference between true donor site pain and the addition of donor site to a general pain syndrome may be difficult to distinguish.[66]

Serious injury to adjacent neural structures may lead to chronic pain and significant morbidity. These may include injury to the lateral femoral cutaneous nerve, ilioinguinal nerve, cluneal nerves, and sciatic or superior gluteal nerves. Stauffer reported 2 of 75 patients with transient lateral femoral cutaneous nerve palsy.[181] Neuropraxia is the most common injury and is usually due to retraction rather than division of the nerve. Most of these injuries recover with time. The course of the lateral femoral cutaneous nerve is variable, and careful dissection is essential to avoid injury. The graft should not be taken within 2 cm of the anterosuperior iliac spine to avoid injury to the lateral femoral cutaneous nerve. The cluneal nerves are at risk during posterior harvest of bone. Dissection should remain within 7–8 cm of the posterosuperior iliac spine to avoid direct injury. In a series of over 500 posterior iliac crest grafts for spinal fusion, Goldstein[78] reported negligible problems associated with occasionally cutting the cluneal nerves. These patients did have complaints of some sensory loss over the buttocks. The development of neuromas may necessitate surgical excision. A midline or vertical approach to the posterior iliac crest is felt by some authors to avoid injury to the cluneal nerves,[42,107] whereas others[109,110] advocate the use of a separate lateral oblique incision to obtain greater exposure and more graft. Fernyhough et al[66] demonstrated, in a limited cadaveric dissection, no significant difference in harvested bone graft volume when comparing a midline versus a lateral approach to the iliac crest. They felt that a more vertical incision within 7-8 cm of the posterosuperior iliac crest will avoid possible injury to the superior cluneal nerves. There are no known reports of injury to the sciatic or femoral nerves; however, placement of a retractor too deeply or slippage of an instrument in the sciatic notch can lead to serious injury to the sciatic nerve. Avoidance of the notch is the best treatment.

Arterial injury is less common but may have catastrophic results. A case of a traumatic superior gluteal arteriovenous fistula formation and ureteral injury complicating a posterior iliac crest harvest was reported by Escalas et al.[61] This resulted from the slippage of a Taylor retractor into the sciatic notch with subsequent moderate bleeding. The fistula was documented by an arteriogram 2 weeks later. Kurz et al[110] noted three additional cases of injury to the superior gluteal artery with significant hemorrhage deep in the donor site wound. The artery should be explored in any questionable case and control obtained by ligation of the stump. Bone removal from the sciatic notch may be required to gain vascular control.

Hematoma formation is a common problem with either anterior or posterior iliac crest harvesting. DePalma[50] noted a 9% incidence of hematoma after harvest of the anterior iliac crest. Sacks[157] reported four wound hematomas after 150 procedures on the anterior iliac crest. Dick[51] noted 3 hematomas in 11 anterior wounds compared to 1 hematoma in 24 posterior wounds. He felt that posteriorly the large gluteal muscle mass may tamponade the bleeding vessels providing local hemostasis. Such a muscle mass is absent anteriorly and may account for the higher rate of hematoma formation seen in this position. Stauffer and Coventry[181] reported on 5 of 164 patients after bicortical graft harvest from the posterior iliac crest that required aspiration or drainage. Local hemostasis should be obtained through the use of bone wax, gelatin foam, or microcrystalline collagen. The judicious use of drains for 24–48 hours has reduced the incidence of hematomas to less than 1%.[110]

Although less common, other complications of bone grafting can be avoided with careful dissection and meticulous technique. Reported complications include symptomatic instability from harvesting partial or full-thickness grafts,[110,181] gross sacroiliac joint dislocation,[115] gait disturbance,[110] herniation of abdominal contents,[108,109] lumbar hernias,[46] peritoneal perforation,[109,110] and postoperative wound infections with osteomyelitis.[218] These complications can lead to significant patient morbidity and present a source of chronic pain to the patient. The use of local autologous bone for spinal fusions to minimize graft site morbidity has been reported by Keene and McKinley[101] in spinal fusions for traumatic thoracolumbar injuries. This technique has not been reported on in the cervical spine.

Alternatives to the use of autogenous grafts usually involve some form of cadaveric allograft, which avoids the problems of donor site morbidity, but may not facilitate healing unless it is placed under compression. Disadvantages of the use of allograft include its cost and its lack of osteoinductive properties. A newer recognized risk, although rare, is the transmission of fatal infectious diseases. There has been one reported transmission of HIV via a cadaveric graft.[194] This occurred in bone which was not freeze-dried or treated with ethylene oxide.

COMPLICATIONS OF SURGERY IN INFLAMMATORY DISEASES

Surgical treatment for rheumatoid arthritis and ankylosing spondylitis can be very satisfying for the patient and the surgeon, but may be wrought with complications if adequate preoperative planning and attention to detail are not carried through. The specific deformity needs to be addressed and the appropriate surgical procedure performed on the appropriate patient.

Rheumatoid Arthritis

Rheumatoid arthritis can affect any level of the cervical spine and may result in atlantoaxial subluxation, atlantoaxial subluxation combined with subaxial subluxation, isolated subaxial subluxation, and superior migration of the odontoid. The occiput–C1–C2 articulations are most commonly involved. Development of neurologic symptoms may occur, but in fact, is uncommon preoperative occurrence. With development of significant cervical instabilities and/or neurologic involvement in the rheumatoid patient, surgical decompression and stabilization are indicated. Most of these problems can be addressed with straightforward posterior arthrodesis. Atlantoaxial subluxation is the most common problem seen in rheumatoid patients, requiring surgical stabilization. Preoperative reduction of this deformity should be attempted through traction or patient positioning. Operative reduction should be avoided as it is associated with a higher rate of neurologic injury and potential mortality.[68,75,200] Neurologic deterioration may result from attempted passage of sublaminar wires. Clark et al[36] reported a case of transient hemiparesis secondary to passage of a sublaminar wire. Routine employment of somatosensory evoked potentials is recommended during these procedures. Generally these deformities are reduced before the operation, by placing the patient in a halo device with a C-ring. Once stabilized, the patient can be safely positioned and surgery performed. Perioperative mortality was of significant concern in early studies, but is now felt to be related more to the underlying disease process and not directly to the surgical procedure. Zoma and colleagues,[219] reporting on 40 procedures in 32 patients, noted a 35% failure rate, and an 8% incidence of perioperative death. These patients had severe preoperative neurologic deficits. Other complications in this series included nine graft failures and four infections. Heywood et al[92] reported on 30 surgical procedures in 26 patients and noted 12 successful fusions in 15 attempted atlantoaxial arthrodeses. There was also an 8% mortality rate in this study. Early surgical intervention with improved perioperative management and advances in anesthetic technique have resulted in lower mortality rates.[44,47,65,111,112,145,193]

Pseudoarthrosis is a not uncommon complication at the C1–C2 articulation. Bohlman[13] reported 10 unions in 17 patients with atlantoaxial subluxation. Ferlic and associates[65] reported a 50% fusion rate using the Gallie-type fusion. Conaty and Mongan[44] reported 67% satisfactory results in their patients. Clark and associates,[36] reporting on a series of 41 consecutive but variable types of cervical arthrodeses, noted an overall fusion rate of 88%. However, all non-unions occurred in attempted atlantoaxial fusions. A 15% non-union rate was noted by Clark and associates[36] using a Brooks-type fusion with methylmethacrylate augmentation. SantaVirta and associates[160] reported only two non-unions in 13 patients treated with a Gallie-type fusion.

Occipitocervical fusions have been reported to be more successful and require meticulous decortication with abundant iliac crest graft, stable fixation, and postoperative halo immobilization. Conaty and Mongan[44] reported only one non-union in 14 patients they reviewed; Clark and associates[36] reported 16 unions in 16 patients with occipitocervical fusions; Brattstrom and Granholm[22] reported a 58% osseous union rate with an additional 28% obtaining a stable fibrous union.

Progression of previously asymptomatic levels below fused segments may be noticed after surgery. Careful preoperative evaluation should rule out any other instabilities before fusion. Late subaxial subluxation has been reported following cervical fusion.[28,47] Clark and associates,[36] in their series of 41 patients, noted subsequent subluxation and displacement in 13 patients after cervical fusion.

Ankylosing Spondylitis

Unrecognized fractures of the cervical spine in patients with ankylosing spondylitis may lead to a progressive flexion deformity with limited field of vision and difficulty in opening the mouth.[173,174] In Simmons' series, more than a third of patients demonstrated evidence of previous fracture. These fractures typically occur at the C6–T2 region with C7 and T1 being the most common. Simmons has reported his experience in treating 115 patients over the last 24 years and relates a minimum of complications with exceedingly satisfactory results.[175] Fracture non-union occurred in four patients with all requiring an anterior operative stabilizing procedure. Three patients went on to union after anterior cervical fusion using a keystone graft, whereas one required an anterior keystone fusion followed by posterior segmental instrumentation and fusion to obtain union.[173,175]

The most common complication in Simmons' series of cervical osteotomies for fixed flexion deformities has been neurologic impairment. He reported thirteen patients with transient C8 paresthesiae, pain, or weakness, and one patient with a transient ninth and tenth cranial nerve lesion, which resolved spontaneously.[175] Five additional patients had a sustained C8 deficit with one patient requiring further decompression with improvement. All patients improved with no gross functional handicap. No cases of permanent injury to the cord were reported in Simmons' series. One patient developed mild symptoms of central cord syndrome 2 weeks after surgery, and others reported neurologic deficits including a Horner's syndrome.

The importance of performing such operative procedures under local anesthesia cannot be overemphasized. Simmons reported on a patient with intraoperative neurologic changes resulting from dense scarring about the dura caused by previous injury. One patient experienced weakness of both lower limbs and difficulty with speech during midline decompression which responded to splitting of the dura with immediate recovery of function.[175] This phenomenon has been reported previously during laminectomy for cord compression in a patient with a kyphoscoliosis.[129] Extensive splitting of the dura both longitudinally and transversely is recommended to relieve the compression effect of the dura.

Related medical and surgical complications have been reported by Simmons' including fatal and non-fatal pulmonary embolism, intraoperative cardiac arrest, perforated ulcer, and myocardial infarction.[173,174,176]

SUMMARY

In summary, complications in cervical spine surgery can result during any stage of the treatment process. Errors in patient selection, preoperative planning, and surgical technique can lead to significant patient morbidity and mortality. Adherence to careful and detailed preoperative planning, and basic spinal surgical principles will lead to success in most patients. However, complications are inevitable. The surgeon must be aware of their potential. Early recognition and appropriate proper treatment can minimize the associated morbidity.

REFERENCES

1 Albin MS, Carroll RG, Maroun JC. Clinical considerations concerning detection of venous air embolism. *Neurosurgery* **3**: 380–384, 1978.

2 An HS, Evanich C, Nowicki B, Haughton V, Ideal thivkness of Smith–Robinson anterior cervical interbody graft. *Spine* 18: 2043–2047, 1993.

3 An HS, Gordin R, Renner K. Anatomic considerations for plate-screw fixation of the cervical spine. *Spine* **16(10S)**: S548–S551, 1991.

4 Apfelbaum, R. Caspar plating of the cervical spine. In Camins MB, O'Leary PF (eds) *Disorders of the Cervical Spine*, 593–601. Baltimore: Williams & Wilkins, 1992.

5 Argenson C, Francke TP, Sylla S, Dintimille M, Papasian S, Dimarino V. The vertebral arteries. *Anat Clin* **2**: 29–42, 1979.

6 Aronson NI. The management of soft cervical disc protrusion using the Smith-Robinson approach. *Clin Neurosurg* **20**: 253–258, 1973.

7 Baerts WDM, De Lange JJ, Booij LHDJ, et al. Complications of the Mayfield skull clamp. *Anesthesiology* **61**: 460–461, 1984.

8 Bailey RW, Badgely CE. Stabilization of the cervical spine by anterior fusion. *J Bone Joint Surg [Am]* **42**: 565–594, 1960.

9 Baker BB, Wagner JA, Hemenway WG. Succinylcholine-induced hyperkalemia and cardiac arrest. *Arch Otolaryngol* **96**: 464, 1972.

10 Balmaseda MT Jr, Pellioni DJ. Esophagocutaneous fistula in spinal cord injury: a complication of anterior cervical fusion. *Arch Phys Med Rehab* **66**: 783–784, 1985.

11 Bell GD, Bailey SI. Anterior cervical fusion for trauma. *Clin Orthop* **128**: 155, 1977.

12 Bohlman HH. Acute fractures and dislocations of the cervical spine. An analysis of three hundred hospitalized patients and review of the literature. *J Bone Joint Surg [Am]* **61**: 1119–1142, 1979.

13 Bohlman HH. Atlanto-axial dislocations in the arthritic patient: A report of 45 cases. *Orthop Trans* **2**: 197, 1978.

14 Bohlman HH. Cervical spondylosis with moderate to severe myelopathy: A report of seventeen cases treated by Robinson anterior cervical discectomy and fusion. *Spine* **2**: 151–162, 1977.

15 Bohlman HH. Complications of treatment of fractures and dislocations of the cervical spine. In Epps CH Jr (ed) *Complications in Orthopaedic Surgery*, 611–641. Philadelphia: JB Lippincott, 1978.

16 Bohlman HH. Degenerative arthrosis of the lower cervical spine. In Evarts CM (ed) *Surgery of the Musculoskeletal System*, Vol. 2, 4:25–4:55. New York: Churchill Livingstone, 1983.

17 Bohlman HH. The pathology and current treatment concepts of cervical spine injuries. In *Instructional Course Lectures*, American Academy of Orthopaedic Surgeons, Vol. 21, 108. St Louis: CV Mosby, 1972.

18 Bohlman HH. Upper thoracic spine fractures with paralysis: A study of 180 cases. *J Bone Joint Surg [Am]* **56**: 1299, 1974.

19 Bohlman HH, Ducker TB, Lucas JT. Spine and spinal cord injuries. In Rothman RH, Simeone FA (eds) *The Spine*, 729–756. Philadelphia: WB Saunders, 1982.

20 Bohlman HH, Eismont FJ. Surgical techniques of anterior decompression and fusion for spinal cord injuries. *Clin Orthop* **154**: 57–67, 1981.

21 Bohlman HH, Freehafer AA, Dejak JJ. Late anterior decompression of spinal cord injuries: A report of thirty-six cases. *J Bone Joint Surg [Am]* **57**: 1025, 1975.

22 Brattstrom H, Granholm L. Atlanto-axial fusion in rheumatoid arthritis. *Acta Orthop Scand* **47**: 620, 1976.

23 Braunstein EM, Hunter LY, Bailey RW. Long term radiographic changes following anterior cervical fusion. *Clin Radiol* **31**: 201–203, 1980.

24 Brooks AL, Jenkins EB. Atlanto-axial arthrodesis by the wedge compression method. *J Bone Joint Surg [Am]* **60**: 279–283, 1978.

25 Brown MD, Malinin TI, Davis PB. A roentgenographic evaluation of frozen allografts versus autografts in anterior cervical spine fusions. *Clin Orthop* **119**: 231–236, 1976.

26 Bryan WJ, Inglis AE, Sculco TP, Ranawat CS. Methylmethacrylate stabilization for enhancement of posterior cervical arthrodesis in rheumatoid arthritis. *J Bone Joint Surg [Am]* **64**: 1045–1050, 1982.

27 Bucholz RW, Burkhead WZ. The pathological anatomy of fatal atlanto-occipital dislocation. *J Bone Joint Surg [Am]* **59**: 991–1002, 1977.

28 Bulger RF, Rejowski JE, Beatty RA. Vocal cord paralysis associated with anterior cervical fusion: Consideration for prevention and treatment. *J Neurosurg* **62**: 657–661, 1985.

29 Burkus JK. Cervical disc disease. In Chapman MW (ed) *Operative Orthopaedics*, 2045–2054. Philadelphia: JB Lippincott, 1988.

30 Callahan RA, Johnson K, Margolis RN, et al. Cervical facet fusion for control of instability following laminectomy. *J Bone Joint Surg [Am]* **59**: 991–1002, 1977.

31 Capen DA, Garland DE, Waters RL. Surgical stabilization of the cervical spine. A comparative analysis of anterior and posterior spine fusions. *Clin Orthop* **196**: 229–237, 1985.

32 Capen DA, Nelson RW, Zigler JE, et al. Decompressive laminectomy in cervical spine trauma: A review of early and late complications. *Contemp Orthop* **17**: 21, 1988.

33 Caspar W. Anterior stabilization with the trapezoidal osteosynthetic plate technique in cervical spine injuries. In Kehr P, Weidner A (eds) *Cervical Spine*, 198–204. New York: Springer Verlag, 1987.

34 Cattell HS, Filtzer DL. Pseudosubluxation and other normal variations in the cervical spine in children. *J Bone Joint Surg [Am]* **47**: 1295–1309, 1965.

35 Cattell HS, Clark AL. Cervical kyphosis and instability following multiple laminectomies in children. *J Bone Joint Surg [Am]* **49**: 713, 1967.

36 Clark CR, Goetz DD, Menezes AH. Arthrodesis of the cervical spine in rheumatoid arthritis. *J Bone Joint Surg [Am]* **71**: 381–392, 1989.

37 Clark CR, Keggi KJ, Panjabi MJ. Methylmethacrylate stabilization of the cervical spine. *J Bone Joint Surg [Am]* **66**: 40–46, 1984.

38 Clark CR, White AA. Fractures of the dens: A multicenter study. *J Bone Joint Surg [Am]* **67**: 1340–1348, 1985.

39 Cloward RB. New methods of diagnosis and treatment of cervical disc disease. *Clin Neurosurg* **8**: 93–132, 1962.

40 Cloward RB. Treatment of acute fractures and fracture dislocation of the cervical spine by vertebral body fusion: A report of eleven cases. *J Neurosurg* **18**: 201–209, 1961.

41 Cloward RB. Complications of anterior cervical disc operations and their treatment. *Surgery* **69**: 175–182, 1971.

42 Cockin J. Autologous bone grafting complications at the donor site. *J Bone Joint Surg [Br]* **53**: 253, 1971.

43 Coe JD, Wharton KE, Sutterlin CE III, McAfee P. Biomechanical evaluation of cervical spine stabilization methods in a human cadaveric model. *Spine* **14**: 1122–1131, 1989.

44 Conaty JP, Mongan ES. Cervical fusion in rheumatoid arthritis. *J Bone Joint Surg [Am]* **63**: 1218–1227, 1981.

45 Connolly ES, Seymour RJ, Adams JE. Clinical evaluation of anterior cervical fusions for degenerative cervical disc disease. *J Neurosurg* **23**: 431–437, 1965.

46 Cowley SP, Anderson LD. Hernias through donor sites for iliac bone grafts. *J Bone Joint Surg [Am]* **65**: 1023–1025, 1983.

47 Crellin RQ, MacCabe JJ, Hamilton EBD. Severe subluxation of the cervical spine in rheumatoid arthritis. *J Bone Joint Surg [Br]* **52**: 244–251, 1970.

48 Dawson EG, Lotysch M III, Urist MR. Intertransverse process lumbar arthrodesis with autologous bone graft. *Clin Orthop* **154**: 90–96, 1981.

49 DePalma AF, Cooke AJ. Results of anterior interbody fusion of the cervical spine. *Clin Orthop* **60**: 169, 1968.

50 DePalma A, Rothman RH, Lewinnek G, Canale S. Anterior interbody fusion for severe cervical disc degeneration. *Surg Gynecol Obstet* **134**: 755–758, 1972.

51 Dick IL. Iliac-bone transplantation. *J Bone Joint Surg [Am]* **28**: 1–14, 1946.

52 Dillin W, Booth R, Cuckler J, Balderston RA, Simeone FA, Rothman RH. Cervical radiculopathy (A review). *Spine* **11**: 988–991, 1986.
53 Dohn DF. Anterior interbody fusion for treatment of cervical disk conditions. *JAMA* **197**: 897–900, 1966.
54 Dresdale A, Rose EA, Jeevanandam V. Preparation of fibrin glue from single-donor fresh frozen plasma. *Surgery* **97**: 750–754, 1985.
55 Dunn EJ. The role of methylmethacrylate in the stabilization and replacement of tumors of the cervical spine - A project of The Cervical Spine Research Society. *Spine* **2**: 15–24, 1977.
56 Edmunds JO, Goldner JL et al. Arthrodesis of the unstable upper cervical spine for instability with and without myelopathy. *J Bone Joint Surg [Am]* **57**: 1025, 1975.
57 Eismont FJ, Bohlman HH. Posterior atlanto-occipital dislocation with fractures of the atlas and odontoid process. Report of a case with survival. *J Bone Joint Surg [Am]* **60**: 397–9, 1978.
58 Eismont FJ, Bohlman HH. Posterior methylmethacrylate fixation for cervical trauma. *Spine* **6**: 347–53, 1981.
59 Eismont FJ, Wiesel SW, Rothman RH. Treatment of dural tears associated with spinal surgery. *J Bone Joint Surg [Am]* **63**: 1132–1136, 1981.
60 Emery SE, Smith MD, Bohlman HH. Upper airway obstruction after multilevel cervical corpectomy for myelopathy. *J Bone Joint Surg [Am]* **73**: 544–551, 1991.
61 Escalas F, DeWald RL. Combined traumatic arteriovenous fistula and ureteral injury: A complication of iliac bone grafting. *J Bone Joint Surg [Am]* **59**: 270–271, 1977.
62 Esperson JO, Buhl M, Eriksen EF et al. Treatment of cervical disc disease using Cloward's technique, I: General results, effect of different operative methods and complications in 1,106 patients. *Acta Neurochir (Wien)* **70**: 97–114, 1984.
63 Fager CA. Results of adequate posterior decompression in the relief of spondylotic cervical myelopathy. *J Neurosurg* **38**: 684–692, 1973.
64 Fang HSY, Ong GB. Direct anterior approach to the upper cervical spine. *J Bone Joint Surg [Am]* **44**: 1588–1604, 1962.
65 Ferlic DC, Clayton ML, Leidholt JD, Gamble WE. Surgical treatment of the symptomatic unstable cervical spine in rheumatoid arthritis. *J Bone Joint Surg [Am]* **57**: 349–354, 1975.
66 Fernyhough JC, Schimandle JJ, Weigel M, Edwards C, Levine AM. Chronic donor site pain complicating bone graft harvesting from the posterior iliac crest for spinal fusion. *Spine* **17**: 1474–1480, 1992.
67 Fielding JW. The status of arthrodesis of the cervical spine. A current concepts review. *J Bone Joint Surg [Am]* **70**: 1571–1574, 1988.
68 Fielding JW, Hawkins RJ, Ratzan SA. Spine fusion for atlanto-axial instability. *J Bone Joint Surg [Am]* **58**: 400–407, 1976.
69 Fielding JW, Tuul A, Hawkins RJ. 'Ondine's curse.' A complication of upper cervical spine surgery. *J Bone Joint Surg [Am]* **57**: 1000–1001, 1975.
70 Flynn TB. Myelopathy following anterior cervical discectomy and fusion. A case report and discussion of recent literature. *Neurosurgery* **4**: 550, 1979.
71 Flynn TB. Neurologic complications of anterior cervical interbody fusion. *Spine* **7**: 536–539, 1982.
72 Fried LC. Atlanto-axial fracture dislocations. Failure of posterior C1 to C2 fusion. *J Bone Joint Surg [Br]* **55**: 490, 1973.
73 Frymoyer JW, Howe J, Kuhlmann D. The long-term effects of spinal fusion on the sacroiliac joints and ilium. *Clin Orthop* **134**: 196–201, 1978.
74 Galera R, Tovi D. Anterior disc excision with interbody fusion in cervical spondylotic myelopathy and rhizopathy. *J Neurosurg* **28**: 305–310, 1968.
75 Garber JN. Abnormalities of the atlas and axis vertebrae: Congenital and traumatic. *J Bone Joint Surg [Am]* **46**: 1782, 1964.
76 Garfin SR, Botte MJ, Waters RL, Nickel VL. Complications in the use of the halo fixation device. *J Bone Joint Surg [Am]* **68**: 320–325, 1986.
77 Goffart Y, Moreau P, Lenelle J, Boverie J. Traction diverticulum of the hypopharynx following anterior cervical spine surgery. Case report and review. *Ann Otol Rhinol Laryngol* **100**: 852–865, 1991.
78 Goldstein LA, Dickerson RC (eds). Pelvis. In *Atlas of Orthopaedic Surgery*, 450–453. New York: CV Mosby, 1969.
79 Gore DR, Sepic SB. Anterior cervical fusion for degenerated or protruded discs: A review of one hundred forty-six patients. *Spine* **9**: 667–671, 1984.
80 Graham JJ. Complications of cervical spine surgery. In Sherk HH, Dunn EJ, Eismont FJ, et al (eds) *The Cervical Spine*, 2nd ed, 831–837. Cervical Spine Research Society. Philadelphia: JB Lippincott, 1989.
81 Gregory CF. Complications of anterior cervical fusion. *J Bone Joint Surg [Br]* **46**: 715, 1964.
82 Griswold DM, Albright JA, Schiffman E, et al. Atlanto-axial fusion for instability. *J Bone Joint Surg [Am]* **60**: 285–292, 1978.
83 Grob D, Jeanneret B, Aebi M, Markwalder T. Complication of the atlanto-axial fusion with transarticular screw-fixation. Presented at 19th Annual Meeting, Cervical Spine Research Society, December 4–6, 1991, Philadelphia, Pennsylvania.
84 Gronert BA, Theye RA. Effect of succinylcholine on skeletal muscle with immobilization atrophy. *Anesthesia* **40**: 268, 1974.
85 Guity A, Young PH. A new technique for closure of the dura following transsphenoidal and transclival operations. *J Neurosurg* **72**: 824–828, 1990.
86 Haft H, Ransohoff J, Carter S. Spinal cord tumors in children. *Pediatrics* **23**: 1152–1159, 1959.
87 Hamblen DL. Occipito-cervical fusion. Indications, techniques and results. *J Bone Joint Surg [Br]* **49**: 33–45, 1967.
88 Hatchette S. Isolated fracture of the atlas. *Radiology* **36**: 233–235, 1941.
89 Heeneman H. Vocal cord paralysis following approaches to the anterior cervical spine. *Laryngoscope* **83**: 17–21, 1973.
90 Henderson CM, Hennessy RG, Shuey HM, Shackelford EG. Posterior–lateral foraminotomy as an exclusive operative technique for cervical radiculopathy: A review of 846 consecutively operated cases. *Neurosurgery* **13**: 504–512, 1983.
91 Herkowitz HN. A comparison of anterior cervical fusion, cervical laminectomy, and cervical laminoplasty for the surgical management of multiple level spondylotic radiculopathy. *Spine* **13**: 774–780, 1988.
92 Heywood AWB, Learmonth ID, Thomos M. Cervical spine instability in rheumatoid arthritis. *J Bone Joint Surg [Br]* **70**: 702–707, 1988.

93 Highland TR, Salciccioli GG. Is immobilization adequate treatment of unstable burst fractures of the atlas? A case report with long term follow-up evaluation. *Clin Orthop* **201**: 196–200, 1985.

94 Hilgenberg AD, Grillo HC. Acquired nonmalignant tracheoesophageal fistula. *J Thorac Cardiovasc Surg* 1900 **85**: 492–498.

95 Hohf RP. Arterial injuries occurring during orthopaedic operations. *Clin Orthop* **28**: 21–37, 1963.

96 Holness RO, Huestis WS, Howes WJ, Langille RA. Posterior stabilization with an interlaminar clamp in cervical injuries: Technical note and review of the long term experience with the method. *Neurosurgery* **14**: 318–322, 1984.

97 Horwitz NH, Rizzoli HV. Herniated intervertebral discs and spinal stenosis. Postoperative complications in extracranial neurosurgical surgery. In Horwitz NH, Rizzoli HV (eds) *Neurological Surgery*, 30–98. Baltimore: Williams & Wilkins, 1987.

98 Hunter LY, Braunstein EM, Bailey RW. Radiographic changes following anterior cervical fusion. *Spine* **5**: 399–401, 1980.

99 Jenkins DHR. Extensive cervical laminectomy: long term results. *Br J Surg* **60**: 852–854, 1973.

100 Johnson RM, Owen JR, Panjabi MM et al. Biomechanical stability of the cervical spine using a human model. *Orthop Trans* **4**: 46, 1980.

101 Keene JS, McKinley NE. Iliac crest versus spinous process grafts in post-traumatic spinal fusions. *Spine* **17**: 790–794, 1992.

102 Kewalramani LS, Riggins RS. Complications of anterior spondylodesis for traumatic lesions of the cervical spine. *Spine* **2**: 25, 1977.

103 Kitchel SH, Eismont FJ, Green BA. Closed subarachnoid drainage for management of cerebrospinal fluid leakage after an operation on the spine. *J Bone Joint Surg [Am]* **71**: 984–987, 1989.

104 Koop SE, Winter RB, Lonstein JE. The surgical treatment of instability of the upper part of the cervical spine in children and adolescents. *J Bone Joint Surg [Am]* **66**: 403–411, 1984.

105 Kopits SE, Perovic MN, McKusick V, et al. Congenital atlantoaxial dislocations in various forms of dwarfism. *J Bone Joint Surg [Am]* **54**: 1349–1350, 1972.

106 Kraus DR, Stauffer ES. Spinal cord injury as a complication of elective anterior cervical fusion. *Clin Orthop* **112**: 130–140, 1975.

107 Krempen JF, Silver RA, Sotelo A. The removal of iliac bone for bone grafting in back fusion. *Orthop Rev* **8**: 71, 1979.

108 Kuhn JE, Graziano GP. Airway compromise as a result of retropharyngeal hematoma following cervical spine injury. *J Spinal Disorders* **4**: 264–269, 1991.

109 Kurz LT, Garfin SR, Booth RE. Harvesting autogenous iliac bone graft: A review of complications and techniques. *Spine* **14**: 1324–1331, 1989.

110 Kurz LT, Garfin SR, Booth RE. Iliac bone grafting: Techniques and complications of harvesting. In Garfin SR (ed) *Complications of Spine Surgery*, 323–341. Baltimore: Williams & Wilkins, 1989.

111 Lachiewicz PF, Inglis AE, Ranawat CS. Methylmethacrylate augmentation for cervical spine arthrodesis in rheumatoid arthritis. *Orthop Trans* **11**: 7, 1987.

112 Larsson SE, Toolanen G, Fagerlund M. Medullary compression in rheumatoid atlanto-axial subluxation evaluated by computerized tomography. *Acta Orthop Scand* **57**: 262, 1986.

113 Lesoin F, Bouasakao N, Clarisse J, Rousseaux M, Jomin M. Results of surgical treatment of radiculomyelopathy caused by cervical arthrosis based on 1000 operations. *Surg Neurol* **23**: 350–355, 1985.

114 Levine AM, Edwards CC. Complications in the treatment of acute spinal injury. *Orthop Clin North Am* **17**: 183–203, 1986.

115 Lichtblau S. Dislocation of the sacroiliac joint: A complication of bone grafting. *J Bone Joint Surg [Am]* **44**: 193–198, 1962.

116 Lindsey RW, Newhouse KE, Leach J, Murphy MJ. Non union following two-level anterior cervical discectomy and fusion. *Clin Orthop* **223**: 155–163, 1987.

117 Lindskog GE, Liebow AA, Glenn WWL. *Thoracic and Cardiovascular Surgery with Related Pathology*, 439–440. New York: Appleton-Century-Crofts, 1962.

118 Lipscomb PR. Cervico-occipital fusion for congenital and post-traumatic anomalies of the atlas and axis. *J Bone Joint Surg [Am]* **39**: 1289–1301, 1957.

119 Lonstein JE, Winter RB, Bradford DB, et al. Postlaminectomy spine deformity. *J Bone Joint Surg [Am]* **58**: 727, 1976.

120 Lonstein JE. Postlaminectomy kyphosis. *Clin Orthop* **128**: 93–100, 1977.

121 Lunsford LD, Bissonette DJ, Jannetta PJ, et al. Anterior surgery for cervical disc disease. Part I: Treatment of lateral cervical herniation in 253 cases. *J Neurosurg* **53**: 1–11, 1980.

122 Lunsford LD, Bissonette DJ, Zorub DS. Anterior surgery for cervical disc disease, II: Treatment of cervical spondylotic myelopathy in 32 cases. *J Neurosurg* **53**: 12–19, 1980.

123 Magerl F, Grob D, Seeman P. Stable dorsal fusion of the cervical spine (C2–T1) using hook plates. In Kehr P, Weidner A (eds) *Cervical Spine*, 217–221. New York: Springer-Verlag, 1987

124 Maiuri F, Corriero G, Giamundo A, Donati P, Gambardella A. Postoperative cervical pseudomeningocoele. *Neurochirurgia* **31**: 29–31, 1988.

125 Marlin AE, Williams GR, Lee JF. Jefferson fractures in children: Case report. *J Neurosurg* **58**: 277–279, 1983.

126 McAfee PC, Bohlman HH, Ducker TB, Eismont FJ. Failure of methylmethacrylate stabilization of the spine. A retrospective analysis of 24 cases. In Sherk HH, Dunn EJ, Eismont FJ, et al (eds) *The Cervical Spine*, 2nd ed, 838–849. Cervical Spine Research Society. Philadelphia: JB Lippincott, 1989.

127 McAfee PC, Bohlman HH, Eismont FJ. Failure of stabilization of the spine with methylmethacrylate. *J Bone Joint Surg [Am]* **68**: 1145–1157, 1986.

128 McAfee PC, Bohlman HH, Yuan HA. Anterior decompression of traumatic thoracolumbar fractures with incomplete neurologic deficit using a retroperitoneal approach. *J Bone Joint Surg [Am]* **67**: 89–104, 1985.

129 McKenzie KG, Dewar FP. Scoliosis with paraplegia. *J Bone Joint Surg [Br]* 1949; **31**: 162–174.

130 Mclaurin RL, Vernal R, Salmon JH. Treatment of fractures of the atlas and axis by wiring without fusion. *J Neurosurg* **36**: 773–780, 1972.

131 Meyer PR Jr, Rusin JJ, Haak MH. Anterior instrumentation of the cervical spine. In An HS, Cotler JM (eds) *Spinal Instrumentation*, 49–60. Baltimore: Williams & Wilkins, 1992.

132 Mikawa Y, Shikata J, Yamamuro T. Spinal deformity and instability after multilevel cervical laminectomy. *Spine* **12**: 6–11, 1987.

133 Milward FJ. An unusual case of fracture of the atlas. *Br Med J* **1**: 458, 1933.
134 Morgan TH, Wharton GW, Austin GN. The results of laminectomy in patients with incomplete spinal cord injuries. *Paraplegia* **9**: 14–23, 1971.
135 Murphy MJ, Ogden JA, Southwick WO. Spinal stabilization in acute spinal injuries. *Surg Clin North Am* **60**: 1035–1047, 1980.
136 Newhouse KE, Lindsey RW, Clark CR, et al. Esophageal perforation following anterior cervical spine surgery. *Spine* **14**: 1051–1053, 1989.
137 Newman P, Sweetnam R. Occipito-cervical fusion. *J Bone Joint Surg [Br]* **51**: 423–431, 1961.
138 Norrell H. Fractures and dislocations of the spine. In Rothman RH, Simeone FA (eds) *The Spine*, 529–566. Philadelphia: WB Saunders, 1982.
139 Panjabi MM, Hopper W, White AA III, Keggi KJ. Posterior spine stabilization with methylmethacrylate. Biomechanical testing of a surgical specimen. *Spine* **2**: 241–247, 1977.
140 Parks BJ. Postoperative peripheral neuropathies. *Surgery* **74**: 348–357, 1973.
141 Perret G, Greene J. Anterior interbody fusion in the treatment of cervical fracture dislocations. *Arch Surg* **96**: 530–539, 1968.
142 Phillips DG. Surgical treatment of myelopathy and cervical spondylosis. *J Neurol Neurosurg Psychiatry* **36**: 879–884, 1973.
143 Piazza MR, Cotler JM. Graft complications in anterior cervical spine reconstruction. Presented at the Federation of Spine Associations Meeting, February 12, 1989, Las Vegas, Nevada.
144 Piazza MR, Cotler JM, Balderston RA. Complications in cervical spine injury. In Balderston RA, An HS (eds) *Complications in Spinal Surgery*, 105–135. Philadelphia: WB Saunders, 1991.
145 Ranawat CS, O'Leary P, Pellici PM, Tsairis P, Marchisello P, Dorr L. Cervical spine fusion in rheumatoid arthritis. *J Bone Joint Surg [Am]* **61**: 1003–1010, 1979.
146 Randle M, Wolf A, Levi L, Rigamonti D, Mirvis S et al. The use of the anterior Caspar plate fixation in acute cervical spine injury. *Surgical Neurology* **36**: 181–189, 1991.
147 Riley L. Anterior cervical spine surgery. In American Academy of Orthopaedic Surgeons *Instructional Course Lectures*, Vol. 27, 154–158. St Louis: CV Mosby, 1978.
148 Riley LH, Robinson RA, Johnson KA, Walker AE. The results of anterior interbody fusion of the cervical spine. Review of ninety-three consecutive cases. *J Neurosurg* **30**: 127–133, 1969.
149 Rizzoli H. Personal Communication, 1985; in Stambough J, Simeone FA. Vascular complications in spine surgery. In Rothman RH, Simeone FA (eds) *The Spine*, 3rd ed, 1878. Philadelphia: WB Saunders, 1992.
150 Robinson RA, Southwick WO. Surgical approaches to the cervical spine. In American Academy of Orthopaedic Surgeons, *Instructional Course Lectures*, Vol. 17, 299–330. St Louis: CV Mosby, 1960.
151 Robinson RA, Walker AE, Ferlic DC, et al. The results of anterior interbody fusion of the cervical spine. *J Bone Joint Surg [Am]* **44**: 1569–1587, 1962.
152 Roche M, Gilly F, Carret JP, Guibert B, Braillon G, Dejour H. Perforation of the cervical esophagus and hypopharynx complicating surgery by an anterior approach to the cervical spine. *Annales de Chirurgie* **43**: 343–347, 1989.
153 Roger AB, Husser RW, Kenzora JF. Anterior fibular interbody fusion in the treatment of cervical spinal cord injuries. *Surg Neurol* **7**: 55–60, 1977.
154 Rogers WA. Fractures and dislocations of the cervical spine. An end-result study. *J Bone Joint Surg [Am]* **39**: 341–376, 1957.
155 Roy-Camille R, Saillant G, Mazel C. Internal fixation of the unstable cervical spine by a posterior osteosynthesis with plates and screws. In Sherk HH, Dunn EJ, Eismont FJ, et al. *The Cervical Spine*, 2nd ed, 390–403. Cervical Spine Research Society. Philadelphia: JB Lippincott, 1989.
156 Roy-Camille R, Mazel C. Stabilization of the cervical spine with posterior plates and screws. In Camins MB, O'Leary PF (eds) *Disorders of the Cervical Spine*, 577–591. Baltimore: Williams & Wilkins, 1992.
157 Sacks S. Anterior interbody fusion of the lumbar spine. *J Bone Joint Surg [Br]* **47**: 211–223, 1965.
158 Sanders G, Uyeda RY, Karlan MS. Nonrecurrent inferior laryngeal nerves and their association with a recurrent branch. *Am J Surg* **146**: 501–503, 1983.
159 Sang UH, Wilson CB. Postoperative epidural hematoma as a complication of anterior cervical discectomy. *J Neurosurg* **49**: 288–291, 1978.
160 SantaVirta S, Slatis P, Kankaanpaa, U et al. Treatment of the cervical spine in rheumatoid arthritis. *J Bone Joint Surg [Am]* **70**: 658–667, 1987.
161 Saunders RL. Complications of corpectomy. In Tarlov EC (ed) *Complications of Spinal Surgery. Neurosurgical Topics*, 105–113. Park Ridge: American Association of Neurological Surgeons, 1991.
162 Schatzker J, Rorabeck CH, Waddell JP. Fracture of the dens. An analysis of thirty-seven cases. *J Bone Joint Surg [Br]* **53**: 392–405, 1971.
163 Segal LS, Grimm JO, Stauffer ES. Non-union of fractures of the atlas. *J Bone Joint Surg [Am]* **69**: 1423–1434, 1987.
164 Shaffrey CI, Spotnitz WD, Shaffrey ME, Jane JA. Neurosurgical applications of fibrin glue. Augmentation of dural closure in 134 patients. *Neurosurgery* **26**: 207–210, 1990.
165 Shields CL, Stauffer ES. Late instability in cervical spine fractures secondary to laminectomy. *Clin Orthop* **119**: 144, 1976.
166 Shintani A, Zervas NT. Consequence of ligation of the vertebral artery. *J Neurosurg* **36**: 447–450, 1972.
167 Siedentop KH, Harris DM, Sanchez B. Autologous fibrin tissue adhesive. *Laryngoscope* **95**: 1074–1076, 1985.
168 Siegal T, Petah T, Siegal T. Vertebral body resection for epidural compression by malignant tumors. *J Bone Joint Surg [Am]* **67**: 375–382, 1985.
169 Sim FH, Svien HJ, Bickel WH, et al. Swan neck deformity following extensive cervical laminectomy. A review of twenty-one cases. *J Bone Joint Surg [Am]* **56**: 564–580, 1974.
170 Simeone FA, Rothman RH. Cervical disc disease. In Rothman RH, Simeone FA (eds) *The Spine*, 2nd ed, 440–499. Philadelphia: WB Saunders, 1982.
171 Simeone FA, Dillin WA. Treatment of cervical disc disease: Selection of operative approach. *Contemp. Neurosurg* **8**: 1–6, 1986.
172 Simmons EH, Bhalla SK. Anterior cervical discectomy and fusion. A clinical and biomechanical study with eight year follow-up. *J Bone Joint Surg [Br]* **51**: 225–232, 1969.

173 Simmons EH. The surgical correction of flexion deformity of the cervical spine in ankylosing spondylitis. In Sherk HH, Dunn EJ, Eismont FJ, et al. *The Cervical Spine*, 2nd ed, 573–598. Cervical Spine Research Society. Philadelphia: JB Lippincott, 1989.

174 Simmons EH. Surgery of the spine in rheumatoid arthritis and ankylosing spondilitis. In Evarts CM (ed) *Surgery of the Musculoskeletal System*, Vol. 2, 4:85–4:151. New York: Churchill Livingstone, 1983.

175 Simmons EH. Ankylosing spondylitis. Surgical considerations. In Rothman RH, Simeone FA (eds) *The Spine*, 2nd ed, 1447–1511. Philadelphia: WB Saunders, 1982.

176 Simmons EH. Surgery of the spine in ankylosing spondylitis and rheumatoid arthritis. In Chapman M (ed.) *Operative Orthopaedics*, 2077–2114. Philadelphia: JB Lippincott, 1988.

177 Smith MD, Emery SE, Dudley A, Murray KJ, Leventhal M. Iatrogenic vertebral artery injuries during anterior cervical spine procedures. A report of ten patients. Presented at 9th Annual Cervical Spine Research Society Meeting, December 4–6, 1991, Philadelphia, Pennsylvania.

178 Stabler CL, Eismont FJ, Brown MD et al. Failure of posterior cervical fusions using cadaveric bone graft in children. *J Bone Joint Surg [Am]* **67**: 370–375, 1985.

179 Stambough JL, Simeone FA. Vascular complications in spine surgery. In Rothman RH, Simeone FA (eds) *The Spine*, 3rd ed, 1877–1885. Philadelphia: WB Saunders, 1982.

180 Standefer M, Bay JW, Trusso R. The sitting position in neurosurgery: A retrospective analysis of 488 cases. *Neurosurgery* **14**: 649–658, 1984.

181 Stauffer RN, Coventry MB. Anterior interbody lumbar spine fusion. *J Bone Joint Surg [Am]* **54**: 756–768, 1972.

182 Stauffer ES, Kelly EG. Fracture-dislocations of the cervical spine. Instability and recurrent deformity following treatment by anterior interbody fusion. *J Bone Joint Surg [Am]* **59**: 45–48, 1977.

183 Stauffer ES, Wood RW, Kelly EG. Gunshot wounds of the spine: The effects of laminectomy. *J Bone Joint Surg [Am]* **61**: 389–392, 1979.

184 Stuck RM. Anterior cervical disc excision and fusion – Report of 200 consecutive cases. *Rocky Mountain Med J* **60**: 25–30, 1963.

185 Suderman VJ, Crosby ET, Lui A. Elective oral tracheal intubation in cervical spine-injured adults. *Canadian J Anaesth* **38**: 185–189, 1991.

186 Sugar O. Spinal cord malfunction after anterior cervical discectomy. *Surg Neurol* **15**: 4–8, 1981.

187 Summers BN, Eisenstein SM. Donor site pain from the ilium. *J Bone Joint Surg [Br]* **71**: 677–680, 1989.

188 Sundareson N, Galicich JH, Lane BM, Bains MS, McCormack P. Treatment of neoplastic epidural cord compression by vertebral body resection and stabilization. *J Neurosurg* **63**: 676–684, 1985.

189 Tachdijian MO, Matson DD. Orthopaedic aspects of intraspinal tumors in infants and children. *J Bone Joint Surg [Am]* **47**: 223–248, 1965.

190 Tew JM Jr, Mayfield FH. Surgery of the anterior cervical spine: Preventions of complications. In Dunsker SB (ed) *Cervical Spondylosis*, 191–208. New York: Raven Press, 1981.

191 Tew JM, Mayfield FH. Complication of surgery of the anterior cervical spine. *Clin Neurosurg* **23**: 424–434, 1976.

192 Thomas AN. The lateral decubitus position. In Martin JT (ed) *Positioning in Anesthesia and Surgery*, 116–124. Philadelphia: WB Saunders, 1978.

193 Thompson RC Jr, Meyer TJ. Posterior surgical stabilization for atlanto-axial subluxation in rheumatoid arthritis. *Spine* **10**: 597–601, 1985.

194 Transmission of HIV through bone transplantation: Case report and public health recommendations. *JAMA* **260**: 2487–2488, 1988.

195 Troll GF, Dohrmann GJ. Anaesthesia of the spinal cord injured patient. Cardiovascular problems and their management. *Paraplegia* **13**: 162, 1975.

196 U HS, Wilson CB. Postoperative epidural hematoma as a complication of anterior cervical discectomy; report of three cases. *J Neurosurg* **49**: 288–291, 1978.

197 van Berge Henegouwen DP, Roukema JA, de Nie JC, van der Werken C. Esophageal perforation during surgery on the cervical spine. *Neurosurgery* **29**: 766–768, 1991.

198 Van Petegham PK, Schweigel JF. The fractured cervical spine rendered unstable by anterior cervical fusion. *J Trauma* **19**: 110–114, 1979.

199 Verbiest H. A lateral approach to the cervical spine: Technique and indications. *J Neurosurg* **30**: 191–203, 1967.

200 Wadia NH. Myelopathy complicating congenital atlanto-axial dislocation. A study of 28 cases. *Brain* **90**: 449–472, 1967.

201 Weidner A. Internal fixation with metal plates and screws. In Sherk HH, Dunn EJ, Eismont FJ, et al (eds) *The Cervical Spine*, 2nd ed, 404–421. Cervical Spine Research Society. Philadelphia: JB Lippincott, 1989.

202 Weisel SW. Neurologic complications in lumbar laminectomy: A standardized approach to the multiply operated lumbar spine. In Garfin SR (ed) *Complications of Spine Surgery*, 65–74. Baltimore: Williams & Wilkins, 1989.

203 Welsh LW, Welsh JJ, Chinnici JC. Dysphagia due to cervical spine surgery. *Ann Otol Rhinol Laryngol* **96**: 112–115, 1987.

204 Wertheim SB, Bohlman HH. Occipitocervical fusion: Indications, technique and long term results in thirteen patients. *J Bone Joint Surg [Am]* **69**: 833–836, 1987.

205 White AA III, Panjabi MM, Thomas CL. The clinical biomechanics of kyphotic deformities. *Clin Orthop* **128**: 8–17, 1977.

206 White AA III, Southwick WO et al. Practical biomechanics of the spine for the orthopaedic surgeon. In American Academy of Orthopaedic Surgeons, *Instructional Course Lectures*, Vol. 23, 62. St Louis: CV Mosby, 1974.

207 White AA III, Southwick WO, DePonte RJ, Gainar JW, Hardy R. Relief of pain by anterior cervical fusion for spondylosis. A report of sixty-five patients. *J Bone Joint Surg [Am]* **55**: 525–534, 1973.

208 Whitecloud TS III. Complications of anterior cervical fusion. In American Academy of Orthopaedic Surgeons, *Instructional Course Lectures*, Vol. 27, 223–227. St Louis: CV Mosby: 1978.

209 Whitecloud TS, LaRocca H. Fibular strut graft in reconstructive surgery of the cervical spine. *Spine* **1**: 33–43, 1976.

210 Whitehill R, Richman JA, Glaser JA. Failure of immobilization of the cervical spine by the halo vest. *J Bone Joint Surg [Am]* **68**: 326–332, 1986.

211 Whitehill R, Sirna EC, Young DC, Cantrell RW. Late esophageal perforation from an autogenous bone graft. Report of a case. *J Bone Joint Surg [Am]* **67**: 644–645, 1985.

212 Wilder BJ. Hypothesis: The etiology of midcervical quadriplegia after operation with the patient in the sitting position. *Neurosurgery* **11**: 530–531, 1982.
213 Williams JL, Allen MB Jr, Harness JW. Late results of cervical discectomy and interbody fusion: Some factors influencing the results. *J Bone Joint Surg [Am]* **50**: 227–286, 1968.
214 Willison HJ, Gale AN, McLaughlin JE. Creutzfeldt-Jacob disease following cadaveric dura mater graft. *J Neurol Neurosurg Psychiat* **54**: 940, 1991.
215 Yonenobu K, Okada K, Fuji T, Fujiwara K, Yamashita K, Ono K. Causes of neurologic deterioration following surgical treatment of cervical myelopathy. *Spine* **11**: 818–823, 1986.
216 Yonenobu K, Hosono N, Iwasaki M, Asano M, Ono K. Neurologic complicatons of surgery for cervical compression myelopathy. *Spine* **16**: 1277–1282, 1991.
217 Young ML, Smith DS, Murtagh F, et al. Comparison of surgical and anesthetic complications in neurosurgical patients experiencing venous air embolism in the sitting position. *Neurosurgery* **18**: 157–161, 1986.
218 Younger EW, Chapman MW. Morbidity at bone graft donor sites. *J Orthop Trauma* **3**: 192–195, 1989.
219 Zoma A, Sturrock RD, Fisher WD, et al. Surgical stabilization of the rheumatoid cervical spine. *J Bone Joint Surg [Br]* **69**: 8–12, 1987.

Index